Spasticity

Spasticity
Diagnosis and Management

Allison Brashear, MD
Professor and Chair
Department of Neurology
Wake Forest University School of Medicine
Wake Forest Baptist Medical Center
Winston-Salem, North Carolina

Elie Elovic, MD
Professor and Chief
Physical Medicine and Rehabilitation
University of Utah School of Medicine
Salt Lake City, Utah

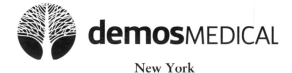

demosMEDICAL

New York

Acquisitions Editor: Beth Barry
Cover Design: Joe Tenerelli
Compositor: The Manila Typesetting Company
Printer: Bang Printing

Visit our website at www.demosmedpub.com

Medicine is an ever-changing science. Research and clinical experience are continually expanding our knowledge, in particular our understanding of proper treatment and drug therapy. The authors, editors, and publisher have made every effort to ensure that all information in this book is in accordance with the state of knowledge at the time of production of the book. Nevertheless, the authors, editors, and publisher are not responsible for errors or omissions or for any consequences from application of the information in this book and make no warranty, express or implied, with respect to the contents of the publication. Every reader should examine carefully the package inserts accompanying each drug and should carefully check whether the dosage schedules mentioned therein or the contraindications stated by the manufacturer differ from the statements made in this book. Such examination is particularly important with drugs that are either rarely used or have been newly released on the market.

Library of Congress Cataloging-in-Publication Data

Spasticity : diagnosis and management / [edited by] Allison Brashear, Elie Elovic.
       p. ; cm.
Includes bibliographical references and index.
ISBN 978-1-933864-51-8
1. Spasticity. I. Brashear, Allison. II. Elovic, Elie.
[DNLM: 1. Muscle Spasticity—diagnosis. 2. Muscle Spasticity—therapy. 3. Extremities—physiopathology. 4. Motor Neuron Disease.
5. Muscle Spasticity—etiology. WE 550 S7368 2011]
RC935.S64S627 2011
616.8'56—dc22

2010024464

Special discounts on bulk quantities of Demos Medical Publishing books are available to corporations, professional associations, pharmaceutical companies, health care organizations, and other qualifying groups. For details, please contact:

Special Sales Department
Demos Medical Publishing
11 W. 42nd Street, 15th Floor
New York, NY 10036
Phone: 800–532–8663 or 212–683–0072
Fax: 212–941–7842
E-mail: specialsales@demosmedpub.com

Made in the United States of America
13 14   5 4

We dedicate this book to our families for their unconditional support, and to our professors, colleagues, students and patients who continue to humble us with their strength and challenge us to improve the care of those with spasticity.

Contents

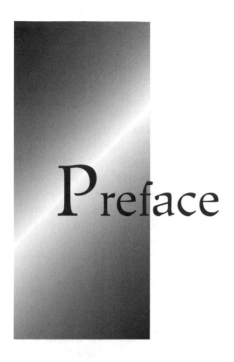

Preface

Spasticity: Diagnosis and Management is the first book solely dedicated to the diagnosis and treatment of spasticity. Arguably, this text could have been titled *Upper Motor Neuron Syndrome*, as spasticity is just one of many components of the constellation of conditions that make up the upper motor neuron syndrome (UMNS). Other authors use the phrase "muscle overactivity" to describe these conditions, but since the term most commonly used by physicians, therapists, patients, and caregivers is *spasticity*, we chose this as our title while the actual focus of the book is about the broader context of UMNS and how it leads to disability.

Spasticity is only part of the UMNS as is so eloquently described by Dr Mayer in Chapter 3. UMNS occurs when damage to the brain or spinal cord results in a constellation of signs and symptoms that may include spasticity or increase in tone, rigidity, and flexor spasms superimposed on any combination of weakness, paralysis, and/or decreased dexterity. The varied clinical characteristics of UMNS must be taken into account when developing a treatment plan. In Chapter 8, Dr Elovic discusses the importance of evaluating the patient, their support systems, and the clinical manifestation of the UMNS so that clinicians can set realistic and obtainable treatment goals. The editors' objective in the development of this book were to clearly define the process for the diagnosis of spasticity, the basic science behind its pathophysiology, the measurement tools used for evaluation, and the available treatment options.

This text is designed to bring the reader up-to-date on the demographics of disorders of tone, with a detailed discussion on epidemiology by Dr McGuire in Chapter 2 and an eloquent description of pathphysiology of the UMNS by Dr Mayer in Chapter 3. In Chapter 4, Dr Ivanhoe and colleagues review concerns of the patient with spasticity that are often overlooked, including bowel and bladder function. In Chapter 5, Dr Elovic discusses the assessment tools for upper and lower extremity spasticity and Drs Watanabe and Esquenazi review the assessment of upper and lower extremity spasticity in Chapters 6 and 7.

Part III of the text focuses on treatment and outlines the many tools available to physicians such as oral medication, intrathecal baclofen, and chemodenervation in Chapters 9 through 11. Chapters 10 and 11 are specifically dedicated to the use of botulinum toxin in adults, with in-depth coverage of chemodenervation treatment protocols for upper and lower extremity spasticity. Drs Truong and Pathak provide a detailed artistic rendering in Chapter 12 of the important muscles and landmarks in spasticity management. Chapter 13 focuses on nonmedical therapeutic modalities and highlights the role of therapists as an important part of the management team. Dr Flanagan's discussion of the role of the emerging technologies in Chapter 14 highlights the continued evaluation of the treatment of spasticity for patients. In Chapters 15 and 16, Drs Meythaler and Saulino, discuss the role of oral medication and more invasive treatments such as intrathecal baclofen. In Chapter 17, Dr Fuller discusses the important and often overlooked option of neuro-orthopedic intervention in the management of spasticity.

Part IV of the book is devoted to the evaluation and management of individual diseases involving spasticity, which reinforces the importance of disease diagnosis and management in the patient with spasticity and reemphasizes the need to establish an accurate diagnosis before embarking on treatment. Amyotrophic lateral sclerosis, multiple sclerosis, poststroke spasticity, traumatic brain injury, and spinocerebellar ataxia (discussed in Chapters 20–24) are very different conditions, even though each may present with spasticity. Accurate diagnosis is paramount in designing the appropriate treatment plan for these distinct diseases. Chapters 25 and 26 are devoted to the unique challenges involved in diagnosing and managing spasticity in children with detailed discussions of chemodenervation and surgery. Finally, Chapter 27 reviews the

basic science and the role of animal models in better understanding the underlying mechanisms of spasticity in patients with spinal cord injury.

Until the advent of oral medications, intrathecal baclofen, and botulinum toxin, the treatment of disorders of tone as part of the UMNS was often frustrating for the patient, caregiver, and physician. With the development of effective therapies and a team approach to management of these disorders, we have sought to address the diagnosis and treatment of spasticity in an integrated, clinically useful text. Our charge was to provide a one-stop resource for physicians, therapists, and other healthcare providers who serve the complex needs of these patients with the goal of offering the highest level of care and improving outcomes.

Allison Brashear, MD
Elie Elovic, MD

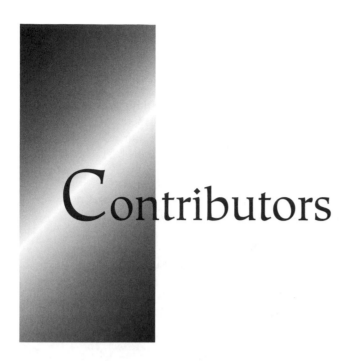

Contributors

Allison Brashear, MD
Professor and Chair
Department of Neurology
Wake Forest University School of Medicine
Wake Forest Baptist Medical Center
Winston-Salem, North Carolina

Surendra Bandi, MS (Orthopaedics), MRCS
Specialist Registrar, Rehabilitation Medicine
North Staffordshire Rehabilitation Centre
University Hospital of North Staffordshire
Stoke-On-Trent, United Kingdom

John W. Chow, PhD
Methodist Rehabilitation Center
Jackson, Mississippi

Stephanie Co
Spaulding Rehabilitation Hospital
Harvard Medical School
Boston, Massachusetts

Edward R. Dabrowski, MD
Division Chief of Physical Medicine and
    Rehabilitation
Department of Pediatrics
Medical Director of Rehabilitation Services
Childrens Hospital of Michigan
Assistant Professor of Pediatrics
Department of Pediatrics
Assistant Professor Physical Medicine and
    Rehabilitation
Wayne State University
Detroit, Michigan

Rachel M. Dolhun, MD
Instructor
Department of Neurology
Vanderbilt University Medical Center
Nashville, Tennessee

Peter D. Donofrio, MD
Department of Neurology
Vanderbilt University Medical Center
Nashville, Tennessee

Elie Elovic, MD
Professor and Chief
Physical Medicine and Rehabilitation
University of Utah School of Medicine
Salt Lake City, Utah

Alberto Esquenazi, MD
Chairman
Department of Physical Medicine and
    Rehabilitation
Director
Gait and Motion Analysis Laboratory
MossRehab
Elkins Park, Pennsylvania

Steven R. Flanagan, MD
Professor and Chairman of Rehabilitation Medicine
New York University School of Medicine
New York, New York

John Frino, MD
Assistant Professor
Wake Forest University School of Medicine
Winston-Salem, North Carolina

David A. Fuller, MD
Assistant Professor of Orthopaedic Surgery
University of Medicine and Dentistry of New Jersey
Camden, New Jersey

Omar Gomez-Medina, MD
Faculty Member
Department of Physical Medicine and
    Rehabilitation
San Pablo Hospital
Bayamón, Puerto Rico

Lawrence J. Horn, MD, MRM
Professor
Department of Physical Medicine and
    Rehabilitation
Wayne State University School of Medicine
Medical Director Neuroscience
Rehabilitation Institute of Michigan
Detroit, Michigan

Cindy B. Ivanhoe, MD
Neurorehabilitation Specialists
Houston, Texas

Jonathan H. Kinzinger, DPT, NCS
Rehabilitation Services
University of Utah Health Care
Salt Lake City, Utah

Steven Kirshblum, MD
Medical Director
Director of Spinal Cord Injury Services
Professor
Kessler Institute for Rehabilitation
Department of Physical Medicine and
    Rehabilitation
New Jersey Medical School
University of Medicine and Dentistry of
    New Jersey
West Orange, New Jersey

Patrick Harvey Kitzman, PhD, MSPT
Department of Rehabilitation Sciences
University of Kentucky
Lexington, Kentucky

Kat Kolaski, MD
Assistant Professor
Wake Forest University School of Medicine
Winston-Salem, North Carolina

L. A. Koman, MD
Professor
Department of Orthopaedic Surgery
Wake Forest University School of Medicine
Winston-Salem, North Carolina

Scott Kowalski, DO
Department of Physical Medicine and
    Rehabilitation
Wayne State University School of Medicine
Rehabilitation Institute of Michigan
Detroit, Michigan

Ian Maitin, MD, MBA
Associate Professor and Chair
Department of Physical Medicine and
    Rehabilitation
Temple University School of Medicine
Philadelphia, Pennsylvania

Nathaniel H. Mayer, MD
Professor Emeritus
Physical Medicine and Rehabilitation
Temple University School of Medicine
Philadelphia, Pennsylvania
Director
Motor Control Analysis Laboratory
MossRehab
Elkins Park, Pennsylvania

Donald McCorquordale, III, BSc
John T. Hussman Institute for Human Genomics
University of Miami Miller School of Medicine
Miami, Florida

John R. McGuire, MD
Associate Professor
Department of Physical Medicine and
    Rehabilitation
Medical College of Wisconsin
Milwaukee, Wisconsin

Jay M. Meythaler, MD, JD
Professor-Chair
Department of Physical Medicine and
    Rehabilitation
Wayne State University School of Medicine
Detroit, Michigan

Elizabeth Moberg-Wolff, M.D.
Children's Hospital of Wisconsin
Medical College of Wisconsin
Milwaukee, Wisconsin

Mayank Pathak, MD
The Parkinson's and Movement Disorder Institute
Fountain Valley, California

Ira Rashbaum, MD
Clinical Professor of Rehabilitation Medicine
New York University School of Medicine
New York, New York

Michael Saulino, MD, PhD
Assistant Professor
Department of Physical Medicine and
 Rehabilitation
MossRehab
Elkins Park, Pennsylvania

Anjali Shah, MD
Assistant Professor
Department of Physical Medicine and
 Rehabilitation
University of Texas Southwestern Medical Center
Dallas, Texas

Robert Shingleton, PT, DPT, MBA
Physical Therapist and Spasticity Management
 Program Coordinator
Therapy Services, Physical Medicine and
 Rehabilitation
University Health Care
Salt Lake City, Utah

Geoffrey Sheean, MD
Professor of Neurosciences
Director of Neuromuscular Program
University of California, San Diego
San Diego, California

Gurtej Singh, MD
Physical Medicine and Rehabilitation
Wayne State University School of Medicine
Rehabilitation Institute of Michigan
Detroit, Michigan

Anath Srikrishnan
Spaulding Rehabilitation Hospital
Harvard Medical School
Boston, Massachusetts

Dobrivoje S. Stokic, MD, DSc
Center for Neuroscience and Neurological Recovery
Methodist Rehabilitation Center
Jackson, Mississippi

Ann Tilton, MD
Professor of Neurology and Pediatrics
Louisiana State University Health and Sciences
 Center
New Orleans, Louisianna

Daniel Truong, MD
The Parkinson's and Movement Disorder Institute
Fountain Valley, California

Heather W. Walker, MD
Assistant Professor
Department of Physical Medicine and
 Rehabilitation
University of North Carolina at Chapel Hill
Chapel Hill, North Carolina

**Anthony B. Ward, BSc, MD, FRCPEd, FRCP,
 SFEBPRM**
Professor of Rehabilitation Medicine
North Staffordshire Rehabilitation Centre
University Hospital of North Staffordshire
Stoke on Tent, United Kingdom

Thomas Watanabe, MD
Clinical Director
Drucker Brain Injury Center
MossRehab at Elkins Park
Elkins Park, Pennsylvania

Stuart A. Yablon, MD
Director of Rehabilitation Research
Baylor Institute for Rehabilitation
Dallas, Texas

Ross Zafonte
Spaulding Rehabilitation Hospital
Harvard Medical School
Boston, Massachusetts

Stephan Züchner, MD
Associate Professor for Human Genetics and
 Neurology
University of Miami Miller School of Medicine
Miami Institute for Human Genomics
Miami, Florida

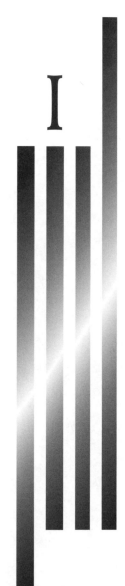

I

GENERAL OVERVIEW

Why Is Spasticity Important?

Allison Brashear
Elie Elovic

Increased tone or spasticity is the tightness that patients and/or caregivers report with passive movement of the limb. In more scientific language, spasticity is a motor disorder characterized by a velocity-dependent increase in the tonic stretch reflex. A clinical finding on the neurologic examination, spasticity together with increased tone, brisk reflexes with incoordination, and weakness represents the upper motor neuron syndrome. So why is spasticity important and why does it merit a textbook?

This textbook is dedicated to the diagnosis and management of these conditions. In an age where imaging is often used more than the physical examination, diagnosis and treatment of spasticity rely solely on the physician's examination of the patient. When many question the enduring role of history and physical examination, spasticity and the resulting impact on the patient and caregiver can only be assessed thru this means. The assessment of spasticity requires that a physician perform a neurologic assessment of the patient, including the tone, reflexes, strength, and coordination. Clinical skills are at the heart of the profession of medicine, and the diagnosis and treatment of spasticity reinforce the importance of these skills.

Regardless of its cause, spasticity causes significant disability. An estimated 4 million individuals are stroke survivors in the United States, and as many as one third may have spasticity with sufficient disability to require treatment. According to the Centers for Disease Control, 1.4 million people in the United States sustain a traumatic brain injury each year, and additional patients develop spasticity after spinal cord injury. The result of any brain or spinal cord injury is a variable pattern of increased tone with weakness and discoordination that leads to significant disability in many patients.

The treatment of spasticity relies on the physician's assessment of the individual treatment together with conversations with the caregiver. Patients' inability to perform simple activities of daily living for themselves and the adverse effects on the caregiver drives physicians to find ways to decrease tone, build strength, and improve coordination. The team approach is a cornerstone of a successful treatment, and interaction of the patient, the caregiver, the therapist, and the physicians works best to provide a care plan that addresses functional impairment and plots a course to treat the problems.

Spasticity is a clinically relevant medical problem when it interferes with function or care of the patients. The evolution of the upper motor neuron syndrome may take days to months after a central nervous system injury. Moreover, the presentation in one patient may differ from another despite them having similar central nervous system lesions. The lesion alone does not predict the amount or impact of the spasticity. Other factors such as medications, stress, medical illness, timing of therapy, and so on impact the clinical presentation. As a result, each patient must be assessed individually with his or her caregiver, noting the concerns that impair the performance of activities of daily living or other deficits. No matter how much we learn about stroke, traumatic brain injury, multiple sclerosis, and spinal cord injury, the assessment of spasticity and the effect of tone on function will remain unique to each individual patient's circumstance.

Although neurologic examination is essential for the diagnosis of spasticity, the management of spasticity has many paths for treatment depending on the disability and goals of the patient and caregiver. One patient may benefit from a combination of tools for spasticity, including interventions such as botulinum toxin injections and intrathecal baclofen, whereas others may require a more conservative route such as splinting or oral medications. The informed physician should know how to assess the amount of spasticity,

determine the functional limitations it creates, and then be able to develop a management plan for that individual patient.

How to assess the complicated picture of spasticity and when to intervene is the focus of this text. Our co-authors define for you why spasticity is important and detail the diagnosis and management options, but the goal is to provide the reader with the best options for the physician's individual patient. As editors, we aim to explore the diagnosis and management of the many different types of patients with spasticity and to open the door to the different treatment paradigms for patients with spasticity.

So why is spasticity important? The answer is because it often causes disability and impairs function in our patients. The goal of this book is to provide the foundation for excellent care of our patients facing these disabilities.

Epidemiology of Spasticity in the Adult and Child

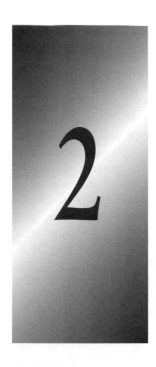

John R. McGuire

Despite the extensive work done to develop improved treatments for muscle overactivity in patients with upper motor neuron (UMN) lesions, there are only a limited number of studies on the incidence and prevalence of spasticity. Most likely, this is due to the lack of consistent definitions and reliable measures of spastic hypertonia. Compounding the difficulties in the literature is that the few prevalence studies that have been performed rely primarily on patient surveys or clinical measures of spasticity, which lack sensitivity for quantifying abnormal muscle activation (1). More importantly, there are fewer studies on the prevalence of problematic or significant spasticity. A final issue is that different authors use dissimilar definitions for the condition. Some of the descriptions have included spasticity that requires medication or physiotherapy (2–4), causes pain, (5) interferes with activities of daily living (ADL) (6–10), or has an Ashworth score of 2 or higher or 3 (11, 12).

The actual incidence of spasticity depends on the cause of the UMN lesion. After damage to central motor pathways above T12, there is initial paralysis followed by adaptive changes in the brain and spinal cord that develop over time, which result in a complex set of motor behaviors (13–17). Paresis, soft tissue contracture, and muscle overactivity are the 3 major mechanisms of motor impairment (18). Although spasticity is often used as an umbrella term, it is just one component of the muscle overactivity that

contributes to the upper motor neuron syndrome (UMNS) (16, 19, 20). Reliable assessments are complicated by the fact that spasticity can vary throughout the day, change with different positions, and increase with any noxious stimulus, such as pressure sores, urinary tract infection, deep venous thrombosis, ingrown toenails, joint pain, or constipation (15, 16, 21).

In a large population-based study initiated by the Christopher & Dana Reeve Foundation Paralysis Resource Center (PRC) and researchers at the University of New Mexico's Center for Development and Disability that was performed from 2006 to 2008, more than 33,000 households across the country were surveyed for any disability (22). From this review, they estimated that nearly 1 in 50 people or approximately 6 million people in the United States are living with paralysis. The leading etiologies for this condition were stroke, spinal cord injury (SCI), multiple sclerosis (MS), and cerebral palsy (CP) (Table 2.1) (22). It should be noted that the prevalence of paralysis noted in people with SCI and MS from this survey is significantly higher than those found previously.

Additional important questions that need to be answered are what are the conditions that cause problematic spasticity and what is the number of people who require treatment? Data collected from the adult spasticity management clinic at the Medical College of Wisconsin (MCW) during a 6-month period in 2008 may give some answers to these questions. The number

TABLE 2.1
Prevalence of Paralysis in the United States
(n = 5,596,000)

CAUSE	n	%
Stroke	1,608,000	29
SCI	1,275,000	23
MS	939,000	17
CP	412,000	7
Postpolio syndrome	272,000	5
TBI	242,000	4
Neurofibromatosis	212,000	4
Other	636,000	11

Paralysis Resource Center, Christopher & Dana Reeve Foundation, 2009 (22).

and diagnosis of the patients treated with intrathecal baclofen (ITB) or botulinum neurotoxin (BoNT) is shown in Table 2.2. Spinal cord injury, CP, and MS were the most common diagnoses treated with ITB, whereas stroke, CP, and SCI were the most common conditions treated with BoNT. This suggests that patients with these conditions may have the highest prevalence of problematic spasticity.

When discussing the conditions in children, data from the work of Hutchison et al. (23) may shed some light. The most common causes of spasticity in 341 children seen at some of the clinics at the Royal Children's Hospital in Melbourne, Australia, in 1998 were CP (79%), traumatic brain injury (TBI; 6%), spina bifida (5%), and SCI (2%).

STROKE

Each year, approximately equal to 795,000 people in the United States experience a new (about 610,000) or recurrent stroke (185,000) (24). The prevalence of stroke in the United States is 2.6 million for men and 3.9 million for women (24), with an annual incidence rate of 183 per 100,000 (25). There are significant differences in the prevalence of stroke by race/ethnicity, education level, and state/area of residence (26). Blacks have a higher incidence of stroke than whites, especially among the young, and the rate increases with age regardless of race (24). In Europe, the annual standardized incidence for stroke is 113 per 100,000 per year (27). In Sweden, with a population of 9 million, about 30,000 patients are hospitalized every year because of stroke, of which 20,000 are a first-ever event (28).

Four studies evaluated the prevalence of spasticity after a stroke and are summarized in Table 2.3. They are all from Europe, with the prevalence of spasticity ranging from 17% to 38%. Each identified the arm and leg spasticity using the Modified Ashworth Scale (MAS) score (29) and used the Barthel Index (BI) (30, 31) as functional measure. In a cross-sectional survey 1 year poststroke, Lundstrom et al. (2) identified 140 people with their first event from a national stroke registry. Arm and leg spasticity were measured using the MAS, and disability was measured with the modified Rankin Scale (32) and the BI. Disabling spasticity (DS) was defined as spasticity in need of an intervention, for example, intensive physiotherapy, orthosis, or pharmacologic treatment. The observed prevalence of any spasticity was 17% and of DS 4%. Patients with DS scored significantly worse on the modified Rankin Scale and the BI than those with no DS. Disabling spasticity was more frequent in the upper extremity and correlated positively with other indices of motor impairment and inversely with age. Although the prevalence of DS after a first-ever stroke from this study was low, in the context of the large number of stroke survivors, the number became more significant.

In a Swedish cohort study, Sommerfeld et al. (33) evaluated 95 patients with a first-ever stroke within 1 week of their stroke (mean, 5.4 days) and 3 months after their event. The authors measured spasticity by obtaining the MAS for the arm and leg, as well as self-reported muscle stiffness, tendon reflexes, several motor impairment measures, and the BI as a disability measure. Of the 95 patients studied, 64 were hemiparetic, 18 were spastic, 6 reported muscle stiffness, and 18 had increased tendon reflexes 3 months after

TABLE 2.2
Patients Treated for Spasticity at the
Medical College of Wisconsin With ITB
or BoNT From January 2008 to July 2008

DIAGNOSIS	ITB PATIENTS	BoNT PATIENTS
SCI	43 (30%)	50 (14%)
CP	34 (24%)	74 (20%)
MS	30 (21%)	23 (6%)
TBI	17 (12%)	37 (10%)
Stroke	6 (4%)	133 (37%)
Anoxic encephalopathy	3 (2%)	43 (12%)
Other	11 (7%)	3 (1%)
Total	144	363

TABLE 2.3
Prevalence of Spasticity After First Stroke

STUDY	NO. OF PATIENTS	TIME POSTSTROKE	SPASTICITY DIAGNOSIS	LOCATION	PREVALENCE OF SPASTICITY	PROBLEMATIC SPASTICITY
Lundstrom et al. 2008 (2)	140	1 year	MAS	Sweden	17%	4%[a]
Welmer et al. 2006 (34)	66	18 months	MAS	Sweden	20%	NR
Sommerfield et al. 2004 (33)	95	<1 week 3 months	MAS	Sweden	21% 19%	NR
Watkins et al. 2002 (10)	106	12 months	MAS-elbow TAS Combined	UK	27% 36% 38%	67%[b]

NR, not reported; Combined, MAS and TAS.
[a]Spasticity that requires an intervention, for example, physiotherapy, orthosis, pharmacologic.
[b]Patients with arm and leg spasticity (67%) had 50% lower Barthel score than patients with no spasticity.

stroke. Nonspastic patients (77) had statistically significantly better motor and activity scores than spastic patients (18). However, the correlations between muscle tone and disability scores were low, and severe disabilities were seen in almost the same number of nonspastic and spastic patients. They concluded that severe disabilities were seen in almost the same number of nonspastic and spastic patients and suggested that the importance of spasticity may be overstated. There were several limitations to this study including the small number of participants and the investigators' reliance on the use of the MAS as the only means of identifying if a person has spasticity. As a result, they may have missed patients with spasticity or other components of the UMN syndrome (10). In addition, the sample of patients only had a limited amount of motor deficits because 67% were hemiparetic at 3 months. Of this group, 28% had spasticity (33). In an 18-month follow-up study with the same cohort of patients, Welmer et al. (34) evaluated the frequency of spasticity and its association with functioning and health-related quality of life (HRQL) (35). Of the 66 patients studied, 38 were hemiparetic; of these, 13 displayed spasticity, 12 had increased tendon reflexes, and 7 reported muscle stiffness 18 months after stroke. Although there was a weak correlation between spasticity and HRQL, the hemiparetic patients without spasticity had significantly better BI functioning scores and significantly better HRQL health scales than patients with spasticity. This follow-up study suggests that spasticity may have a negative impact on functional improvement in patients who have had stroke in the long term.

Watkins et al. (10) evaluated 106 consecutive community-dwelling stroke survivors in Liverpool, UK, who were 12 months poststroke. They measured spasticity at the elbow using the MAS and at several joints and in the arms and legs using the Tone Assessment Scale (TAS) (36); they also assessed disability using the BI. The prevalence of spasticity in their study depended on the metric used. Using the MAS, 29 (27%) of the 106 patients had spasticity, whereas 38 (36%) were identified as spastic using the TAS. Forty (38%) was spastic when including those who were identified as having tone by either metric. Those with spasticity had significantly lower BI scores at 12 months, whereas those with arm and leg involvement had a BI 50% of those without spasticity.

Of the 4 studies that addressed the prevalence of spasticity in stroke survivors, 3 suggest that it is associated with greater motor impairments and has a negative impact on functional capabilities. The low prevalence of spasticity in these reports is most likely due to the lack of sensitivity of the measures used to assess it and the mild motor impairments of the samples studied. The study of more involved patients can be undertaken by looking at prevalence of spasticity from an inpatient rehabilitation unit. Francisco (4) performed this type of study when he presented a retrospective review of 204 stroke admissions to a freestanding rehabilitation hospital in 2002. The mean duration of stroke to admission was 5.76 days (range,

1.2–48 months), and 78% of the patients had hemorrhagic strokes. Seventy percent had spastic hypertonia (MAS ≥1), and 50% had clinically significant spasticity that required treatment. The larger prevalence of problematic spasticity in this group supports the notion that more severe spasticity is associated with greater impairments, as many of the patients included in this investigation also had severe motor, language, and cognitive impairments.

Two studies used electrophysiologic measures to evaluate the prevalence of spasticity after a stroke. O'Dwyer et al. (37) evaluated 24 hemiparetic stroke patients 1 to 13 months (mean, 5.3 months) after their event for upper limb spasticity and contracture. The motor impairment was graded mild to severe based on item 6 of the Motor Assessment Scale (38). They studied stretch-induced electromyographic activity of the biceps muscle at different velocities of stretch and found tonic stretch reflexes in 5 patients (21%). Of the 24 patients, 13 had a flexion contracture from 2° to 22°, suggesting that contracture may be more important than spasticity in this population. Although this study had similar prevalence data to the studies in Table 2.3, there were a limited number of patients in this study and they only tested 1 muscle for spasticity. In a larger study, Malhotra et al. (1) evaluated wrist spasticity in 100 patients 1 to 6 weeks (mean, 3 weeks) after their first stroke with severe weakness (scored 0 in the grasp section of the Action Research Arm Test) (39). Spasticity was evaluated using the MAS and biomechanical and neurophysiological measures. The MAS was abnormal in 44 patients, and 87 patients had abnormal involuntary muscle activation using a novel portable device with an electrogoniometer, force transducer, and surface bipolar electromyographic electrodes. This suggests that neurophysiological measures for spasticity are more sensitive than clinical ones and that assessing prevalence with clinical metrics may result in an underestimate. Additional studies with more objective measures of spasticity are needed to more accurately determine the prevalence of spasticity in patients who have had stroke.

SPINAL CORD INJURY

The estimated annual incidence of SCI in the United States, not including those who die at the scene of the accident, is approximately 40 cases per million or approximately 12,000 new cases each year (40). The estimated prevalence of SCI in the United States for 2008 was approximately 259,000 persons, with studies reporting within a range of 229,000 to 306,000

persons (40). The PRC reports a much higher estimate of SCI prevalence of approximately 1,275,000 people in the United States, with the most common cause of SCI being motor vehicle accidents followed by falls and acts of violence (22). Sports-related spinal cord injuries occur more commonly in children and teenagers, whereas work-related injuries are more common in adults. Most people with SCI are in their teens or twenties, and 78% are male (41). The male preponderance of SCI decreases after age 65, at which point, the most common mechanism of SCI is falls. More than half of all SCI occur at the cervical level, almost a third in the thoracic level, and the remainder in the lumbar area (41).

Table 2.4 summarizes the studies that assessed the prevalence of spasticity in patients with SCI. Of the 7 studies reviewed, 3 of the studies used clinical assessments to identify patients with spasticity, whereas 3 used patient questionnaires. The prevalence of spasticity ranged from 40% to 78% (average, 68%), with the higher prevalence noted in the studies that used a clinical scale. The prevalence of problematic spasticity was addressed in 5 of the studies. The criteria used to define it was if the patient required medication for treatment and if their spasticity interfered with ADL, was painful, or both. Using these measures, the prevalence of problematic spasticity ranged from 12% to 49%, with an average of 33%.

In the first of 2 epidemiologic studies, Maynard et al. (3) evaluated the occurrence of spasticity and its severity in 96 patients at one SCI center. Spasticity was considered present if the patient had increased deep tendon reflexes, muscle tone during passive movements, or involuntary muscle spasms. Severity of spasticity was determined if they were taking antispasticity medication and if they had satisfactory treatment. Treatment was indicated if the spasticity was interfering with ADL and sleep or caused pain that prevented or interfered with activities. By this definition, 67% of the patients had spasticity at the time of their discharge (average, 118 days) and 37% were taking antispasticity medication. The incidence of spasticity was higher among groups with cervical and upper thoracic levels of injury compared with groups with other levels of injury. At their 1-year follow-up, the percent of patients with spasticity increased to 78% and 49% of them required medication. The second part of the study analyzed the presence of spasticity severe enough to require treatment in 466 subjects with SCI from 13 different SCI centers. From this patient population, 26% of the patients received antispasticity treatment at the time of discharge (average, 105 days), and the percentage increased to 46% at their 1-year follow-up. Spasticity treatment was more common in cervical and

TABLE 2.4
Prevalence of Spasticity After SCI

Study	No. of Patients	Time Post Injury	Spasticity Diagnosis	Location, Duration	Prevalence of Spasticity	Problematic Spasticity
Maynard et al. 1990 (3) Study 1	96	DC, 1 year	CS	MI, 1985–1988	67% 78%	37%[a] 49%
Maynard et al. 1990 (3) Study 2	466	DC, 1 year	CS	USA	NR	26% 46%
Anson et al. 1996 (46)	191	1 to >15 years	NR	Atlanta	62%	12%[b]
Johnson et al. 1998 (44)	853	1 years 3 years 5 years	PSR	Colorado	NR	35%[c] 32% 28%
Sköld et al. 1999 (5)	354	12 months	MAS	Sweden, 1997	65%	30%[d]
Noreau et al. 2000 (47)	482	12 months	PSR[e]	Quebec	40%	NR
Walter et al. 2002 (45)	99	NR	PSR[f]	Chicago Hines VA	53%	40%[a]

CS, Clinical Scale (spasticity present if deep tendon reflexes increased, increased muscle tone during passive movements, or involuntary muscle spasms); DC, discharge from hospital; NR, not reported; PSR, patient self-report.
[a]Spasticity that required medication.
[b]Spasticity that interfered with ADLs.
[c]Problematic spasticity.
[d]Spasticity that was painful, restricting ADLs, or both.
[e]PSR: "Over the past 12 months have you developed or suffered from spasticity?"
[f]PSR: "Are you having a problem with spasticity?"

upper thoracic patients with incomplete injuries. The percentage of patients requiring spasticity treatment with Frankel grades B (sensory incomplete, motor complete) and C (motor incomplete, nonfunctional) was 50% and 52% (42), respectively, whereas the percentage of patients requiring spasticity treatment with Frankel grades A (sensory and motor complete) and D (motor incomplete, functional) was 27% and 29%, respectively. Little et al. (43) reported similar findings in 26 patients with SCI, where the patients with Frankel grade C had greater flexor withdrawal responses and extensor spasms, more pain, and interference with sleep than those with Frankel grades A and D. These findings suggest that increased time after injury and motor incompleteness of SCI may contribute to the increased severity of spasticity.

Johnson et al. (44) investigated the frequency of both medical and nonmedical complications reported to the Colorado Spinal Cord Injury Early Notification System for patients with SCI. They interviewed each patient by telephone at 1, 3, and 5 years after injury. They noted a decrease in the prevalence of spasticity from year 1 (35%) to year 5 (28%), which may have

been due to reduced sample size at year 5 (50% of year 1). They also noted that spasticity had a variable impact on quality of life and productivity measures. They recommended that follow-up needs to be longer than 5 years (decades rather than years) to gauge the full impact of each SCI complication. Using both physical examination and patient self-report, Sköld et al. (5) found abnormal MAS in only 60% of the patients reporting significant spasticity, whereas 97% of patients with abnormal MAS report spasticity. This study underscores the importance of using both clinical measures and patient self-report when evaluating problematic spasticity. The other studies using patient self-report, which are summarized in Table 2.4, support the need for patient questionnaires to ask sufficient questions to determine the full impact of spasticity and the other components of UMNS on the patient's daily activities (45–47).

Traumatic Brain Injury

In 2003, an estimated 1,565,000 people in the United States experienced TBI, a rate of 538.2 per 100,000

TABLE 2.5
Prevalence of Spasticity After TBI

STUDY	NO. OF PATIENTS	TIME POST INJURY	SPASTICITY DIAGNOSIS	COUNTRY	PREVALENCE OF SPASTICITY	PROBLEMATIC SPASTICITY
Wedekind and Lippert-Gruner 2005 (52)	32	1 year	PE	Germany	34%	NR

PE, physical examination (measure not reported); NR, not reported.

population with 230,000 hospitalizations as a result (48). Although almost 90% of all TBI are mild and cause no lasting impairment, TBI of any severity has the potential to cause significant long-term disability (49, 50). An estimated 5.3 million people are living in the United States with disability related to TBI (51). Based on these estimates, one might expect that the number of TBI patients with paralysis (242,000) reported from the PRC may be an underestimate (Table 2.5). Using the prevalence data from the PRC and based on the prevalence of problematic spasticity of 30% to 50% from other conditions (Table 2.6), there could be more than 100,000 TBI patients with problematic spasticity. This number is consistent with the number of patients treated in the spasticity clinic at MCW, where TBI is the fourth most common diagnosis treated with ITB or BoNT (Table 2.2). However, there is no study that demonstrates this number.

Despite the number of patients with TBI, there has been very little work that has attempted to quantify the problem of spasticity in people with this condition. In a retrospective study, Wedekind and Lippert-Gruner (52) investigated the 1-year outcome of 32 survivors with severe TBI. They divided the patients into 2 groups: those with brainstem injury (midbrain and pons, $n = 15$) and those without brainstem lesions ($n = 17$). At 1 year, 8 of the 15 (53%) in the brainstem injury group and 3 of the 17 (18%) in the nonbrainstem group had spasticity. The authors failed to mention how they assessed spasticity. However, patients with a brainstem lesion had lower Functional Independence Measure scores and lower disability rating scale (53) and were unable to return to work even with support. It is difficult to determine from this small study what impact, if any, spasticity had on the negative long-term outcome. Elovic and Zafonte (54) reported that 25% of the patients admitted to the Traumatic Brain Injury Model Systems had evidence of increased tone while undergoing inpatient rehabilitation. Unfortunately, the nature of the system data did not allow an identification if the spasticity was problematic. More recently, consecutive admissions with the diagnosis of TBI to the Kessler Institute for Rehabilitation were assessed for the presence of spas-

TABLE 2.6
Estimated Prevalence of Spasticity and Problematic Spasticity in the United States

CONDITION	ESTIMATE US PATIENTS	PREVALENCE OF SPASTICITY[a]	PREVALENCE OF PROBLEMATIC SPASTICITY[a]
Stroke	6,500,000	1,495,000 (23%)	448,500 (30%)
TBI	5,300,000	NA	NA
CP	764,000	649,400 (85%)	382,000 (50%)
MS	400,000	268,000 (67%)	152,000 (38%)
SCI	259,000	172,040 (68%)	83,490 (33%)

NA, insufficient data from published reports.
[a]Average percent from referenced population-based studies.

ticity. In total, 161 were evaluated and 45 (27.9%) of them were noted to have increased tone on evaluation. Clearly, more research is needed on the impact and prevalence of spasticity in the TBI population. In addition, better outcome measures are needed for the assessment of spasticity in patients with TBI (55).

MULTIPLE SCLEROSIS

Hirtz et al. (25) estimate that in the general population the 1-year prevalence for MS is 0.9 per 1000. In the United States, there are approximately 400,000 people with MS, and 200 more people are diagnosed every week (56). This number is nearly two and a half times less than the estimated number of patients with MS with paralysis from the PRC (22). Worldwide, MS is thought to affect more than 2.5 million people. It occurs with greater frequency above the 40° latitude, is more common among whites, and is 2 to 3 times more common in women than in men (56). Although most people are diagnosed between the ages of 20 and 50, MS is also diagnosed in children and adolescents. Estimates suggest that 8000 to 10,000 children (<18 years old) in the United States have MS, and another 10,000 to 15,000 have experienced at least one symptom suggestive of MS (56).

Table 2.7 summarizes the 3 studies on the prevalence of spasticity in patients with MS. These reports relied primarily on patient self-report for determining severity of spasticity, and one study used the MAS. Two studies (6, 12) suggest that MS-related spasticity was not adequately treated. Barnes et al. (12) conducted a random sample of 100 people with MS (from a total of 260 patients) in the city of Newcastle upon Tyne in the north of England. From a total of 68 patients who participated in the study, 45 (67%) were women with a mean age of 49 years (range, 28–73). The mean time from diagnosis was 10.2 years (range, 0–48 years). Spasticity for each limb was assessed using the MAS, and the worst joint score was recorded. Ninety-seven percent of the patients had detectable leg spasticity (MAS ≥1), and 50% had arm spasticity. The 32 (47%) patients with significant spasticity (MAS ≥2) had more severe disability as measured by the Kurtzke Functional Systems Scale (57), the Newcastle Independence Assessment Form (58), and the motor subscale of the Functional Independence Measure (59), suggesting that spasticity is one factor that may play an important role in the overall disability in MS and effective intervention may reduce disability. Unfortunately, 50% of the patients from this study needed oral medications, which were either not prescribed or were dosed suboptimally.

In a survey of 493 patients with MS from the Northern California Chapter of the National Multiple Sclerosis Society, 168 patients (34%) returned completed questionnaires (6). Fifty-eight percent rated

TABLE 2.7
Prevalence of Spasticity in Patients With MS

STUDY	NO. OF PATIENTS	DURATION OF SURVEY	SPASTICITY DIAGNOSIS	COUNTRY	PREVALENCE/SEVERITY OF SPASTICITY, NO. (%)
Goodin, 1999 (6)	168	1997	PSR[a]	USA	None: 50 (30) Mild: 64 (38) Moderate/severe: 54 (32)
Barnes et al. 2003 (12)	68	1998–1999	MAS	UK	MAS <2: 36 (53) MAS ≥2: 32 (47)[b]
Rizzo et al. 2004 (7)	20,380	1996–2003	PSR[c]	USA	None: 3196 (16) Minimal/mild: 10,248 (50) Moderate: 3494 (17) Severe/total: 3440 (17)

MAS, Modified Ashworth Scale; PSR, patient self-report.

[a]PSR: none, mild, moderate, or severe spasticity and/or spasms for each arm and leg.

[b]Fifty percent needed spasticity medication.

[c]PSR: 0 = normal (no symptoms of spasticity), 1= minimal (some problems with spasticity, but does not interfere with activities), 2 = mild (spasticity occasionally forces me to change some of my activities, for example, once a week or less), 3 = moderate (spasticity frequently affects some of my activities, for example, several times a week), 4 = severe (every day, spasticity problems force me to modify my daily activities), 5 = total (every day, spasticity problems prevent me from doing many of my daily activities).

themselves as partially or totally disabled, and 65% felt that their disability was in part or in whole due to fatigue. Seventy percent of the patients had mild, moderate, or severe spasticity. Spasticity was rated for each arm and leg as none, mild, moderate, or severe spasticity and/or spasms (60). Unfortunately, the survey did not correlate spasticity with their measures of disability. Only 67% of the patients with moderate or severe spasticity and 44% of those with mild spasticity had received any treatment. The obvious limitations of this study are the subjective metrics used to assess spasticity and the limited (34%) response rate that suggests that this may not have had a representative sample of the population sampled.

In a much larger cross-sectional study from the Patient Registry of the North American Research Committee on Multiple Sclerosis, Rizzo et al. (7) published the most extensive review of the prevalence and severity of spasticity in patients with MS. More than 20,000 patients were enrolled for the study between 1996 and 2003. In the survey, spasticity was described for the patients as "unusual tightening of muscles that feels like leg stiffness, jumping of legs, a repetitive bouncing of the foot, muscle cramping in legs or arms, legs going out tight and straight or drawing up." A 0-to-5 (0 = normal, 5 = total) spasticity scale that reflected severity and frequency of spasticity on the patients' daily activities was used. Eighty-four percent of the respondents had some degree of spasticity, of which 63% had problematic spasticity that at least occasionally forced them

to alter some of their daily activities. Patients with more severe spasticity were more likely to be older, male, disabled, or unemployed; had a longer duration of disease; and had more relapses and worsening MS symptoms in the months before the survey. Only 1.1% of the respondents had the ITB pump, and 78% of the patients with severe/total spasticity were using any medication for it. This suggests that poor tolerance or undertreatment may be a problem. A weakness of this study was the use of a subjective patient self-report measure of spasticity, which may have resulted in an overestimation of the prevalence of spasticity (5). Nevertheless, the patient self-report may be a more accurate reflection of problematic spasticity for the patient.

CEREBRAL PALSY

Cerebral palsy is the most common cause of motor disability in childhood (61–64). It is an umbrella term covering a group of nonprogressive but often changing motor impairment syndromes secondary to lesions or anomalies of the brain, arising at any time during brain development (61). Population-based studies have reported the prevalence of CP to range from 1.5 to 3.0 cases per 1000 children (25, 62–64). The number of people with CP in the United States is estimated at 764,000 (64). The estimated number of CP patients with paralysis is more than 400,000 according to the PRC (Table 2.1). It is the second most common

TABLE 2.8
Prevalence of Spasticity in Children With CP

STUDY	NO. OF CP	AGE (YEARS)	DIAGNOSIS	COUNTRY	PREVALENCE OF SPASTICITY	DISABLING SPASTICITY
Yeargin-Alisop et al., 2008 (66)	416	8	CR	USA, 2002	All: 80.6% Di: 93 (22%) Tri: 5 (1%) Tet: 104 (25%) Hem: 94 (22%)	NR
Wichers et al., 2005 (8)	127	6–19	PE	Netherlands, 1977–1988	All: 93.7% Di: 30 (25%) Tri: 12 (9%) Tet: 29 (24%) Hem: 48 (38%)	40%[a] 58% 93% 8%

CR, Clinician review and *International Classification of Disease* codes; NR, not reported; PE, physical examination; Di, spastic diplegia; Tri, spastic triplegia; Tet, spastic tetraplegia (quadriplegia); Hem, spastic hemiplegia.
[a]Percentage of severe motor disability: not able to walk independently by the age of 5.

condition treated with ITB or BoNT at the MCW (Table 2.2), suggesting a higher prevalence of problematic spasticity.

In a recent meta-analysis, Himpens et al. (65) reported that the prevalence of CP decreased significantly with increasing gestational age category: 14.6% at 22 to 27 weeks' gestation, 6.2% at 28 to 31 weeks, 0.7% at 32 to 36 weeks, and 0.1% in term infants. The significant decrease in the prevalence started after a gestational age of 27 weeks, with spastic CP the most common in preterm infants. In term infants, the nonspastic form of CP was more prevalent. Bilateral spastic CP (includes diplegia, triplegia, and tetraplegia) was the most prevalent in both preterm and term infants. There was no reported relationship between the severity of CP and gestational age.

The two most recent studies on the prevalence of spasticity in patients with CP are summarized in Table 2.8. Using methods developed by the Centers for Disease Control and Prevention Metropolitan Atlanta Developmental Disabilities Surveillance Program, and the Autism and Developmental Disabilities Monitoring Network, Yeargin-Allsopp et al. (66) conducted a survey on 8-year-old children with CP living in northern Alabama, metropolitan Atlanta, and southeastern Wisconsin in 2002 ($N = 114,897$). *International Classification of Disease* codes (67) and multiple nonschool sources were used to identify patients, and the data were linked to birth certificate and census files information. The average prevalence of CP across the 3 sites was 3.6 cases per 1000, with similar site-specific prevalence estimates (3.3 cases per 1000 in Wisconsin, 3.7 cases per 1000 in Alabama, and 3.8 cases per 1000 in Georgia). At all sites, prevalence was higher in boys (overall boy/girl ratio, 4:1). In addition, at all sites, the prevalence of CP was highest in black non-Hispanic children and lowest in Hispanic children. Spastic CP was the most common subtype (77% of all cases), with bilateral CP the most common in the spastic group (70%).

In a population-based study on prevalence of CP in Dutch children, Wichers et al. (8) examined 170 reported patients with a preliminary diagnosis of CP and excluded 43 (25%) because they did not meet criteria. Motor disability was classified as mild if by the age of 5 the child was able to ambulate independently (with or without assistive device) or severe if by age 5 the child had not been able to ambulate independently. This study reported that the spastic subtype accounted for more than 90% of all CP cases, and spastic hemiplegia was the largest individual clinical subtype (Table 2.8). Two thirds of the patients with bilateral spastic CP and more than 90% of the patients with spastic tetraplegia had severe motor deficits, suggesting that spasticity has a negative impact on independent ambulation. This study also highlighted the importance of patient examination to confirm diagnosis.

CONCLUSION

Several studies in this review support the notion that spasticity is associated with greater motor impairments and has a negative impact on functional capabilities. Although it may be difficult to accurately estimate the prevalence of spasticity and problematic spasticity in the United States, the author's best estimate is summarized in Table 2.6. Unfortunately, there are insufficient data on patients with TBI to address the issue in this condition. A recent survey by PRC suggests that the number of patients with disabling conditions related to MS and SCI may be significantly underestimated. Clearly, additional study is needed to clarify the prevalence of problematic spasticity in the adult and child with UMNS. This information would help direct resources to the populations that need it the most, as a significant number of patients may be undiagnosed and undertreated (6, 7, 12). A combination of clinical, biomechanical, and electrophysiogic measures of both active and passive activity and functional and quality of life measures are all needed to gauge the full impact of spasticity for each patient and to assess treatment benefits (1, 9, 55). Clarifying and treating problematic spasticity remain critical to improving outcomes in patients with UMNS. Although the remainder of this book revolves around the issues of diagnosis and treatment, it is important to understand the scope of the problem.

References

1. Malhotra S, Cousins E, Ward A, et al. An investigation into the agreement between clinical, biomechanical and neurophysiological measures of spasticity. *Clin Rehabil.* 2008;22:1105–1115.
2. Lundstrom E, Terent A, Borg J. Prevalence of disabling spasticity 1 year after first-ever stroke. *Eur J Neurol.* 2008;15:533–539.
3. Maynard FM, Karunas RS, Waring WP. Epidemiology of spasticity following traumatic spinal cord injury. *Arch Phys Med Rehabil.* 1990;71:566–569.
4. Francisco GE. How common is spastic hypertonia during stroke rehabilitation? *Arch Phys Med Rehabil.* 2002;83:A21. Abstract.
5. Sköld C, Levi R, Seiger Å. Spasticity after traumatic spinal cord injury: nature, severity, and location. *Arch Phys Med Rehabil.* 1999;80:1548–1557.
6. Goodin DS. A questionnaire to assess neurological impairment in multiple sclerosis. *Mult Scler.* 1998;4:444–451.

7. Rizzo MA, Hadjimichael OC, Preiningerova J, Vollmer TL. Prevalence and treatment of spasticity reported by multiple sclerosis patients. *Mult Scler.* 2004;10:589–595.

8. Wichers MJ, Odding E, Stam HJ, van Nieuwenhuizen O. Clinical presentation associated disorders and aetiological moments in cerebral palsy: a Dutch population–based study. *Disabil Rehabil.* 2005;27:583–589.

9. Mayer N, Esquenazi A. Muscle overactivity and movement dysfunction in the upper motoneuron syndrome. *Phys Med Rehabil Clin N Am.* 2003;14:855–883.

10. Watkins CL, Leathley MJ, Gregson JM, Moore AP, Smith TL, Sharma AK. Prevalence of spasticity post stroke. *Clin Rehabil.* 2002;16:515–522.

11. Ashworth B. Preliminary trial of carisoprodol in multiple sclerosis. *Practitioner.* 1964;192:540–542.

12. Barnes MP, Kent RM, Semlyen JK, McMullen KM. Spasticity in multiple sclerosis. *Neurorehabil Neural Repair.* 2003;17:66–70.

13. Denny-Brown D. *The cerebral control of movement.* Liverpool: Liverpool University Press; 1966;170–184.

14. Burke D. Spasticity as an adaptation to pyramidal tract injury. *Adv Neurol.* 1988; 47: 401–422.

15. Little JW, Massagli TL. Spasticity and associated abnormalities of muscle tone. In DeLisa JA. *Rehabilitation medicine: principles and practice.* Philadelphia: Lippincott Co; 1993:666–680.

16. Mayer N. Clinicophysiologic concepts of spasticity and motor dysfunction in adults with an upper motoneuron lesion. *Muscle Nerve.* 1997;6:S1–S13.

17. Sheean G. The neurophysiology of spasticity. In: Barnes MP, Johnson GR. *Upper motor neurone syndrome and spasticity.* 2nd ed. New York: Cambridge University Press; 2008: 9–63.

18. Gracies JM. Pathophysiology of spastic paresis. II: emergence of muscle overactivity. *Muscle Nerve.* 2005;31:552–571.

19. Lance J. Symposium synopsis in spasticity. In: Feldman R, Young R, Koella W. *Disordered motor control.* Chicago: Year Book Medical Publishers; 1980:487–489.

20. Katz RT, Rymer WZ. Spastic hypertonia: mechanisms and measurement. *Arch Phys Med Rehabil.* 1989;70:144–155.

21. McGuire J, Rymer W. Spasticity: mechanisms and management. In: Green D. *Medical management of long-term disability.* Newton: Butterworth-Heinemann; 1996:277–288.

22. http://www.christopherreeve.org/site/c.mtKZKgMWKwG/b.5184189/k.5587/Paralysis_Facts__Figures.htm Jan 2009.

23. Hutchison R, Graham HK. Management of spasticity in children. In: Barnes MP, Johnson GR. *Upper motor neurone syndrome and spasticity.* 2nd Ed. New York: Cambridge University Press; 2008:214–239.

24. Lloyd-Jones D, Adams R, Carnethon M, et al. Heart disease and stroke statistics—2009 update: a report from the American Heart Association Statistics Committee and Stroke Statistics Subcommittee. *Circulation.* 2009;119;e71–e82.

25. Hirtz D, Thurman DJ, Gwinn-Hardy K, Mohamed M, Chaudhuri AR, Zalutsky R. How common are the "common" neurologic disorders? *Neurology.* 2007;68:326–337.

26. Neyer JR, Greenlund KJ, Denny CH, Keenan NL, Casper M, Labarthe DR, Croft JB, Div for Heart Disease and Stroke Prevention, National Center for Chronic Disease Prevention and Health Promotion, CDC. Prevalence of stroke—United States, 2005. *JAMA.* 2007;298:279–281.

27. Bejot Y, Benatru I, Rouaud O, et al. Epidemiology of stroke in Europe: geographic and environmental differences. *J Neurol Sci.* 2007;262:85–88.

28. Appelros P, Nydevik I, Seiger A, Terént A. High incidence rates of stroke in Orebro, Sweden: further support for regional incidence differences within Scandinavia. *Cerebrovasc Dis.* 2002;14:161–168.

29. Bohannon RW, Smith MB. Interrater reliability on a Modified Ashworth Scale of muscle spasticity. *Phys Ther.* 1987;67:206–207.

30. Mahoney FI, Barthel DW. Functional evaluation: the Barthel Index. *Md State Med J.* 1965;14:61–65.

31. Wade DT, Hewer RL. Functional abilities after stroke: measurement, natural history and prognosis. *J Neurol Neurosurg Psychiatry.* 1987;50:177–182.

32. Rankin J. Cerebral vascular accidents in patients over the age of 60: prognosis. *Scott Med J.* 1957;2:200–215.

33. Sommerfeld DK, Eek EU, Svensson AK, Holmqvist LW, von Arbin MH. Spasticity after stroke: its occurrence and association with motor impairments and activity limitations. *Stroke.* 2004;35:134–140.

34. Welmer AK, von Arbin M, Widen Holmqvist L, Sommerfeld DK. Spasticity and its association with functioning and health-related quality of life 18 months after stroke. *Cerebrovasc Dis.* 2006;21:247–253.

35. Guyatt GH, Feeny DH, Patrick DL. Measuring health-related quality of life. *Ann Intern Med.* 1993;118:622–629.

36. Barnes SA, Gregson JM, Leathley MJ, Sharma AK, Smith TL, Watkins CL. Development and inter-rater reliability of an assessment scale to measure abnormal tone in adult, hemiplegic stroke patients. *Physiotherapy.* 1999;85:405–409.

37. O'Dwyer NJ, Ada L, Neilson PD. Spasticity and muscle contracture following stroke. *Brain.* 1996;119:1737–1749.

38. Carr JH, Sheperd RB, Nordholm L, Lynne D. Investigation of a new Motor Assessment Scale for stroke. *Phys Ther.* 1985;65:175–180.

39. Lyle A. A performance test for assessment of upper limb function in physical rehabilitation treatment and research. *Int J Rehabil Res.* 1981;4:483–492.

40. http://www.spinalcord.uab.edu/show.asp?durki=119513 Jan 2009.

41. http://www.christopherreeve.org/atf/cf/%7B3d83418f-b967-4c18-8ada-adc2e5355071%7D/Spinal%20Cord%20Injury%206-09.PDF Jan 2009.

42. Frankel HL, Hancock DO, Hyslop G, et al. The value of postural reduction in the initial management of closed injuries of the spine with paraplegia and (part I) tetraplegia. *Paraplegia.* 1969;7:179–192.

43. Little JW, Micklesen P, Umlauf R, Britell C. Lower extremity manifestations of spasticity in chronic spinal cord injury. *Am J Phys Med Rehabil.* 1989;68:32–36.

44. Johnson RL, Gerhart KA, McCray J, Menconi JC, Whiteneck GG. Secondary conditions following spinal cord injury in a population-based sample. *Spinal Cord.* 1998;36:45–50.

45. Walter JS, Sacks J, Othman R, et al. A database of self-reported secondary medical problems among VA spinal cord injury patients: its role in clinical care and management. *J Rehabil Res Dev.* 2002;39:53–61.

46. Anson CA, Shepherd C. Incidence of secondary complications in spinal cord injury. *Int J Rehabil Res.* 1996;19:55–66.

47. Noreau L, Proulx P, Gagnon L, Drolet M, Laremee M. Secondary impairments after spinal cord. *Am J Phys Med Rehabil.* 2000;79:526–535.

48. Rutland-Brown W, Langlois JA, Thomas KE, Xi YL. Incidence of traumatic brain injury in the United States, 2003. *J Head Trauma Rehabil.* 2006;21:544–548.

49. Brown AW, Leibson CL, Malec JF, Perkins PK, Diehl NN, Larson DR. Long-term survival after traumatic brain injury: a population-based analysis. *NeuroRehabilitation.* 2004;19: 37–43.

50. Brown AW, Elovic EP, Kothari S, Flanagan SR, Kwasnica C. Congenital and acquired brain injury. 1. Epidemiology, pathophysiology, prognostication, innovative treatments, and prevention. *Arch Phys Med Rehabil.* 2008;89:S3–S8.

51. Thurman DJ, Alverson C, Dunn KA, Guerrero J, Sniezek JE. Traumatic brain injury in the United States: a public health perspective. *J Head Trauma Rehabil.* 1999;14:602–615.

52. Wedekind C, Lippert-Gruner M. Long-term outcome in severe traumatic brain injury is significantly influenced by brainstem involvement. *Brain Inj.* 2005;19:681–684.

53. Rappaport M, Hall KM, Hopkins K, Belleza T, Cope DN. Disability rating scale for severe head trauma: coma to community. *Arch Phys Med Rehabil.* 1982;63:118–123.

54. Elovic E, Zafonte R. Spasticity management of traumatic brain injury. *State of the Art Review of Rehabilitation.* 2001;15: 327–348.

55. Elovic EP, Simone LK, Zafonte R. Outcome assessment for spasticity management in the patient with traumatic brain injury: the state of the art. *J Head Trauma Rehabil.* 2004;19:155–177.

56. http://www.nationalmssociety.org/about-multiple-sclerosis/who-gets-ms/epidemiology-of-ms/index.aspx. Jan 2009.

57. Kurtzke JF. Rating neurologic impairment in multiple sclerosis: an expanded disability status scale (EDSS). *Neurology.* 1983;33:1444–1452.

58. Semlyen JK, Hurrell E, Carter S, Barnes MP. The Newcastle Independence Assessment Form (Research): development of an alternative functional measure. *J Neurol Rehabil.* 1996; 10:251–257.

59. Keith RA, Granger CV, Hamilton VV, Sherwin FS. The Functional Independence Measure: a new tool for rehabilitation. In: Eisenberg MG, Grzesiak RC, eds. *Adv Clin Assess.* 1997;1:6–18.

60. Goodin DS. A questionnaire to assess neurological impairment in multiple sclerosis. *Mult Scler.* 1998;4:444–451.

61. Mutch L, Alberman E, Hagberg B, Kodama K, Perat MV. Cerebral palsy epidemiology: where are we now and where are we going? *Dev Med Child Neurol.* 1992;34:547–551.

62. Paneth N, Hong T, Korzeniewski S. The descriptive epidemiology of cerebral palsy. *Clin Perinatol.* 2006;33:251–267.

63. SCPE Collaborative Group. Surveillance of cerebral palsy in Europe: a collaboration of cerebral palsy surveys and registers. *Dev Med Child Neurol.* 2000;42:816–824.

64. Krigger KW. Cerebral palsy: an overview. *Am Fam Physician.* 2006;73:91–100.

65. Himpens E, Van den Broeck C, Oostra A, Calders P, Vanhaesebrouck P. Prevalence, type, distribution, and severity of cerebral palsy in relation to gestational age: a meta-analytic review. *Dev Med Child Neurol.* 2008;50:334–340.

66. Yeargin-Allsopp M, Braun KV, Doernberg NS, Benedict RE, Kirby RS, Durkin MS. Prevalence of cerebral palsy in 8-year-old children in three areas of the united states in 2002: a multisite collaboration. *Pediatrics.* 2008;121: 547–554.

67. US Department of Health and Human Services. *International classification of siseases, ninth revision, clinical modification [CDROM].* 5th ed. Washington, DC: US Government Printing Office; 2006.

Spasticity and Other Signs of the Upper Motor Neuron Syndrome

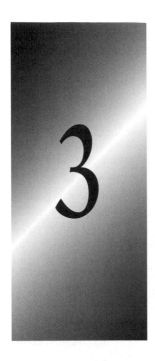

Nathaniel H. Mayer

The noted 19th century neurologist John Hughlings Jackson was one of the first to recognize that a lesion of the central nervous system could *simultaneously* result in the development of positive and negative signs, although he did not believe that the lesion directly caused the observed signs. In humans, a lesion of the descending corticospinal motor system is capable of producing the negative sign of muscle weakness during voluntary effort and, at the same time and in the same muscle, the positive sign of increased resistance to passive stretch. The combination is the key feature of muscle spasticity, although it is important to recognize that spasticity is only one of a number of positive signs that materialize after an upper motor neuron (UMN) lesion. The aggregate of positive and negative signs after a UMN lesion comprises the upper motor neuron syndrome (UMNS).

Jackson conceptualized the central nervous system as a hierarchical system operating across a number of levels. He believed that negative signs represented dissolution of the highest, most flexible, most volitional level of neural function, whereas positive signs resulted from less flexible, more stereotypic levels of neural circuitry that became excessively excited or released from higher-level inhibitory controls (1). Negative signs reflected a loss of a particular capacity ordinarily controlled by the lesioned area of the brain, whereas positive signs reflected release phenomena, abnormal or exaggerated behaviors, that were stereotypic

in nature and potentially explained by withdrawal of inhibition from neural tissue normally mediating that behavior. A loss of inhibition resulted in positive signs, manifested clinically by stereotypic movements and postures that were generated by stereotypic linkages of overactive muscle groups. Positive and negative signs interact often at the same time.

Inequalities of muscle weakness and muscle overactivity within and across muscle groups often lead to a net balance of muscle torques acting across joints shared in common by these groups. For example, a positive behavior such as an associated reaction may promote involuntary elbow and finger *flexion* in a hemiplegic patient. Because the lesion in this example also impairs voluntary elbow and finger *extension*, the patient is unable to actively extend elbow and fingers to reverse the flexed joint attitude produced by the associated reaction. Based on clinical experience, passive stretching exercises do not fend off the persistence of UMNS postural patterns. In time, this combination of unidirectional, unreversed flexion of elbow and fingers leads to stereotyped flexion postures in our patient. Thus, the stereotypy inherent in UMN release phenomena gives rise to movements and postures familiar to clinicians (eg, flexed elbow, clenched fist, equinovarus foot) (2). These movement patterns and postures, generated by various positive signs and unreversed by negative signs, often have detrimental consequences for patient care and require treatment. For example, persistent posturing often creates overlapping skin folds, underneath which maceration, erythema, and malodor flourish. Fixed, excessive postures can cause stretch injury of nerves. Fingernails can dig into the palm, causing pressure, pain, and laceration. Moreover, clinical experience reveals that UMN patterns are more diverse than perhaps commonly noted. For example, a flexed elbow is very common, but an extended elbow is also found. A flexed wrist is common, but an extended wrist is also seen. No matter the diversity of pattern, it still reflects an underlying net balance of torques brought on by positive sign stereotypy and deficient voluntary reversal of negative signs.

In summary, a lesion of the descending motor system according to Jackson's hierarchical notion produced higher-level neural dysfunction or frank absence of voluntary movement (negative signs) and simultaneous (although not necessarily instantaneous) stereotypic behaviors (positive signs) that reflect released lower-level, premorbidly inhibited behaviors of an involuntary nature. In a sense, the influence of a UMN lesion, variable in its severity, can cause any given muscle to behave variably in 2 ways: a negative way (loss of volitional command) and a positive way (acquisition of involuntary behaviors). As a result, the interaction between positive and negative signs, the aggregate effect of a UMN lesion on *all muscles* surrounding a joint, makes the analysis of joint movement and limb function complicated. What follows is a clinical description of the features of the UMNS with respect to negative and positive signs. For the sake of brevity, this chapter will focus primarily on upper limb examples.

NEGATIVE SIGNS

Impairment of Meaningful Action

With patients commonly complaining of weakness, loss of strength is considered the premier negative sign of UMNS, and voluntary strength testing can be significantly reduced. Studies at the physiological level have shown that reduced motor unit recruitment and frequency contribute importantly to the clinical effect of weakness (3). Against increasing loads, the orderly recruitment of small to larger units may also be impaired (4). Nevertheless, many patients retain considerable strength, especially if tested isometrically. In some cases, it is striking how much forward push a patient can develop against an examiner's hand isometrically while being unable to reach forward even an inch isotonically. This observation raises questions

regarding the value and validity of the testing of muscle strength in this population. On further reflection, weakness does not seem to be the best description of impaired volition in UMNS. Two features stand out. The first is a loss of selective control, that is, a loss of independent joint movement and inability to perform separate movements of individual joints or to operate and control several joints selectively as a unit at will. Instead of autonomous control, the patient with UMNS, attempting to make selective joint movement, makes multijoint obligatory patterns of movement that reflect obligatory muscle activations within and across joints. A patient of mine with UMNS after 7 years following a head injury reported to me the recovery of selective control of thumb, index, and long fingers. When he sat down at the piano one morning, he was able to strike keys separately with his thumb, index, and long fingers. However, when he attempted to selectively strike a key with the ring or little fingers, they coupled together and 2 keys were struck. He was unable to operate the ring and little fingers selectively no matter how much voluntary effort was made.

The commonest example of obligatory linkages across jointed limb segments during a movement effort is the so-called flexor synergy pattern (see Figure 3.1): scapular retraction, shoulder abduction and external rotation, elbow flexion, and forearm supination. When asked to perform a task such as reaching forward to

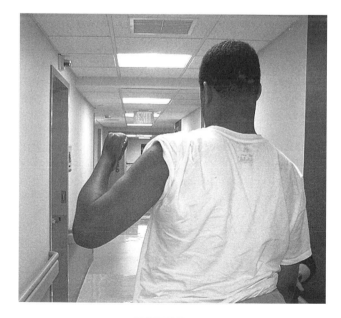

FIGURE 3.1

Flexor synergy pattern. Note: Shoulder (scapular) retraction, relative shoulder abduction and external rotation, elbow flexion and forearm supination.

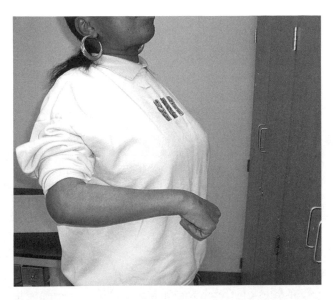

FIGURE 3.2

Effort by a hemiparetic patient to reach forward and grasp a door handle does not produce the intended movement pattern but only components of flexor synergy (shoulder retraction, abduction, elbow flexion).

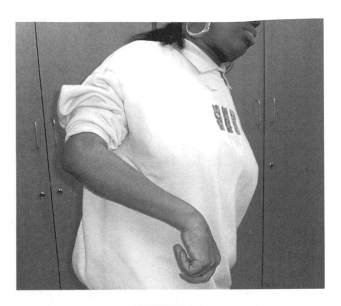

FIGURE 3.3

Effort by the same hemiparetic patient to touch her chin, a totally different task from reaching forward to grasp a door handle, produces a similar meaningless stereotypy of movement as in Figure 3.2.

grasp an object (see Figure 3.2), the patient dominated by flexor synergy reveals many, if not all, of these joint movements. When asked to perform a totally different task (see Figure 3.3), the flexion "synergy-bound" patient produces a similar stereotyped behavior. The patient is locked into an obligatory movement pattern that is initiated (and terminated) by volitional effort. It is beyond the scope of this chapter to discuss the nature of voluntary movement, but for now, we note that a number of voluntary features are retained by a patient with UMNS during synergy production, including initiation, termination, and varying the speed of synergy pattern movement. The key characteristic of an obligatory flexor or extensor synergy pattern is that it is meaningless with respect to the task at hand. Upon seeing repeated flexion synergy patterns of movement, for example, a remote observer would become puzzled about the patient's intended actions since the movement pattern would be very similar across differently intended tasks. No intent can be discerned, no outcome of the movement effort makes sense, and analogous to aphasia in the language system, the obligatory flexion synergy pattern seems to produce an inscrutable "aphasic" response or meaningless behavior. The stereotypic behavior of a flexor synergy pattern is without apparent meaning from the point of view of intentional action. The patient dominated

by flexor synergy pattern seems unable to generate an appropriate set of task-related instructions for transmission to muscles of the upper limb in order to produce meaningful motor behaviors that reflect different intentions. Extrapolating from Jackson's hierarchical model, high-level neural entities that assemble and organize the movements comprising an action task are seemingly absent in the synergy-bound patient. Lacking higher-level, task-related neural function—a negative consequence of UMNS—what becomes manifest clinically with volitional effort is released positive lower-level neural activity, neural circuits with fixed muscle linkages across limb segments, resulting clinically in the stereotypic behavior of obligatory synergy patterns. The behavior starts and stops by volitional effort, but its content is not meaningfully related to an intention-driven task, its instructional set is empty, and the resulting stereotypic behavior ends up as a kind of released default pattern. In the synergy-bound patient, an attempt to produce meaningful action ends up initiating the same repetitive default pattern, time after time. Chronic unidirectional joint movements with little, if any, redirection or reversal of joint movement are a source of recognizable UMNS patterns, generated by persistence of stereotypic, positive or release behaviors resulting from higher-level dissolution of nervous control, Jackson's negative sign.

STRETCH SENSITIVE POSITIVE SIGNS

Stretch Reflexes

Spasticity is a term linked to sensitivity of a muscle to stretch. Clinically, stretch sensitivity results in exaggerated stretch reflexes. Spasticity as a phenomenon has a specific definition, but it is often used (confusingly) as a collective term for all positive signs of UMNS, many of which are not based on sensitivity of a muscle to stretch. Strictly speaking, spasticity is a clinical behavior based on increased excitability of phasic and tonic stretch reflexes that are present in many patients with a UMN lesion. In normal individuals, passive stretch, including rapid passive stretch of a muscle group, does not produce noteworthy resistance. Electromyographically, little, if any, activity is generated (see Figure 3.4), and when present, the electromyographic (EMG) activity is brief, reminiscent of a tendon jerk response, and typically produced only by the most rapid of stretches.

In a spastic patient, however, once the threshold of the EMG activity is triggered at a given degree of muscle stretch, the EMG activity persists until stretch is relinquished (see Figure 3.5). The examiner experiences increased resistance shortly after threshold activity begins, and resistance persists and usually continues to increase until stretch is released. Starting from a position of maximal muscle shortening and "rest" (ie, the patient eschews voluntary effort), the defining characteristic of spasticity as experienced by an examiner doing the stretching is a velocity sensitive increase in resistance. Velocity sensitivity means the following:

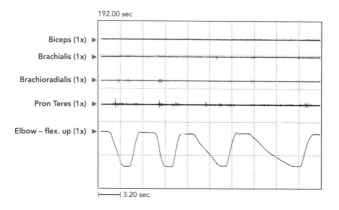

FIGURE 3.4

In normal individuals, passive stretch generates little, if any, EMG activity. When EMG is present, the activity is of short duration, reminiscent of a tendon jerk response, and typically only produced by the most rapid of stretches.

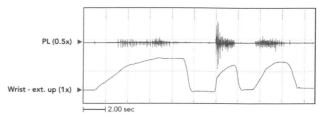

FIGURE 3.5

This patient with UMNS shows different EMG thresholds (ie, onset of EMG activity) at different wrist angles and different amounts of EMG activity as a function of the initial velocity of stretch (slowest rate in the left record, fastest rate in the middle record).

the examiner performs several trials of stretch at different rates of stretch for each trial. The target muscle group is stretched through the full (available) range of joint motion at different rates of stretch, for example, slow, moderate, fast, and very fast rates of limb segment motion. If the patient is spastic, resistance to stretch will be felt by the examiner beginning at some joint angle during the stretch maneuver, and the intensity of resistance will increase the faster the examiner stretches the muscle group in each subsequent trial. An increased tendon jerk reflex is also considered a manifestation of muscle stretch sensitivity and is discussed below.

The character of the stretch reflex was first identified by Sherrington's seminal studies of the cat's myotatic reflex (5, 6). Before his studies, clinicians were well aware of tendon jerk responses, but they thought the jerk phenomenon was a local response generated by *muscle*. Sherrington's studies demonstrated that stretch responses could be abolished by cutting the relevant dorsal roots. By doing so, he established the afferent-efferent nature of the stretch reflex, a circuit that required transmission through the central nervous system, and he established a basis for understanding later descriptions of clinical reflex phenomena. One of my favorites is the succinct description of the clinical characteristics of spastic stretch reflexes by Peter Nathan (7): "Spasticity is a condition in which stretch reflexes that are normally latent become obvious. In spasticity, the tendon reflexes have a lowered threshold to tap, the response of the tapped muscles is increased, and additional muscles besides the tapped one respond; tonic stretch reflexes are affected in the same way" (7).

Spasticity and muscle tone are often confused. Tonus or tone of a system generally refers to *baseline* physiologic activity of a system. For example, normal bowel sounds reflect baseline peristalsis in the intestinal tract. Historically, muscle tonus, like baseline activity in other bodily systems, was originally thought to be an active phenomenon, the result of a small degree of physiologic muscle contraction occurring "at rest." When electromyography became available, no EMG activity was found in normal muscle at rest, and baseline muscle tone could not be explained as an active contraction phenomenon. It was then realized that normal muscle tone was more likely a product of its inherent rheologic (elastic, viscous, and plastic) properties. As described above, passive stretch of normal (in vivo) muscle tissue produces little, if any, EMG response and normal muscle shows little stretch sensitivity (see Figure 3.4). The tone or resistance felt by an examiner when passively stretching normal muscle is rheologic (related to the physical properties of muscle tissue) and not dynamic or actively contractile. The problem arises when a muscle develops stretch sensitivity after a corticospinal system lesion. Passive stretch of a stretch-sensitive muscle results in dynamic contraction generated by the stretch reflex. In theory, spastic muscle at rest (if there is no associated increased tone) is silent (a finding demonstrated as early as 1941 by Hoefer and Putnam (8)), but a spastic muscle develops active contraction after stretching has begun and stretch reflex activity has been elicited. Muscle tonus, that is, baseline tone of muscle as an organ (like baseline peristalsis of the intestinal tract) cannot be measured by stretching because a stretched UMNS muscle is no longer at baseline, with reflex tension typically developing when it is stretched. Logically, baseline tone of a spastic muscle needs to be measured *before* it is stretched to avoid generating stretch reflex tension. We note that nerve blocks can eliminate reflex contraction (a variation on Sherrington's "dorsal root" strategy) and reveal the state of muscle tone freed from reflex contraction. Many studies have shown a change in rheologic properties of the UMNS muscle and have found that noncontractile hypertonia can be considerable (9). Nevertheless, clinicians seem to ignore this contradiction and prefer to equate muscle tone with muscle sensitivity to passive stretch, that is, the degree of resistance elicited by an examiner during passive muscle stretch, often sorting patients into "high tone" and "low tone" categories. If one prefers to use resistance to passive stretch as a measure of tone, it is important to realize that it has neural and nonneural components. The neural component produces stretch reflex activity. The nonneural component comes from rheologic or physical properties intrinsic to muscle and other soft tissues. Patients early in recovery may start with increased muscle tone on a neural (spastic) basis, only to develop advanced stiffness and contracture later, resulting in a similar finding of increased muscle

resistance that now has a nonneural basis (10). Such nonneural stiffness may be associated with reduced tonic stretch reflex and tendon jerk activity. Under circumstances of advanced stiffness and contracture, separating neural from nonneural contributions to muscle tone may be very difficult at the bedside. This distinction is not merely academic because treatment of muscle overactivity by drugs such as botulinum toxin and dantrolene sodium depends on mechanisms that block muscle contraction, not mechanisms that mitigate rheologic properties. In particular, the presence of contracture (fixed shortening of soft tissues) reflects an end-stage condition for the nonneural component and typically requires physical strategies such as serial casting or surgery.

Returning to Peter Nathan's description of stretch reflexes, he refers to an increase in phasic stretch reflexes (tendon jerks) and tonic stretch reflexes (progressive passive stretch). Generally, the term *phasic* implies time varying, whereas *tonic* is relatively time-invariant. Neilson (11) identifies the tonic stretch reflex as a reflex whose response can be described as a linear transformation of the stimulus waveform (progressive passive stretch). On the other hand, the reflex mechanism of a tendon jerk is one that generates a triggered response, having little or no relationship to the mechanical waveform of the tendon strike. Latash (12) identifies the term *phasic stretch reflex* with the response to a *change* in the level of a stimulus specific to muscle stretch receptors. When an examiner performs a tendon tap, the joint angle and, hence, muscle length are held at a steady level of tautness (ie, stretch) before the tendon strike. A sudden tap of the taut tendon produces a sudden *change* in muscle length, resulting in a jerk response. Phasic behavior usually represents a brief excitation of muscle that leads to a twitchy movement, a tendon jerk being one example. In this respect, all monosynaptic reflexes are phasic. Tonic stretch reflexes, on the other hand, respond to the *level of a stimulus* and lead to sustained muscle contraction for the duration of the stimulus. For example, passive stretch of a muscle, that is, progressive lengthening of the muscle, generates a change in the level of the stimulus (muscle length), and in spastic patients, once the threshold of excitation is reached, sustained reflex contraction is produced until stretch is relinquished. Some authors use "phasic" and "tonic" to describe the nature of the *input* stimulus, whereas others describe the *output* response of the system as either "phasic" or "tonic." Lance (13) characterized spasticity as an increase in velocity-dependent *tonic* stretch reflexes with exaggerated tendon jerks. In Lance's consensus definition, "tonic" stretch reflexes referred to the output response of a muscle group that was stretched at different velocities. In our view, the 2 bedside ways of assessing phasic and tonic stretch reflexes are tendon taps and passive muscle lengthening at different rates of stretch, respectively. From a Jacksonian perspective, phasic and tonic stretch reflexes are stereotypic positive signs. Patients with a stable UMNS have phasic and tonic stretch reflexes that do not vary much from day to day at the bedside.

Phasic Stretch Reflexes and Clonus

A phasic jerk response is produced by briskly tapping a tendon held taut by the examiner. In this way, stretch of the tendon-muscle system occurs virtually at the instant of tap. Stretch of extrafusal muscle fibers is detected by the muscle spindle and transmitted to the central nervous system by Ia afferents that project through the dorsal roots and make a number of connections in the spinal cord. These include monosynaptic excitatory connections with homonymous alpha motor neurons that innervate the tapped muscle group and from which afferent outflow originates, along with monosynaptic, excitatory connections to heteronymous synergists. The clinical observation of reflex radiation to muscles other than the one whose tendon has been tapped is explained by Burke (14) as the result of muscle spindles excited by spreading vibrations originating from the site of tap. Monosynaptic connections are also made to the Ia inhibitory interneuron that projects to alpha motor neurons of antagonist muscles. Consequently, when a muscle is stretched, motor neurons innervating antagonist muscles are inhibited. The pattern of simultaneous inhibition of antagonists and excitation of homonymous and heteronymous motor neurons underlies the mechanism of reciprocal inhibition. Interneuronal circuitry, therefore, plays an important role in regulating segmental spinal reflex activity. After a UMN lesion, a net loss of inhibition impairs descending control over motor neurons. A loss of inhibitory control over interneuronal pathways in the spinal cord also occurs. As a result, there is enhancement of the central excitatory state, and tonic and phasic stretch reflexes become manifest clinically.

Clonus is a low-frequency rhythmic oscillation observed in one or more limb segments. It may be generated by rapid stretch and hold of a muscle group. It may also be patient-generated when a muscle group is stretched during limb positioning or passive exercise. Clonus may also be triggered during voluntary movement, for example, during a reaching effort when voluntary elbow extension triggers clonus in elbow flexors. Electrophysiologically, clonus represents short-duration electrical activity of involved muscles

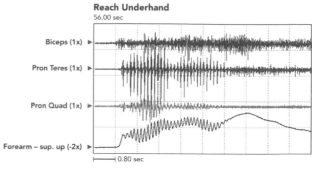

FIGURE 3.6

Clonus at a frequency of 7 Hz developed in both pronators during voluntary underhand reaching performed by a patient with UMNS.

that occur at typical frequencies of 6 to 8 Hz (see Figure 3.6). Figure 3.6 shows forearm pronator clonus in a patient with stroke and left hemiparesis of 4 years duration. Clonic bursts of EMG develop in both pronators at a rate of about 8 Hz. Clonus can be sustained or unsustained, and it can be stopped by repositioning clonic muscles to a shorter length. Clonus is usually associated with other hyperexcitable phasic stretch reflexes. In addition to rapid stretch, various cutaneous stimuli, especially cold or noxious stimulation, may give rise to ipsilateral or even contralateral clonus (15). Clonus may represent self reexcitation of stretch reflexes in a hyperexcitable stretch reflex loop (16). Rack et al. (17) viewed clonus as a self-sustaining oscillation of the stretch reflex pathway, with the frequency of clonus being determined by physical parameters rather than central mechanisms. On the other hand, others felt that a central oscillator was operating (18, 19).

Tonic Stretch Reflexes

The defining characteristic of clinical spasticity is excessive resistance of muscle to passive stretch, a resistance that intensifies as the examiner increases the rate of stretch in subsequent stretch maneuvers. Slow stretch may offer modest resistance, but fast stretch can result in a suddenly intensified resistance that may even catch the examiner off guard. Increased EMG activity of the stretched muscle accompanies different clinical rates of stretch (see Figure 3.7). Contractile tension generated by the stretch reflex opposes the examiner's act of stretching. If reflex tension is high, it can decelerate the examiner's rate of stretch so that a constant "velocity of stretch" cannot be maintained by the examiner. Studies that use machines to apply a

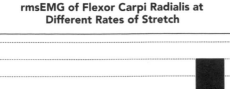
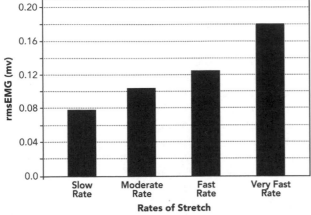

FIGURE 3.7

Using root mean square EMG activity as a quantitative measure, an increase in root mean square EMG activity is observed with increasing rates of stretch, from slow to very fast stretch, applied by a clinical examiner to a patient with spastic wrist flexors.

constant velocity of stretch do not simulate what clinicians experience because clinicians, unlike machines, cannot maintain a constant stretch velocity when spastic tension runs high. Figure 3.8 illustrates spasticity of wrist flexors in an adult with spinal cord injury of 2 years' duration. The EMG responses to stretch of wrist flexors at 2 different rates of stretch are dis-

played. Note an increase of EMG in the faster stretch record on the right. Differential muscle responses to stretch can occur within a group as illustrated in Figure 3.9 and likely signifies a lack of homogeneity in the central lesion or in its reorganization. When using focal treatments delivered to individual muscles, it is important to identify whether all or only some muscles of a group are spastic. When a spastic muscle is stretched, reflex activity, once triggered, commonly continues until the examiner stops stretching and immediately releases the muscle group. In some patients, reflex activity persists if the examiner continues to hold the muscle statically in a stretched state after dynamic stretch has ended. Such activity has been referred to as a static stretch reflex. The static stretch reflex has been attributed to secondary muscle spindle endings; primary endings of the muscle spindle are known to have dynamic or velocity sensitivity.

It remains unclear what operational mechanisms underlie exaggerated stretch reflex activity in the UMNS. Proprioceptive afferent activity generated by muscle stretch is not increased above baseline, and so far, evidence for the theory of increased fusimotor drive has been lacking (20). Evidence seems to favor a reduction in the threshold of the tonic stretch reflex, namely, less afferent input is necessary to trigger stretch

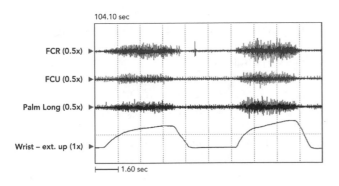

FIGURE 3.8

Passive stretch of wrist flexors in a patient with spinal cord injury. Note that a constant velocity of stretch is not maintained by the examiner. As the amplitude of stretch increases, stretch reflex activity superimposed on the tension length curve of muscle creates increasing resistance that counters the examiner's stretching force, causing the rate of stretch to slow down.

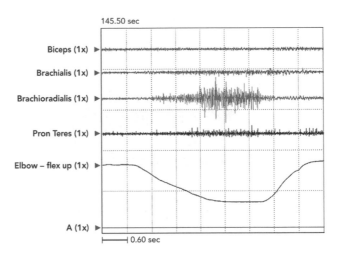

FIGURE 3.9

Differential muscle responses can occur within a muscle group as illustrated in this record of passive stretch of elbow flexors in a patient with clinical spasticity. Note considerable stretch-induced activity in brachioradialis with minimal responses in brachialis and pronator teres and no response in biceps. When using focal treatments for spasticity, it would be important to identify which muscles in a group are actually spastic.

reflex activity in the presence of a UMN lesion. Increased stretch reflex activity resulting from increased gain in the system, that is, more output reflex activity for the same amount of afferent input ("more bang for the buck") is a less favored view. Mechanisms of reduced presynaptic and postsynaptic inhibition and impaired recurrent inhibition in the Renshaw system are likely to contribute to the handling of afferent input by a reorganized spinal cord (21). Herman (22) expressed the view that enhanced reciprocal inhibition is characteristic of spastic hemiplegia, whereas reduced reciprocal inhibition is more characteristic of spastic paraplegia.

Stretch Sensitive Cocontraction

Cocontraction in the UMNS is seen during voluntary effort. Cocontraction is the simultaneous activation of agonist and antagonist muscles. The key feature of cocontraction is that it occurs during *voluntary* effort and that it is generated by simultaneous supraspinal motor drive to agonist and antagonists (23, 24) (see Figure 3.10).

Physiologically, Humphrey and Reed (25) found cocontraction to be activated and deactivated at a cortical level. Although cocontraction can be a normal mechanism to provide joint stability under particular circumstances, cocontraction in the UMNS refers to inappropriate antagonist activation that blunts or even reverses agonist-driven movement. Cocontraction, because it originates supraspinally, may occur during isometric effort when antagonist muscle stretch does

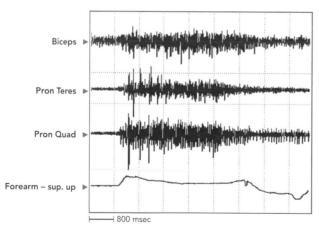

FIGURE 3.10

Activity at the onset of movement is seen in both pronator muscles in this record of a voluntary effort to supinate the forearm, made by a patient with UMNS. Note how pronator cocontraction eventually limits, even reverses, forearm movement.

not occur (26). However, antagonist muscles are being stretched during isotonic movements driven by agonists. Therefore, stretch-sensitive antagonist muscles may be subject to stretch reflex activity superimposed on the supraspinal drive of cocontraction, and hence, the term *spastic* cocontraction has been applied to such antagonist activity. Essentially, the antagonists have 2 sources of efferent input: supraspinal motor drive and segmental stretch driven reflex activity. It is difficult to make practical clinical distinction between supraspinal and segmental stretch reflex drives going to an antagonist muscle. Such a distinction is not vital to medications with a peripheral mechanism of action, but theoretically, drugs that have relevant central mechanisms of action could have a differentiating effect. Clinically, patients with spastic cocontraction often move with slowness and with great effort. Problems arise when patients experience a restraining or braking action produced by antagonist cocontraction during voluntary isotonic movements. When cocontraction is present, the performance of alternating voluntary movements about a joint will reveal temporal asymmetry. For example, during alternating flexion and extension movements about the elbow, elbow flexion is typically quicker, whereas elbow extension is typically slower because flexors cocontract during extension phase. The cocontracting elbow flexors restrain elbow extension, causing temporal asymmetry. The amplitude of elbow extension may also be altered.

Stretch Sensitive Dystonia

Denny-Brown (27) used the term *dystonia* to describe a variety of postural reactions developed by monkeys after ablations of the cerebral cortex were performed. Lesions were independent of, or in addition to, damage to the pyramidal tract. Holding the monkeys in different spatial positions led to a variety of different postural reactions of the limbs, and these limb postures remained persistent in their attitude. Any attempt by an examiner to pull a limb away from its persistent position was met by an increased resistance of springy quality. The limb would fly back to its original posture when released. Denny-Brown called this fixed attitude *dystonia*, a term signifying a persistent posture *maintained by muscular contraction*. He revealed the active nature of dystonia in these monkeys by demonstrating continuous EMG activity in relevant limb muscles. In addition, he showed the dystonia to be efferent. It did not depend on afferent input from the limb because it persisted even after the dorsal roots were cut.

Like Jackson's thinking regarding the effects of brain lesions, Denny-Brown thought that dystonia after cortical ablations represented released motor be havior generated by parts of the motor mechanism that had direct access to alpha motor neurons (28). Of interest in the present context, he pointed out that monkeys who underwent various cortical ablations did not have spastic features, such as tendon jerk hyperreflexia. Efferent drive at rest was supraspinal in origin and seemingly was unrelated to afferent-efferent stretch reflex arcs. However, Denny-Brown also indicated that the dystonia of his monkeys was affected by the degree of stretch placed on a muscle, and in humans with UMNS, dystonic (at rest) activity in a muscle can be modified by prolonged stretch (29, 30). The presence of muscle activity at rest (ie, without obvious source of afferent input, phasic stretch, or volitional effort), sensitive to prolonged (tonic) stretch, has been called *spastic dystonia*. For example, Figures 3.11 and 3.12 illustrate a patient with right hemiparesis secondary to a stroke sitting quietly at rest.

Persistent EMG activity was recorded from the pectoralis major, and a lesser level of activity is also noted in long head of triceps. The clinical posture of an adducted/internally rotated shoulder is noted in the figure. The shoulder adductors were spastic on passive stretch. Range of motion exercises with sustained

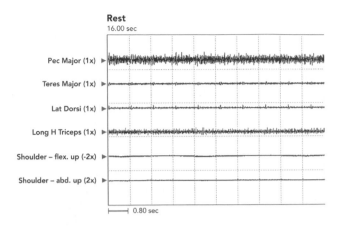

FIGURE 3.12

At rest, persistent dystonic EMG activity was recorded from the pectoralis major, and a lesser level of activity was also present in long head of triceps. The patient was asked to sit quietly and relax. Pectoralis major is an adductor and internal rotator of the shoulder (correlate with Figure 3.11).

stretching eased her clinical complaint of shoulder stiffness, but passive stretching had to be repeated frequently. Dystonia "sensitive to stretch" can result in a *lessening* of the dystonic activity as a result of sustained stretch. Phasic or brief duration stretch can elicit a spastic (resistive) reaction. Some are of the opinion that delayed relaxation after voluntary contraction characterized by continuous firing of motor units is also a form of spastic dystonia (31).

If available, EMG equipment can help identify persistent muscle activity that is potentially consistent with the dystonic form of muscle overactivity. However, without using this confirmation method, it may be risky to assume that all patients with persistent limb postures have underlying muscle activity that sustains the posture. Passive tissue stiffness alone may be sufficient to hold a posture. Stretching a muscle group may elicit a spastic response that brings the stretched muscle back to its equilibrium position at which it will remain in equilibrium, balanced by the passive rheologic properties of muscles and other soft tissues surrounding the joint. Muscle contracture, that is, fixed shortening, holds a limb in a fixed posture as does heterotopic ossification. Activity generated by an unnoticed associated reaction could mimic dystonic posturing, for example, standing "quietly at rest" while actually weightbearing on a cane with the contralateral limb could promote ipsilateral elbow flexor activity and a flexed elbow posture. Associated reactions in UMNS are described in the next section. Their essential feature is that voluntary activity in one part of the body accompanies involuntary activity in another.

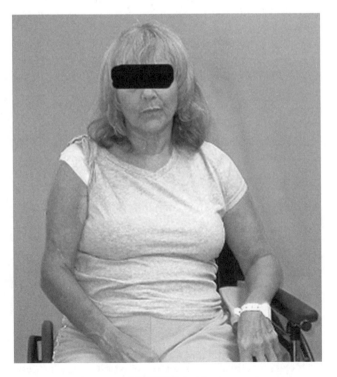

FIGURE 3.11

Note an adducted, internally rotated shoulder at rest in this hemiparetic patient due to stroke.

POSITIVE SIGNS THAT ARE NOT STRETCH-SENSITIVE

Flexor and Extensor Spasms

A characteristic feature of the UMNS, according to Lance (32), is the release of flexor reflex afferent activity. The flexor reflex is a polysynaptic reflex that results in contraction of flexor muscles across several limb segments. It is generated by afferent stimuli collectively known as flexor reflex afferents. These afferents may include cutaneous receptors responding to touch, temperature, and pressure and nociceptors responding to painful stimuli, secondary endings from muscle spindles (group II afferents), and free nerve endings scattered diffusely in skeletal muscles. The polysynaptic flexor reflex has a long latency (twice the latency of a monosynaptic tendon jerk) due to slow afferent conduction into the cord and to central delay. Flexor reflex afferent activity ascends and descends in the cord, synapsing in the internuncial pool, a system of spinal interneurons influenced by inputs from peripheral as well as central sources. Compared with segmental stretch reflexes, the time course of polysynaptic flexor reflexes is slower, and unlike segmental stretch reflexes, flexor reflexes represent coordinated activity of groups of motor neurons spanning many segments. Polysynaptic reflexes result in muscle contraction across multiple joints, sometimes bilaterally. Recruitment of flexor muscles across a number of joints is an example of an interjoint reflex that can protect tissues subject to noxious stimulation. Extensor reflexes are also polysynaptic and may contribute to body support functions. Flexor and extensor reflexes may be the substrate for more complex coordinative patterns, such as locomotor stepping generators.

After a UMN lesion, particularly after a spinal cord lesion, disinhibition of the flexor reflex becomes more prominent clinically. Flexor reflexes can range from the familiar Babinski sign to a mass triple flexion reflex involving the hip, knee, and ankle. A patient may call the flexor reflex a muscle "spasm." but a careful history will reveal that the patient refers to multijoint activity rather than focal spasm of a single muscle group crossing one joint. Flexor reflex afferents from limbs and enteroceptors from bladder and bowel can singly or in combination promote polysegmental reflex activity with contraction of muscles about the ankle, knee, hip, abdominals, even paraspinals. A large, sudden rise in intra-abdominal pressure caused by contraction of the rectus abdominis can result in urinary incontinence as part of the phenomenon. In UMN lesions, the onset threshold of the flexor reflex is reduced, contraction intensity is increased, and more muscles and more joints are recruited. Flexor spasms are more common in patients with lesions of the spinal cord than patients with supraspinal hemiplegia. The studies of Herman (33) indicated that the manner in which afferent activity was transmitted through the spinal cord was diffferent for paraplegic and hemiplegic patients.

Associated Reactions

An associated reaction is another form of involuntary muscle overactivity seen in the UMNS. An associated reaction refers to involuntary activity in one limb that is associated with a voluntary movement effort made in another limb. Figure 3.13(A)-(C) shows the sequence of right elbow motion in a right hemiplegic patient moving from a sitting position to a standing position. Body motion including voluntary arm and leg movements on the uninvolved left side was most active during the stand up phase in the middle photo. Note how an associated reaction of the right elbow flexors developed on the hemiparetic side and produced an increase in right elbow flexion in the middle photo compared with elbow flexion during sitting (left photo) and during the subsequent standing equilibrium phase (right photo). Associated reactions were first described by Walshe in 1923 (34).

Following Jackson's release phenomena formulation, Walsh referred to associated reactions as "released postural reactions deprived of voluntary control." Associated reactions may be due to disinhibited spread of voluntary motor activity into a limb affected by the UMN syndrome. Figure 3.14 shows a patient with right hemiparesis throwing a ball with the left upper limb. The patient did not involve the right upper limb with the throw, having no volitional control of this limb. Figure 3.14 reveals the presence of EMG activity in the right-sided shoulder muscles associated with the patient's effort to throw the ball with her left hand. The intensity of an associated reaction in the limb with UMN may depend on how much effort is made by the voluntary limb. Dewald and Rymer (35) thought that impaired descending supraspinal commands were involved in generating an associated reaction. They hypothesized that unaffected bulbospinal motor pathways may have taken over the role of transmitting descending voluntary commands when the other UMN tracts were damaged.

Although clinicians often seem more concerned about spasticity than other positive phenomena of the UMNS, the clinical impact of spasticity may be less than advertised when one ponders how often patients and caregivers might actually stretch spastic muscles at rates that would elicit intense resistance. We have

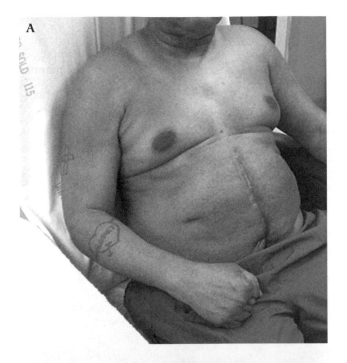

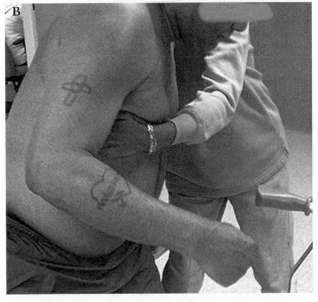

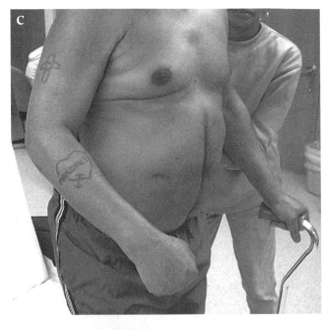

FIGURE 3.13

Note changes in elbow angle as the patient moves through the sequence: (A) sitting, (B) standing up, (C) maintaining a standing position. The photos illustrate an associated reaction of involuntary right elbow flexion during the standing up phase (B) as voluntary movement efforts in other limbs are taking place.

observed patients and caregivers performing limb manipulations at slow rates of stretch to avoid or minimize rate-sensitive spastic resistance. We also note that what often passes for spastic resistance is, in large measure, decreased tissue compliance due to changes in the intrinsic rheologic properties of muscle. Associated reactions, on the other hand, may be unavoidable because voluntary movement efforts of a patient with UMNS must necessarily go on throughout the day (36).

High-intensity voluntary efforts required during transfers, gait, and many activities of daily living

might be expected to provide ample opportunity for the development of muscle overactivity generated by associated reactions.

Muscle Rheology

Although Jackson conceived of positive and negative signs of the UMNS with respect to nervous system production of motor behavior, others subsequently became cognizant of how changes in peripheral soft tissue could also affect extremity movements. Changes in the rheological properties of soft tissues, especially muscle, are

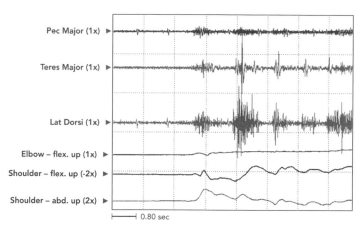
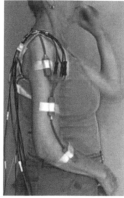

FIGURE 3.14

A patient with right hemiparesis throwing a ball with her left hand. The patient did not involve the right upper limb with the throw, having no volitional control of this limb. The figure reveals EMG activity in right-sided shoulder muscles as an associated reaction to the patient's voluntary ball throw with her left upper limb. Note that these right-sided muscles, pectoralis major, teres major, and latissimus dorsi, are adductors and internal rotators. The patient presented clinically with the UMN pattern of an adducted/internally rotated shoulder.

important clinically (37). Muscle contracture, a physical shortening of muscle length, limits the operating range of joint motion and, as such, has a broad influence on the performance of activities of daily living and mobility. Muscle contracture is often accompanied by physical shortening of other soft tissues such as fascia, nerves, blood vessels, and skin. (Muscle *contracture*, an invariant physical state of fixed tissue shortening, is not to be confused with muscle *contraction*, a dynamic, variable state of internal shortening produced by the sliding action of actin and myosin filaments within a muscle fiber. Contracture implies that muscle length remains the same even if one were to block all muscle contraction by local or general anesthesia.)

The development of contracture is promoted by a number of processes that start when an acute UMN lesion occurs: (1) paresis impairs cycles of shortening and lengthening of agonist and antagonist muscles caused by everyday muscle use; (2) the force of gravity generates positional effects on limb segments and joints; (3) positional effects are also created by a net balance of static soft tissue forces traversing joints; and (4) the various involuntary UMN motor behaviors described above lead to a net balance of dynamic limb torques acting across joints, resulting in the development of chronic 1-way positioning of joints that typically leads to stiffness and contracture. Because muscle relaxant medications affect dynamic muscle contraction only, a clinical picture dominated by contracture will not respond to such drugs. Physical methods are necessary to undo contractures. Distin-

guishing between dynamic tension of muscle overactivity and static rheologic tension can be difficult. O'Dwyer et al. (38) suggested that what appears clinically as spasticity after stroke is really increased muscle stiffness and muscle contracture. They suggested that mechanical and biological changes in soft tissues played a major role in resistance to both passive and active movements. Muscles immobilized in a shortened position for long periods became shorter and stiffer. When muscle overactivity developed in these shortened muscles, tension was generated at shorter lengths. A lack of voluntary contraction in the antagonists of these shortened muscles prevented their natural reextension, leading to a continuation of the process of stiffness and fixation. In the upper limb, muscles that typically shorten include shoulder adductors/internal rotators, forearm pronators, and elbow, wrist, and finger flexors. In the lower limb, muscles that typically shorten include ankle plantar flexors, toe flexors, and hip and knee flexors. The position of any given joint results from a net balance of static and dynamic torques of muscles acting across the joint, as well as rheologic properties of related soft tissues. Variability in central lesion recovery and reorganization can lead to other types of UMN patterns such as the intrinsic plus hand and the hyperextended wrist.

Based on studies of patients with cerebral palsy (CP), contractures are thought to arise from muscle fibers that have fewer sarcomeres in series and, therefore, are shorter than normal (39). Sarcomere lengths are greater than normal when muscle fibers with fewer sarcomeres in series are stretched during normal movement. These longer sarcomeres are thought to be the main reason that muscles of patients with CP have excessive passive tension. Similar processes might conceivably account for elevated passive tension in adults with UMNS. However, Friden and Lieber (40), reexamining the issue of excessive passive tension in CP, have described the mechanical properties of isolated muscle fiber segments obtained from spastic patients with CP undergoing surgical correction of flexion contractures. They found that single fibers developed passive tension at significantly shorter sarcomere lengths than fibers taken from subjects without spasticity. Muscle fibers of patients were almost twice as stiff as controls, and resting sarcomere lengths were shorter. Friden and Lieber also found that the cross-sectional area of spastic fibers was less than one third of normal fibers. This resulted in greater stress forces when spastic fibers were passively stretched. Their study suggested that sarcomeres in CP do not have to be stretched beyond normal lengths to develop excessive passive tension. From this perspective, their study challenges the assumption that tendon lengthenings or even stretching exercises that aim to allow a muscle to achieve normal sarcomere lengths will lessen passive tension to normal levels. The study of Friden and Lieber points to a process of considerable structural remodeling of spastic muscle tissue components. In that regard, their study challenges the current theoretical framework suggesting that muscle-tendon lengths need to be appropriately adjusted by therapeutic exercise or surgical lengthening. Current theory believes that sarcomeres operating over a more normal range will result in a reduction in passive tension along with better force generation if the muscle-tendon length is adjusted appropriately. The study of Friden and Lieber suggests that this view may have to be altered.

MALADAPTIVE CONSEQUENCES OF THE UMNS

We have offered the argument that the interaction between stereotypic positive and negative signs of the UMNS results in chronic 1-way joint attitudes giving rise to common patterns of UMN dysfunction. Mechanical and biological changes in soft tissues, such as muscle, play an important role in resistance to passive and active movements. Generated by the various forms of positive signs, muscle overactivity, superimposed on emerging soft tissue changes, contributes to a net balance of torques that promotes and maintains tissue shortening and chronic 1-way positioning of upper and lower limb joints (see Figure 3.15). The negative sign of impaired limb usage and weak voluntary contraction of the antagonists of shortened muscles prevents range of motion in the opposite direction, contributing to the continuation of the process of postural fixation and its maladaptive consequences for patient care. Stereotypic movement patterns and

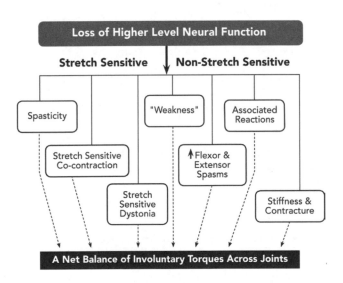

FIGURE 3.15

This figure illustrates the concept that UMN postural and movement patterns reflect a net balance of torques generated by combinatorial interactions of various positive and negative UMN signs.

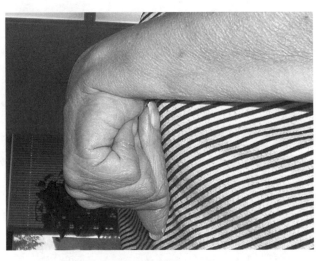

FIGURE 3.16

Clenched fist and flexed wrist deformities in this hemiparetic patient illustrate the potential for maceration, organism overgrowth, and malodor as moisture accumulates and persists between fingers in contact with palm and in redundant tissue folds at the wrist.

postures, generated by positive signs and not reversed because of negative signs, promote maladaptive UMNS consequences (41) under the following personal health categories exemplified for the upper limb:

Skin Integrity: Clenched fist (see Figure 3.16) and redundant skin folds lead to moisture accumulation, bacterial and fungal overgrowth, malodor, skin irritation, skin breakdown, ulceration, and skin and nail bed infections.

Bone and Joint Integrity: Shoulder and wrist subluxation, adhesive capsulitis, impingement syndrome, osteoporosis, and joint contracture.

Physical Pressure and Injury: Thumbnail and fingernails digging into the skin of the palm (see Figure 3.17); fist and finger pressure against chest, breast, throat, chin or face; traction on the ulnar nerve in the cubital tunnel by a chronically flexed elbow; pressure on the median nerve in the carpal tunnel by a chronically flexed wrist.

Soft Tissue Integrity: Stiffness and contracture of muscle, skin, nerve, and blood vessels.

Personal Care Integrity: Patients and caregivers having difficulty manipulating limbs encumbered by static and dynamic torques during the delivery of personal hygiene, dressing, grooming, and bathroom care.

Body Image Integrity: Embarrassing "claw" hand, unsightly flexed elbow, bent wrist, clenched fist, and thumb-in-palm with frequently present malodor.

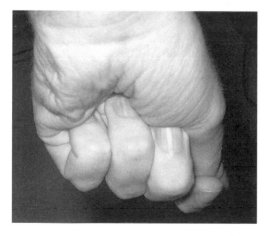

FIGURE 3.17

Note potential for skin laceration by fingernails digging into palmer skin due to overactive flexor digitorum profundus.

CONCLUSIONS

Skeletal muscle is a key effector organ of the nervous system. Skeletal muscle develops torque about a joint in response to efferent neural activity coming from the central nervous system. Normally, everyday voluntary movements are sufficient to take joints through significant portions of their range of motion, and they are also sufficient to maintain skin and musculoskeletal integrity. After a UMN lesion, 2-way voluntary motion across a given joint is impaired by a reduction of voluntary capacity, the negative sign of UMNS, combined with released positive signs that promote unidirectional movements and postures, ultimately affecting skin and musculoskeletal integrity. A UMN lesion alters the net balance of efferent activity to skeletal agonist and antagonist muscles. As a consequence, limbs develop postures and movements according to the net balance of individual muscle torques acting across their joints. The development of mechanical and biological changes in compliance of soft tissues, especially of skeletal muscle, adds to the neurally driven phenomena of UMNS that lead to clinical problems. By forcing joints into undesired static positions or into stereotypic dynamic movements, sometimes with injurious potential, the combined effects of negative and positive signs lead to many maladaptive skin and musculoskeletal consequences (38, 41). From this perspective, individual muscles can be thought of as units of structure and function in the production of movement and posture—a concept that may be exploited by focal therapies.

References

1. Pearce J. Positive and negative cerebral symptoms: the roles of Russell Reynolds and Hughlings Jackson. *J Neurol Neurosurg Psychiatry.* 2004;75(8):1148.
2. Patterns of UMN Dysfunction from WE MOVE.
3. Whitlock JA. Neurophysiology of spasticity. In: Glen MB, Whyte J, eds. *The practical management of spasticity in children and adults.* Philadelphia: Lea & Febiger; 1990;8–33.
4. Sheean G. The pathophysiology of spasticity. *Eur J Neurol.* 2002;9(suppl 1):3–9.
5. Sherrington CS. *The integrative action of the nervous system.* New Haven: Yale University Press; 1947.
6. Stuart DG. Integration of posture and movement: contributions of Sherrington, Hess, and Bernstein. *Hum Mov Sci.* 2005; 24:621–643.
7. Nathan P. Some comments on spasticity and rigidity. In: Desmedt JE, ed. *New developments in electromyography and clinical neurophysiology.* Basel: Karger; 1973;13–14.
8. Hoefer PFA, Putnam TJ. Action potentials of muscles in "spastic" conditions. *Arch Neurol Psychiatry.* 1940;43:1–22.
9. Herman R. The myotatic reflex. *Brain.* 1970;93:273–312.
10. Dietz V, Trippel M, Burger W. Reflex activity and muscle tone during elbow movements in patients with spastic paresis. *Ann Neurol.* 1991;30:767–779.

11. Neilson PD. Tonic stretch reflex in normal subjects and in cerebral palsy. In: Gandevia SC, Burke D, Anthony M, eds. *Science and practice in clinical neurology*. Cambridge, England: Cambridge University Press; 1994: 169–190.

12. Latash M. *Neurophysiological basis of movement*. 2nd ed. Champaign, IL: Human Kinetics, 2008.

13. Lance JW. Symposium synopsis. In: Feldman RG, Young RR, Koella WP, editors. *Spasticity: disordered motor control*. Chicago: Yearbook Medical; 1980:485–494.

14. Burke D. Spasticity as an adaptation to pyramidal tract injury. In: Waxman SG, editor. *Functional recovery in neurological disease, advances in neurology*. New York: Raven Press; 1988:401–423.

15. Miglietta O: Effect of dantrolene sodium on muscle contraction. *Amer J Phys Med*. 1977;56:293–299.

16. Pedersen E: Clinical assessment in pharmacological therapy of spasticity. *Arch Phys Med Rehabil*. 1974;55:344–354.

17. Rack PMH, Ross HF, Tillman AF. The ankle stretch reflexes in normal and spastic subjects. *Brain* 1984;107:637–654

18. Dimitrijevic MR, Nathan PW, and Sherwood AM: Clonus: the role of central mechanisms. *J Neurol Neurosurg Psychiatry*. 1980; 43:329–332

19. Walsh EG, Wright GW. Patellar clonus: an autonomous central generator. *J Neurol Neurosurg Psychiatry*. 1987;50(9):1225–1227

20. Burke D: Critical examination of the case for or against fusimotor involvement in disorders of muscle tone. In Desmedt JE, ed. *Motor control mechanisms in health and disease*. New York:Raven Press, 1983;133–150.

21. Delwaide PJ OE. Pathophysiological aspects of spasticity in man. In: Benecke R CB, Marsden CD, eds. *Motor disturbances*. London: Academic Press; 1987.

22. Herman RF, W. Meeks, S.M. Physiological aspects of hemiplegic and paraplegic spasticity. In: Desmedt JE, editor. *New developments in electromyography and clinical neurophysiology*. Basel: Karger, 1973;579–588.

23. Gracies JM, Wilson L, Gandevia SC, Burke D. Stretch position of spastic muscles aggravates their co-contraction in hemiplegic patients. *Ann Neurol*. 1997; 42(3):438–439.

24. Damiano DL. Reviewing muscle co-contraction: is it a developmental, pathological, or motor control issue. *Phys Occup Ther Pediatr*. 1993;12:3–20.

25. Humphrey DR, Reed DJ. Separate cortical systems for control of joint movement and joint stiffness: reciprocal activation and co-activation of antagonist muscles. In: Desmedt JE, ed. *Motor control mechanisms in health and disease*. New York: Raven Press, 1983;347–372.

26. Fellows SJ, Klaus C, Ross HF, Thilmann AF. Agonist and antagonist EMG activation during isometric torque development at the elbow and spastic hemiparesis. *Electroencephalogr Clin Neurophysiol*. 1994;93:106–112.

27. Denny-Brown D. *The cerebral control of movement*. Liverpool: University Press; 1966.

28. Denny-Brown, D. and Gilman, S., Dystonic posture in relation to various levels of decerebration. *Trans Am Neurol Assoc*. 1966;91:69–70.

29. Denny-Brown D. Historical aspects of the relation of spasticity to movement. In: Feldman RG, Young RR, Koella WP, eds. *Spasticity: disordered motor control*. Chicago: Yearbook Medical, 1980;1–15.

30. Sheean G. Neurophysiology of spasticity. In: Barnes M, Garth RJ, eds. *Upper motor neurone syndrome*. 2nd ed. Cambridge, England: Cambridge University Press, 2008:9–63.

31. Gracies JM. Pathophysiology of spastic paresis. II: emergence of muscle overactivity. *Muscle Nerve*. 2005;31(5):552–571.

32. Lance JW. Pyramidal and extrapyramidal disorders. In: Shahani DT, ed. *Electromyography in CNS disorders: central EMG*. Boston: Butterworth, 1984;1–19.

33. Herman RM, Freedman W, Meeks SM. Physiological aspects of hemiplegic and paraplegic spasticity. In: Desmedt JE, editor. *New developments in electromyography and clinical neurophysiology*. Basel: Karger; 1973;579–588.

34. Walshe FMR. On certain tonic or postural reflexes in hemiplegia with special reference to the so-called 'associated movements'. *Brain*. 1923;46:1–37.

35. Dewald JPA, Rymer WZ. Factors underlying abnormal posture and movement in spastic hemiparesis. In: Thilmann AF, Burke DJ, Rymer WZ, eds. *Spasticity: mechanisms and management*. Berlin: Springer-Verlag, 1993;123–138.

36. Dickstein R, Heffes Y, Abulaffio N. Electromyographic and positional changes in the elbows of spastic hemiparetic patients during walking. *Electroencephalogr Clin Neurophysiol*. 1996;101:491–496.

37. Goldspink G, Williams PE. Muscle fibre and connective tissue changes associated with use and disuse. In: Ada A, Canning C, eds. *Foundations for practice: topics in neurological physiotherapy*. London: Heinemann, 1990;197–218.

38. O'Dwyer N, Ada L, Neilson PD. Spasticity and muscle contracture following stroke. *Brain*. 1996;119:1737–1749.

39. Tardieu C, Huet de la Tour E, Bret MD, Tardieu G. Muscle hypoextensibility in children with cerebral palsy. I: clinical and experimental observations. *Arch Phys Med Rehabil*. 1982;63:97–102.

40. Friden J, Lieber RL. Spastic muscle cells are shorter and stiffer than normal cells. *Muscle Nerve*. 2003;26:157–164.

41. Mayer NH, Esquenazi A. Upper limb skin and musculoskeletal consequences of the upper motor neuron syndrome. In: Jankovic J et al, eds. *Botulinum toxin: therapeutic clinical practice & science*. Philadelphia:Saunders Elsevier, 2009;131–147.

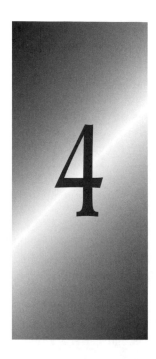

Ancillary Findings Associated With Spasticity

4

Cindy B. Ivanhoe

It is challenging to describe the "ancillary features and associated findings" connected with spasticity and the upper motor neuron syndrome (UMNS). Aside from the usual problems we think about in terms of spasticity, muscle overactivity also has the potential to affect a wide range of body systems and functions. How these interactions, directly and indirectly, will affect an individual is determined by a range of factors. These factors include diagnosis, duration, age of onset, and chronicity. Inherent in this discussion is how the UMNS affects function across organ systems. For example, skin is affected by positioning and external interventions, such as orthotics and casts. Skin lesions, such as pressure sores, will further affect the presentation of tone because they present a noxious stimulus. Swallowing and breathing are affected by positioning, weakness, tone, and coordination. Cognition and socialization can be affected by postures and dysarthria. The integrated effects of the UMNS coalesce to create individual functional issues. Treatment approaches to one feature of the presentation consequently affect other aspects of overall functioning.

Although the term *spasticity* is often used to describe a symptom complex that includes but is not limited to spasticity, it is important to untangle the effects of spasticity from other components of the UMNS, for example, negative features (weakness, decreased dexterity, etc.) and sensory cognitive and behavioral changes. Separating the effects of spasticity without incorporating these other features creates an artificial divide (1).

Another consideration is how spasticity affects the body system being discussed, that is, does it directly affect the end organ or is the muscle overactivity reducing function in the body system? Both options must be considered. Detrusor-sphincter dyssynergia would be an illustration of the direct effects of spasticity on an end organ, whereas difficulty with toileting may occur from impaired posture, balance, and motor control. Drooling may be the result of decreased oromotor control from spasticity, weakness, incoordination, or dystonia (Figure 4.1). Sedation due to medications may increase these baseline impairments even if they reduce tone.

Lastly, in some situations, the combination of spasticity effects on multiple body systems impairs higher-order functional states. Sexuality may be affected by restricted muscle movement or contracture, aside from cognitive concerns and psychological issues. Depression, altered body image, change in role, and self-esteem significantly affect the overall function level in this realm.

The following chapter covers a variety of symptoms, complexes, and body systems that are affected by and are associated with UMNS. Oral medications have their place in the management of UMNS; however, they have limitations due to their side-effect profiles, including effects on endurance and cognition.

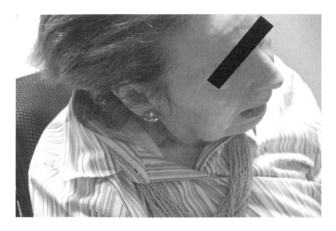

FIGURE 4.1

Cervical dystonia untreated.

Botulinum toxin injections, motor point blocks, nerve blocks, and intrathecal baclofen (ITB) therapy coupled with therapies and an understanding of each individual's goals and potential combine to allow for maximal functional improvement. Gains achieved are frequently noted by patients, caregivers, and clinicians, although they may remain undetected by commonly used assessment scales (2).

SENSORY DISTURBANCES

One cannot address UMNS without considering the associated sensory issues. Spasticity, a sensorimotor disorder, may be associated with disorders of proprioception, spatial orientation, and other sensory disturbances.

Pain is one of the noxious sensory issues associated with spasticity. The mechanisms of pain associated with UMNS and spasticity are not clearly understood. One hypothesis is that prolonged muscle contraction or activation of the motor pathways stresses the vascular supply or consumes oxygen, leading to ischemia. Nociceptor fibers are activated and contribute to the maintenance of flexor reflex. Neurotransmitters that contribute to pain are also released. This is one area where botulinum toxin injections may act to decrease pain in spasticity, not just via a decrease in muscle contraction but via a decrease in the release of neurotransmitters associated with pain (3). Pain is a complication of UMNS that has implications for spasticity, mood, cognition, sexuality, and overall function. It is a noxious stimulus that can lead to increased spasticity. Unfortunately, it is a sometimes overlooked clinical consideration, especially when the scenario involves someone unable to express his or her own needs.

Pain can arise from stresses on the musculoskeletal system (4). It can be related to weakness and immobility that result from the disease causing UMNS, leading to spasticity and dystonia. Fortunately, interest in assessing and treating pain is becoming increasingly recommended and mandated by regulatory agencies.

Oral medications are the most commonly used interventions for spasticity and may have some mild analgesic effects as well, although there is only limited evidence pertaining to the effectiveness of baclofen, dantrolene, diazepam, and tizanidine in facilitating functional gains (5). They do reduce spasticity, often at the cost of alertness, strength, and cognition. In multiple sclerosis, there is no evidence that ITB has a direct impact on pain, although baclofen has been suggested to have some analgesic properties. In multiple sclerosis, however, ITB therapy improves activity. By limiting pressure sores in less mobile individuals, it can indirectly prevent another potential source of pain. In one study that looked at the prevalence and treatment of spasticity in multiple sclerosis, respondents reported less spasticity and fewer painful spasms when treated with ITB therapy compared with those treated with oral medications alone (6). Satisfaction was greater with ITB therapy when compared to oral medications. The performance scales measured included mobility, hand function, vision, fatigue, cognition, bladder/bowel, sensory, and spasticity (Figure 4.2).

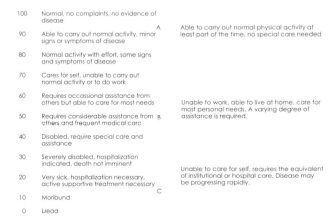

FIGURE 4.2

Performance scales (sensory). (*Journal of the National Medical Association.* Vol 96. No 12. December 2004).

Cerebral palsy (CP) contributes to deformities in the growing child due to abnormal forces on joints, reduced activity levels, and inefficient biomechanics. These factors are compounded by weakness and balance disturbances, again with resultant pain (7).

Severe spasticity can lead to complete immobility. This in turn brings with it a decline in body systems, ultimately leading to pressure sores, bladder and bowel complications, respiratory compromise, and decreased cognitive interaction.

Botulinum toxin injections into spastic, painful muscles have long been noted to decrease pain. The first open-label study that actually used pain as the primary outcome measure with spasticity considered secondarily was conducted in 2000 (3). There is now a body of literature addressing the effects of botulinum toxins on neurotransmitters that contribute to pain (8).

Pain can primarily be neuropathic and/or musculoskeletal in nature. Complex regional pain syndrome (CRPS), whether type 1 or type 2, can significantly impair function, sleep, and mood. Complex regional pain syndrome type 1 involves the sympathetic nervous system, whereas CRPS type 2 involves a specific injury to a nerve. Both syndromes exhibit pain beyond the distribution of the original injury. Medications need to be chosen judiciously to avoid side effects that can further negatively impact function. Complex regional pain syndrome was formally known as "reflex sympathetic dystrophy." It is associated with disabling pain, swelling, vasomotor instability, sudomotor abnormality, and impairment of motor function (9). Varied treatments consist of mobilization, antidepressants, steroids, anticonvulsants, and sympathetic blocks. Plastic changes have been reported in the sensory and motor pathways in patients with CRPS (10).

Central pain syndrome, also known as thalamic pain, can occur after any lesion to the central nervous system (CNS), particularly somatosensory pathways, thalamus, thalamocortical connections, and cortex. Pain is typically constant, of moderate to severe in intensity, and often made worse by touch, movement, emotions, and temperature changes. Burning pain is the most common presentation, although other descriptions include "pins and needles"; pressing, lacerating, or aching pain; and brief bursts of sharp pain similar to the pain. Individuals may have numbness in the areas affected by the pain. The burning and loss of touch sensations are usually most severe on distant parts of the body, such as the feet or hands. Central pain syndrome often begins shortly after the causative injury or damage but may be delayed by months or even years, especially if it is related to poststroke pain. Diffuse peripheral neuropathies and nerve compressions may arise from trauma and/or repetitive trauma and may need to be distinguished from other pain syndromes. Medication suggestions for these syndromes are relatively interchangeable with variable effects.

Early in the rehabilitation process, focus should be placed on interventions that will limit pain acutely and later down the rehabilitation road. For example, prevention of spasms can limit plantar flexion contractures and shearing injury to the skin. Positioning patients with extensor tone, with their legs over a wedge, can help break up synergy patterns,

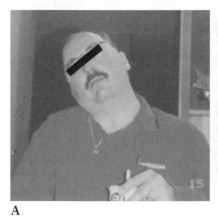 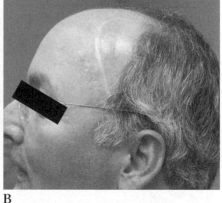 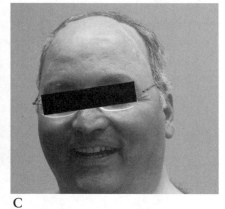

A   B   C

FIGURE 4.3

(A) Before picture, 10 years post injury with recurrent episodes of "asthma." (B and C) After treatment with ITB therapy and Botox A every 3 months, patient sees improvement and no longer aspirates and is without "asthmatic" episodes. Patient begins coughing during eating 2 to 3 weeks before next injection, demonstrating efficacy of treatment.

maintaining range and limiting discomfort. Methods such as standing programs and bed positioning programs, regardless of the nature of the injury, serve to decrease hypertonia and the tendency toward more discomfort from deformity, spasms, and the like. This allows for improved stretch, range of motion, pressure relief, bladder and bowel management, muscle strength, and overall well-being (Figure 4.3).

Tone can be affected by positioning and should be a primary assessment task when starting the evaluation of the clinical presentation and treatment plan. Appropriate positioning programs are difficult to maintain in many rehabilitation venues and take the enlistment of the nursing staff (11). Tonic neck and vestibular reflexes modulate tone and can be incorporated into a bed positioning program to modulate abnormal, functionally limiting postures. Casting and positioning can diminish tone as can heat or cold. Stretching can diminish tone, albeit temporarily, but casting a joint to a painful extreme becomes a noxious stimulus of combined physical and emotional pain (Figure 4.4). There are short-term and longer-term benefits to be considered. In spinal cord injury, incomplete lesions are more likely to be associated with

pain. Nerve root entrapment and direct deafferentation also contribute to pain. Complex regional pain syndrome may be associated with any of the causes of UMNS, as well as with peripheral injuries. Carpal tunnel syndrome can develop as a result of overuse or the subsequent deformities that develop from spasticity. Botulinum toxin A has been shown to reduce capsaicin-induced pain and neurogenic vasodilatation without affecting the transmission of thermal pain modalities as measured by the Visual Analog Scale (Table 4.1) (12).

Pain in CP is mostly associated with musculoskeletal deformities and conditions related to overuse and arthritis. A combination of fatigue, pain, and weakness develops over time and can be related to deformities, weakness, and nerve entrapments. Positioning programs, energy conservation, analgesics, and therapy modalities of heat and stretching can provide relief. Early intervention with the goal of decreasing these complications while decreasing tone is preferable. Selective dorsal rhizotomy, ITB therapy, botulinum toxin injections, orthotics, and therapies are all best delivered through a team approach based on the goals of the interventions.

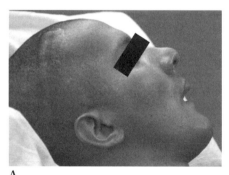

A

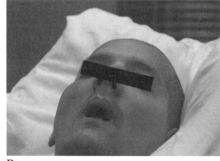

B

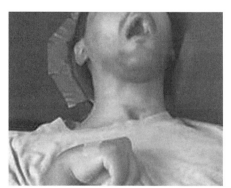

C

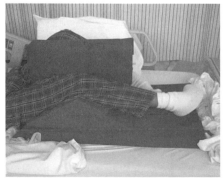

D

FIGURE 4.4

(A and B) Spasticity intervention began 5 years post injury. Patient's oropharyngyl swallow intact. Face remains "stuck" with lips and cheeks in constant contracture. (C) First attempt at lower extremity (LE) positioning program. Patient did not tolerate due to restlessness of left LE; patient was constantly rubbing against his right LE. Right LE was unable to be flexed. Theraband component was added to the device due to constant adduction over his right LE. The head was unable to be safely positioned to prevent left rotation, as the patient would continually push through anything that was attempted and cry out when it was in place. (D) Second attempt at LE positioning. Patient is tolerating his LE and head position; no restlessness, no crying out, no resistance to devices. Able to get about 30° to 40° of right knee flexion.

Some common causes of pain that are more specific in the acute neurorehabilitation setting include fractures, therapy interventions, skin breakdown, and urinary tract infections. In one prospective study, 25% of high-risk patients developed adhesive capsulitis. Adhesive capsulitis is associated with impaired consciousness, hemiparesis, duration of postoperative intravenous infusion, age, and depressive personality (13). Although consumption of analgesics in poststroke spasticity associated with shoulder pain does not appear to decrease significantly with botulinum toxin injection, the decrease in pain is statistically significant. In addition, despite injections being limited to the shoulder, there can be a significant decrease in tone in the finger flexors (14). This is suggestive of the contribution of pain to the presentation of spasticity and/or the overflow or decrease in tone associated with the effect of spasticity.

VOICE, SPEECH, AND SWALLOWING

When therapy is considered for a patient with UMNS, it is most commonly physical and occupational; the role of speech and language pathology is often overlooked, although treating the deficits of UMNS also falls within the realm of the speech and language pathologist. Features of spasticity, dysphagia, and oromandibular dystonia need to be addressed in this population. Again, the positive and negative signs of UMNS come into play, leading to issues with weakness, coordination, hypertonia, and pain.

Dysphagia

Dysphagia can present with deficits along different phases of swallowing. If not addressed, complications of aspiration, fevers, and social isolation become significant. Swallowing assessments can be performed at the bedside or radiographically. Bedside evaluations do not allow for assessment of the pharyngeal phase of swallowing but provide information about oral motor functioning, ability to understand and follow directions, postural concerns, and performance. Specific structures that can be assessed at the bedside include the lips, tongue, palate, larynx, pharynx, and facial musculature. Sensation can also be assessed. Many patients may have difficulty initiating jaw opening to take in bolus or displaying a tonic bite reflex or a sensory defensive response. Poor oral hygiene and thrush can further compromise swallowing.

Fluoroscopic swallowing evaluations or modified barium swallow is commonly performed to allow for a clear definition of the oral and pharyngeal phases of swallowing. The patient is given different consistencies of food, such as thin liquids, pudding, or cookie consistency. Swallowing is monitored for signs of aspiration. Appropriate techniques to work on compensating for or correcting dysphagia in the individual patient can be identified.

Compensatory strategies for managing dysphagia include postural changes that alter the position of the structures of the oropharynx, thermal stimulation, textural stimuli, tongue base exercises, different swallowing techniques, and alterations in diet consistency (15).

Oromandibular dystonia presents with involuntary sustained contractions of assorted muscles of the craniopharyngeal area, leading to deviation of the jaw, jaw opening, jaw clenching, abnormal movements, and positions of the tongue. These contribute to difficulties with dysphagia, articulation, pain, and distraction. Like the limb muscles, the facial, pharyngeal, and cervical muscles can become shortened, tightened, and painful. Although underestimated, these conditions have been noted in 20% of acutely brain-injured patients (16). Bruxism may be seen as part of the presentation as well (17).

Botulinum toxin injections can be quite effective as a therapeutic intervention, although dosing must be based on the clinical considerations of aspiration risk, associated dysphagia, and alternative means of providing hydration and nutrition, if necessary.

Considerations in the management also include muscle relaxants, Beckman exercises for stretch and range of motion, positioning techniques, and botulinum toxin. Indications for treatment or treatment goals can include pain reduction, improvement in oral hygiene, and facilitation of progress in the areas of communication and eating (Figure 4.5).

Dysarthrias

The range of dysarthrias, or motor speech disorders, varies with the diagnosis and the affected locations in the CNS. Spastic dysarthria is characterized by a strangled quality of voice and a decreased rate of speech. Hyperkinetic dysarthria is characterized by impairments in rate and rhythm. Prosody is variable with disturbances in pitch and volume. Hypokinetic dysarthrias are those associated with a soft breathy vocal quality and pressured, short rushes. Flaccid dysarthria presents as a breathy and hypernasal tone with nasal emissions. Inspiration may also be audible. Ataxic dysarthria is characterized by decreased tone and impaired articulation with inaccurate force and

TABLE 4.1
Visual Analog Scale

Information Point: Visual Analogue Scale (VAS)	A Visual Analogue Scale (VAS) is a measurement instrument that tries to measure a characteristic or attitude that is believed to range across a continuum of values and cannot easily be directly measured. For example, the amount of pain that a patient feels ranges across a continuum from none to an extreme amount of pain. From the patient's perspective this spectrum appears continuous—their pain does not take discrete jumps, as a categorization of none, mild, moderate and severe would suggest. It was to capture this idea of an underlying continuum that the VAS was devised.
	Operationally, a VAS is usually a horizontal line, 100 mm in length, anchored by word descriptors at each end. The patient marks on the line the point that they feel represents their perception of their current state. The VAS score is determined by measuring in millimetres from the left-hand end of the line to the point that the patient marks.
	How severe is your pain today? Place a vertical mark on the line below to indicate how bad you feel your pain is today.
	No pain l_____l Very severe pain
	Figure 1. Effects of the interpersonal, technical, and communication skills of the nurse on the effectiveness of treatment.
	There are many other ways in which VAS have been presented, including vertical lines and lines with extra descriptors. Wewers and Lowe (1990) provide an informative discussion of the benefits and shortcomings of different styles of VAS.
	As such an assessment is clearly highly subjective, these scales are of most value when looking at change within individuals, and are of less value for comparing across a group of individuals at one time point. It could be argued that a VAS is trying to produce interval/ratio data out of subjective values that are at best ordinal. Thus, some caution is required in handling such data. Many researchers prefer to use a method of analysis that is based on the rank ordering of scores rather than their exact values to avoid reading too much into the precise VAS score.
Further reading	Wewers M.E. & Lowe N.K. (1990) A critical review of visual analogue scales in the measurement of clinical phenomena. *Research in Nursing and Health* 13, 227–236. NICOLA CRICHTON

Patient Name: _____ Date: _____

Visual Analog Scale (VAS)*

l--l

No   Pain as bad
Pain   as it could
                            possibly be

*A 10-cm baseline is recommended for VAS scales.

From: Acute Pain Management: Operative or Medical Procedures and Trauma, Clinical Practice Guideline No. 1. AHCPR Publication No. 92-0032; February 1992. Agency for Healthcare Research & Quality, Rockville, MD; pages 116-117.

TABLE 4.1
(*Continued*)

Visual Analog Scale

|--|

NO   WORST
PAIN   PAIN

Directions: Ask the patient to indicate on the line where the pain is in relation to the two extremes. Measure from the left hand side to the mark.

timing. Mixtures of these presentations are not unusual, particularly in traumatic brain injury, intracerebral hemorrhages, multiple sclerosis, and other disease processes that can affect more diffuse areas of the CNS.

As with swallowing, the techniques and interventions to assist in the recovery or improvement of articulation deficits include compensatory and restorative strategies. Positioning also plays a role in these techniques. There are specialized techniques to improve the relaxation of spastic and dystonic muscles of articulation, just as of the extremities. Other aspects of

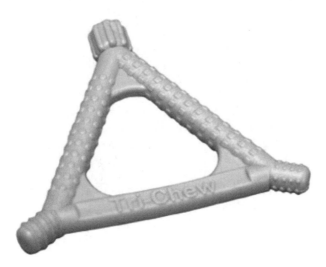

FIGURE 4.5

Beckman exercises (dysphagia).

speech therapy are geared toward targeting articulation, strengthening, and self-awareness.

Botulinum toxin is used for spasmodic dysphonia and other focal dystonic presentations. Intrathecal baclofen therapy has led to demonstrated improvement in communication and speech in children with CP (18). The Lee Silverman Voice Treatment, which was originally developed for Parkinson disease, is being expanded to other neurologic patient populations, with some positive, sustainable effects (19). The short-term and long-term effectiveness of the Lee Silverman Voice Treatment for dysarthria after traumatic brain injury and stroke is demonstrating promise (Figure 4.6) (20).

Quality of speech is also a symptom that cannot be ignored or minimized in the treatment of spasticity. There are social effects and limitations imposed by dysarthria. It has been suggested that speech therapy should be more involved in community activities and psychosocial considerations (21).

BOWEL AND BLADDER

Changes in the autonomic and somatic reflexes are seen in varying degrees with injuries of the CNS (22). Spasticity, weakness, lack of coordination, atrophy, and hyperactive reflexes affect bladder and bowel function directly and indirectly. Issues with balance contribute to considerations of functional positioning for toileting. Transfers may be difficult, and adductor tone is notorious for limiting access for perineal care.

SYMPTOMS VOICE DISORDERS
Inconsistent voice production
Vocal fatigue
Decreased ability to project one's voice
Decreased volume
Throat clearing
Hoarse, labored or breathy vocal quality
Decreased articulation or slurring of words

COMMUNICATION SCREENING (Y or N)
Do people ask you to repeat?
Does your voice sound hoarse scratchy or breathy?
Does your family say you talk too softly?
Does your voice fatigue easily?
Does your voice sound strong on some days; weak on others?

If you answered "yes" to any of these questions, may indicate
Lee Silverman Voice Treatment as potential treatment options.

FIGURE 4.6

Screening and symptoms treated by Lee Silverman Voice Treatment.

Extensor spasms can make wheelchair transfers actually dangerous. Mobility and hand function are significant features in the successful completion of bladder and bowel programs.

Individuals with CP often have spastic-type bladder function, even when continence is achieved, leading to a risk of elevated intravesicular pressures and resultant upper tract damage (23). This can be true of patients with other UMNS presentations. Depending on the diagnosis and the length of time bladder dysfunction is present, care setting in bladder training programs can be particularly difficult to develop. Long-term monitoring and follow-up of bladder dysfunction is more common in patients with spinal cord injury than those with other CNS conditions, but should be monitored in other diagnostic scenarios as well.

Botulinum toxin injections have shown promising effects in detrusor overactivity and in overactive bladder. This indication was first suggested in 2000. Thus far, there is a growing body of evidence that botulinum toxin works to treat detrusor overactivity and overactive bladder by both sensory and motor pathways and may have a positive effect on bladder wall structure and fibrosis (24, 25).

Changes in voiding patterns after ITB have been noted incidentally in a small percentage of patients. These are generally temporary and manifested by urinary retention. Initially decreasing the ITB dose has been effective for short-term management. Retention does not return in patients who have had stroke even when the dose is gradually returned to the initial higher dose (26). Preimplant voiding issues must also be taken into consideration, as well as cognitive and behavioral concerns.

If tone is fairly well managed but a sudden increase or change occurs, it remains prudent to search for causes that may be contributing to the change in presentation. In most neurologic diagnoses, urinary tract infections remain a common cause of increased tone, especially if the presentation had been stable and increases for no apparent reason. Other causes should be assessed, nonetheless. In one such case, an increase in tone was attributed to multiple bladder calculi, but ultimately, it was due to an acute dislodgement of an ITB catheter in a spinal cord–injured patient (27). This underscores the need for thorough evaluations whenever there is a clinical change.

Impaired sphincter control and mobility deficits contribute to the overall functioning of the genitourinary system. Adequate and appropriate genitourinary functions involve the coordination of the parasympathetic, sympathetic, and somatic nerves in concert with coordination of the brain. Factors include voluntary relaxation of the puborectalis muscle and the external anal sphincter and physiologically appropriate intra-abdominal pressure. The striated muscle of the external anal sphincter is normally under voluntary control, which can be affected by neurologic injury, leading to difficulty with relaxation.

Bowel problems in the neurologically impaired population are frequently multifactorial (28). Constipation affects 60% of stroke patients in rehabilitation. Fecal incontinence can occur as a result of constipation. The upper motor neuron (UMN) bowel can manifest as nausea, vomiting, constipation, impaction, abdominal distension, and/or the perception of discomfort or pain.

Basic considerations in a bowel program begin with diet, fiber, and fluid content, along with consideration of the type of injury. A program can include stool softeners, enemas, mini enemas, and supposito-

TABLE 4.2
Basic Considerations in Bladder and Bowel Programs

FACTORS	CONSIDERATIONS
Timing	Is the patient/caregiver physically and emotionally prepared to begin a bladder/bowel program?
Premorbid function	Was the patient at a functional level, premorbid, to adequately follow a bladder/bowel program?
Comorbid conditions	Are there any comorbid conditions that need to be addressed when planning the bladder/bowel program?
Medications	Is the patient taking any medications that would inhibit, disturb, or make difficult a bladder/bowel program?
Diet (fiber, hydration)	Is the patient receiving adequate nutritional intake to allow a bladder/bowel program to be possible?
Hand function	Does the patient have adequate hand function to toilet properly?
Transfer status	Are there any transfer issues (bed to toilet or chair to toilet) that need to be assessed before beginning bladder/bowel program?
Caregiver ability	Is the caregiver physically and emotionally able to assist in the bladder and bowel program?

ries. Medications can be liquid or tablet, oral, per rectum, or via a feeding tube. Positioning and timing of bowel movements are useful considerations in terms of administration of agents to maximize evacuation. Individualizing the bowel program may be more realistic in a home setting than in a hospital.

Long-standing bowel dysfunction can contribute to other gastrointestinal complications, such as megacolon and early diverticuli. Fear of awkward social situations can have a profound effect on quality of life (29). The life expectancy of persons with CP has risen, but it is difficult for adults with CP to access appropriate health care, particularly outsiders of urban communities, and this needs to be addressed further (30). It has been observed that the conditions in this patient population represent comorbidities found in the neurologic populations at large. They include chronic constipation, nutritional deficiencies, pressure ulcers, joint deformities, urologic disorders, and of course, spasticity (Table 4.2).

SLEEP

Sleep disorders are notoriously underdiagnosed in the general population, as well as in the neurologically impaired population. Sleep disorders can be premorbid or related to CNS disorders. The actual prevalence of sleep disorders, for example, after traumatic brain injury, is unknown (31).

The Diagnostic and Statistical Manual of Mental Disorders, Fourth Edition classifies sleep disorders into parasomnias and dyssomnias. Parasomnias are abnormal events that occur during sleep, such as nightmares and sleepwalking. Dyssomnia refers to disturbances in the quality, quantity, and timing of sleep. Insomnia would fall into this category. Considerations in managing sleep disorders can vary with the stage of illness and setting. A thorough understanding of the contributing factors will lead to a more effective treatment plan.

Daytime hypersomnia is common with many neurologic disorders for a multitude of reasons. Medications that are used for spasticity and UMNS can have positive and negative effects. Oral baclofen alters the sleep architecture and oxygen saturations in subjects without neurologic injuries but with underlying obstructive sleep apnea. Baclofen has been shown to cause a minor decrease in oxygen saturation but not an increase in apneic periods. Baclofen is sedating, but daytime sedating effects are not quantified collected (32). There is an increased incidence of sleep apnea in tetraplegic patients, which is believed to be due to a combination of paralyzed intercostal and abdominal musculature, impaired diaphragmatic function, and elevated airway resistance. Sleep posture, antispasmodic medications, periodic limb movements of sleep, spasticity, pain, and insomnia have all been implicated in sleep disturbances (33). Also of note, there are correlations between periodic leg movements and myoclonus during sleep in paraplegic adults before and after acute physical activity (34).

Insomnia after traumatic brain injury has been associated with brainstem injury, psychiatric disorders, pain, headaches, medications, and environmental elements as precipitating factors. Perpetuating issues include psychosocial factors, pain, and daytime fatigue with naps (35). Sleep, or the lack thereof, can also affect the presentation of the features of the UMNS. Poor sleep can contribute to an increase or decrease in muscle tone. In addition, the relaxation of sleep can help maintain range of motion because the abnormal tone diminishes. Positioning devices and orthotics may be better tolerated as well. Conversely, assessing a patient who is fatigued during the day may mask the full effect of the spasticity experienced when that person is well rested, awake, alert, and performing functional activities. Muscle fatigue sometimes increases with activity, so that clonus not visible initially increases with activity.

Bed positioning programs provide a means for patients to reap passive benefits of their therapy program when they are resting. Patients can be placed in positions that allow lengthening of shortened muscle groups. Bolsters can be used to position patients on their side, stretching the contralateral side of the trunk. Positioning programs should work toward breaking up painful synergistic tone patterns. For example, a towel roll placed in the thoracic area limits the detrimental effects of a prolonged amount of time with internally rotated shoulders. This can have beneficial effect on respiration, which can subsequently have beneficial effects on speech. Not all patients will be able to tolerate and maintain the positions while maintaining sleep.

There does not appear to be a study looking specifically at sleep apnea or sleep disorders and spasticity (36).

However, it is not difficult to extrapolate potential sleep issues related to overactive muscles, phrenic nerve injuries, spasms, and positional issues. Many patients may complain of an increase in their lower extremity spasms at night when they are trying to sleep or that wake them from sleep. It is important to distinguish spasticity from restless leg syndrome (RLS). Restless leg syndrome is characterized by unpleasant sensations in the legs and an uncontrollable urge to move. The sensations associated with RLS are described as "burning," "creeping," "tugging," or like insects crawling inside the legs. Restless leg syndrome is often associated with periodic limb movement disorder, which is also associated with leg jerking and twitching that interfere with sleep. This is more common than RLS. Once they develop, these sleep disorders are generally lifelong. Pharmacologic treatments include ropinirole (a D2 and D3 agonist), benzodiazepines, and other dopaminergic agents. Aside from the potential effects of sleep disturbances on spasticity and of spasticity on sleep, other symptoms that may be exacerbated include pain, cognition, endurance, and mood. These are all implications for a negative effect on the rehabilitation process and on function.

Psychosocial Issues

The impact of spasticity per se cannot be separated from the overall concerns of disability when considering the psychosocial considerations of the UMNS. There is generally a poor to modest correlation between the Ashworth Scale and the patients' self-report in assessing the effects of spasticity in our patients' lives with clinical measures (Figure 4.7). Assessments should be supplemented by patients' subjective report. The impact of spasticity on psychosocial functioning again demonstrates how many aspects of disability combine to create a presentation specific to the individual.

First, it should be acknowledged that patients associate other sensations with spasticity (37). For many with spasticity, dystonia, and other aspects of UMNS, pain is a daily or constant presence impacting their daily experience. There is interplay among pain, psychological factors, and disability. Mood issues in general and with disability in particular are multifactorial. Mood can also contribute to increases in tone. Many patients experience an increase in their tone, such as increased synergy postures, with extremes of emotion. In many patients with brain injury, tone and posturing increase in the presence of emotional family members, much as a calming environment can decrease the presentation of their spasticity. In patients with higher-level brain injury, cognitive-behavioral therapy is one avenue for addressing the psychological component of pain, including attitudes, coping skills, and relaxation techniques. Biofeedback, hypnosis, and meditation are used as coping strategies just as in the "able bodied" population.

There is a proven and expected link between depression and higher costs of health care in the general population (38). Depressive symptoms can predict medical care utilization in a population-based sample of patients (38). Depression is linked to higher health care costs. It has been suggested that effective management of secondary and other health care needs of women with physical disabilities could reduce

Name		Date

Modified Ashworth Scale

R/L	Muscle under stretch	Score

Modified Ashworth Scale for Grading Spasticity

Grade	Description
0	No increase in muscle tone
1	Slight increase in muscle tone, manifested by a catch and release, or by minimal resistance at the end of the range of motion when the affected part(s) is moved in flexion or extension
1+	Slight increase in muscle tone, manifested by a catch, followed by minimal resistance throughout the remainder (less than half) of the range of movement (ROM)
2	More marked increase in muscle tone through most of ROM, but affected part(s) easily moved
3	Considerable increase in muscle tone, passive movement difficult
4	Affected part(s) rigid in flexion or extension

Joint Range of Motion, Active and Passive

R/L	Flex/Ex	Joint to be tested	Passive ROM	Active ROM	ROM range of movement
					Degrees from extension

Muscle Strength

R/L	Muscle	Score

MRC score

0. No movement
1. Palpable contraction, no visible movement
2. Movement but only with gravity eliminated
3. Movement against gravity
4. Movement against resistance but weaker than normal
5. Normal power

FIGURE 4.7

Ashworth Scale (psychosocial). Bohannon RW, Smith MB. Interrater Reliability of a Modified Ashworth Scale of Muscle Spasticity; Phys Ther. 1987 Feb;67(2):206–7.

SIP

The SA-SIP30

Body Care and Movement
1. I make difficult moves with help, for example getting into or out of cars, bathtubs

2. I move my hands or fingers with some limitation or difficulty

3. I get in and out of bed or chairs by grasping something for support or using a cane or walker

4. I have trouble getting shoes, socks, or stockings on

5. I get dressed only with someone's help

Social Interaction
6. I show less interest in other people's problems, for example, don't listen when they tell me about their problems, don't offer to help

7. I often act irritable to those around me, for example, snap at people, give sharp answers, criticize easily

8. I show less affection

9. I am doing fewer social activities with groups of people

10. I talk less to those around me

Mobility
11. I stay home most of the time

12. I am not going into town

13. I do not get around in the dark or in unlit places without someone's help

Communication
14. I carry on a conversation only when very close to the other person or looking at him

15. I have difficulty speaking, for example, get stuck, stutter, stammer, slur my words

16. I do not speak clearly when I am under stress

Emotional Behavior
17. I say how bad or useless I am, for example, that I am a burden on others

18. I laugh or cry suddenly

19. I act irritable and impatient with myself, for example, talk badly about myself, swear at myself, blame myself for things that happen

20. I get sudden frights

Household Management
21. I am not doing any of the maintenance or repair work that I would usually do in my home or yard

22. I am not doing any of the shopping that I would usually do

23. I am not doing any of the house cleaning that I would usually do

24. I am not doing any of the clothes washing that I would usually do

Alertness Behavior
25. I am confused and start several actions at a time

26. I make more mistakes than usual

27. I have difficulty doing activities involving concentration and thinking

Ambulation
28. I do not walk up or down hills

29. I get around only by using a walker, crutches, cane, walls, or furniture

30. I walk more slowly

FIGURE 4.8

Sickness Impact Profile. Source: van Straten, A., de Haan, R. J., Limburg, M Schuling, J., Bossuyt, P.M., van den Bos, G.A.M. (1997). A Stroke-Adapted 30-item Version of the Sickness Impact Profile to Asses Quality of Life (SA-SIP30). Stroke, 28, 2155-2161.

depressive symptoms and health care costs (39).Evidence shows that the UMNS affecting communication is associated with social stigma from the resultant communication deficits, dysphagia, and facial disfigurement (40). Quality of life can be affected by various medications and their side-effect profiles. For instance, oral baclofen may have negative effects on motor function and in some cases can worsen quality of life (41). Intrathecal baclofen therapy can contribute to benefits of growth, with a gain in weight and height. Weight is considered a sensitive measure of spasticity management because there is a decrease in caloric expenditure when involuntary muscle activity is decreased (42). Weight gain is often of noted importance, indicating improved feeding and decreased metabolism. The decrease in spasticity in a population often associated with being underweight, such as CP, helps with appropriate weight gain (43).

Ultimately, clinical decisions need to be based on the realities of each individual's circumstances and beliefs. Adults with CP are prone to overuse syndromes, chronic pain, and deterioration in motor function over time. It is important to remember that adults with CP have experienced their disabilities all their lives. At times, the interventions prescribed by well-meaning medical professionals may not add anything useful to the person's quality of life. The goals of treatment must be discussed and understood by all parties for an optimal outcome to treatment and patient satisfaction.

In stroke, ITB has been shown to improve quality of life in the areas of physical and psychosocial functioning. Improvements have been seen in body care and movement, mobility, emotional behavior, social interest, communication, sleep, rest, and recreation (44). There is good evidence that ITB improves function, along with quality of life, as measured by the Sickness Impact Profile (Figure 4.8) (44).

There are the considerations of the behavioral component of neurologic motor function. Included in this arena is the phenomenon of "learned nonuse." Arising from animal studies in behavioral research is a school of thought in rehabilitation referred to as "constraint-induced movement therapy." Constraint-induced movement therapy has gained an increased following and has been applied to patients immediately after stroke and among patients with chronic illness. It is shown to be effective when administered 3 to 9 months poststroke, resulting in statistically significant and clinically relevant improvements in upper extremity function during year 1 compared to that achieved by participants undergoing more traditional forms of therapy (45).

In addition, there is the suggestion that behavioral mechanisms contribute to the "hemineglect phenomena," as well as to structural damage. There tends to be a preference for the use of the less-involved limb and for less spontaneous movement even when the involved limb is more functional than it would appear (46). Aside from the behavioral considerations in motoric abilities, there are psychosocial and interpersonal considerations. It is likely that adjustment to the changes of a wide variety of chronic diseases is best when family is involved in counseling, not just the person directly affected (47).

Case Study

J.T. is a patient who sustained a right middle cerebral artery stroke with resultant spastic right-sided hemiparesis and aphasia. He went on to develop CRPS in his right upper extremity and clonus of his leg with ambulation. Medications for his pain had a negative effect on his speech. Pain had a negative effect on his sleep and participation in therapy and to a lesser degree on his speech. He was not a candidate for a stellate ganglion block because he could not be taken off anticoagulation. Spasticity would get worse when he went 2 days without a bowel movement. Sexual activity was affected by his positional issues, spasms, pain, mood, and relationship issues that grew from the psychosocial impact of his lifestyle changes. Eventually, an improved balance of benefits and risks was found with oral medications for CRPS, botulinum toxin injections, ITB therapy, and therapy interventions. The time course for his treatments involved multiple inpatient rehabilitation admissions and outpatient therapies.

CONCLUSIONS

There are short-term and long-term considerations in the approach to treating the "ancillary" conditions associated with the UMNS. They are parts of the whole clinical and functional presentation. Separating these issues according to medical and psychosocial is really an artificial divide. The parts of the puzzle should be considered together in a plan to create the most functional and holistic approach to identifying and accomplishing rehabilitation and life goals. When therapies and interventions are looked at in isolation for the sake of research purity, the art of treating patients is potentially lost. Measures that are available and accepted can miss the mark, not adequately valuing the nuances of how therapies and interventions contribute to functional improvements. It is exceedingly important to realize that spasticity is one part of UMNS and that treatment needs to be directed toward the complexities of each individual. Ultimately, treatment approaches and outcomes are most significant when observed or measured from the perspective of the person treated.

References

1. Mayer, NH. Functional management of spasticity after head injury. *Neurorehabil Neural Repair.* 1991;5(5):S1–S4.
2. Francisco GE, Latorre JM, Ivanhoe CB. Intrathecal baclofen therapy for spastic hypertonia in chronic traumatic brain injury. *Brain Inj.* 2007;21(3):335–338.
3. Wissel J, Müller J, Dressnandt J, et al. Management of spasticity associated pain with botulinum toxin A. *J Pain Symptom Manage.* 2000;20(1):44–49.
4. Newrick PG, Langton-Hewer R. Pain in motor neuron disease. *J Neurol Neurosurg Psychiatry.* 1985;48(8):838–840.
5. Beard S, Hunn A, Wight J. Treatments for spasticity and pain in multiple sclerosis: a systematic review. *Health Technol Assess.* 2003;7(40):iii, ix-x, 1–111.
6. Rizzo MA, Hadjimichael OC, Preiningerova J, Vollmer TL. Prevalence and treatment of spasticity reported by multiple sclerosis patients. *Mult Scler.* 2004;10(5):589–595.
7. Graham HK, Selber P. Musculoskeletal aspects of cerebral palsy. *J Bone Joint Surg Br.* 2003;85-B(2):157–166.
8. Argoff CE. A focused review on the use of botulinum toxins for neuropathic pain. *Clin J Pain.* November-December 2002;18(6 suppl):S177–S181.
9. Albazaz R, Wong YT, Homer-Vanniasinkam S. Complex regional pain syndrome: a review. *Ann Vasc Surg.* 2008;22(2):297–306.
10. Raja SN. Motor dysfunction in CRPS and its treatment. *Pain.* May 2009;143(1-2):3–4.
11. Jones A, Carr EK, Newham DJ, Wilson-Barnett J. Positioning of stroke patients: evaluation of a teaching intervention with nurses. *Stroke.* 1998;29(8):1612–1617.
12. Tugnoli V, Capone JG, Eleopra R, et al. Botulinum toxin type A reduces capsaicin-evoked pain and neurogenic vasodilatation in human skin. *Pain.* 2007;130(1–2):76–83.
13. Bruckner FE, Nye CJS. A prospective study of adhesive capsulitis of the shoulder ('frozen shoulder') in a high risk population. *Q J Med.* 1981;50(198):191–204.
14. Yelnik AP, Colle FM, Bonan IV, Vicaut E. Treatment of shoulder pain in spastic hemiplegia by reducing spasticity of the subscapular muscle: a randomised, double blind, placebo controlled study of botulinum toxin A. *J Neurol Neurosurg Psychiatry.* 2007;78(8):845–848.
15. Logeman JA. *Evaluation and Treatment of Swallowing Disorders.* 2nd ed. Austin, TX: Pro-Ed; 1998.
16. Lo SE, Rosengart AJ, Novakovic RL, et al. Identification and treatment of cervical and oromandibular dystonia in acutely brain-injured patients: a pilot study using botulinum toxin. *Neurocrit Care.* 2005;3(2):139–145.
17. Ivanhoe CB, Lai JM, Francisco GE. Bruxism after brain injury: successful treatment with botulinum toxin-A. *Arch Phys Med Rehabil.* 1997;78(11):1272–1273.
18. Awaad Y, Tayem H, Munoz S, Ham S, Michon AM, Awaad R. Functional assessment following intrathecal baclofen therapy in children with spasticity cerebral palsy. *J Child Neurol.* 2003;18(1):26–34.
19. Wenke RJ, Theodoros D, Cornwell P. The short- and long-term effectiveness of the LSVT for dysarthria following TBI and stroke. *Brain Inj.* 2008;22(4):339–352.
20. Solomon NP, Makashay MJ, Kessler LB, Sullivan KW. Speech-breathing treatment and LSVT for a patient with hypokinetic-spastic dysarthria after TBI. *J Med Speech Lang Pathol.* 2004;12(4):213–219.
21. Dickson S, Barbour RS, Brady M, Clark AM, Paton G. Patients' experience of disruption associated with post stroke dysarthria. *Int J Lang Commun Disord.* 2008;43(2):135–153.
22. Frost F, Nanninga J, Penn R, Savoy S, Wu Y. Effect on bladder management programs in patients with myelopathy. *Am J Phys Med Rehabil.* June 1989;68(3):112–115.
23. Farmer JP, Sabbagh AJ. Selective dorsal rhizotomies in the treatment of spasticity related to cerebral palsy. *Childs Nerv Syst.* 2007;23(9):991–1002.
24. Nitti, VW. Botulinum toxin for the treatment of idiopathic and neurogenic overactive bladder: state of the art. *Rev Urol.* 2006;8(4):198–208.
25. Gharajeh A, Steele S, Siemens DR. Botulinum toxin in bladder and for a continence urinary diversion for relief of voiding discomfort and abdominal pain. *Can Urol Assoc J.* 2008:2(4)417–419.
26. Meythaler JM, Guin-Renfroe S, Brunenr RC, Hadley MN, Francisco GE. Intrathecal baclofen for spastic hypertonia from stroke. *Stroke.* 2001;32(9):2099.
27. Vaidyanathan S, Soni BM, Oo T, et al. Bladder stones—red herring for resurgence of spasticity in a spinal cord injury patient with implantation of Medtronic Synchromed pump for intrathecal delivery of baclofen—a case report. *BMC Urol.* 2003;3:3.
28. Harari D, Norton C, Lockwood L, Swift C. Treatment of constipation and fecal incontinence in stroke patients: randomized controlled trial. *Stroke.* 2004;35(11):2549–2555.
29. Stiens SA, Bergman SB, Goetz LL. Neurogenic bowel dysfunction after spinal cord injury: clinical evaluation and rehabilitative management. *Arch Phys Med Rehabil.* 1997;78(3 suppl):S86–S102.
30. Wood DL, Kantor D, Edwards L, James H. Health care transition for youth with cerebral palsy. *Northeast Florida Medicine.* 2008;44(59):44–47.
31. Castriotta RJ, Wilde MC, Lai JM, Atanasov S, Masel BE, Kuna ST. Prevalence and consequences of sleep disorders in traumatic brain injury. *J Clin Sleep Med.* 2007;3(4):349–356.
32. Finnimore AJ, Roebuck M, Sajkov D, McEvoy RD. The effects of the GABA agonist, baclofen, on sleep and breathing. *Eur Respir J.* 1995;8(2):230–234.
33. Stockhammer E, Tobon A, Michel F, et al. Characteristics of sleep apnea syndrome in tetraplegic patients. *Spinal Cord.* 2002;40(6):286–294.
34. Mello MT, Silva AC, Rueda AD, Poyares D, Tufik S. Correlation between K complex, periodic leg movements (PLM), and myoclonus during sleep in paraplegic adults before and after an acute physical activity. *Spinal Cord.* 1997;35(4):248–252.
35. Ouellet MC, Savard J, Morin CM. Insomnia following traumatic brain injury: a review. *Neurorehabil Neural Repair.* 2004;18(4):187–198.
36. Sahlin C, Sandberg O, Gustafson Y, et al. Sleep apnea is a risk factor for death in patients with stroke: a 10-year follow-up. *Arch Intern Med.* 2008;168(3):297–301.
37. Lechner HE, Fortzler A, Eser P. Relationship between self- and clinically rated spasticity in spinal cord injury. *Arch Phys Med Rehabil.* 2006;87(1):15–19.
38. Rowan PJ, Davidson K, Campbell JA, Dobrez DG, Maclean DR. Depressive symptoms predict medical care utilization in a population-based sample. *Psychol Med.* 2002;32(5):903–908.
39. Morgan RO, Byrne MM, Hughes RB, et al. Do secondary conditions explain the relationship between depression and health care cost in women with physical disabilities? *Arch Phys Med Rehabil.* 2008;89(10):1880–1886.
40. Bhattacharyya N, Tarsy D. Impact on quality of life of botulinum toxin treatments for spasmodic dysphonia and oromandibular dystonia. *Arch Otolaryngol Head Neck Surg.* 2001;127(4):389–392.
41. Vargus-Adams JN, Michaud LJ, Kinnett DG, McMahon MA, Cook FE. Effects of oral baclofen on children with cerebral palsy. *Dev Med Child Neurol.* 2004;46(11):787.

42. Bottanelli M, Rubini G, Venturelli V, et al. Weight and height gain after intrathecal baclofen pump implantation in children with spastic tetraparesis. *Dev Med Child Neurol.* 2004;46(11):788.

43. Armstrong RW, Steinbok P, Cochrane DD, Kube SD, Fife SE, Farrell K. Intrathecally administered baclofen for treatment of children with spasticity of cerebral origin. *J Neurosurg.* 1997;87(3):409–414.

44. Ivanhoe CB, Francisco GE, McGuire JR, Subramanian T, Grissom SP. Intrathecal baclofen management of poststroke spastic hypertonia: implications for function and quality of life. *Arch Phys Med Rehabil.* 2006;87(11):1509–1515.

45. Wolf S, Winstein C, Miller J, et al. The EXCITE Trial: retention of improved upper extremity function among stroke survivors receiving CI movement therapy. *Lancet Neurol.* 2008;7(1):33–40.

46. Sterr A, Freivogel S, Schmalohr D. Neurobehavioral aspects of recovery: assessment of the learned nonuse phenomenon in hemiparetic adolescents. *Arch Phys Med Rehabil.* 2002;83(12):1726–1731.

47. Martire LM, Schultz R. Involving family in psychosocial interventions for chronic illness. *Curr Dir in Psychol Sci.* 2007;16(2):90–94.

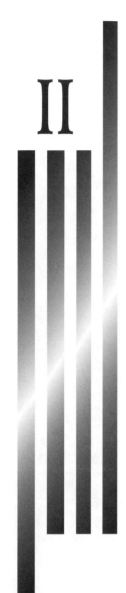

II

ASSESSMENT TOOLS

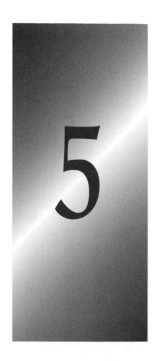

5

Measurement Tools and Treatment Outcomes in Patients With Spasticity

Omar Gomez-Medina
Elie Elovic

Numerous forces have changed the face of rehabilitation over the last decade. Some of them include a greater emphasis on evidence-based medicine, a tighter control of medical services by payers, and a greater importance being placed on functional outcome metrics. Pierson (1, 2) stated that the driving force behind the development of objective measurements is pressure from academic medical centers and insurance companies. As a result, objective and functional measures are being used to evaluate the efficacy of spasticity interventions. Past assessment efforts have focused on specific impairments (e.g., range of motion [ROM], tone, and velocity-dependent resistance to passive stretch), and they have been used widely in the spasticity literature. The correlation between improvements in these parameters and overall function has not been well documented, and there is a need to further explore means of assessing outcomes to further develop research and clinical assessment. Although objective information is important, the correlation with functional improvements remains critical. As was stated so eloquently by Taricco et al. (3) in their *Cochrane Database Review*, "No matter how difficult these latter measurements could be, evidence based clinical practice should be primarily based on patient oriented outcomes."

Spasticity Outcome Measures—What Is a Useful Outcome Measure?

Spasticity is a derivative of the Greek word "spasticus," which means to pull (4). Young and Wiegner (5) defined spasticity as a velocity-dependent hyperreflexia, whereas the definition most often quoted is by Lance (6), "A motor disorder characterized by a velocity-dependent increase in tonic stretch reflexes with exaggerated tendon reflexes, resulting from excitability of the stretch reflex." The next question is what is meant by the term *outcome*. A text written by Finch et al. (7) was dedicated to the subject of rehabilitation outcome assessment. They described it as "a characteristic or construct that is expected to change owing to the strategy, intervention or program." The authors gave the reader further useful advice when they gave recommendations regarding the choice of an appropriate outcome metric. They suggested that one should choose a measure that is likely to be sensitive to the changes that may occur as a result of the intervention. In addition to clinical skills, awareness of the potential positive and negative results from an intervention and a keen awareness of the patient and his or her clinical situation are required to appropriately choose an outcome measure. Ideally, outcome measures should facilitate the clinicians' efforts in the determination of condition severity and treatment efficacy. Using an appropriate metric to assess treatment efficacy is critical to logically decide when to modify a treatment protocol or when to stop treatment.

What are useful outcome measures? To some extent, it depends on the prospective of the observer. For many clinicians and rehabilitation scientists, intrarater and interrater reliability is critical. Ideally, a measure should be objective because subjective ones may depend on the skill set of the rater and certainly may reflect the examiner's bias. For scientific purposes, objective metrics have a clear advantage over subjective ones. For the insurance companies, significant functional changes, level of care required, and pharmacoeconomics matters may be the most important. For the patient and family, function and the demands on caregivers are essential. Although clinicians may be happy with reduced tone and increased ROM, the patient may be pleased if an arm is easier to wash and move passively even if no active function is recovered from an intervention. This issue will become even more important as the cost of health care is debated. Is reducing perceived tightness in a hand without active or passive function worth injections with botulinum toxin 4 times a year? This question is not one that has to be answered by clinicians but more likely will be answered by society, insurance, and government bodies.

An Organized Approach to Spasticity Outcomes

To fully understand the different metrics that can be used to evaluate spasticity outcomes, it is important to organize the material to facilitate understanding. The first categorization of outcome metrics is if they are subjective or objective. The Ashworth Scale used to assess tone and the Disability Assessment Scale (DAS) are examples of subjective measures, as the judgment of the evaluators plays an important part in the assignment of scores. This is true despite the fact that intrarater and interrater reliability has been demonstrated with both of these metrics. On the other hand, the measurement of ROM around a joint and the 6-minute walk test are examples of objective measures. Another way to divide the means of outcome assessments is to group them by what they measure. Revising earlier work performed by the authors (8), they are proposing 6 separate categories of metrics in a hierarchical progression to stratify outcome goals from spasticity interventions. They are physiological measurements (H/M ratios), measures of passive activity (eg, Ashworth Scale and passive ROM), measures of voluntary activity (ie, Fugl-Meyer, nine-hole

peg test [9-HPT]), measurements of passive (ability to don a shirt) and active function (25-foot walk), and quality of life (QOL) measures (36-Item Short Form [SF-36]). Clinicians treating the patients can set goals at multiple levels. Ideally, addressing goals at the highest level would be the most desirable, but a patient's clinical presentation may require that the bar be set lower initially.

At the lower end of the spectrum, specific musculoskeletal and physiological measures are evaluated, whereas at the higher end, function, performance of volitional tasks, and how a person perceives his or her life are evaluated. Patients do not often present to a clinician's office asking for changes based solely on achieving changes in physiological measures. Their desires often reflect improvement in their ability to interact and function within the world. Although initially clinicians must often set short-term goals that are more limited in scope, ultimately when possible, it is important that the issue of function be addressed. As Finch et al. (7) stated, "While rehabilitation efforts target many different substrates that include impairments, activity limitation, and decreased participation, outcome assessment efforts should be directed at an individual's ability to be active and to participate in life as he/she wishes."

It is problematic for clinicians and researchers to measure changes in function and QOL in people who are undergoing treatment for spasticity. Although there are many reasons for this, some of the more common ones are the heterogeneity of the population served, other impairments that are often associated with spasticity (eg, weakness, incoordination, and sensory deficits) that complicate function, and finally, "fixing" muscle overactivity may not directly result in improved QOL. Elovic et al. (9) was one of the first groups that were able to demonstrate improvements in QOL with repeated open-label injections of botulinum neurotoxin in the upper extremity in people with upper extremity spasticity secondary to stroke. However, much further work needs to be done.

PHYSIOLOGICAL MEASURES

When one uses the term *physiological outcome measure*, it often refers to electrophysiologic information that has been correlated with muscle overactivity. Some examples of these include measuring the excitability of the motor neuronal pool or measuring the decrease in length that is seen in muscle cells when spasticity is evident (10). Other items that have been used as outcome metrics include the vibratory inhibitory reflex and the Hmax/Mmax ratio, as they have been noted to be abnormal in people with spasticity. Stokic and Yablon (11) have evaluated the efficacy on intrathecal and its relationship to the H reflex. The question remains that although these findings may be true, they are at best correlated with spasticity and at this time have not yet been shown to be directly related to function. One fact that is in favor of physiologic assessments is that the data collected are objective in nature, which is different than many of the measures commonly used by rehabilitation professionals. It is possible that these measures will be of benefit to researchers and assist both clinicians and researchers in understanding the pathophysiology of muscle overactivity.

Measures of Passive Activity

For this category of assessment metrics, few things are asked from the person being examined, except possibly to relax. It is the clinician or researcher who performs the activity. Some examples of this work include evaluating resistance to movement using a scale such as the Ashworth Scale or Tardieu Scale if a velocity component to stretch resistance is assessed. Biomechanical devices where torque is applied and measured also fall into this category. Metrics such as the Ashworth and Tardieu scale are somewhat subjective in nature, whereas some of the torque measurement devices give more objective feedback.

Measures of Voluntary Activity

The assessment metrics in this group differ from the previous one because they involve measurements taken while the person is actively involved. These measures are not actually addressing real-life functional tasks. Examples of this include items such as 9-HPT or the Fugl-Meyer. These tests evaluate motor function and may well be correlated to real-life function, but they are not real-life tasks by themselves. Another example is pedobarography (measurement of foot pressures during weight-bearing activities). This could be accomplished during a timing walking task. The velocity of walking is a true active functional measure; however, the pressures on the foot are not functional themselves. When gait analysis is performed, measures of both true function and voluntary activity (kinematics, pressures, electromyographic [EMG] cycle) are often collected simultaneously.

Passive and Active Function

In the rehabilitation environment, function is commonly defined as one's ability to perform important activities such as hygiene, walking, or dressing. Commonly used scales include the Functional Independence Measure (FIM) and the Berg Balance Scale, which can be somewhat subjective in nature. The timed 25-foot and 6-minute walk are more objective functional measures that are assessed commonly in the neurologic population. After a neurologic event, the word *function* is often further subdivided into passive and active functional tasks. Examples of passive function include the ability to perform hygiene in the hand that can be complicated by muscle overactivity or the ability to perform a straight catherization that is complicated by adductor spasticity. The difference between active and passive function is that in the passive arena, something is done to the area versus active movement by the area being assessed.

Quality of Life Measures

Ideally as clinicians, one would like to intervene and improve the QOL of the people we treat, as that would imply that our efforts improve our patients' satisfaction with life. However, this task can be somewhat challenging because improving muscle overactivity may be inadequate to accomplish this, as so many factors affect QOL in the populations with spasticity. Elovic et al. (9) was able to demonstrate that repeated injections with neurotoxin did make a statistical difference in the QOL of people with stroke-related spasticity. This study was limited by its open-label design but should give clinicians and researchers some hope for the future.

Choosing an Outcome Measure to Assess Intervention Effectiveness

How does one choose an appropriate outcome metric to assess clinical efficacy? This may be a challenging exercise because one must pick a metric that is relevant to the intervention being provided and at a minimum correlates with a desirable outcome. Taricco et al. (3) called for "more clinically relevant measures of treatment effects to be able to realistically assess clinically relevant end points dealing with functional recovery." This statement was a result of the fact that after they performed a comprehensive review of the medication interventions for the management of muscle overactivity, they found a paucity of functional metrics being reported. The DAS that was originally introduced in 2002 (12, 13) is an attempt to develop subjective measures of functional improvement/reduced impairment. Rehabilitation scientists are also working to objectify and investigate the changes and relationships in motor impairment, disability, and real-life function (14–16).

Engineering solutions that can address the issues of developing objective quantifiable outcome metrics are also being developed (17, 18).

Because there are differences in every patient's presentation, condition, current level of functioning, diagnosis, pathophysiology, comorbidities, and residual function, it is hard to predict with 100% accuracy what changes will be noted after an intervention. However, the outcome and, therefore, the choice of appropriate metrics are clearly products of the factors mentioned above and the modality/modalities that are being used for treatment. Evaluations must be performed by skilled clinicians, and goal setting should be reality-based. A single intervention can demonstrate changes at multiple levels depending on the patient being treated.

A good example of this issue is the management of hip adductor spasticity. This condition can be a result of numerous etiologies and can manifest itself very differently depending on the clinical presentation. In some very severe cases of multiple sclerosis–related spasticity, the patient is bedridden and the entire purpose for intervening is to improve hygiene and ability to perform straight catherization, whereas in other patients, the muscle overactivity results in a narrow-based gait and the reason to treat is to improve ambulation, although increased ROM and decreased tone can be goals in both cases. In the former case, the goals at the highest level are primarily a passive functional one, whereas in the later gait, speed and stability may be the active functional goals that are strived for.

Types of Assessment Methods and Tools

Up to this point, the authors have discussed the categories in general. They will now turn their attention to the individual outcome assessment metrics. In Table 5.1, many of the metrics that are commonly used in the assessment of spasticity are listed, along with their classification as proposed by the authors and whether they are subjective or objective in nature.

Measures of Physiological Activity

Measures Utilizing Nerve Conductions

Electrophysiologic measures have often been used in the assessment of spasticity. In particular, the Hmax, the ratio of the Hmax/Mmax, F response, and vibratory inhibition of the H reflex have been used by investigators as metrics evaluating spasticity (18). The H reflex is elicited by a stimulation of the sciatic nerve at

gradually increasing frequency at a relatively low current that stimulates the Ia sensory fibers which then antidromically stimulates some of the motor neurons. It appears with an approximately 30-millisecond time delay. As one increases the strength of the stimulation, the H reflex disappears and the M wave that reflects the activity of the total pool of motor neurons firing appears. The H reflex is mediated through the Ia sensory fiber, and because these fibers have increased activity when spasticity is present, it is increased when muscle overactivity is present. As a result of this fact, the ratio of Hmax/Mmax reflects the physiology that is seen in spasticity. The M response reflects the total pool of motor neurons that can be excited by stimulation, whereas the H reflects only the motor neurons that can be excited by antidromic stimulation mediated through the Ia fibers (18). Because the excitability of the Ia fibers is intimately involved with spasticity, the ratio of Hmax/Mmax measures the underlying physiology associated with spasticity (18–21). The ratio ranges between 5% and 35% in normals and is higher than that when spasticity is present (22, 23) and has been used frequently in various populations by authors quantifying spasticity (24–27), as well as a component for the evaluation of treatment efficacy (28–32). The readers are cautioned to be aware that this is not a true measure of spasticity but instead its electrophysiologic correlate, which is not diagnostic by itself.

Another electrophysiologic measure that results from antidromic stimulation of the motor neuron is the F wave. Similar to the H reflex, it has also been shown to be increased when spasticity is present or there is hyperexcitability of the motorneuronal pool (18, 33–35). Changes in the amplitude of the F-wave amplitude has been used as a potential outcome metric for different treatments of spasticity in different patient populations. Again, the caution mentioned above regarding the clinical relevance of these electrophysiologic metrics must be noted. In fact, Pauri et al. (36) demonstrated that although patients treated with botulinum toxin demonstrated clinical changes, there was not a comparable change in these electrophysiologic measures.

Vibration reduces the H reflex, and the classic measure used to evaluate this is the Vibratory Inhibitory Index, which is standardized to be applied at 100 Hz to the Achilles tendon, which then in turn inhibits the H reflex (18, 37, 38). In young normals, the vibration reduces the Hmax to roughly 40% of the nonvibratory state; however, it is elevated in patients with spastic hemiplegia (39). Investigators have shown that inhibitive casting lowers this ratio (40).

TABLE 5.1
Examples of Outcome Measures for the Assessment of Spasticity

OUTCOME	CATEGORY	SUBJECTIVE VS OBJECTIVE
Muscle activity	1 – Physiological measures	Objective
Vibratory Inhibitory Index	1 – Physiological measures	Objective
Hmax/Mmax ratio	1 – Physiological measures	Objective
Tendon reflex gain	1 – Physiological measure	Objective
Intrinsic properties: inertia, viscosity, elasticity	2 – Measures of passive activity	Objective
Joint angle, angular velocity (ROM)	2 – Measures of passive activity	Objective
Stretch reflex properties	2 – Measures of passive activity	Objective
Reflex threshold angle	2 – Measures of passive activity	Objective
Muscle tone or "stiffness"	2 – Measures of passive activity	Objective
Torque (eg, using force transducers)	2 – Measures of passive activity	Objective
Pendulum test	2 – Measures of passive activity	Either
Ashworth, MASs, and Modified Ashworth Scales	2 – Measures of passive activity	Subjective
Tardieu Scale	2 – Measures of passive activity	Subjective
Passive ROM	2 – Measures of passive activity	Subjective
Dynamic foot pressure (pedobarographs)	3 – Measures of voluntary activity	Objective
Fugl-Meyer	3 – Measures of voluntary activity	Subjective
Movement smoothness	3 – Measures of voluntary activity	Either
Movement elements (via motion analysis)	3 – Measures of voluntary activity	Either
9-HPT	3 – Measures of voluntary activity	Objective
TTT	3 – Measures of voluntary activity	Objective
Jebsen-Taylor Hand Function tests	3 – Measures of voluntary activity	Objective
BBT	3 – Measures of voluntary activity	Objective
ARAT	3 – Measures of voluntary activity	Subjective
Kinetic and kinematic patterns of walking	3 – Measures of voluntary activity	Objective
Caregiver performs passive ROM	4 – Passive Functional measures	Subjective
Likert scale to describe ease of performing hygiene on person	4 – Passive Functional measures	Subjective
Caregiver performs catheterization, hygiene tasks	4 – Passive Functional measures	Subjective
VAS	Could be 4 or 5 depending on what construct is being measured	Subjective
Berg Balance Scale	5 – Active Functional measures	Subjective
FIM	5 – Active Functional measures	Subjective
Likert scale used to quantify ability to straight catherization	5 – Active Functional measures	Subjective
Ability to perform self-catheterization	5 – Active Functional measures	Subjective
Assessment of motor and process skills	5 – Active Functional measures	Objective
Standing balance	5 – Active Functional measures	Either
Emory Functional Ambulation Profiles	5 – Active Functional measures	Objective
Frenchay Arm Test	5 – Active Functional measures	Subjective
DASs	5 – Active Functional measures	*Subjective
Timed walking test	5 – Active Functional measures	Objective
Barthel Index	5 – Active Functional measures	Subjective
Disability Rating Scale	5 – Active Functional measures	Subjective
Craig Handicap Assessment and Reporting Technique	5 – Active Functional measures	Subjective
Kinetic and kinematic pattern of walking	5 – Active Functional measures	Objective
SWLS	6 – QOL measures	Subjective
SF-36 health survey	6 – QOL measures	Subjective

Tendon Reflex

To obtain quantitative information regarding reflex activity, it is necessary to be able to apply reproducible and measurable stress, stretch, and perturbations to muscles and tendons. Advances in technology have enabled researchers to perform these actions to obtain a better understanding of the stretch reflex and joint mechanics. As a result, reflex gain and threshold have been explored. Gain is defined as the slope of the stretch reflex amplitude plotted against angular velocity, whereas threshold is defined as the angular velocity when the stretch reflex is first evoked. When compared with normal controls, people with spasticity have a much steeper slope of the stretch reflex amplitude and a much lower threshold (41). Reinkensmeyer et al. (42) created a device to assess and treat a person's arm after neurologic injury. It assesses one's muscle overactivity and is also a therapeutic device. Its mechanism for assessment is to measure a reflex response after the application of small perturbation. Potentially, this device could also be effective in monitoring response to treatment.

Reflex excitability can be estimated by a series of devices that tap the tendon and elicit reflex activity at the knee. When the stimulus is applied, reflex torque is measured and EMG activity is recorded from the soleus, gastrocnemius, and tibialis anterior. One group (43) mounted a force sensor on either the patellar or Achilles tendon to measure both the stimulation tap and subsequent response. Further work by these scientists in a sample of people with multiple sclerosis–related quadriceps increased tone noted a decreased tapping threshold necessary to elicit a response of an increased torque that was related to increased spasticity (44). These type of devices have the ability to objectify and quantify hyperreflexia. It is worth noting that increased reflexes are often related to spasticity but can be separate constructs that can be found either together or by themselves (45).

Measures of Passive Activity

This group of metrics consists of measurements that are performed upon a person who remains passive throughout and whose spasticity is being assessed. These include passive ROM, the assessment muscle tone (Ashworth Scale) or spasticity (Tardieu) as examples. In an engineering sense, this includes the assessment of torque, stiffness, and viscosity. The later groups of assessment are often used as quantifiable correlates of common clinical measures.

Ashworth, Modified Ashworth, and Modified Modified Ashworth Scales

Despite enormous criticism, most spasticity papers have used either Ashworth or Modified Ashworth Scales (MASs) as a primary or secondary outcome metric. First published in 1964 (46), the Ashworth Scale is probably the most universally recognized metric (1, 2). Subjectively, the examiner assigns a score ranging from 0 to 4 based on the amount of increased resistance that he or she perceives while passively moving the person's joint through its available ROM. As seen in Table 5.2, the scores range from 0 when no increased tone is perceived to a level of 4 when the limb is rigid (46). For the upper extremity stroke patient, Brashear et al. (12, 47) demonstrated there was good intrarater and interrater reliability in the assessment of spasticity at the wrist, fingers, and elbows. However its use and reliability in the lower extremity are more questionable. A group that studied the Ashworth Scale for plantar flexor tone secondary to traumatic brain injury (TBI) classified it as "minimally adequate" because of marginal intrarater and interrater reliability (48). A similar study evaluated the Ashworth in plantar flexors of patients with stroke (49). They found questionable interrater reliability, with the best correlation noted with the score of 0.

The MAS (see Table 5.3) was purposed by Bohannon and Smith (50) in an attempt to strengthen the original Ashworth Scale by adding a 1+ measure, differentiating it from a 1 by the presence or absence of increased tone after the initial catch was appreciated. The authors reported that for elbow flexor tone secondary to acquired brain injury, there was good interrater reliability. Ansari et al. (51) raise further questions regarding the interrater reliability of both the Ashworth and the MAS. Instead, they propose the

TABLE 5.2 *Ashworth Scale*	
SCORE	DESCRIPTION
0	No increase in muscle tone
1	Slight increase in muscle tone manifested at end ROM
2	More marked increase in tone, through most of the ROM, but joint easily moved
3	Considerable increase in muscle tone, passive movement is difficult
4	Affected part is rigid in flexion or extension

TABLE 5.3
Modified Ashworth Scale

SCORE	DESCRIPTION
0	No increase in muscle tone
1	Slight increase in muscle tone manifested by a catch and release at end ROM
1+	Slight increase in muscle tone manifested by a catch, followed by minimal resistance throughout the reminder (less than ½) of the ROM
2	More marked increase in tone, through most of the ROM, but joint easily moved
3	Considerable increase in muscle tone, passive movement is difficult
4	Affected part is rigid in flexion or extension

TABLE 5.5
Tardieu Scale

SCORE	DESCRIPTION
0	No resistance throughout the course of the passive movement
1	Slight resistance throughout the course of the passive movement with no clear catch at precise angle
2	Clear catch at a precise angle, interrupting the passive movement, followed by a release
3	Fatigable clonus, less than 10 seconds when maintaining the pressure, appearing at a precise angle
4	Nonfatigable clonus, more than 10 seconds when maintaining the pressure, at a precise angle

Modified Modified Ashworth Scale (see Table 5.4), which they report has good better interrater reliability in both the elbow and wrist (52, 53).

In summary, the Ashworth and its cousin the Modified Ashworth are well known, are easy to perform, and have a long history of use. Their effectiveness as metrics has always been questionable. The place for the new Modified Modified Ashworth Scale is not yet known, and further studies will hopefully answer these questions. Clinicians and scientist should be aware of the strengths and weaknesses of these measures.

TABLE 5.4
Modified Modified Ashworth Scale

SCORE	DESCRIPTION
0	No increase in muscle tone
1	Slight increase in muscle tone manifested at end ROM
2	Marked increase in muscle tone manifested by a catch in the middle range and resistance throughout the remainder of the ROM, but affected part(s) easily moved
3	Considerable increase in muscle tone, passive movement is difficult
4	Affected part is rigid in flexion or extension

Tardieu Scale

The Tardieu Scale has been suggested as a suitable and reliable alternative to the Ashworth for the use in the measurement of muscle spasticity (54–56) It was first published in 1954 (57) and has an advantage over the Ashworth group of metrics because it truly incorporates velocity into the assessment. Although first published in 1954, it has undergone 2 modifications. The first was by Held and Pierrot-Deseilligny in 1969 (58). A further update was published in 1999 and was called the Modified Tardieu Scale. Items addressed by the scale include intensity of the resistance to muscle stretch, the angle at which the catch is first noticed, the presence of clonus (fatigable vs nonfatigable), and the differences noted when a muscle is ranged at different velocities (see Table 5.5).

Gracies (59) has been championing this metric and demonstrated its ability to assess spasticity, its reliability, and its potential to document changes secondary to interventions. There are certainly potential problems with the scale, including its reliance on clonus may make it difficult to interpret at the higher ends of tone. In addition, clonus can worsen as a person's ROM increases after an intervention, and as a result, although there may be clinical improvement, the Tardieu Score could worsen (8). The literature regarding the reliability of the Modified Tardieu Scale has been mixed, and there are studies that show both good (60) and poor (61) intrarater and interrater reliability. Ansari et al. (62) showed that the inexperienced raters resulted in poor interrater reliability.

In summary, the Tardieu and Modified Tardieu are appearing more often in the spasticity literature, and it is useful for evaluators to be aware of these instruments. However, it is essential to reiterate that there is no concrete evidence demonstrating that they are clinically superior to the Ashworth scale. In addition, there has been no correlation demonstrated between changes on the Tardieu scale and functional activity.

Range of Motion

Range of motion measurements have been used as an outcome measure for spasticity intervention for many years. They are ubiquitous because they are relatively easy to perform. The information can be obtained by manually using a goniometer and brute strength for a tight ankle or by using electrogoniometry (the electrical measurement of joint angles), which can deliver more accurate and precise measurements. The technology needed for electrogoniometry can be accomplished using precision rotary potentiometers, rotary variable differential transformers, flexible strain gauges, and noncontact magnetic and capacitive technologies (17). Range of motion is often measured along with the stretch reflex utilizing the same assessment device. Three-dimensional (3D) motion analysis can capture ROM kinematics during functional task performance (63). There are potential problems with these devices, and it is critical that torque remain uniform for these devices to be accurate (64). There remains the continuing problem regarding functional significance. Changes in function were not always seen when there were changes in MAS and ROM brought about by spasticity intervention (65).

Stiffness and Muscle Tone

With the desire to obtain objective data regarding the assessment of muscle tone, it is natural that engineers and scientists addressed this with technological advances. These devices can measure stiffness, muscle tone, and reflex activity and provide quantitative data related to the qualitative information obtained from the subjective assessment of tone. In addition, a properly maintained device can eliminate the issues of test-retest variability and interrater differences that plague the Ashworth. These devices can measure torque, angular velocity, and EMG simultaneously. Torque is defined as force that tends to produce a rotation and is the product of force × distance. Torque is the tendency of a force to rotate an object around an axis and is produced when a force is applied at a distance from the point of rotation. Many authors and researchers have advocated the use of the torque versus angle relationship at a joint as the most appropriate assess-

ment of spasticity based on its similarity to the clinical quantitative assessments and definition of spasticity. The most common outcome measure for comparisons and correlations has been the MAS (17, 66–69). However, a change in muscle tone from a spasticity intervention does not necessarily correspond to functional improvement.

Stretch and Stretch Reflexes

The observed behaviors of spasticity and hyperreflexia are actually a result of the combination of the intrinsic mechanical properties of the soft tissue and the reflex activity itself. By varying the rates at which a joint is stretched, investigators have made progress into studying these parameters separately. When a joint is stretched at a relatively slow rate of between 2° and 12° per second, the effects of limb inertia are relatively minor and an assessment of the nonneurologic components of tone and stiffness can be obtained, whereas when a joint is put at stretch at a much higher rate (greater than 14°-35° per second), the stretch reflexes are initiated and can be assessed (70, 71).

Engineers developed a portable device that measured angular velocity around the knee that resulted from a force applied to the ankle (72). When using the device, the evaluator flexes and extends the knee at different speeds. While this is being performed, plots of the force-angle-velocity are recorded. Spasticity was quantified as a regression slope of the linear fit to the peak force/angular velocity data.

Spasticity can be evaluated using computer-controlled foot plates operating in a ramp-and-hold mode or sinusoidal motion mode. Resistive force is measured at the ankle joint as it moved through its available ROM as speed is varied. Resistance force is recorded as the joint is moved through a ROM at different speeds. Graphs of this data are created with the resultant resistance curves serving as a quantitative measure of spasticity (73, 74). The use of the ramp-and-hold module at assessing spasticity at the elbow was demonstrated by Dewald et al. (70), whereas Wang et al. (75) utilized the technique as an effective measure of the treatment efficacy of surface stimulation on the spinal cord on hemiplegia-related spasticity. Pandyan et al. (17) were unsuccessful in their efforts to use this technology to quantify the difference between 1 and 1+ on the MAS.

The Pendulum Test Models

The pendulum test is a biochemical method of evaluating muscle tone by using gravity to provoke muscle stretch reflexes during passive swinging of the lower limb. The leg is fully extended, released, and then allowed to swing freely. The resultant oscillating swing pattern of alternating flexion and extension is observed. With muscle overactivity/spasticity, there is a characteristic pattern of significant reciprocal movement that is greater than the nonspastic patient (76). Bohannon (77) suggests that a rest interval of 15 seconds should be allowed to prevent erroneous results. Fowler et al. (78) stated that the best information could be obtained from the first swing, as it is the most sensitive outcome metric. When initially reported by Wartenburg in 1951 (76), it was performed as a simple observational metric. Mathematical modeling has changed this as simulations have been developed to describe the oscillatory patterns in the elbow and knees allowing other components of the system to be evaluated, including the stretch reflex pathway (time delay, threshold, and gain), limb dynamics, musculotendon actuators, and neural activation (79). Fee et al. (80) singled out this measure because of its "sensitivity to small changes in spasticity."

As testing goes, this one is extremely easy to perform, and it also has the advantage of being noninvasive. Work with a small group of 3 children with a diagnosis of cerebral palsy has suggested that the pendulum test has a high test-retest validity (81). However, a more recent study with 21 children casts some doubt on this fact because the investigators found that while as a group there was not a significant difference between trials, with individual participants, the relaxation index could differ to a large extent. This could create a significant limitation toward the use of the pendulum test's viability as a metric to follow a person before and after an intervention (82). An additional concern with this metric from the engineering standpoint is that posture, muscle length, starting angle, subject relaxation, and position of the individual during the test can affect the measurement of the stretch reflexes, as the force velocity and the force length relationships in the muscle are nonlinear (18, 79, 83). Clinicians who treat spasticity on a regular basis are aware that the findings of spasticity disappear as a result of general and local anesthesia. In a similar fashion, when people with spasticity are under the effects of anesthesia, the results of their pendulum test approach those of normal age-matched controls (80).

Reflex Threshold Angle

Although the amount of EMG activity does not always correlate well with the severity of spasticity that is appreciated (70), exploring the relationship between this activity and the increase in torque that is generated during passive stretch can provide an estimate of the stretch reflex threshold (84) and/or angular threshold (85). Allison and Abraham (85) evaluated the change in plantar flexor spasticity as a result of cryotherapy. They were able to demonstrate the change in the correlation between change in torque and onset of EMG activity. On the other hand, Kim et al. (86) were unable to replicate these findings. They evaluated ankle spasticity in 20 normal controls and 20 people with stroke-related hemiplegia. In the stroke group, there were significantly higher measurements in the peak torque, threshold angle, work, and EMG activity as compared with the controls. As angular velocity was increased, there was an increase in the EMG activity and the threshold ankle; however, the peak torque and work did not increase in the stroke group. Finally, they found that peak torque, work, and the threshold angle were significantly correlated to the MAS, whereas the EMG was not.

MEASURES OF VOLUNTARY ACTIVITY

Isolated Voluntary Time Movement Tests

The box and block test (BBT) and the 9-HPT are 2 clinical metrics that are used to assess the function of the upper extremity. The BBT takes approximately 5 minutes to administer including setup. It was designed to evaluate gross manual dexterity of adults. During the performance of this test, the person being evaluated is given 1 minute to move 1-in cube blocks from one side of the box to another with a partition separating the 2 sides. The subject is required to use one hand to grasp one block at a time and transport it over the partition and release it on the opposite side (7). Mathiowetz et al. (87) were the original group to collect normative data on this metric, and the BBT has been shown to be a sensitive metric for detecting changes in people with a diagnosis of multiple sclerosis (88). The BBT has also been used to assess the efficacy of hand function in the stroke population (89). Sorinola et al. (90) investigated the relationship between increased stretch reflex activity, clinical assessments of spasticity, and numerous clinical assessment metrics including the BBT. They demonstrated a significant decrease in function as measured by these metrics and increased spastic reflex activity.

The 9-HPT is another metric that assesses dexterity and finger and hand movement. It is a component of the National MS Society's Multiple Sclerosis Functional Composite and can be administered in less than 10 minutes. When a subject performs this test, he or she is seated at a table that has a small, shallow container holding 9 pegs and a block. The subject is then tasked to insert each peg, one at a time, into holes in the block. Once that task is completed, he or she then removes them, and the total time to complete the task is recorded (91). The 9-HPT has been shown to be potentially useful in populations other than those with multiple sclerosis, as it has been shown to have good test-retest reliability in people who have had a stroke (92). One of the potential limitation of the 9-HPT is that it requires significant fine motor dexterity, which often limits its utility because many patients are unable to perform it (92). Efforts at using it as an outcome metric for people with stroke-related spasticity have been largely unsuccessful. Rousseaux et al. (93) were unable to demonstrate statistical significance after treating hemiplegia, whereas another group reported that too few people evaluated were capable of completing the task successfully (94).

Different timed instruments have been developed to test one's ability to perform different skills needed to perform activities of daily living. These instruments include the Jebsen Taylor Hand Function Tests and the Minnesota Rate of Manipulation. The Jebsen evaluates the motor control of motions used in daily activities, whereas the Minnesota Rate of Manipulation Test assesses hand-eye coordination and gross motor skills, such as speed and accuracy of hand and arm movements. The quantitative nature of these measures makes them ideal for the design and development of robotic systems that mimic normal human performance and movement. The ultimate goal of this work is to enhance the motor recovery and control of individuals with disabilities (95).

Timed performance tasks can also be of value in the assessment of lower extremity function. One example of these metrics is the timed toe tapping (TTT). In this test, the subject is instructed to tap his toe on a wedge as rapidly as possible for 15 seconds (7). Allison and Abraham (96) evaluated the efficacy of cryotherapy in 26 subjects with ankle spasticity. They used numerous measures to assess changes in spasticity both before and after treatment, whereas TTT was used as a functional metric. Although improvements were noted in the spasticity parameters, no change was noted in TTT. A simple explanation could be that there was no improvement in motor control so a reduction in tone did not increase volitional function.

Performance-Based Measures

The term *performance-based measures* is used to describe the set of metrics that focuses on an individual's ability to execute movement and motor tasks. Some examples of these include the motor components of the Fugl-Meyer (97, 98) or the Assessment of Motor and Process Skills (99). Although these tests do assess the ability to perform movement and motor control, which may be correlated with overall function, this has never been demonstrated. Other scales that assess true function, which will be discussed later in the chapter, may be better designed to assess true functional benefit.

Another metric that is commonly used in research to assess motor function and control is the Action Research Arm Test (ARAT) (100), particularly in the stroke population, with good intrarater and interrater reliability having been demonstrated (101, 102). The ARAT is composed of 19 items that assess hand function, which are grouped into 4 categories; grasp, grip, pinch, and gross movement. Each subscale is arranged into a hierarchical manner, with the individual receiving a score ranging from 0 to 3 in each subtest, with a perfect score being 57. In the past, this scale has been used to assess changes in hand function after electrical stimulation in the management of poststroke hemiplegia (103, 104), although it is presently being used to assess the efficacy and cost-effectiveness of botulinum toxin therapy in the management of spasticity (105).

Pedobarography

Pedobarography is the study of the pressures experienced on the plantar surface of the foot and their interaction with the weight-bearing surface. Rather than being concerned with the components of the gait cycle, measurements of where and how much pressure is being applied to the different areas of the plantar surface of the foot during the stance phase of gait are taken. Observed patterns are compared to known normal patterns for identification of dysfunction. Examples of pathology observed include initial foot pressures at areas other than the heel secondary to plantar flexor muscle overactivity or an increased pressure on the lateral surface of the foot due to valgus deformity. Pedobarography is uniquely suited to study gait on uneven surfaces, such as ramps and uneven pavement, and is an area currently being investigated by the senior author of this chapter. Equipment that records this information provides objective and quantitative information that correlates with a clinical description or observation. Park et al. (106) demonstrated the use of pedobarography in the quantification of the benefit of surgical management of hindfoot valgus deformity in patients with cerebral palsy.

Detection of Movement

For motor movement to be effective, it is not sufficient to just be able to move a joint. The ability to stop and start as well as change, velocity, acceleration, and direction are all very important for appropriate limb control. Therefore, acceleration and deceleration are critical, and measures of the ability to perform these actions play an important part in describing and evaluating movement. Researchers have categorized complex motions into a series of "movement elements," which consist of events of acceleration or deceleration (8). Although the number and type of movement elements can be used to classify movements, subjective acceleration and deceleration thresholds are required to define an event, especially when spasticity is present (107).

Accelerometers are devices that are capable of measuring and recording the length and intensity of an activity. At present, the technology has advanced that these devices can be quite inexpensive, lightweight, and portable and can be worn very comfortably, allowing for the collection of objective outcome data in the community. Therefore, as a result, they can be used to assess if an individual increases his or her overall activity after an intervention (108). There are various algorithms for these devices. Some of them are designed to specifically evaluate arm movements (109–111), whereas others assess trunk movement (112) during gait.

The smoothness of movement is evaluated by measuring the change in acceleration of the body part being evaluated, which is calculated from 3D position data. The rate of change in acceleration is defined mathematically by the term *jerk* and is the third derivative of position. Feng and Mak (113) evaluated both the average jerk and standard deviation in path trajectory for voluntary movements in normal controls and in people with spasticity. They found that those with spasticity had more shifts in acceleration and deceleration as compared with the controls. This evaluation can be performed for any type of movement task. The utilization of these instruments may allow researchers and clinicians to develop a better understanding of what is required to perform certain passive and active functions and potentially can aid in outcome prediction and in measuring the effectiveness of a particular intervention.

Gait

Gait analysis commonly involves the measurement of the movement of the body in space, kinematics, EMG, and forces involved in producing these movements. It has been used in various populations for both adults and children and especially in different neurologic conditions, such as cerebral palsy, stroke, and TBI. This kind of analysis encompasses description and quantification of various parameters of gait, such as walking speed, foot-floor contact, and stride length. Subjective reports and observational gait analysis are now been supplemented with quantifiable changes in joint angle and movements (114, 115).

Objective assessment of these metrics both before and after an intervention may assist both the clinician and scientist to assess what is abnormal in someone's function as well as true changes that result from an intervention (116–118). For the best results, it is important to normalize data based on height and time to properly analyze limb strides (119, 120). It may also be useful in to evaluate changes in gait that result from spasticity intervention in the upper extremities. The work of Esquenazi et al. (121) demonstrated a small but statistically significant improvement in gait velocity after botulinum toxin treatment was administered to the elbow flexors.

Perry et al. (120) demonstrated that the use of force plate data could obtain data that were important in the stratification of peoples' performance. They found that by studying ankle and knee motion, internal moments with EMG for exploring muscular demands, they could differentiate ambulatory status. Perry's group was able to use these data and a commercial stride analyzer during toe walking to differentiate community from household ambulators.

It is also important to obtain physiological EMG data while performing 3D gait analysis. This allows the clinicians and scientist to identify normal and abnormal muscle patterns during actual function rather than during isolated muscle movement. These data cannot be recorded by any other means and are particularly important when planning for surgical interventions (122). Recognizing an abnormal pattern and identification of the dynamic deformity that creates it facilitate the proper treatment selection and give one the best chance for am optimal outcome (123, 124). Used properly, gait analysis can give very valuable information in the assessment of motor function. However, significant skill is needed to run an evaluation properly. Errors in marker placement, improper lead placement for EMG data collection, and improper determination of the different components of the gait cycle can all lead to significant errors (125).

Balance

It is commonly known by clinicians that spasticity can negatively affect one's balance. If fact, Rousseaux et al. (126) demonstrated that improving spasticity with a tibial neurotomy resulted in improved balance in the long term. Balance is often assessed in a relative standing position. Some authors have questioned the relationship between standing balance and actual dynamic walking balance (127). Some feel that the Tinetti may be a better measure for walking balance, but it has limitations secondary to its approximation of results. The Berg Balance is another subjective metric where up to 14 different skills are assessed and are scored on a 4-point scale for a potentially maximal score of 56. However, the lack of true differentiation and small changes with interventions limit its utility (128). A mechanism of measuring balance and response to perturbations in a standing position is the use of posturography with the response to perturbations and change in sensory input, potentially giving information regarding reaction time and motor control secondary to changes in the surface experienced. Patients with significant pathology can have problems in motor control, vestibular, coordination, cognition, visual deficit or proprioceptive issues, or some combination or all of these issues. In individuals with TBI (129), up to 80% may experience symptoms of dizziness or vestibular dysfunction. Posturography is an effective means to evaluate people with suspected balance dysfunction. This is regardless of the source. While undergoing this evaluation, standing balance is evaluated with different sensory challenges and changes in the surface experienced. One example of what can be done with posturography is the manipulation of the visual input with either no visual stimulus or false information. Another is the adjustment of the proprioceptive input. The floor can be tilted to have the patient stand at an angle, or it can be translated. Different outcomes can be analyzed, such as balance reactions, reaction time, position of the center of gravity, and sway. Khademi et al. (130) tested a single patient before and after performance of a tibial nerve block and demonstrated an improvement in the person's center of gravity and sway after the intervention. Not all interventions have demonstrated improvement, as many other etiologies can account for the balance disturbance in addition to spasticity (131–133).

Body Segment Analysis

The utilization of motion analysis and mathematical modeling to the upper extremity can provide significant information regarding the distribution of forces at the joints, muscles, and ligament structures during the performance of simple functional tasks such as gripping, pinching, and lifting. Although for normal individuals these tasks are trivial, they can be quite challenging for an individual with an upper motor neuron syndrome. This analysis and modeling may be helpful in both the planning of treatment and the analysis of the effects of interventions. A force trans-

ducer with 6 degrees of freedom has been developed to measure the forces applied to at the hand's interphalangeal joint during the performance of activities of daily living (134). To better exploit the potential of this device, versions incorporating this device into jars, keys in a lock, tap, and jug have been developed (135). Currently, efforts are underway to develop 3D models of the wrist and shoulder during free movement while performing grasping, pointing, and reaching (136–140). The potential to develop a better understanding of motor control of both normal controls and those with the upper motor neuron syndrome has significant potential to improve both our understanding and treatment of conditions involving the upper extremity.

FUNCTIONAL MEASURES

In this section, measures are used to assess how a person performs functionally in real life. This will include both passive functions, where after the intervention it is easier for the person to have something performed to it, and measures where after treatment it is easier for the person to actively perform an activity secondary to a change from treatment. Examples of passive function include ease of hygiene in an area such as the elbow, hand, or perineum after treatment or greater ease in donning a glove or jacket after the spasticity is treated effectively. Examples of active function include walking speed, better balance, improved ability to reach with an arm, or decreased falls. There are many ways to measure these quantities, and the examples that will follow will be discussed more as food for thought rather than an exhaustive list.

Visual Analog Scale and Likert Scale

Both the Visual Analog Scale (VAS) (Figure 5.1) and the Likert Scale (Table 5.6) are measures that ask the person to subjectively report on a characteristic or the benefit from an intervention. The VAS is designed to assess a characteristic that is believed to range across

VISUAL ANALOG SCALE—Perineal Hygiene

Please mark and "X" on the number line which describes difficulty in performance of perineal hygiene.

Effortless _____ Unable to Perform

FIGURE 5.1

Visual Analog Scale.

TABLE 5.6
Likert Scale to Assess Difficulty in Performing Perineal Hygiene

SCORE	DESCRIPTION
1	Can be performed without difficulty
2	Can be performed with little difficulty
3	Can be performed with moderate difficulty
4	Can be performed with great difficulty
5	Cannot be performed

a continuum of values (141). Originally, it was developed to assess pain, but since its introduction, it has been used far more widely and has been validated for other uses throughout rehabilitation. It has been used frequently as a metric for spasticity and the efficacy of interventions (142–147). Fleuren et al. (148) used the VAS to evaluate the discomfort experienced by patients with spinal cord injury (SCI) with increased tone. Attempts to correlate the VAS with other spasticity measures (surface EMG, Modified Tardieu Scale) have been unsuccessful up to this point (146, 147).

The Likert Scale (Table 5.6) is an instrument commonly used for subjective reporting of outcomes. It uses a 5-point scale that can be a measure how much the person agrees with a particular statement or how they have changed from an intervention where 1 = much worse, 3 = the same, and 5 = much better. Gruenthal et al. (149) used this scale to evaluate the effect of gabapentin on spasticity of spinal cord etiology.

Timed Ambulation Tests

If one wishes to examine a person's ability to walk, there are a whole host of metrics used in the rehabilitation community. The 2 most commonly used are the 6-minute walk and the 10-meter walk. These tests are chosen because of their ability to predict real-life function. If one has the ability to walk effectively for 6 minutes, this normally qualifies one to be a community ambulator. The 10-meter walk test is important because a satisfactory performance on that test predicts how well a person can cross the street. These tests over level ground are easy to perform and are simple and are useful low-budget functional metrics that reflect real-life function (150). These tests have been used in numerous populations including those with stroke (151), multiple sclerosis (152), and SCI (153).

People with neurologic deficits and spasticity do not routinely experience their greatest difficulties when ambulating on level surfaces. As a result, some researchers have tried to make their testing metrics more closely reflect real life with nonlevel surfaces, including uneven surfaces, steps, stepping over obstacles, sidewalk curbs, and ramps (154–158). One of the better known ambulation metrics on different surfaces is the Emory Functional Ambulation Profile, which records timed walking on 5 different scenarios including hard floor, walk over carpet, time up and go, standardized obstacle course, and ascending and descending 5 steps. It was found to have good reliability, validity, and responsiveness for assessing walking function and recovery in patients with stroke (159). Current work is investigating if there is a correlation between higher scores and improvements in community and household ambulation (160). A similar walk test is the Means et al. (161) obstacle course. This measure focuses on functional mobility tasks experienced during activities of daily living, including different floor textures, graded surfaces, stairs, and object negotiation. Testing on both of these courses is easy to administer and relatively inexpensive.

Functional Performance Measures

There are numerous metrics that clinicians and scientists use to evaluate functional performance and in particular specific functional tasks. In this section, the authors will discuss several metrics that have been used in the spasticity literature. Specifically this will include the FIM, the Frenchay Arm Test, the Modified Frenchay, the DAS, and the Pediatric Evaluation of Disability Inventory (PEDI).

The FIM is a commonly used metric in the rehabilitation population where 18 items are subjectively scored as to a person's ability to perform them (162). Items are graded between 1 (dependent) and 7 (totally independent). Components that are evaluated by the FIM include self-care, mobility, eating, grooming, dressing, toileting, transfers, walking, and stair climbing. Many of the subsections of the FIM may well respond to spasticity intervention. Some literature have demonstrated improvements on the FIM secondary to spasticity interventions. Francisco et al. (163) reported on a small case series of 3 patients who received intrathecal baclofen therapy for their spasticity and reported that improvements in functional domains such as gait, transfers, and sitting were noted. Cardoso et al. (164) reported that on a larger series of 20 patients who were treated with botulinum toxin A for the management of their stroke-related spasticity, significant improvement was noted in the motor components of the FIM with treatment.

In the evaluation of the Frenchay Arm Test, the person examined performed 5 tasks that were rated in a pass-fail manner. The items included stabilizing a ruler and drawing a straight line, grasping a cylinder, drinking from a half-full glass of water, replacing a clothes' peg, and combing one's hair (165). One study used it as one of the outcome metrics to demonstrate the efficacy of botulinum toxin type A intervention for the management of upper extremity spasticity in patients with stroke and it did demonstrate change from the intervention (166). A modified version of the Frenchay has been developed where rather than grading pass-fail, the examiner assigns a numerical score between 1 and 10. This metric was used as part of a study comparing tizanidine to botulinum toxin A for the management of upper extremity spasticity (167); however, the authors will publish that data separately at a later time.

The DAS was first developed to assess and quantify disability perceived in people with stroke-related spasticity. There are 4 separate areas that are evaluated by the DAS, including personal hygiene, dressing, pain, and position. The grading ranges from 0 to 3, with a grade of 0 = there is no disability, 1 = mild, 2 = moderate, and 3 = severe disability. It was the functional metric that was used in Brashear et al. (13); the double blinded, placebo-controlled trial evaluated the efficacy of botulinum neurotoxin for upper extremity spasticity, with the toxin treatment group having statistically superior improvement on the DAS as compared with placebo. The intrarater and interrater reliability for the DAS was demonstrated in another study (12). Elovic et al. (9), in a study looking at repeated injections with open-label toxin, were also able to show consistent long-term improvement with decreased disability as assessed with the DAS.

The Barthel Index is a scale that measures performance in basic activities of daily living, particularly mobility and personal hygiene (168). These are 2 areas that can be especially sensitive to muscle overactivity and may show improvement after intervention. It takes between 5 and 20 minutes to administer, and the scoring is based on a person's performance on 10 tasks, including feeding, donning of a brace, dressing, grooming, hygiene, toileting, transfers, and mobility. Several studies have documented improvement in this measure after specific spasticity interventions, including intrathecal baclofen (169) and acupuncture (170). Efforts at using the Barthel as a metric for chemodenervation with botulinum toxin intervention have been more interesting, with a large multicenter study using it as one of the outcome metrics (105), another study showing changes on the Barthel Index in only 1 of 18 patients (171), and a third study showing some changes with a combination of toxin treatment and a course of occupational therapy (172).

The Pediatric Evaluation of Disability Inventory

The PEDI was developed to provide a comprehensive clinical assessment of key functional capabilities and performance in children between the ages of 6 months and 7 years. It was designed to serve as a descriptive measure of the child's current functional performance, as well as a method for tracking change across time. The PEDI measures both capability and performance of functional activities in self-care, mobility, and social function (173). It was validated in 1990 by Feldman et al. (173) to identify disabilities in this population. It has been used to assess changes in disability after different spasticity interventions, such as botulinum toxin type A injections, oral medications intrathecal baclofen, and selective dorsal rhizotomy. However, after intervention, no change in function and disability as measured by the PEDI was noted (65, 174–177). Ohata et al. (178) demonstrated a lack of correlation between the PEDI and the MAS. However, what can be learned from this is questionable because similar statements can be made in the adult population as well. In view of these results, it is reasonable to assume that the metrics measured by the PEDI might not be sensitive enough to evaluate from spasticity interventions of multiple types.

Quality of Life Measures

As mentioned earlier, what matters most to a person is how he or she is functioning and his or her overall satisfaction with life. It has been for many different reasons for clinicians and researchers to show that their interventions for spasticity make a difference in this important area. However, this may well be a critical area to pursue because the health care environment in the United States changes. A complete discussion of all metrics that assess QOL is beyond the scope of this chapter. Instead the authors will discuss some of the more commonly used metrics in the rehabilitation community.

36-Item Short Form Health Survey

The SF-36 is a multipurpose, short-form health survey with 36 questions. It yields an 8-scale profile of functional health and well-being scores and mental and health summary measures. It is frequently used, and more than 1000 articles using it suggest its utility in various populations (179). This includes the populations of patients with TBI (180), SCI (181, 182), and stroke (183, 184). In both populations of patients with hemiplegia and SCI spasticity, it has been cor-

TABLE 5.7
Satisfaction With Life Scale

Score	Description
1	In most ways my life is close to ideal
2	The conditions of my life are excellent
3	I am satisfied with my life
4	So far I have gotten the important things I want in life
5	If I could live my life over, I would change almost nothing

In some cases this could reflect passive function, as improvement could result from ease of passive activity performed (ie, ease of hygiene secondary to reduced muscle over-activity).

related with lower QOL. In fact, individuals with hemiplegia, 18 months after the event, have a higher level of QOL if they do not have spasticity, as measured by the physical functioning domain of the 36-SF health survey (184). However, efforts of Childers et al. (183) to evaluate QOL changes from intervening with botulinum toxin to manage upper extremity spasticity failed to demonstrate any changes on the SF-36. It is easy to blame the sensitivity of the metric, but it could just as easily be a result of the intervention's inability to make a real-life change.

Satisfaction With Life Scale

The Satisfaction With Life Scale (SWLS) was first described by Diener et al. (185), and it attempts to assess a person's overall life satisfaction. This scale consists of 5 separate statements that reflect their current state for which they reply with a number from 1 to 7 to express how strongly they agree or disagree with each statement (Table 5.7).

This metric has been used as an instrument to assess QOL for adults who had sustained an SCI as a child (186). Their conclusion was that spasticity negatively impacted a person's QOL as measured on the SWLS. The SWLS has not been used in any other population to evaluate the effect of spasticity on life, but it has been used in 2 separate studies to evaluate peoples' overall satisfaction after their recovery from a TBI (187, 188).

The EuroQol

The EuroQol or EQ-5D is a standardized instrument that measures health outcome and QOL and can be applicable in a wide range of health conditions and treatments. It provides a simple descriptive profile and a single index value for health status. This measure was first described by the EuroQol Group in 1990 (189). The EQ-5D was originally designed to complement other instruments but is now increasingly used as a "stand alone" measure. It consists of 2 components: the EQ-5D descriptive system and the EQ VAS. In the EQ-5D descriptive system, the respondent is asked to indicate his or her health state by marking the box next to the most appropriate statement in each of the 5 dimensions. In the EQ VAS, the respondent rates his or her health state by drawing a line from the box marked "Your health state today" to the appropriate point on the EQ VAS. It was used in a study that demonstrated the effectiveness of botulinum toxin treatment in the management of upper extremity spasticity (9). In addition, a large multicenter is using this as one of the metrics to assess outcome from upper extremity botulinum neurotoxin treatment for spasticity (105). Although this is a relatively new use for the metric, it may have ever increasing use because clinicians are charged to find meaningful measures for improvement in a person's condition beyond less tightness.

CONCLUSIONS

The authors of this chapter have presented an overview of many, but not all, of the metrics used by clinicians and scientists in the assessment of spasticity and the results of interventions. In addition, the issues of subjectivity and objectivity and the strengths and weaknesses of these assessments strategies were discussed. The similarities and differences between these measures are discussed paying particular attention between subjective measures and their objective cousins. Finally, the authors have attempted to provide structure, organization, and hierarchy for determining the results of a clinical treatment or a research trial. Ideally, the perfect metric reflects the potential results, can be collected objectively, and measures a substrate that is truly meaningful to all parties involved. The group that needs to be satisfied is the patient, the clinician, the caregivers, and in these times, the source of reimbursement. The authors call on clinicians and scientists to emphasize proving the efficacy of new treatments and the treatment results of current treatments using meaningful assessment metrics. New metrics that are to be developed in the future should emphasize some of the deficiencies that have been highlighted in this chapter.

References

1. Pierson SH. Outcome measures in spasticity management. *Muscle Nerve Suppl.* 1997;6:S36–S60.
2. Pierson SH. Outcome measures in spasticity management. In: Mayer NH, Simpson DM, editors. *Spasticity: etiology, evaluation, management and the role of botulinum toxin.* New York, New York: We Move; 2002:27–43.
3. Taricco M, Adone R, Pagliacci C, Telaro E. Pharmacological interventions for spasticity following spinal cord injury. *Cochrane Database Syst Rev.* 2000;(2):CD001131.
4. Elovic E, Zafonte RD. Spasticity management in traumatic brain injury. *State of the Art Review of Rehabilitation.* 2001; 15(2):327–348.
5. Young RR, Wiegner AW. Spasticity. *Clin Orthop.* 1987;219: 50–62.
6. Lance JW. The control of muscle tone, reflexes, and movement: Robert Wartenberg Lecture. *Neurology.* 1980;30(12):1303–1313.
7. Finch E, Brooks D, Stratford PW, Mayo NE. *Physical rehabilitation outcome measures: a guide to enhanced clinical decision making.* 2nd ed. Hamilton, Ontario: BC Decker; 2002.
8. Elovic EP, Simone LK, Zafonte R. Outcome assessment for spasticity management in the patient with traumatic brain injury: the state of the art. *J Head Trauma Rehabil.* 2004;19(2): 155–177.
9. Elovic EP, Brashear A, Kaelin D et al. Repeated treatments with botulinum toxin type a produce sustained decreases in the limitations associated with focal upper-limb poststroke spasticity for caregivers and patients. *Arch Phys Med Rehabil.* 2008;89(5):799–806.
10. Friden J, Lieber RL. Spastic muscle cells are shorter and stiffer than normal cells. *Muscle Nerve.* 2003;27(2):157–164.
11. Stokic DS, Yablon SA. Neurophysiological basis and clinical applications of the H-reflex as an adjunct for evaluating response to intrathecal baclofen for spasticity. *Acta Neurochir Suppl.* 2007;97(Pt 1):231–241.
12. Brashear A, Zafonte R, Corcoran M et al. Inter- and intrarater reliability of the Ashworth Scale and the Disability Assessment Scale in patients with upper-limb poststroke spasticity. *Arch Phys Med Rehabil.* 2002;83(10):1349–1354.
13. Brashear A, Gordon MF, Elovic E et al. Intramuscular injection of botulinum toxin for the treatment of wrist and finger spasticity after a stroke. *N Engl J Med.* 2002;347(6):395–400.
14. Chae J, Yang G, Park BK, Labatia I. Muscle weakness and cocontraction in upper limb hemiparesis: relationship to motor impairment and physical disability. *Neurorehabil Neural Repair.* 2002;16(3):241–248.
15. Chae J, Labatia I, Yang G. Upper limb motor function in hemiparesis: concurrent validity of the Arm Motor Ability test. *Am J Phys Med Rehabil.* 2003;82(1):1–8.
16. Sietsema JM, Nelson DL, Mulder RM, Mervau-Scheidel D, White BE. The use of a game to promote arm reach in persons with traumatic brain injury. *Am J Occup Ther.* 1993;47(1): 19–24.
17. Pandyan AD, Price CI, Rodgers H, Barnes MP, Johnson GR. Biomechanical examination of a commonly used measure of spasticity. *Clin Biomech* (Bristol, Avon) 2001;16(10): 859–865.
18. Sehgal N, McGuire JR. Beyond Ashworth. Electrophysiologic quantification of spasticity. *Phys Med Rehabil Clin N Am.* 1998;9(4):949–979, ix.
19. Angel RW, Hoffmann WW. The H reflex in normal, spastic and rigid subjects. *Arch Neurol.* 1963;9:591–596.
20. Iles JF, Roberts RC. Presynaptic inhibition of monosynaptic reflexes in the lower limbs of subjects with upper motoneuron disease. *J Neurol Neurosurg Psychiatry.* 1986;49(8): 937–944.
21. Matthews WB. Ratio of maximum H reflex to maximum M response as a measure of spasticity. *J Neurol Neurosurg Psychiatry.* 1966;29(3):201–204.
22. Eisen A. Electromyography in disorders of muscle tone. *Can J Neurol Sci.* 1987;14(3 Suppl):501–505.
23. Little JW, Halar EM. H-reflex changes following spinal cord injury. *Arch Phys Med Rehabil.* 1985;66(1):19–22.
24. Artieda J, Quesada P, Obeso JA. Reciprocal inhibition between forearm muscles in spastic hemiplegia. *Neurology.* 1991;41(2 (Pt 1)):286–289.
25. Cahan LD, Kundi MS, McPherson D, Starr A, Peacock W. Electrophysiologic studies in selective dorsal rhizotomy for spasticity in children with cerebral palsy. *Appl Neurophysiol.* 1987;50(1-6):459–462.
26. Ongerboer De Visser BW, Bour LJ, Koelman JH, Speelman JD. Cumulative vibratory indices and the H/M ratio of the soleus H-reflex: a quantitative study in control and spastic subjects. *Electroencephalogr Clin Neurophysiol.* 1989;73(2): 162–166.
27. Pisano F, Miscio G, Del CC, Pianca D, Candeloro E, Colombo R. Quantitative measures of spasticity in post-stroke patients. *Clin Neurophysiol.* 2000;111(6):1015–1022.
28. Feve A, Decq P, Filipetti P et al. Physiological effects of selective tibial neurotomy on lower limb spasticity. *J Neurol Neurosurg Psychiatry.* 1997;63(5):575–578.
29. Milanov IG. Mechanisms of baclofen action on spasticity. *Acta Neurol Scand* 1992;85(5):305–310.
30. Panizza M, Castagna M, di SA, Saibene L, Grioni G, Nilsson J. Functional and clinical changes in upper limb spastic patients treated with botulinum toxin (BTX). *Funct Neurol.* 2000;15(3):147–155.
31. Remy-Neris O, Denys P, Daniel O, Barbeau H, Bussel B. Effect of intrathecal clonidine on group I and group II oligosynaptic excitation in paraplegics. *Exp Brain Res.* 2003;148(4): 509–514.
32. Roujeau T, Lefaucheur JP, Slavov V, Gherardi R, Decq P. Long term course of the H reflex after selective tibial neurotomy. *J Neurol Neurosurg Psychiatry.* 2003;74(7):913–917.
33. Bischoff C, Schoenle PW, Conrad B. Increased F-wave duration in patients with spasticity. *Electromyogr Clin Neurophysiol.* 1992;32(9):449–453.
34. Eisen A, Odusote K. Amplitude of the F wave: a potential means of documenting spasticity. *Neurology.* 1979;29(9 Pt 1):1306–1309.
35. Fisher MA. F/M ratios in polyneuropathy and spastic hyperreflexia. *Muscle Nerve.* 1988;11(3):217–222.
36. Pauri F, Boffa L, Cassetta E, Pasqualetti P, Rossini PM. Botulinum toxin type-A treatment in spastic paraparesis: a neurophysiological study. *J Neurol Sci.* 2000;181(1-2):89–97.
37. Hagbarth KE, Eklund G. The effects of muscle vibration in spasticity, rigidity, and cerebellar disorders. *J Neurol Neurosurg Psychiatry.* 1968;31(3):207–213.
38. Lance JW. The reflex effects of muscle vibration. *Proc Aust Assoc Neurol.* 1966;4:49–56.
39. Milanov I. A comparative study of methods for estimation of presynaptic inhibition. *J Neurol.* 1992;239(5):287–292.
40. Childers MK, Biswas SS, Petroski G, Merveille O. Inhibitory casting decreases a vibratory inhibition index of the H-reflex in the spastic upper limb. *Arch Phys Med Rehabil.* 1999;80(6): 714–716.
41. Powers RK, Campbell DL, Rymer WZ. Stretch reflex dynamics in spastic elbow flexor muscles. *Ann Neurol.* 1989;25(1): 32–42.
42. Reinkensmeyer DJ, Kahn LE, Averbuch M, McKenna-Cole A, Schmit BD, Rymer WZ. Understanding and treating arm movement impairment after chronic brain injury: progress with the ARM guide. *J Rehabil Res Dev.* 2000;37(6):653–662.
43. Zhang, LQ. Xu D. Liao W, Rymer,WZ. A quantitative and convenient method of evaluating tendon reflex and spasticity: Proceedings of the First Joint BMES/EMBS Conference Serving Humanity, Advancing Technology 1999.

44. Zhang LQ, Wang G, Nishida T, Xu D, Sliwa JA, Rymer WZ. Hyperactive tendon reflexes in spastic multiple sclerosis: measures and mechanisms of action. *Arch Phys Med Rehabil.* 2000;81(7):901–909.

45. Sherman SJ, Koshland GF, Laguna JF. Hyper-reflexia without spasticity after unilateral infarct of the medullary pyramid. *J Neurol Sci.* 2000;175(2):145–155.

46. Ashworth B. Preliminary trial of carisoprodal in multiple sclerosis. *Practitioner.* 1964;192:540–542.

47. Brashear A, Zafonte R, Corcoran M et al. Inter- and intra-rater reliability of the Ashworth Scale and the Disability Assessment Scale in patients with upper-limb poststroke spasticity. *Arch Phys Med Rehabil.* 2002;83(10):1349–1354.

48. Allison SC, Abraham LD, Petersen CL. Reliability of the Modified Ashworth Scale in the assessment of plantarflexor muscle spasticity in patients with traumatic brain injury. *Int J Rehabil Res.* 1996;19(1):67–78.

49. Blackburn M, van VP, Mockett SP. Reliability of measurements obtained with the Modified Ashworth Scale in the lower extremities of people with stroke. *Phys Ther.* 2002;82(1):25–34.

50. Bohannon RW, Smith MB. Interrater reliability of a Modified Ashworth Scale of muscle spasticity. *Phys Ther.* 1987;67(2):206–207.

51. Ansari NN, Naghdi S, Moammeri H, Jalaie S. Ashworth Scales are unreliable for the assessment of muscle spasticity. *Physiother Theory Pract.* 2006;22(3):119–125.

52. Naghdi S, Ansari NN, Azarnia S, Kazemnejad A. Interrater reliability of the Modified Modified Ashworth Scale (MMAS) for patients with wrist flexor muscle spasticity. *Physiother Theory Pract.* 2008;24(5):372–379.

53. Ansari NN, Naghdi S, Hasson S, Mousakhani A, Nouriyan A, Omidvar Z. Inter-rater reliability of the Modified Modified Ashworth Scale as a clinical tool in measurements of post-stroke elbow flexor spasticity. *NeuroRehabilitation.* 2009;24(3):225–229.

54. Patrick E, Ada L. The Tardieu Scale differentiates contracture from spasticity whereas the Ashworth Scale is confounded by it. *Clin Rehabil.* 2006;20(2):173–182.

55. Haugh AB, Pandyan AD, Johnson GR. A systematic review of the Tardieu Scale for the measurement of spasticity. *Disabil Rehabil.* 2006;28(15):899–907.

56. Scholtes VA, Becher JG, Beelen A, Lankhorst GJ. Clinical assessment of spasticity in children with cerebral palsy: a critical review of available instruments. *Dev Med Child Neurol.* 2006;48(1):64–73.

57. Tardieu G. A la recherche d'une technique de mesure de la spasticite. *Rev Neurol.* 1954;91:143–144.

58. Held JP, Pierrot-Deseilligny E. Rèèducation Motrice des Affections Neurologiques. Paris: JB Baillere et Fils. 1969;31–42.

59. Gracies JM, Marosszeky JE, Renton R, Sandanam J, Gandevia SC, Burke D. Short-term effects of dynamic lycra splints on upper limb in hemiplegic patients. *Arch Phys Med Rehabil.* 2000;81(12):1547–1555.

60. Fosang AL, Galea MP, McCoy AT, Reddihough DS, Story I. Measures of muscle and joint performance in the lower limb of children with cerebral palsy. *Dev Med Child Neurol.* 2003;45(10):664–670.

61. Mackey AH, Walt SE, Lobb G, Stott NS. Intraobserver reliability of the modified Tardieu scale in the upper limb of children with hemiplegia. *Dev Med Child Neurol.* 2004;46(4):267–272.

62. Ansari NN, Naghdi S, Hasson S, Azarsa MH, Azarnia S. The Modified Tardieu Scale for the measurement of elbow flexor spasticity in adult patients with hemiplegia. *Brain Inj.* 2008;22(13-14):1007–1012.

63. Van Bogart J, McGuire J., Harris GF;. Upper extremity motion assessment in adult ischemic stroke patients: a 3-D kinematic model. Engineering in Medicine and Biology Society, 2001 Proceedings of the 23rd Annual International Conference of the IEEE 2001; 2:1190–1192.

64. Zhang LQ, Chung SG, Lin AF, van Ray EM, Bai Z, Grant EH. A portable intelligent stretching device for treating spasticity and contracture with outcome evaluation. Proceedings of the Second Joint EMBS/MBES Conference 2002.

65. Hurvitz EA, Conti GE, Brown SH. Changes in movement characteristics of the spastic upper extremity after botulinum toxin injection. *Arch Phys Med Rehabil.* 2003;84(3):444–454.

66. Malhotra S, Cousins E, Ward A et al. An investigation into the agreement between clinical, biomechanical and neuro-physiological measures of spasticity. *Clin Rehabil.* 2008; 22(12):1105–1115.

67. Pandyan AD, Vuadens P, van Wijck FM, Stark S, Johnson GR, Barnes MP. Are we underestimating the clinical efficacy of botulinum toxin (type A)? Quantifying changes in spasticity, strength and upper limb function after injections of botox to the elbow flexors in a unilateral stroke population. *Clin Rehabil.* 2002;16(6):654–660.

68. Given JD, Dewald JP, Rymer WZ. Joint dependent passive stiffness in paretic and contralateral limbs of spastic patients with hemiparetic stroke. *J Neurol Neurosurg Psychiatry.* 1995;59(3):271–279.

69. Ghika J, Wiegner AW, Fang JJ, Davies L, Young RR, Growdon JH. Portable system for quantifying motor abnormalities in Parkinson's disease. *IEEE Trans Biomed Eng.* 1993;40(3):276–283.

70. Dewald JP, Given JD, Rymer WZ. Long-lasting reductions of spasticity induced by skin electrical stimulation. *IEEE Trans Rehabil Eng.* 1996;4(4):231–242.

71. Lee HM, Huang YZ, Chen JJ, Hwang IS. Quantitative analysis of the velocity related pathophysiology of spasticity and rigidity in the elbow flexors. *J Neurol Neurosurg Psychiatry.* 2002;72(5):621–629.

72. Hughes TAT, Westem BJ, Thomas M, van Deursen RWM, Griffiths H. An instrument for the bedside quantification of spasticity: a pilot study. Engineering in Medicine and Biology Society, 2001 Proceedings of the 23rd Annual International Conference of the IEEE, 2001.

73. Hershler C, Colotla I. Romilly DP, Computer controlled measurement of spasticity. Electrical and Computer Engineering, 1993 Canadian Conference 1993;2:1299–1300.

74. Yeh ,CY. Tsai KH. Chen, JJ, Development of a device for prolonged muscle stretch treatment and for quantitative assessment of spasticity. Proceedings of the 22nd Annual Conference of the IEEE Engineering in Medicine and Biology Society. 2000; 3:1856–1858.

75. Wang RY, Tsai MW, Chan RC. Effects of surface spinal cord stimulation on spasticity and quantitative assessment of muscle tone in hemiplegic patients. *Am J Phys Med Rehabil.* 1998;77(4):282–287.

76. Wartenburg R. Pendulousness of the legs as a diagnostic test. *Neurology.* 1951;1:18–24.

77. Bohannon RW. Variability and reliability of the pendulum test for spasticity using a Cybex II isokinetic dynamometer. *Phys Ther.* 1987;67(5):659–661.

78. Fowler EG, Nwigwe AI, Ho TW. Sensitivity of the pendulum test for assessing spasticity in persons with cerebral palsy. *Dev Med Child Neurol.* 2000;42(3):182–189.

79. He J. Stretch reflex sensitivity: effects of postural and muscle length changes. *IEEE Trans Rehabil Eng.* 1998;6(2):182–189.

80. Fee JW. The leg drop pendulum test under anesthesia, part II: normal vs limbs with spasticity. Proceedings of the Second Joint EMBS/EMBE conference. 2002.

81. White H, Uhl TL, Augsburger S, Tylkowski C. Reliability of the three-dimensional pendulum test for able-bodied children and children diagnosed with cerebral palsy. *Gait Posture.* 2007;26(1):97–105.

82. Syczewska M, Lebiedowska MK, Pandyan AD. Quantifying repeatability of the Wartenberg pendulum test parameters in children with spasticity. *J Neurosci Methods* 2009;178(2):340–344.

83. Fleuren JF, Nederhand MJ, Hermens HJ. Influence of posture and muscle length on stretch reflex activity in poststroke patients with spasticity. *Arch Phys Med Rehabil.* 2006;87(7): 981–988.

84. Powers RK, Campbell DL, Rymer WZ. Stretch reflex dynamics in spastic elbow flexor muscles. *Ann Neurol.* 1989;25(1): 32–42.

85. Allison SC, Abraham LD. Sensitivity of qualitative and quantitative spasticity measures to clinical treatment with cryotherapy. *Int J Rehabil Res.* 2001;24(1):15–24.

86. Kim DY, Park CI, Chon JS, Ohn SH, Park TH, Bang IK. Biomechanical assessment with electromyography of post-stroke ankle plantar flexor spasticity. *Yonsei Med J.* 2005;46(4): 546–554.

87. Mathiowetz V, Volland G, Kashman N, Weber K. Adult norms for the box and block test of manual dexterity. *Am J Occup Ther.* 1985;39(6):386–391.

88. Goodkin DE, Hertsgaard D, Seminary J. Upper extremity function in multiple sclerosis: improving assessment sensitivity with box-and-block and nine-hole peg tests. *Arch Phys Med Rehabil.* 1988;69(10):850–854.

89. Alon G, Sunnerhagen KS, Geurts AC, Ohry A. A home-based, self-administered stimulation program to improve selected hand functions of chronic stroke. *NeuroRehabilitation.* 2003;18(3):215–225.

90. Sorinola IO, White CM, Rushton DN, Newham DJ. Electromyographic response to manual passive stretch of the hemiplegic wrist: accuracy, reliability, and correlation with clinical spasticity assessment and function. *Neurorehabil Neural Repair.* 2009;23(3):287–294.

91. National MS Society. Measures for use in clinical studies of MS 9 hole peg test (9-HPT). http://www.nationalmssocietyorg, 2003 (Accessed December 31, 2007).

92. Chen HM, Chen CC, Hsueh IP, Huang SL, Hsieh CL. Test-Retest reproducibility and smallest real difference of 5 hand function tests in patients with stroke. *Neurorehabil Neural Repair.* 2009;23(5):435–440.

93. Rousseaux M, Kozlowski O, Froger J. Efficacy of botulinum toxin A in upper limb function of hemiplegic patients. *J Neurol.* 2002;249(1):76–84.

94. Richardson D, Edwards S, Sheean GL, Greenwood RJ, Thompson AJ. The effect of botulinum toxin on hand function after incomplete spinal cord injury at the level of C5/6: a case report. *Clin Rehabil.* 1997;11(4):288–292.

95. Pernalete N, Gottipati R, Yu WDR. Telerobotic haptic system to enhance the performance of vocational tests by motion impaired users. *Int J Hum Friendly Welf Robotic Syst.* 2003;4(1).

96. Allison SC, Abraham LD. Sensitivity of qualitative and quantitative spasticity measures to clinical treatment with cryotherapy. *Int J Rehabil Res.* 2001;24(1):15–24.

97. Fugl-Meyer AR. Post-stroke hemiplegia assessment of physical properties. *Scand J Rehabil Med Suppl.* 1980;7:85–93.

98. Fugl-Meyer AR, Jaasko L, Leyman I, Olsson S, Steglind S. The post-stroke hemiplegic patient. 1. A method for evaluation of physical performance. *Scand J Rehabil Med.* 1975;7(1): 13–31.

99. Fisher AG. *Assessment of motor and process skills.* 2 ed. Fort Collins,CO: Three Star Publication; 1997.

100. Lyle RC. A performance test for assessment of upper limb function in physical rehabilitation treatment and research. *Int J Rehabil Res.* 1981;4(4):483–492.

101. van der Lee JH, De G, V, Beckerman H, Wagenaar RC, Lankhorst GJ, Bouter LM. The intra- and interrater reliability of the Action Research Arm Test: a practical test of upper extremity function in patients with stroke. *Arch Phys Med Rehabil.* 2001;82(1):14–19.

102. van der Lee JH, Beckerman H, Lankhorst GJ, Bouter LM. The responsiveness of the Action Research Arm Test and the Fugl-Meyer Assessment Scale in chronic stroke patients. *J Rehabil Med.* 2001;33(3):110–113.

103. Sullivan JE, Hedman LD. Effects of home-based sensory and motor amplitude electrical stimulation on arm dysfunction in chronic stroke. *Clin Rehabil.* 2007;21(2):142–150.

104. Turk R, Burridge JH, Davis R et al. Therapeutic effectiveness of electric stimulation of the upper-limb poststroke using implanted microstimulators. Arch Phys Med Rehabil 2008;89(10):1913–1922.

105. Rodgers H, Shaw L, Price C et al. Study design and methods of the BoTULS trial: a randomised controlled trial to evaluate the clinical effect and cost-effectiveness of treating upper limb spasticity due to stroke with botulinum toxin type A. *Trials.* 2008;9:59.

106. Park KB, Park HW, Lee KS, Joo SY, Kim HW. Changes in dynamic foot pressure after surgical treatment of valgus deformity of the hindfoot in cerebral palsy. *J Bone Joint Surg Am.* 2008;90(8):1712–1721.

107. Feng CJ, Mak AF. Three-dimensional motion analysis of the voluntary elbow movement in subjects with spasticity. *IEEE Trans Rehabil Eng.* 1997;5(3):253–262.

108. Bouten CV, Koekkoek KT, Verduin M, Kodde R, Janssen JD. A triaxial accelerometer and portable data processing unit for the assessment of daily physical activity. *IEEE Trans Biomed Eng.* 1997;44(3):136–147.

109. Bernmark E, Wiktorin C. A triaxial accelerometer for measuring arm movements. *Appl Ergon.* 2002;33(6):541–547.

110. Uswatte G, Taub E, Morris D, Vignolo M, McCulloch K. Reliability and validity of the upper-extremity Motor Activity Log-14 for measuring real-world arm use. *Stroke.* 2005;36(11): 2493–2496.

111. Uswatte G, Giuliani C, Winstein C, Zeringue A, Hobbs L, Wolf SL. Validity of accelerometry for monitoring real-world arm activity in patients with subacute stroke: evidence from the extremity constraint-induced therapy evaluation trial. *Arch Phys Med Rehabil.* 2006;87(10):1340–1345.

112. Mizuike C, Ohgi S, Morita S. Analysis of stroke patient walking dynamics using a tri-axial accelerometer. *Gait Posture.* 2009;30(1):60–64.

113. Feng CJ, Mak AFT, Neuromuscular model for the stretch reflex in passive movement of spasticity elbow joint. *Engineering in Medicine and Biology Society.* 1998;5:2317–2320

114. Ubhi T, Bhakta BB, Ives HL, Allgar V, Roussounis SH. Ran domised double blind placebo controlled trial of the effect of botulinum toxin on walking in cerebral palsy. *Arch Dis Child.* 2000;83(6):481–487.

115. Chua KS, Kong KH. Alcohol neurolysis of the sciatic nerve in the treatment of hemiplegic knee flexor spasticity: clinical outcomes. *Arch Phys Med Rehabil.* 2000;81(10):1432–1435.

116. Caty GD, Detrembleur C, Bleyenheuft C, Deltombe T, Lejeune TM. Effect of simultaneous botulinum toxin injections into several muscles on impairment, activity, participation, and quality of life among stroke patients presenting with a stiff knee gait. *Stroke.* 2008;39(10):2803–2808.

117. Cole GF, Farmer SE, Roberts A, Stewart C, Patrick JH. Selective dorsal rhizotomy for children with cerebral palsy: the Oswestry experience. *Arch Dis Child.* 2007;92(9):781–785.

118. Papadonikolakis AS, Vekris MD, Korompilias AV, Kostas JP, Ristanis SE, Soucacos PN. Botulinum A toxin for treatment of lower limb spasticity in cerebral palsy: gait analysis in 49 patients. *Acta Orthop Scand.* 2003;74(6): 749–755.

119. Van der Linden ML, Aitchison AM, Hazlewood ME, Hillman SJ, Robb JE. Effects of surgical lengthening of the hamstrings without a concomitant distal rectus femoris transfer in ambulant patients with cerebral palsy. *J Pediatr Orthop.* 2003;23(3):308–313.

120. Perry J, Burnfield JM, Gronley JK, Mulroy SJ. Toe walking: muscular demands at the ankle and knee. *Arch Phys Med Rehabil.* 2003;84(1):7–16.

121. Esquenazi A, Mayer N, Garreta R. Influence of botulinum toxin type A treatment of elbow flexor spasticity on hemiparetic gait. *Am J Phys Med Rehabil.* 2008;87(4):305–310.

122. Perry J. The use of gait analysis for surgical recommendations in traumatic brain injury. *J Head Trauma Rehabil.* 1999;14(2):116–135.

123. Preiss RA, Condie DN, Rowley DI, Graham HK. The effects of botulinum toxin (BTX-A) on spasticity of the lower limb and on gait in cerebral palsy. *J Bone Joint Surg Br.* 2003;85(7):943–948.

124. Winters TF, Jr., Gage JR, Hicks R. Gait patterns in spastic hemiplegia in children and young adults. *J Bone Joint Surg Am.* 1987;69(3):437–441.

125. Gage JR. Con: Interobserver variability of gait analysis. *J Pediatr Orthop.* 2003;23(3):290–291.

126. Rousseaux M, Buisset N, Daveluy W, Kozlowski O, Blond S. Long-term effect of tibial nerve neurotomy in stroke patients with lower limb spasticity. *J Neurol Sci.* 2009;278(1-2): 71–76.

127. Shimada H, Obuchi S, Kamide N, Shiba Y, Okamoto M, Kakurai S. Relationship with dynamic balance function during standing and walking. *Am J Phys Med Rehabil.* 2003;82(7):511–516.

128. Yelnik A, Bonan I. Clinical tools for assessing balance disorders. *Neurophysiol Clin.* 2008;38(6):439–445.

129. Maskell F, Chiarelli P, Isles R. Dizziness after traumatic brain injury: overview and measurement in the clinical setting. *Brain Inj.* 2006;20(3):293–305.

130. Khademi A, Elovic EP, Strax T. Treatment of post-traumatic brain injury balance disorder with percutaneous posterior tibial nerve block measured with posturography: a case report. *Arch Phys Med Rehabil.* 1995;76:1084-1085.

131. Basford JR, Chou LS, Kaufman KR et al. An assessment of gait and balance deficits after traumatic brain injury. *Arch Phys Med Rehabil.* 2003;84(3):343–349.

132. O'Neill DE, Gill-Body KM, Krebs DE. Posturography changes do not predict functional performance changes. *Am J Otol.* 1998;19(6):797–803.

133. Wade LD, Canning CG, Fowler V, Felmingham KL, Baguley IJ. Changes in postural sway and performance of functional tasks during rehabilitation after traumatic brain injury. *Arch Phys Med Rehabil.* 1997;78(10):1107–1111.

134. Fowler NK, Nicol AC. Measurement of external three-dimensional interphalangeal loads applied during activities of daily living. *Clin Biomech.* 14(9):646–652.

135. Fowler NK, Nicol AC. A force transducer to measure individual finger loads during activities of daily living. *J Biomech.* 1999;32(7):721–725.

136. Rash GS, Belliappa PP, Wachowiak MP, Somia NN, Gupta A. A demonstration of validity of 3-D video motion analysis method for measuring finger flexion and extension. *J Biomech.* 1999;32(12):1337–1341.

137. Schmit BD, Dhaher Y, Dewald JP, Rymer WZ. Reflex torque response to movement of the spastic elbow: theoretical analyses and implications for quantification of spasticity. *Ann Biomed Eng.* 1999;27(6):815–829.

138. Tseng Y, Scholz JP, Schoner G. Goal-equivalent joint coordination in pointing: affect of vision and arm dominance. *Motor Control.* 2002;6(2):183–207.

139. Wang X. Three-dimensional kinematic analysis of influence of hand orientation and joint limits on the control of arm postures and movements. *Biol Cybern.* 1999;80(6):449–463.

140. Wright M, Van der Linden ML, Kerr AM, Burford B, Arrowsmith G, Middleton RL. Motion analysis of stereotyped hand movements in Rett syndrome. *J Intellect Disabil Res.* 2003;47(Pt 2):85–89.

141. Wewers ME, Lowe NK. A critical review of Visual Analogue Scales in the measurement of clinical phenomena. *Res Nurs Health.* 1990;13(4):227–236.

142. Skold C. Spasticity in spinal cord injury: self- and clinically rated intrinsic fluctuations and intervention-induced changes. *Arch Phys Med Rehabil.* 2000;81(2):144–149.

143. Skold C, Lonn L, Harms-Ringdahl K et al. Effects of functional electrical stimulation training for six months on body composition and spasticity in motor complete tetraplegic spinal cord–injured individuals. *J Rehabil Med.* 2002;34(1):25–32.

144. Al-Khodairy AT, Gobelet C, Rossier AB. Has botulinum toxin type A a place in the treatment of spasticity in spinal cord injury patients? *Spinal Cord.* 1998;36(12):854–858.

145. Fleuren JF, Snoek GJ, Voerman GE, Hermens HJ. Muscle activation patterns of knee flexors and extensors during passive and active movement of the spastic lower limb in chronic stroke patients. *J Electromyogr Kinesiol.* 2009;19(5): e301–e310.

146. Voerman GE, Fleuren JF, Kallenberg LA, Rietman JS, Snoek GJ, Hermens HJ. Patient ratings of spasticity during daily activities are only marginally associated with long-term surface electromyography. *J Neurol Neurosurg Psychiatry.* 2009;80(2): 175–181.

147. Vles GF, de Louw AJ, Speth LA et al. Visual Analogue Scale to score the effects of botulinum toxin A treatment in children with cerebral palsy in daily clinical practice. *Eur J Paediatr Neurol.* 2008;12(3):231–238.

148. Fleuren JF, Voerman GE, Snoek GJ, Nene AV, Rietman JS, Hermens HJ. Perception of lower limb spasticity in patients with spinal cord injury. *Spinal Cord.* 2009;47(5):396–400.

149. Gruenthal M, Mueller M, Olson WL, Priebe MM, Sherwood AM, Olson WH. Gabapentin for the treatment of spasticity in patients with spinal cord injury. *Spinal Cord.* 1997;35(10):686–689.

150. Richardson D, Sheean G, Werring D et al. Evaluating the role of botulinum toxin in the management of focal hypertonia in adults. *J Neurol Neurosurg Psychiatry.* 2000;69(4):499–506.

151. Michael KM, Allen JK, Macko RF. Reduced ambulatory activity after stroke: the role of balance, gait, and cardiovascular fitness. *Arch Phys Med Rehabil.* 2005;86(8):1552–1556.

152. Nilsagard Y, Lundholm C, Gunnarsson LG, Denison E. Clinical relevance using timed walk tests and 'timed up and go' testing in persons with multiple sclerosis. *Physiother Res Int.* 2007;12(2):105–114.

153. Barbeau H, Elashoff R, Deforge D, Ditunno J, Saulino M, Dobkin BH. Comparison of speeds used for the 15.2-meter and 6-minute walks over the year after an incomplete spinal cord injury: the SCILT Trial. *Neurorehabil Neural Repair.* 2007;21(4):302–306.

154. Brown M, Sinacore DR, Binder EF, Kohrt WM. Physical and performance measures for the identification of mild to moderate frailty. *J Gerontol A Biol Sci Med Sci.* 2000;55(6): M350–M355.

155. Lamoureux EL, Sparrow WA, Murphy A, Newton RU. The relationship between lower body strength and obstructed gait in community-dwelling older adults. *J Am Geriatr Soc.* 2002;50(3):468–473.

156. Medell JL, Alexander NB. A clinical measure of maximal and rapid stepping in older women. *J Gerontol A Biol Sci Med Sci.* 2000;55(8):M429–M433.

157. Spaulding SJ, Livingston LA, Hartsell HD. The influence of external orthotic support on the adaptive gait characteristics of individuals with chronically unstable ankles. *Gait Posture.* 2003;17(2):152–158.

158. Sun J, Walters M, Svensson N, Lloyd D. The influence of surface slope on human gait characteristics: a study of urban pedestrians walking on an inclined surface. *Ergonomics.* 1996;39(4):677–692.

159. Liaw LJ, Hsieh CL, Lo SK, Lee S, Huang MH, Lin JH. Psychometric properties of the modified Emory Functional Ambulation Profile in stroke patients. *Clin Rehabil.* 2006;20(5):429–437.

160. Baer HR, Wolf SL. Modified Emory Functional Ambulation Profile: an outcome measure for the rehabilitation of post-stroke gait dysfunction. *Stroke.* 2001;32(4):973–979.

161. Means KM, Rodell DE, O'Sullivan PS. Use of an obstacle course to assess balance and mobility in the elderly. A validation study. *Am J Phys Med Rehabil.* 1996;75(2):88–95.

162. Dodds TA, Martin DP, Stolov WC, Deyo RA. A validation of the Functional Independence Measurement and its perfor-

mance among rehabilitation inpatients. *Arch Phys Med Rehabil.* 1993;74(5):531–536.

163. Francisco GE, Latorre JM, Ivanhoe CB. Intrathecal baclofen therapy for spastic hypertonia in chronic traumatic brain injury. *Brain Inj.* 2007;21(3):335–338.

164. Cardoso E, Pedreira G, Prazeres A, Ribeiro N, Melo A. Does botulinum toxin improve the function of the patient with spasticity after stroke? *Arq Neuropsiquiatr.* 2007;65(3A): 592–595.

165. Heller A, Wade DT, Wood VA, Sunderland A, Hewer RL, Ward E. Arm function after stroke: measurement and recovery over the first three months. *J Neurol Neurosurg Psychiatry.* 1987;50(6):714–719.

166. Lagalla G, Danni M, Reiter F, Ceravolo MG, Provinciali L. Post-stroke spasticity management with repeated botulinum toxin injections in the upper limb. *Am J Phys Med Rehabil.* 2000;79(4):377–384.

167. Simpson DM, Gracies JM, Yablon SA, Barbano R, Brashear A. Botulinum neurotoxin versus tizanidine in upper limb spasticity: a placebo-controlled study. *J Neurol Neurosurg Psychiatry.* 2009;80(4):380–385.

168. Mahoney FI, Barthel DW. Functional evaluation: the Barthel Index. *Md State Med J.* 1965;14:61–65.

169. Boviatsis EJ, Kouyialis AT, Korfias S, Sakas DE. Functional outcome of intrathecal baclofen administration for severe spasticity. *Clin Neurol Neurosurg.* 2005;107(4):289–295.

170. Zhao JG, Cao CH, Liu CZ et al. Effect of acupuncture treatment on spastic states of stroke patients. *J Neurol Sci.* 2009;276(1-2):143–147.

171. Ashford S, Turner-Stokes L. Goal attainment for spasticity management using botulinum toxin. *Physiother Res Int.* 2006;11(1):24–34.

172. Rampazo FM, Bianchin MA, Oliveira FN, Lucato RV, Jr. Comparative analysis of occupational therapy benefits in spastic patients with hands involvement before and after botulinum toxin infiltration. *Rev Neurol.* 2009;48(9): 459–462.

173. Feldman AB, Haley SM, Coryell J. Concurrent and construct validity of the Pediatric Evaluation of Disability Inventory. *Phys Ther.* 1990;70(10):602–610.

174. Chu ML, Sala DA. The use of tiagabine in pediatric spasticity management. *Dev Med Child Neurol.* 2006;48(6):456–459.

175. Yang TF, Fu CP, Kao NT, Chan RC, Chen SJ. Effect of botulinum toxin type A on cerebral palsy with upper limb spasticity. *Am J Phys Med Rehabil.* 2003;82(4):284–289.

176. Campbell WM, Ferrel A, McLaughlin JF et al. Long-term safety and efficacy of continuous intrathecal baclofen. *Dev Med Child Neurol.* 2002;44(10):660–665.

177. Nordmark E, Josenby AL, Lagergren J, Andersson G, Stromblad LG, Westbom L. Long-term outcomes five years after selective dorsal rhizotomy. *BMC Pediatr.* 2008;8:54.

178. Ohata K, Tsuboyama T, Haruta T, Ichihashi N, Kato T, Nakamura T. Relation between muscle thickness, spasticity, and activity limitations in children and adolescents with cerebral palsy. *Dev Med Child Neurol.* 2008;50(2):152–156.

179. Ware JE, Jr. SF-36 health survey update. *Spine.* 2000;25(24): 3130–3139.

180. Findler M, Cantor J, Haddad L, Gordon W, Ashman T. The reliability and validity of the SF-36 health survey questionnaire for use with individuals with traumatic brain injury. *Brain Inj.* 2001;15(8):715–723.

181. Noonan VK, Kopec JA, Zhang H, Dvorak MF. Impact of associated conditions resulting from spinal cord injury on health status and quality of life in people with traumatic central cord syndrome. *Arch Phys Med Rehabil.* 2008;89(6): 1074–1082.

182. Westgren N, Levi R. Quality of life and traumatic spinal cord injury. *Arch Phys Med Rehabil.* 1998;79(11):1433–1439.

183. Childers MK, Brashear A, Jozefczyk P et al. Dose-dependent response to intramuscular botulinum toxin type A for upper-limb spasticity in patients after a stroke. *Arch Phys Med Rehabil.* 2004;85(7):1063–1069.

184. Welmer AK, von AM, Widen HL, Sommerfeld DK. Spasticity and its association with functioning and health-related quality of life 18 months after stroke. *Cerebrovasc Dis.* 2006;21(4): 247–253.

185. Diener E, Emmons RA, Larsen RJ, Griffin S. The Satisfaction With Life Scale. *J Pers Assess.* 1985;49(1):71–75.

186. Vogel LC, Krajci KA, Anderson CJ. Adults with pediatric-onset spinal cord injuries: part 3: impact of medical complications. *J Spinal Cord Med.* 2002;25(4):297–305.

187. Cicerone KD, Azulay J. Perceived self efficacy and life satisfaction after traumatic brain injury. *J Head Trauma Rehabil.* 2007;22(5):257–266.

188. Arango-Lasprilla JC, Ketchum JM, Gary K et al. Race/Ethnicity differences in satisfaction with life among persons with traumatic brain injury. *NeuroRehabilitation.* 2009;24(1):5–14.

189. EuroQol—a new facility for the measurement of health-related quality of life. The EuroQol Group. *Health Policy.* 1990;16(3):199–208.

Assessment of Spasticity in the Upper Extremity

6

Thomas Watanabe

A comprehensive assessment of the patient with spasticity is critical to maximize outcome in the treatment of upper extremity spasticity. Although a number of key components to this evaluation comprise this evaluation, the most important component is the identification of appropriate goals. Once the treatment goals are identified, the clinician can then look for barriers to achieving them. These barriers may be identified through physical examination. This evaluation may lead to the need for further diagnostic testing. Awareness of concomitant pathological processes, which may or may not be related to the condition that has led to complications of the upper motor neuron syndrome (UMNS), may lead to the identification of other barriers to achieving goals. Knowledge of functional anatomy, including neurologic and muscular action, will aid in the evaluation and development of an appropriate treatment plan. The arm must be assessed in the context of other needs and goals of the individual, since interventions targeting the arm may affect function or alter the ability to intervene elsewhere. If intervention for spasticity has already been initiated, the assessment also must include an evaluation of the efficacy of prior interventions. The goal of this chapter is to provide the reader with tools to carry out a comprehensive assessment of the individual with upper extremity spasticity and demonstrate how this assessment can aid in the development of a successful treatment plan.

IDENTIFYING GOALS IN UPPER EXTREMITY ASSESSMENT

Depending on the situation, it may be important to solicit information from a number of different individuals to identify goals. Whenever appropriate, the patient should be the primary person who identifies the goals, but clearly, there are situations in which the patient cannot provide much, if any, information. The patient's family or other caregivers may be able to identify important goals. Other treating clinicians, including therapists, nurses, aides, or other physicians, may also be useful sources of information regarding goals. As these goals are identified, the clinician will need to make some determination regarding the appropriateness of the goals. There will be times when it will not be possible to determine appropriateness with confidence, but this may become clearer with subsequent evaluations associated with ongoing treatment.

Goal setting is important because goals encourage the treatment team to evaluate and address spasticity, not by its presence or absence but rather by determining whether spasticity is a barrier to achieving the stated goal. There will be occasions where this is not the case and, in fact, the presence of spasticity to a degree may be beneficial in achieving a goal. Spasticity is also only one component of deficits related to upper motor neuron dysfunction, so it is important to assess which aspects of the UMNS are the primary barriers to attaining goals. Taking this approach will help the clinician make decisions regarding what treatment modality or modalities to use. For example, a determination may be made that the most appropriate goal for an individual with severe finger flexor spasticity is positioning to prevent breakdown of skin in the palm. In such a situation, the clinician may choose more aggressive or longer-acting interventions such as surgery if it is determined that there is minimal likelihood of functional use of the hand.

Different goals that can be generated when assessing upper extremity spasticity are infinite depending on how specific the clinician wants them to be. For patients with a greater degree of impairment, goals may be more related to decreasing the amount of care that providers need to deliver or preventing complications related to relative immobility. Such goals could include maintaining hygiene, improving ease of care for activities of daily living, helping with positioning, preventing breakdown of skin, and minimizing pain. More active goals may be helping the patient to participate in dressing, eating, grooming, or other daily activities. Goals may also be related to improving finer motor activities, such as writing or playing the piano. If feasible, it is important to encourage all participants in the goal-setting process to think about goals that may positively affect activity and participation, rather than the more traditional goals that tend to focus on body functions and structure.

Finally, it is important to identify goals because achievement of these goals is one of the most, if not the most, important measure of efficacy in a spasticity management program. The reevaluation of goals and the setting of new goals should be the focal points of follow-up visits.

ANATOMIC CONSIDERATIONS IN ASSESSING THE UPPER EXTREMITY

A proper understanding of the anatomy of the upper limb is essential for assessment of upper extremity spasticity. Although there are a number of stereotypical patterns seen in any arm as part of the UMNS (1), these patterns may involve a number of different muscles or combinations of muscles as seen in Table 6.1. Many muscles carry out more than one function or movement, and this must be taken into account, for instance, when one is considering focal chemodenervation. Otherwise, efforts to address a problem related to movement or positioning at one joint may alter function pertaining to a different movement. In addition, changes in the position of the limb at one joint may have direct effects on function and movement at another joint, such as with tenodesis.

TABLE 6.1 *Common Patterns of Muscle Overactivity Seen in the UMNS*	
Shoulder adduction and internal rotation	Pectoralis major, subscapularis, latissimus dorsi, teres major
Elbow flexion	Biceps brachii, brachialis, brachioradialis
Forearm pronation	Pronator teres, pronator quadrates
Wrist flexion	Flexor carpi radialis, flexor carpi ulnaris, FDS, and profundus
Wrist extension	Extensor carpi radialis longus and brevis, extensor carpi ulnaris, long finger extensors
Finger flexion	Flexor digitorum superficialis and profundus (can target specific fascicles)
Thumb-in-palm	FPL and brevis, adductor pollicis, FPL

UMNS, upper motor neuron syndrome.

ASSESSMENT OF THE SHOULDER

The shoulder joint is inherently very unstable. This instability allows for a greater degree of range of motion. As seen in Table 6.1, a number of different muscles are involved in various movements of the shoulder. This makes the evaluation of the shoulder at times quite complex. The initial assessment should include a discussion of problems related to the shoulder, addressing function, ease of care, and other issues, such as pain. The initial examination of the shoulder should include inspection of the joint and skin, identification of areas of tenderness and swelling, and, as appropriate, an assessment of strength and active and passive range of motion. This assessment, which should also be undertaken for the joints discussed below, will help the process of identification of goals and will also identify problems that may impair joint function including those not necessarily related to UMNS.

A common pattern seen in the UMNS is the adducted and internally rotated shoulder (1). This position may lead to poor hygiene, breakdown of skin and the axilla, difficulties with dressing and positioning, and pain in the shoulder. Although there are a number of muscles that may contribute to adduction and internal rotation, the pectoralis major, latissimus dorsi, subscapularis, and teres major are the most commonly involved. In trying to determine the relative contributions of these or other muscles in the adducted and internally rotated shoulder, it may be helpful to remember some of the other actions of each of these muscles. For instance, the latissimus dorsi is also a shoulder extensor as is the teres major. Therefore, when shoulder extension is also noted, one might consider focusing on these muscles. Recall also that the latissimus dorsi is an important shoulder depressor and is important when using crutches. Other muscles that may contribute to excessive shoulder extension include the long head of the triceps, posterior deltoid, wound, and sternocostal portion of the pectoralis major. Cocontraction of shoulder extensors may inhibit the patient's ability to voluntarily flex the shoulder (Figure 6.1).

If, on the other hand, shoulder flexion is seen along with internal rotation and adduction, one might anticipate that the pectoralis major is relatively more active, as the clavicular portion assists in flexing the arm. Other muscles that may contribute to excessive shoulder flexion include the anterior deltoid, coracobrachialis, and biceps brachii. Because these muscles all have other functions, this is another example of the need to consider all of the actions of a particular muscle when considering focal chemodenervation. The sub-

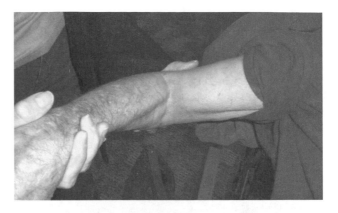

FIGURE 6.2

This patient demonstrates a flexed elbow and pronated forearm. Shoulder adductor tone is also present.

scapularis also deserves mention, as it is in many cases the primary internal rotator of the shoulder, although the pectoralis major, latissimus dorsi, anterior deltoid, and teres major may also contribute (2).

ASSESSMENT OF THE ELBOW

The general assessment of the elbow is similar to that of the shoulder. Discussion with the patient and caregiver may identify problems, such as poor hygiene in the flexor crease, difficulties with reaching and hand-to-mouth activities, dressing, and pain. The functional examination of the elbow may be more straightforward than the shoulder, as there are only 2 movements to consider: flexion/extension and pronation/supination. The more common pattern seen in the UMNS is excessive flexion and pronation (1). It is easy to understand how this position would lead to the problems identified above (Figure 6.2). Severe flexion may cause maceration and skin breakdown in the flexor crease.

The 3 main flexors of the elbow are the biceps brachii, brachialis, and brachioradialis. There may also be small contributions from the extensor carpi radialis and pronator teres. In determining the role to contributions of the 3 main flexors, it may be worthwhile to note whether the forearm is supinated or not. Remember that the biceps brachii is the primary supinator. In the nonpathological state, flexion in the pronated position is carried out primarily by the brachialis. A related consideration is that in the case of excessive flexion and pronation, sparing the biceps, when addressing elbow flexion, may help address the pronation. The brachioradialis on the other hand may contribute to the excessive pronation.

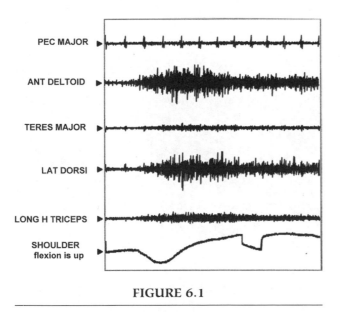

FIGURE 6.1

Dynamic electromyography demonstrating the cocontraction of the latissimus dorsi as well as the long head of the triceps when the patient is reaching forward, flexing the shoulder. These 2 shoulder extensors may be targets for focal chemodenervation to improve voluntary shoulder flexion. A third shoulder extensor, the teres major, demonstrates minimal cocontraction. (Used with permission from Dr. Nathaniel Mayer.)

The 2 main pronators of the forearm are the pronator teres and the pronator quadratus. The flexor carpi radialis may also assist in pronation if the wrist is flexed. In the UMNS, it is often difficult to distinguish the relative contributions of the pronator teres and pronator quadratus. It has been suggested that the pronator quadratus may be isolated if pronation in the distal forearm is identified when the forearm is fixed in supination at its midpoint. Clearly, this cannot always be achieved. This is one of many situations in which a diagnostic block may be appropriate.

ASSESSMENT OF THE WRIST

Hyperflexion of the wrist is the more common position seen in UMNS, although hyperextension of the wrist is not rare. Problems seen with exaggerated wrist flexion include difficulties with dressing and pain. Regarding pain, carpal tunnel syndrome is often associated with excessive wrist flexion and therefore should be a consideration in the evaluation (3). The position of the wrist is crucial for hand function, and conversely, changes in tightness of the long finger flexors will affect positioning of the wrist. This is an important concept and may affect surgical decision making as well (4). Excessive extension of the wrist may lead to passive tightness of the finger flexors (tenodesis). It is, therefore, important to incorporate finger positioning in the evaluation of range motion and function of the wrist and vice versa.

The primary wrist flexors are the flexor carpi radialis and flexor carpi ulnaris. The palmaris longus and abductor pollicis longus may also contribute. As mentioned above, the long finger flexors (flexor digitorum superficialis [FDS] and flexor digitorum profundus [FDP]) can also participate in wrist flexion, especially when the fingers are extended. If the wrist is also ulnarly deviated, one may surmise that the flexor carpi ulnaris is more involved (as well as the extensor carpi ulnaris). Flexion with radial deviation may suggest that the flexor carpi radialis is more involved, although there are several other muscles that may contribute to radial deviation, including the abductor pollicis longus, extensor carpi radialis and brevis, and extensor pollicis longus and brevis.

Excessive wrist extension may also be seen in the UMNS. Muscles that may contribute include extensor carpi radialis longus, extensor carpi radialis brevis, and extensor carpi ulnaris. As with wrist flexion, extension may be affected by the long finger muscles, such as extensor digitorum, extensor indices, extensor pollicis longus, and extensor digiti minimi.

Lower motor neuron processes may also affect function in the position of the wrist, as well as the fingers. For example, a lower plexus injury will affect wrist flexion and may therefore lead to excessive wrist extension. Alternatively, a radial nerve injury could lead to or exacerbate excessive wrist flexion. Such problems would be more likely encountered in certain UMNS etiologies, such as traumatic brain injury (TBI) with multiple trauma. For example, radial nerve injuries may be associated with humeral fractures, and there are a number of other traumatic injuries that are associated with specific nerve injuries affecting the wrist or other parts of the upper extremity (5). The evaluation of the wrist and hand should include a consideration of these complications.

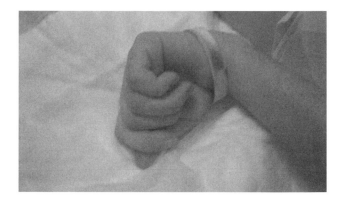

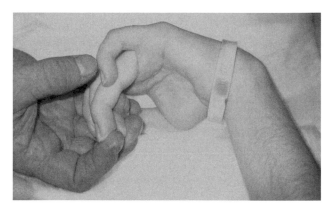

FIGURE 6.3

This patient appeared to have significant finger flexor overactivity. Further examination reveals that the fingers can actually be extended fairly easily with minimal flexor activity being noted. Because of the severe wrist flexor contracture, surgery will be required to allow the wrist to achieve a more neutral position to aid in basic activities of daily living. This surgery will need to address the long finger flexors, as the digits will otherwise become even more flexed due to tenodesis.

ASSESSMENT OF THE FINGERS

In the arm, UMNS typically leads to a clenched fist. Excessive finger flexion may prevent or at least limit functional use of the hand. Serious complications may arise, including maceration of the palmar surface of the hand. This is due to the inability to clean the palm and the trapping of moisture. Inability to access the fingernails will also contribute to tissue damage. This condition can be very painful, and the pain can exacerbate the excessive flexion. It is worth reviewing the contribution of wrist position to finger flexion. That is, some improvements in finger *extension* may be made if the wrist can be placed in a more flexed position. Alternatively, excessive wrist extension may contribute to worsening of finger flexion (Figure 6.3).

A number of different muscles, as well as specific fascicles within muscles, can contribute to the clenched fist deformity. The FDS and FDP are commonly implicated. It may be possible to differentiate the contribution of these 2 muscles to the clenched fist depending on whether the distal interphalangeal (DIP) joints are extended or not. Because the FDP inserts in the distal phalanx, if it is involved, then the DIP will be flexed, whereas if the FDS is involved, then the DIP will be extended, as the FDS inserts on the middle phalanx of the fingers. Often, not all fingers demonstrate excessive flexion. Therefore, the clinician may choose to target specific fascicles of the FDS and/or FDP for chemodenervation (Figure 6.4). In addition to the FDS and FDP, the lumbricals and interossei also contribute to flexion

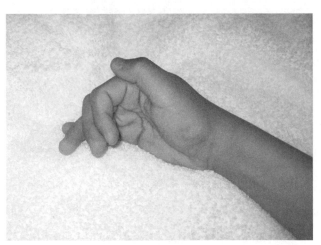

FIGURE 6.4

As demonstrated here, not all of the muscle slips of the long finger flexors may need to be treated for muscle overactivity. The clinician may choose to target only some of the fascicles of the flexor digitorum superficialis and/or FDP.

at the metacarpal joints. These intrinsic muscles also contribute to extension at the proximal interphalangeal (PIP). When the wrist and long finger flexors are lengthened, one may see an intrinsic plus position, characterized by excessive flexion of the metacarpophalangeal joint and extension at the PIP.

The thumb is often flexed within the palm in UMNS. Because the thumb is such an important component of hand function, appropriately addressing spasticity of the thumb may lead to significant functional improvement. The primary muscles involved in this position are the flexor pollicis brevis (which also assist with opposition and adduction), the adductor pollicis (which adducts and flexes the thumb), and the flexor pollicis longus (FPL). Because the FPL originates in the forearm and crosses ventral the wrist, its role in the deformity may be suspected if improvement in thumb extension is noted when the wrist is flexed.

FUNCTIONAL CONSIDERATIONS IN ASSESSMENT OF THE UPPER EXTREMITY

To achieve the goals identified, it is important that the assessment and treatment plan identify and address as many barriers as possible. Pain, difficulties with limb movement, loss of range of motion, and other problems are seen as part of the UMNS, but the relative role of spasticity differs from patient to patient. Movement disorders other than spasticity, such as rigidity, dystonia, or tremor, may be present and may require different interventions. It is essential that the clinician look for nonneurologic causes of loss of upper extremity function. These may or may not be related to the disease process that precipitated the UMNS. In addition, the evaluation should consider the duration of the condition because this may affect the course of treatment, as conditions such as hypertonicity and weakness are not static and may change significantly, especially in the more acute phase, as part of the natural history of the underlying disease process.

Loss of passive range of motion may be a result of spastic cocontraction, but a number of other processes must also be considered. Agonist/antagonist cocontraction is best demonstrated by using dynamic electromyography, where the muscle activity of both groups can be demonstrated simultaneously (Figure 6.5). Improvement in passive range of motion in response to diagnostic blocks to the antagonists is another way to demonstrate this process. If there is no improvement with the diagnostic block, cocontraction cannot be ruled out. However, it is likely that one or more other processes that affect range of motion in a joint are also present.

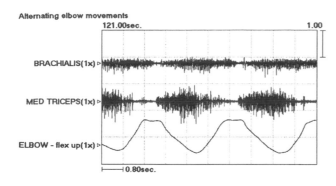

FIGURE 6.5

Poor reciprocal activation of the medial triceps and brachialis is demonstrated by dynamic electromyography. Note that the brachialis remains active during voluntary extension of the elbow. (Used with permission from Dr. Nathaniel Mayer.)

Soft tissue contracture will lead to loss of range of motion, and changes in connective tissue that are a major component of the development of contractures may occur rapidly (6). In the absence of hypertonicity or other pathological processes, preservation of joint range of motion is reported to be achievable by ranging the joint through its full range at least once a day. In the presence of hypertonia, however, intermittent range of motion may have fairly minimal effect. Techniques that maintain muscles and tendons at their functional length, such as splints and casting, may be of more use (7). Muscles and tendons that remain in a shortened position lose length, and therefore, range of motion across the joint is also lost. There are also changes in the properties of the soft tissue within the joint itself that contribute to loss of range of motion (8).

It may be difficult to determine the contribution of these soft tissue changes to loss of range of motion (9). Generally, methods used to provide prolonged static stretching, such as serial casting, will restore some range of motion, so a positive response to this intervention is supportive of the presence of contracture. Because contracture formation occurs over a period of time and in joints with limitations in mobility, it will be suspected when the condition is more chronic and function of the limb has been more severely compromised (Figure 6.6). Ongoing spasticity will contribute to this process, so treatment may need to include measures to treat spasticity in addition to stretching. If the condition is severe, surgical intervention may be required to restore adequate range of motion (10), but even in these cases, continued treatment will likely be required to prevent recurrence.

Orthopedic complications in a joint may also be seen, which may or may not be related to the un-

derlying disease process. Heterotopic ossification is a condition seen after TBI and spinal cord injury. Although the process is not well understood, it appears to be related to alterations in osteoblast and osteoclast activity and results in bone being formed across joints (11). The reported incidence ranges from 11% to 20% in TBI (12) and 13% to 57% after spinal cord injury (13). Joints typically affected include the hips, knees, shoulders, and elbows. Clinically, it presents as progressive loss of range of motion in a joint and pain with range of motion and is often warm and tender to palpation. It may be diagnosed radiographically or by triple-phase bone scan. Surgical excision may be required if loss of range of motion leads to significant dysfunction, but it is often delayed until the bone has matured (14).

Patients with spasticity may also have preexisting degenerative joint processes that affect range of motion at a joint. There is also evidence that persons who sustained a TBI may have an increased incidence of arthritis as they age (15). The presence of an arthritic joint may be identified when the history is taken on examination and can also be evaluated radiographically. In addition to loss of range of motion, the examination of the joint may reveal tenderness, warmth, and/or swelling. The presence of spasticity may lead to increased inflammation in the joint, accelerating the degenerative process or increasing the pain. Soft tissue edema related to a number of conditions may also decrease range of motion in a joint.

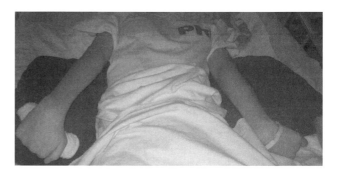

FIGURE 6.6

This patient with a severe traumatic and hypoxic brain injury demonstrates severe extension at the elbows, forearm pronation, and wrist flexion. She had significant paroxysmal autonomic instability with dystonia acutely and was reportedly often in a decerebrate position. Range of motion was very limited at the elbows. Electromyography demonstrated minimal triceps activity bilaterally. It was concluded that the loss of elbow flexion was related to the prolonged decerebrate position and resultant contractures rather than triceps overactivity. This patient subsequently also developed heterotopic ossification of the elbows.

Spastic joints are often painful, both at rest and with passive or active range of motion. The examination may be suggestive of velocity-dependent increased tone, but this may be due to guarding, with the patient being even more guarded or protective when the limb is moved more quickly or through a greater range. The examination may also be complicated by the fact that pain may increase spasticity. In addition, chemodenervation of spastic muscles can decrease poststroke shoulder pain (16). A diagnostic anesthetic block may help elucidate the relative contribution of pain to the loss of active and passive range of motion. Some causes of pain in a joint have already been discussed. In the setting of TBI or stroke, complex regional pain syndrome may also be considered. In the upper limb, the shoulder and metacarpophalangeal joints may be preferentially affected and may be tender to touch or with range of motion. Although there is no "gold standard" for diagnosis, criteria have been proposed (17). A triple-phase bone scan or diagnostic sympathetic blocks may be considered.

Weakness also contributes to loss of functional movement in the upper extremity. Although by definition UMNS implies an upper motor neuron process, other causes of weakness also need to be considered; as for a given individual, these other processes may be more amenable to intervention and/or contributing more to the patient's degree of dysfunction. Central processes may include direct damage to the corticomotor system, difficulties with coordination, neglect, motor planning deficits, and other movement disorders. There may also be concomitant lower motor neuron processes that contribute to weakness. These diagnoses may be related to the event that precipitated the UMNS, may be preexisting, or both. For example, preexisting carpal tunnel syndrome may contribute to functional deficits in the hand caused by an upper motor neuron injury, or in the setting of multiple trauma, mononeuropathies or plexopathies may lead to focal weakness, pain, or other sensory deficits that affect function. More generalized preexisting or injury-related neuropathies must be considered during an evaluation of limitations of upper extremity function. Some patients will have underlying medical conditions that may increase the likelihood of a generalized peripheral polyneuropathy, such as those with diabetes or hypothyroidism. Acutely ill patients may have critical illness polyneuropathy. In general, one would expect these neuropathic processes to diminish some of the positive signs of the UMNS, but some of the negative signs, especially weakness, would be worsened.

Dystonic posturing may be idiopathic or a sequela of upper motor neuron injury. In addition, dystonia may be related to medications, such as dopamine antagonists or anticholinergic agents (18). These etiologies should be considered by reviewing the list of current medications and the medication history. A number of movement disorders may result from hypoxic-ischemic events, so the presence of these should be considered and evaluated for persons who may have had an ischemic brain injury (19). Injury to the basal ganglia is thought to play an important role in many of the posthypoxic movement disorders (20). Differentiating these movement disorders from spasticity may result in improved functional outcome, as treatments among these movement disorders often differ.

It is important to obtain a thorough history as part of the functional assessment. The time course of the functional deficits may help identify reasons for loss of function. The evaluation, differential diagnosis, and treatment of a condition in which upper extremity function appears to be spontaneously improving would likely differ significantly from a condition in which there is rapid loss of arm function. The chronicity of the problem is also an important factor in the functional evaluation and determination of appropriate goals for the patient with upper extremity deficits. In the setting of trauma, knowledge of injuries that may impact upper extremity activity is important to determine the reason(s) for problems and to develop an appropriate treatment plan.

Several aspects of the physical examination that assesses function have already been discussed. The physical examination is, of course, important in terms of evaluating what appears to improve function. The initial examination also provides baseline data from which an assessment of efficacy of subsequent interventions can be determined. A number of resources are available that provide details regarding the assessment of active and passive range of motion (21). Strength can be assessed and reevaluated using a measure such as the Medical Research Council scale. The reader is referred to Chapter 5 which is devoted to discussion of measurement, including ways to assess tone and spasticity.

DEVELOPMENT OF THE TREATMENT PLAN TO ASSESS UPPER EXTREMITY SPASTICITY

Goal setting and anatomic and functional considerations are all important aspects of the evaluation process and assist in the formulation of the treatment plan. However, before making decisions regarding interventions, further evaluation or gathering of information may be necessary. As mentioned previously, diagnostic blocks may aid in the evaluation and determination of further treatment (22). These blocks allow the clinician and patient to evaluate the potential effects of treatment on a temporary basis and are also useful to help differentiate the processes that may be affecting function. Single- or multichannel dynamic electromyography may also be of help in the evaluation of, for example, the relative contributions of different muscles involved in the loss of motion at a joint (23). If there have been prior interventions, it is important to determine how efficacious those interventions have been, and if they have not achieved the desired effect, reasons why not. Prior goals need to be reviewed, and a determination should be made as to whether ongoing interventions are hoping to achieve those goals and whether modifications of existing goals are warranted.

As part of the evaluation process and development of the treatment plan, goals that conflict with other goals may have been identified. For example, aggressive efforts to decrease finger flexor tone to maintain palmar hygiene and prevent skin breakdown may have negative effects on the patient's ability to use the fingers for functional activities requiring flexor strength. In such cases, the clinician and patient may need to prioritize the goals. At a minimum, the clinician may want to counsel the patient and caregivers regarding the potential negative effects of interventions. If there is a question as to the potential outcome, it may make more sense to choose a shorter-acting or less permanent intervention, at least initially.

The development of the treatment plan must also take into account the possible complications related to the intervention. Splinting or serial casting of the upper extremity may lead to skin breakdown, for instance, in situations in which there is significantly increased tone or fluctuations in edema. The evaluation of the upper extremity must include efforts to identify such risks. Interventions to address tone in the arm can also have a more generalized negative functional impact. An example of this would be the use oral medications, which may inadvertently lead to a decline in cognitive function (24). Patients with UMNS due to injuries involving the brain may be at greater risk of developing this side effect of treatment.

The treatment plan for the upper extremity must take into account the arm in the context of the rest of the body. There are several different aspects of this concept. Addressing aspects of the UMNS in the arm may improve function in other areas. For example, there is evidence that decreasing tone and improving motion in the arm can improve ambulation (25, 26). Alternatively, a cast that adds weight and decreases range of motion in the arm may worsen balance and gait. The use of botulinum toxin presents another scenario in which the development of a treatment plan for the arm must take into account needs of the rest of the body. Because there is a limit to how much botulinum toxin can be safely administered at one time, one may need to determine how to most effectively utilize a finite amount of this medication to address hypertonia affecting many muscles.

One other aspect of the evaluation process and development of the treatment plan is to determine the natural history of the underlying disease process. In the acute phase, it may be difficult to predict whether hypertonia will increase, decrease, or remain the same. In such a situation, the clinician may choose to be more conservative regarding the choice of interventions to avoid the potential of worsening function. Weakening muscles that are initially hypertonic may slow functional recovery if the natural course of the disease process is that of diminution of hypertonicity and improvement in isolated voluntary muscle activity. However, severe spasticity, if untreated, may lead to contracture formation or other complications of the UMNS that worsen recovery of function. In a more chronic situation, in which it has been demonstrated that the hypertonicity invariably returns as interventions wear off, more "permanent" interventions may be warranted. There are also diseases, such as multiple sclerosis, in which spasticity and other neurologic deficits may vary over time. In such situations, the clinician must understand that the neurologic condition and therefore function status may vary independent of the spasticity management program. The evaluation in this situation may have less to do with current status and more with attempting to predict neurologic and functional changes related to the disease and, if applicable, effects of interventions for the disease itself.

FOLLOW-UP ASSESSMENTS OF UPPER EXTREMITY SPASTICITY

In most cases, the management of upper extremity dysfunction related to UMNS will be an ongoing process. Often, alterations will need to be made in the initial treatment plan. As noted above, this may be due to the natural history of the underlying disease process. As some barriers to function are addressed, other barriers may take on greater importance. Complications may have resulted from the initial treatment plan, necessitating alternative interventions. Goals may also change. As initial goals are achieved, other goals may become more attainable. Alternatively, some goals may prove to be unrealistic or may need to be scaled back.

It is important to maintain records that allow the clinician to reassess the patient in the context of prior examinations and interventions. Appropriate measures of outcome must be used, although the choice of such measures may change over time, depending on alterations in clinical presentation and goals. Tone and resistance to passive movement can be serially assessed with instruments, such as the Ashworth Scale or the Tardieu Scale (27, 28). Range of motion (active and passive) and strength can also be assessed. Examples of more functional measures are the nine-hole peg test (29) and the Barthel Index (30). More specific outcomes, such as the presence or absence of skin breakdown, may also be appropriate. It may also be appropriate to assess more general outcomes, such as ease of care and pain. As mentioned previously, outcome measures selected should, in general, reflect the goals that the patient and clinician have identified.

SUMMARY

The assessment of the upper extremity in the UMNS must involve more than just the identification of spastic muscles. The assessment process should include the identification of appropriate goals and barriers to goal attainment. The clinician must remember that these barriers are not always due to spastic or hypertonic muscles. It is important to think broadly in terms of etiologies for upper extremity dysfunction in the context of the UMNS. The assessment needs to include an awareness of anatomic considerations regarding upper extremity function. The management team should identify appropriate outcome measures to aid in the initial assessment and subsequent evaluations to determine the efficacy of the treatment plan.

References

1. Mayer NH, Esquenazi A, Childers MK. Common patterns of clinical motor dysfunction. *Muscle Nerve Suppl* 1997;6: 21–35.
2. Chang YW, Hughes RH, Su FV, Itoi E, An, KN. Prediction of muscle force involved in shoulder internal rotation. *J Shoulder Elbow Surg* 2000;9:188–95.
3. Orcut SA, Kramer WG 3rd, Howard MW, et al. Carpal tunnel syndrome secondary to wrist and finger flexor spasticity. *J Hand Surg Am* 1990;15:940–4.
4. Pomerance JF and Keenan MA. Correction of severe spastic flexion contractures in the non-functional hand. *J Hand Surg Am* 1996;21:828–33.
5. Nelson AJ, Izzi JA, Green A, Weiss A-PC, Akelman E. Traumatic nerve injuries about the elbow. *Orthop Clin North Am* 1999;30:91–4
6. Kottke FJ, Pauley DL, Ptak RA. The rationale for prolonged stretching for correction of shortening of connective tissue. *Arch Phys Med Rehabil* 1966;47:345–52.
7. Halar EM, Bell KR. Immobility and inactivity: physiological and functional changes, prevention and treatment. In: DeLisa JA, Gans BM, Walsh NE, eds. *Physical medicine and rehabili-*

8. *tation.* 4th ed. Philadelphia: Lippincott, Williams and Wilkins, 2005:1447–67.
8. Behrens F, Krah EL, Oegema TR Jr. Biochemical changes in articular cartilage after joint immobilization y casting or external fixation. *J Orthop Res* 1989;7:335–43.
9. Ada L, O'Dwyer N, O'Neill E. Relation between spasticity, weakness and contracture of the elbow flexors and upper limb activity after stroke: an observational study. *Disabil Rehabil* 2006;28:891–7.
10. Keenan MA, Mayer NH, Esquenazi A, Pelensky J. A neuro-orthopedic approach to the management of common patterns of upper motoneuron dysfunction after brain injury. *NeuroRehabil* 1999;12:119–43.
11. Kaplan FS, Glaser DL, Hebela N, Shore EM. Heterotopic ossification. *J Am Acad Orthop Surg* 2004;12:116–25.
12. Garland D. A clinical perspective on common forms of heterotopic ossification. *Clin Orthop Relat Res* 1991;263:13–29.
13. Kirshblum S. Rehabilitation of spinal cord injury. In: DeLisa JA, Gans BM, Walsh NE, eds. *Physical medicine and rehabilitation.* 4th ed. Philadelphia: Lippincott, Williams and Wilkins, 2005:1715–51.
14. van Kujik AA, Geurts A. Kuppevelt H. Neurogenic heterotopic ossification in spinal cord injury. *Spinal cord* 2002;40: 313–26
15. Colantonio A, Ratcliff G, Chase S, Vernich L. Aging with traumatic brain injury: long-term health conditions. *Int J Rehabil Res* 2004;27:209–14.
16. Yelnik AP, Colle FM, Bonan IV, Vicaut E. Treatment of shoulder pain in spastic hemiplegia by reducing spasticity if the subscapularis muscle: a randomized, double blind, placebo controlled study of botulinum toxin A. *J Neurol Neurosurg Psychiatry* 2007;78:845–8.
17. Harden RN, Bruehl SP. Diagnosis of complex regional pain syndrome: signs, symptoms, and new empirically derived diagnostic criteria. *Clin J Pain* 2006;22:415–9.
18. Dressler D, Benecke R. Diagnosis and management of acute movement disorders. *J Neurol* 2005;252:1299–1306.
19. Khot S, Tirschwell DL. Long-term neurological complications after hypoxic-ischemic encephalopathy. *Semin Neurol* 2006;26;422–31.
20. Venkatesan A, Frucht S. Movement disorders after resuscitation from cardiac arrest. *Neurol Clin* 2006;24:123–32.
21. *Clinical measurement of joint motion.* Greene WBB, Heckman JD, eds. 1st ed. Rosemont, IL, American Academy of Orthopedic Surgeons, 1994.
22. Wassef MR. Interadductor approach to obturator nerve blockade for spastic conditions of adductor thigh muscles. *Reg Anesth* 1993;18:13–7.
23. Keenan MA, Haider TT, Stone LR. Dynamic electromyography to assess elbow spasticity. *J Hand Surg Am* 1990;15:607–14.
24. Zafonte R, Lombard L, Elovic E. Antispasticity medications: uses and limitations of enteral therapy. *Am J Phys Med Rehabil* 2004;83(Suppl):S50–8.
25. Bakheit AM, Sawyer J. The effects of botulinum toxin treatment on associated reactions of the upper limb on hemiplegic gait—a pilot study. *Disabil Rehabil* 2002;24:519–22.
26. Esquenazi A, Mayer NH, Garreta R. Influence of botulinum toxin type A treatment of elbow flexor spasticity on hemiparetic gait. *Am J Phys Med Rehabil* 2008;87:305–10.
27. Pandayan AD, Johnson GR, Price CI, Curless RH, Barnes MP, Rodgers H. A review of the properties and limitations of the Ashworth and Modified Ashworth Scales as measures of spasticity. *Clin Rehabil* 1999;13:373–83.
28. Haugh AB, Pandayan AD, Johnson GR. A systematic review of the Tardieu Scale for the measurement of spasticity. *Disabil Rehabil* 2006;28:899–907.
29. Mathiowetz V, Weber K, Kashman N, Volland G. Adult norms for the nine hole peg test of finger dexterity. *Occup Ther J Res* 1985;5:24–38.
30. Mahoney FI, Barthel DW. Functional evaluation: the Barthel Index. *Md State Med J* 1965;14:61–5.

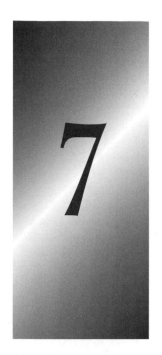

7 Assessment of Spasticity and Other Consequences of the Upper Motor Neuron Syndrome Affecting the Lower Limb

Alberto Esquenazi

A number of clinical assessment strategies are routinely used to evaluate the patient with residual consequences of the upper motor neuron syndrome (UMNS). *Spasticity* is a term that is often used by clinicians, and although frequently used, it can have different meaning in its interpretation and presentation. Spasticity is just one of the many positive signs of the UMNS. The clinical features of the UMNS include negative signs or signs of absence (eg, paresis, loss of dexterity, and selective movement control). Positive signs or signs of presence (eg, different forms of muscle overactivity including the stretch-sensitive and non–stretch-sensitive motor phenomena, such as spastic stretch reflexes, cocontraction, dystonia, enhanced cutaneomotor reflexes, associated reactions, tissue stiffness, and contracture) are a component of the syndrome. Mayer describes in depth these phenomena in Chapter 3 of this text.

The clinical expression of motor dysfunction in the UMNS is strongly influenced by 3 factors: spasticity and other forms of muscle overactivity, contracture, and impaired motor control. The time elapsed between the acute event leading to the upper motor neuron (UMN) signs, and the comprehensive management of the patient (particularly physical treatment) significantly influences the clinical presentation as rheologic changes affecting soft tissue pliability can rapidly occur. A limb with a UMN dysfunction is vulnerable to loss of range of motion (ROM) and skin,

bone, and joint problems resulting in functional impairment that negatively affect activities of daily living and body image.

Although many scales that intend to assess spasticity concentrate on resistance to passive movement as the main construct, spasticity might also lead to other clinically observable phenomena. Therefore, scales that measure associated clinical phenomena in the context of spasticity, that is, passive ROM (PROM), limb position at rest including postural alignment, tendon reflexes, clonus, spasms, or associated reactions, should be included as part of the assessment. Evaluation of a patient with a UMN related movement dysfunction requires a thorough comparison of needs and perceptions reported by the patient and the caregiver with the objective physical examination and, when available, movement evaluation in a motion analysis laboratory. There are many assessment techniques used in the routine clinical examination, and for their simplicity, PROM, motor control, manual muscle strength, Ashworth, and Tardieu are the most frequently used in the clinic.

Because clinical scales are based on ratings, they are prone to subjectiveness. Intrarater and interrater reliability are important characteristics that document the potential of a scale to produce stable results within and across clinicians. It reflects whether a repeated use of the scale can produce stable test results in clinically stable patients. Test-Retest reliability is a prerequisite for scales that are to be used for evaluation particularly when comparative follow-up is to be performed (1).

Passive range of motion can be used to determine the available movement for each joint, but it does not provide information on the cause of range limitations if present. Spasticity, muscle overactivity, contracture, and pain can all play a role in limiting PROM. Goniometric measurements can effectively document the PROM and permits comparison to normalcy (Table 7.1).

It is imperative to understand the effect of biarticular muscles on joint ROM. Manual muscle testing allows grading of available strength if normal motor control is present; the grading is done using The Medical Research Council 6-point scale, where 5 is a normal rating with ability to resist significant force and 0 reflects the inability to generate a muscle contraction (Table 7.2).

The clinician needs to recognize that in subjects with UMNS, testing of strength may be affected by impaired motor control, the presence of synergistic patterns, contractures, and communication or cognitive deficits.

The Ashworth Scale allows assessment of muscle tone; the Modified Ashworth utilizes a 5-point rating scale. The scale has only been validated for the elbow and requires the movement of the joint through its available range in 1 second (3). Ideally, the test should always be done with the subject in the same position and under similar conditions to measure the tone perceived across a joint (4). One disadvantage is that this test does not take into consideration the presence of a contracture or other nonneural components that may limit joint motion (5–7).

The neural component of spastic muscle comes from its stretch reflex activity, whereas the nonneural component comes from rheologic or physical properties intrinsic to muscle and other soft tissues. Many patients with UMNS have a large degree of nonneural resistance whose source is altered viscoelastic and plastic properties of muscle tissue itself (5, 8, 9).

TABLE 7.1
Normal Lower Limb Joint ROM

Ankle	Dorsiflexion/plantar flexion	0-20/0-0
	Inversion/eversion	0-30/0-15
Knee	Extension/flexion	0/135
Hip	Extension/flexion	0/115
	Abduction/adduction	0-50/0-30
	Internal rotation/ external rotation	30/50

TABLE 7.2
The Medical Research Council Scale

0	No evidence of contraction
1	Palpable muscle contraction
2	Limb moves with gravity eliminated
3	Limb moves against gravity
4	Limb moves against resistance
5	Normal

From Medical Research Council of the UK. Aids to the investigation of peripheral nerve injuries. Memorandum No 45. London: Pendragon House; 1976, p. 6–7, with permission.

When spasticity emerges after a UMN lesion, increased muscle tone may be attributed primarily to its neural component. In time, muscle tone receives an enhanced contribution from its nonneural component when rheologic properties of muscle become stiffer resulting in a contracture. Distinguishing neural from nonneural components of muscle tone has important implications for treatment selection.

Muscle contracture refers to physical shortening of muscle length, and it is often accompanied by shortening of other soft tissues such as fascia, nerves, blood vessels, and skin. Contracture is promoted by the acute paresis which develops after UMNS that impairs the normal cycles of shortening and lengthening of agonist and antagonist muscles during everyday voluntary usage; a net balance of contractile forces promotes unidirectional effects on joint position that set the stage for the fixed shortening present in a contracture.

The concept of rheologic change after a UMN lesion has literature support from many studies (10). Herman (5) described changes in the rheologic properties of spastic muscles in a study of 220 hemiplegic patients. Patients with contracture often had *reduced* reflex activity, yet resistance to passive stretch was high because of increased tissue stiffness and contracture.

These studies specify that the understanding of muscle tone should consider the complex interaction between rheologic and spastic properties of muscle because stretch reflexes themselves may be influenced by alterations in the physical properties of muscle. O'Dwyer et al. (11). suggested that what appears clinically as "spasticity" after stroke is actually increased muscle stiffness and in some cases contracture. Herbert, (8) Gossman et al. (12) and Carey and Burghardt (13) suggested that immobility imposed on a patient by the negative signs of UMN can result in soft tissue contracture.

The Tardieu Scale was developed in the mid 1960 as an ordinal rating assessment tool for the pediatric population; it attempts to assess spasticity by

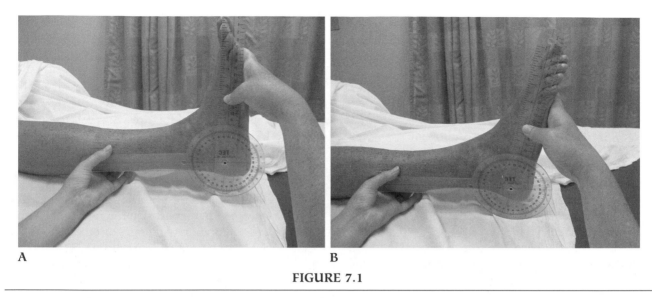

A   B

FIGURE 7.1

Low-velocity (A) and high-velocity (B) PROM of the ankle demonstrate the two positions of the ankle during the different measures of the Tardieu Scale with a resulting spasticity angle of –20°.

varying the speed of joint motion available from very slow (V1) to as fast as possible (V3). The difference between the parameters permits an estimation of the effect of spasticity (velocity dependence) and takes into consideration the joint ROM limitations imposed by contracture (Figure 7.1) (14).

Voluntary capacity and spastic reactivity are examined and interpreted in light of clinical and functional complaints. Not surprisingly, several outcome measures are utilized to attempt to evaluate spasticity, pain, function, and disability in patients with UMN problems; other measures include the Penn spasm frequency ordinal rank scale (15) and Biering-Sorensen postural analysis (16). According to Cohen and Marino (17), functional scales estimate the patients' functional status regardless of the specific underlying impairment. Table 7.3 is a list of the commonly used scales for the assessment of spasticity and associated clinical phenomena.

The selection of outcome measures to assess the functional impact of spasticity is not straightforward, and this is probably a reason why in most studies of spasticity, disability and function have been evaluated using a heterogeneous collection of outcome measures. Global scales measuring activity limitation such as the Functional Independence Measure and the Barthel Index have not shown to be sensitive enough to record change after the use of interventions such as botulinum neurotoxin (BoNT) for lower limb hypertonicity, and generally, they have not demonstrated changes directly related to variations of spasticity (18–20).

Richardson et al. (21) and Johnson et al. (22) have demonstrated functional improvement in mobility us-

ing the Rivermead Motor Assessment Scale. Likewise, one placebo-controlled, randomized control trial using BoNT and electrical muscle stimulation to assist gait

TABLE 7.3
List of Frequently Used Clinical Assessment Tools and the Parameter They Intend to Measure

PARAMETER	NAME OF SCALE
Resistance to PROM	Ashworth Scale
Resistance to PROM	MAS
Resistance to PROM	Velocity corrected MAS
Velocity-dependant resistance to PROM	Tardieu Scale
Resistance to PROM	VAS for tone
Resistance to PROM	Tone Assessment Scale
Hip adductor resistance to PROM	Spasticity score
Ankle resistance to PROM, tendon jerk, clonus	Total spasticity score
ROM	ROM with or without goniometer
ROM	Maximum inter-knee distance
Resting posture	Ankle position at rest
Spasm severity	Spasm Severity Scale
Spasm frequency	Spasm Frequency Scale
Extensor toe sign	Babinsky response
Clonus	Clonus score

Abbreviations: MAS, Modified Ashworth Scale; VAS, Visual Analog Scale.

retraining for spastic foot drop and one prospective case series using BoNT to treat stiff knee syndrome after stroke have been unable to demonstrate changes in health-related quality of life using the 36-Item Short-Form or in social participation using the SATISPART-Stroke (22–25).

The Goal Attainment Scale can be used to grade the achievement of outcomes following treatment with BoNT, with a focus on improvements of function and participation, which are relevant to the patient or their caregivers (26).

More recent publications have reported a link of functional outcomes based on the Physician Global Assessment Scale Score for the upper limb to the Ashworth-based clinical measure of tone (27). Unfortunately, none of them have provided a meaningful correlate to lower limb functional performance of common activities, such as walking velocity, and none have precisely identified the source of the problem impairing function. These deficiencies in part may be due to the fact that most indices quantifying function are ordinal; they merely rank persons with little input into how people function or how they are rehabilitated. For example, a total Functional Independence Measure score is a composite value of the multiple components, and without an item-by-item analysis, the ability to discern where the deficits are and how to intervene to attempt a solution is not possible. Based on our clinical experience, assessment methods based on a functional perspective or functional impairment such as those described later in this chapter may be more helpful in this regard.

Each year in the United States, approximately 700,000 people are affected by a stroke, and many more sustain a traumatic brain injury (TBI). These are the two prevalent forms of acquired brain injury producing an UMNS in the adult population. Acquired brain injury affects a person's cognitive, language, perceptual, sensory, and motor function (28). There are more than 1,700,000 Americans surviving with residual functional impairment after stroke and TBI (29, 30).

Dysfunction in the corticospinal tract and other descending pathways involved in voluntary motor activity is seen frequently. The immediate consequences may include paralysis and joint immobilization, with symptoms such as weakness, stiffness or rigidity, decreased manual dexterity, slowed movement, and fatigue. The loss of inhibitory impulses from higher centers in the central nervous system allows excessive muscle activity. Symptoms that may accompany lower limb spasticity include involuntary muscle spasms, clonus, scissoring of legs, abnormal limb postures, and joint contractures. Recovery is a long process that continues beyond the hospital stay and into the home setting. The rehabilitation process is guided by clinical assessment of motor and cognitive abilities. Accurate assessment of the motor abilities is important in selecting the different treatment interventions available to a patient. Ideally, a team approach to the evaluation of this patient population, their residual deficits, and the resulting limb postures is necessary, as the disabling forms of muscle overactivity affecting patients with UMNS are a widespread problem with functional implications for which a variety of interventions exist to address them. Spasticity is not always harmful; some patients rely on their spasticity for functional activities such as walking or standing. For others, however, spasticity can be painful and distressing (31).

More than half a century ago, Nikolai A. Bernstein suggested that a basic problem of motor control relates to overcoming redundant degrees of freedom in our multijointed skeletal system that allow us to interact with the 3-dimensional world in which we live. Commonly, there are multiple agonists and antagonists muscles called upon for virtually any movement direction. To match a required joint torque even across a single joint, the question regarding which muscles should be activated and how much force will it generate is likely to have a variable answer without an exclusive solution. For a given circumstance, for example, there may be a unique solution in that equinovarus deformity may be solely attributable to an overactive tibialis anterior in one patient, whereas in another, it may be the result of an overactive tibialis posterior (32). Simply put, identifying muscles that produce deforming maladaptive joint movements

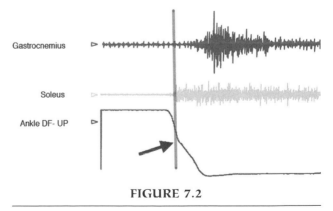

FIGURE 7.2

Ankle Ashworth test with dynamic EMG of ankle plantar flexors recorded with multichannel Motion Lab System and 3-dimensional movement tracing of ankle (black line) ecorded with CODA CX1 (Charnwood Dynamics). Note increase activation of soleus and then gastrocnemius during the passive dorsiflexion phase. Note the gradual slope of the ankle motion curve (the catch) caused by soleus overactivity as marked by the vertical line.

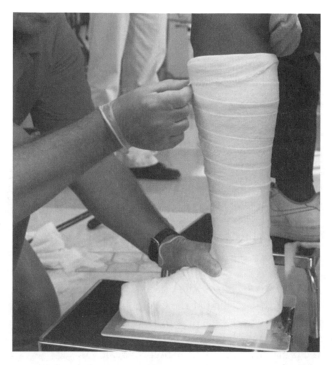

FIGURE 7.3

Patient with left ankle serial casting used to stretch a ROM limitation and reduce the point at which a spastic reaction occurs. The cast will be replaced at 3-day intervals and applied for a total of 9 to 12 days.

and postures statically and dynamically is an important endeavor in aiding clinical interpretation of lower limb dysfunction and its impact on gait and in rationalizing available treatment interventions and assessing the result of such intervention.

Clinical evaluation is useful to the analysis of movement dysfunction, but gait and movement laboratory evaluation using dynamic electromyography (EMG) is often necessary to identify the particular contributions of offending muscles with confidence (Figure 7.2).

The therapies for management of UMNS-related lower limb spasticity and muscle overactivity include exercises for stretching, strengthening, and coordination. Physical modalities such as casting and splinting, the use of focal neurolitic blockades, systemic medications and intrathecal drugs, neuro-orthopedic and neurosurgical interventions, and other forms of therapies are also used (Figure 7.3).

Problems of movement control and limb deformities are common consequences of UMNS. Dynamic EMG, gait analysis, and diagnostic nerve blocks frequently provide the necessary detailed information about specific muscle groups that will guide decision making for treatment. Ideally, all treatment interven-

tions must be patient-focused based on a multidisciplinary assessment that will result in targeted interventions to achieve patient-specific goals. The correct selection of target muscles that contribute to any one pattern of dysfunction may serve as a rational basis for interventions that focus on specific muscles for therapy (focal intervention).

Functional goals may be classified as symptomatic, passive, or active in nature. A symptomatic goal refers to clonus, flexor, or extensor spasms and pain among others as some of the targeted goals. However, it is also important to consider the impact on function. Sheean (33) and Mayer and Esquenazi (34) have proposed a recent update of this useful classification of function for this patient population (Table 7.4).

Application of lower limb orthoses, transfers and standing balance, perineal hygiene or catheterization, facilitation of therapy, and decrease of burden of care are examples of *passive function* (type II), where a carer carries out a task or where the individual tends to the affected limb with the unaffected limb. Options for assessment of passive function include verbal or visual analogue ratings of "ease of care," "timed care tasks" (eg. time taken for dressing), and formal scales that measure dependency or carer burden. Digital photography before and after treatment can provide a useful record of skin breakdown caused by pressure or difficulty with skin hygiene. Some studies have shown improvement in passive functions such as ease of hygiene and dressing after treatment with BoNT or ability to tolerate orthoses (35–37).

Mobility, transfers, activities of daily living, and sexuality are examples of *active function (type III)*, where the individual carries out a functional task (32).

A number of standardized scales can be used to compare outcomes between individuals and groups. The Leeds Adult Spasticity Impact Scale (38) is an example. The reality is that most global scales of independence in activities of daily living are rarely

---

TABLE 7.4
Classification of UMNS-Related Problems for Treatment Goal Development

Type I Symptomatic
Type II Passive Function
   Personal care
   Positioning
   Transfers
Type III Active Function
   Transfers
   Mobility
Type IV Mixed

sensitive to focal interventions for lower limb spasticity. Based on this, the goals for treatment will determine the appropriate scale.

When assessing a patient for development of a treatment plan, the clinician should consider the following:

- Is the presenting problem preventing function or affecting independence?
- Is there limb pain or other symptoms that may impact quality of life?
- The treatment options that have already been employed and what were the results of those interventions (39)?
- Overall health status of the patient and the expected therapeutic goals.
- The severity and scope of the problem, that is, local vs regional vs generalized problems (40).

Combined with clinical information, laboratory measurements of muscle function can provide the degree of detail and confidence necessary to optimize the rehabilitation interventions. Is the muscle resistive to passive stretch? Does the muscle have fixed shortening (contracture)? These questions can be best answered in an evaluation using quantitative instrumentation of the Gait and Motion Analysis Laboratory; dynamic EMG is acquired and examined in reference to simultaneous measurements of joint motion (kinematics) and during walking ground reaction forces (kinetics) obtained from force platforms. These data augment the clinician's ability to interpret whether voluntary function is present in a given muscle and whether that muscle behavior is also out of phase (dyssynergic). Several types of muscle overactivity are found in the UMNS, including the following:

- Exaggerated tonic and phasic stretch reflexes
- Cocontraction of antagonist muscles
- Associated reactions (synkinesia)
- Flexor and extensor spasms
- Spastic dystonia

The use of the International Classification of Functioning, Disability and Health (ICF) framework to underpin the assessment of outcomes in rehabilitation can assist with developing client-centered models of treatment planning (Figure 7.4) (41).

The ICF model identifies 3 domains of human function, which are categorized as impairment of body structure/function, activity limitation, and participation restriction, and sets out 2 contextual factors (environment and social) that may impact on the outcome of interventions, but the ICF does not quantify function.

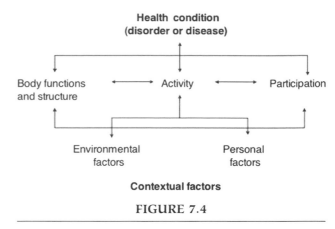

FIGURE 7.4

World Health Organization structural definition of the ICF.

In this scenario, the effects of spasticity are most commonly described at the level of impairment of body function (hypertonicity, associated reactions, limb deformity, etc), which may be assessed through, for example, the previously described Ashworth Scale (3).

Activity assessment can be made through lower limb measures of function such as the 6-Minute Walk test and Timed Up & Go test (Table 7.5).

CLINICAL ASSESSMENT OF SPASTICITY

Understanding the distribution of the presenting problem is of great importance to determine the appropriate assessment tool and treatment strategy. The distribution classification proposed by Esquenazi and Mayer follows with some lower limb examples:

- *Focal*: hyperextend hallux
- *Multifocal*: several joints in the same limb

TABLE 7.5
Possible Treatment Goals
Increased ROM
Decreased spasm frequency
Improved mobility
Improved positioning
Improved cosmesis
Decrease energy expenditure
Improved orthotic fit
Decreased pain
Improved gait
Increased ease of hygiene
Reduce a contracture
Protect skin and soft tissue integrity

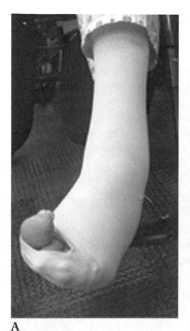 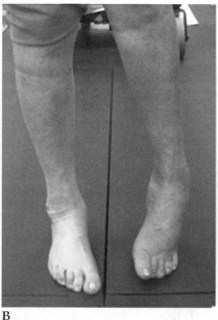 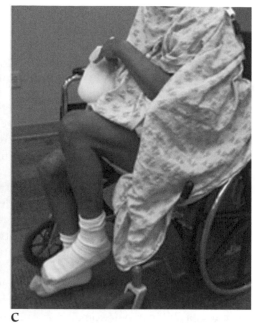

A   B   C

FIGURE 7.5

(A) Focal spasticity with hyperextension of the hallux. (B) Multifocal spasticity involving the lower limb. (C) Regional spasticity involving the right leg and arm.

- *Regional (multilimb)*: spastic diplegia
- *Generalized*: diffuse muscle overactivity, diffuse stiffness, and clonus

Figures 7.5(A), (B), and (C) illustrates examples of focal, multifocal, and regional problem distribution, respectively.

The clinician can use this classification to help rationalize the type of treatment selection. For example, a patient presenting a focal problem such as hyperextension of the hallux may appropriately guide the optimal treatment intervention selection to focal treatment with BoNT chemodenervation. A sensible approach would be to select a more systemic treatment approach to address the regional presentation while using a more focal treatment to address the focal or multifocal problems. Patients who are most likely to benefit from a selective treatment approach are those in whom focal or multifocal limb spasticity is causing harmful effects or making a substantial contribution to a clinical problem (42, 43).

FUNCTIONAL ASSESSMENT OF GAIT TO EVALUATE LOWER LIMB DYSFUNCTION

Gait is a functional task performed by most humans. The three main functional goals of ambulation are to move from one place to another, to move safely, and to move efficiently. These three goals are frequently compromised in the patient with residual UMNS. To identify the potential source of the problem and to focus more appropriately on the essence of multifactorial gait dysfunction, instrumented gait and movement analysis in a laboratory is of great value. Combining clinical evaluation with laboratory measurements will increase the degree of resolution needed to understand the problems affecting the lower limbs and the common patterns of gait dysfunction in the UMN (40) (Table 7.6).

The reader is encouraged to review Chapter 10 for further details of the topic. Gait as a functional outcome is a valuable indicator of function that can be extrapolated to more global functional outcomes which can measure quality of life and even predict participation.

TABLE 7.6
Patterns of Lower Limb UMNS-Related Dysfunction

Equinus or equinovarus foot
Hyperextend hallux
Stiff knee
Flexed knee
Adducted thigh
Flexed hip

Spasticity refers to a velocity-dependent increase in excitability of phasic and tonic muscle stretch reflexes that is present in most patients with UMNS. During walking, spasticity may become apparent and interfere with the task. Furthermore, normally latent stretch reflexes, such as the tonic stretch reflex, become obvious; hyperactivity of phasic stretch reflexes (exaggerated tendon jerks and clonus) have a lowered threshold and the muscle response is increased; and muscles besides the one stretched usually respond (44). Clonus is an exaggerated phasic stretch reflex characterized by repetitive, rhythmic contractions observed in one or more muscles of a single limb segment or multiple limb segments; at times, it may be difficult to identify the source of the spastic response at the joint or muscle level, which may interfere with treatment selection or delivery.

Using dynamic poly-EMG as illustrated in Figure 7.6 can help ascertain the source of the problem. The patient is a 24-year-old woman with residual UMNS from TBI. Left leg clonus during gait was interfering with her stability. Clinical assessment did not provide the particular muscle or joint source for this problem

since she had clonus in the ankle and knee during passive stretch. Lower-limb 3-dimensional motion tracking in conjunction with EMG demonstrates that the source of the clonus affecting the ankle and knee is the soleus followed by activation of the gastrocnemius. The timing of the problem can also be determined from this information (marked by the gray line) as the late stance phase and the instance in which the ankle is stretched because of the need to gain maximal contralateral limb advancement (Figure 7.6).

Muscle overactivity (ie, evidence of a neurogenic component) as the cause of limited ROM should ideally be confirmed with EMG or examination under local nerve block or in some selected cases general anesthesia. Patients in whom the dominant problem is fixed contracture or those with generalized spasticity without a focal source are unlikely to be suitable for management with interventions like botulinum toxin.

The evaluation of treatment outcome for patients with lower limb muscle overactivity and spasticity has focused predominantly on the assessment of changes in impairments, such as hypertonia, range of joint motion, and muscle tone. Increasingly, consumers and third-party funders are requiring evidence for a beneficial effect of therapeutic interventions on activity limitation and participation restriction.

Examples exist in the literature, but more work is needed in this sphere. The 10-meter walk test has been used by a number of investigators to measure functional change after BoNT treatment of calf muscle overactivity (23, 45–49).

Fock et al. (50) in an open-label study, demonstrated improvement in gait velocity, cadence, and stride length using instrumented 10-meter gait evaluation in a small group of patients with spastic equinus deformity after TBI treated with BoNT.

More recently, kinematic and qualitative gait improvements have been demonstrated after BoNT injection for stiff knee gait in adults with hemiplegia secondary to stroke (23, 51, 52) and to reduce associated reactions of the hemiparetic upper extremity (53). Pittock et al. (54) also used reduction in the use of walking aids as an outcome measure.

Differentiating between all of the components of the UMNS contributing to a patient's dysfunction and having the ability to appropriately identify what is the best assessment tool are of great importance in the selection and delivery of appropriate interventions and outcomes measurement. It is important to clearly identify the muscles involved by using a combination of focused clinical examination supplemented by evaluation in the Gait and Motion Analysis Laboratory. Kinematic, kinetic, and dynamic poly-EMG analysis along with diagnostic selective temporary blocks can

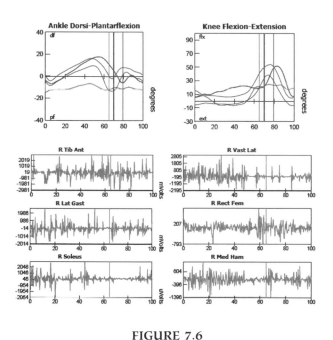

FIGURE 7.6

Three-dimensional motion and poly-EMG representation of the right ankle and knee used to assess clonus during walking. Data were collected with CODA CX1 system (Charnwood Dynamics). Data are normalized where 0 is the beginning of the stance phase and 100 the end of the swing phase. The gray line marks the time when the clonus becomes apparent in the muscle activation, and irregularity of the ankle and knee tracing is also present.

help define spasticity, contracture, and impaired motor control after UMN injury and optimize rehabilitation planning and treatment interventions. Clinical evaluation helps in the analysis of dysfunction, but laboratory evaluation using dynamic EMG and selective diagnostic nerve blocks are often necessary to identify the particular contributions of offending muscles with confidence. The correct selection of target muscles to any one pattern of dysfunction may serve as a rational basis for interventions that focus on specific muscles, including chemodenervation with botulinum toxin, neurolysis with phenol and surgical lengthening, and transfers and releases of individual muscles (55).

References

1. Platz T., Eickhof C., Nuyens G., Vuadens P. Disability clinical scales for the assessment of spasticity, associated phenomena, and function: a systematic review of the literature. *Disabil Rehabil.* 2005;27(1/2):7–18.
2. Medical Research Council of the UK. *Aids to the investigation of peripheral nerve injuries.* Memorandum No 45. London: Pendragon House; 1976, p. 6–7.
3. Ashworth B: Preliminary trial of carisprodol in multiple sclerosis. *Practitioner* 1964;192:540–542.
4. Bohannon RW, Smith MB. Interrater reliability of a Modified Ashworth Scale of muscle spasticity. *Phys Ther* 1987;67:206–207.
5. Herman R. The myotatic reflex. *Brain.* 1970;91:273–312.
6. Katz RT, Rymer WZ. Spastic hypertonia: mechanisms and measurement. *Arch Phys Med Rehabil* 1989;70:144–55.
7. Powers RK, Marder-Meyer J, Rymer WZ. Quantitative relations between hypertonia and stretch reflex threshold in spastic hemiparesis. *Ann Neurol* 1988;23:115.
8. Herbert R. The passive mechanical properties of muscle and their adaptations to altered pattern of use. *Aust J Physiother* 1988;34:141–9.
9. Thilmann AF, Fellows SJ, Ross HF. Biomechanical changes at the ankle joint after stroke. *J Neurol Neurosurg Psychiatry* 1991;54:134–9.
10. Pohl M, Mehrholz J, Rockstroh G, Ruckriem S, Koch R. Contractures and involuntary muscle overactivity in severe brain injury. *Brain Inj* 2007;4:421–432.
11. O'Dwyer N, Ada L, Neilson PD. Spasticity and muscle contracture following stroke. *Brain* 1996;119:1737–49.
12. Gossman MR, Rose SJ, Sahrmann SA, et al. Length and circumference measurement in one-joint and multijoint muscles in rabbits after immobilization. *Phys Ther* 1986;66:516–20.
13. Carey JR, Burghardt DT. Movement dysfunction following CNS lesions: a problem of neurologic or muscular impairment. *Phys Ther* 1993;73:538–547.
14. Tardieu G, Shentoub S, Delarue R. A la recherché d'une technique de mesure de la spasticite. *Rev Neurol* 1954;91:143–144.
15. Penn RD, Savoy SM, Corcos D., et al. 1989. Intrathecal baclofen for severe spinal spasticity. *N Engl J Med* 320, 1517–1521.
16. Biering-Sorensen F., Nielsen JB., Klinge K., 2006. Spasticity-assessment: a review. *Spinal Cord* 44, 708–722.
17. Cohen, ME, Marino RJ, 2000. The tools of disability outcomes research functional status measures. *Arch Phys Med Rehabil* 81 (Suppl. 2), S21–S29.
18. Dodds TA, Martin DP, Stolov WC, Deyo RA. A validation of the Functional Independence Measurement and its perfor-

mance among rehabilitation inpatients. *Arch Phys Med Rehabil* 1993;74(5):531–6.
19. Shah SN, Hornyak J, Urquhart AG. Flexion contracture after total knee arthroplasty in a patient with Parkinson's disease: successful treatment with botulinum toxin type A. *J Arthroplasty* 2005;20(8):1078–80.
20. Hinderer SR, Gupta S. Functional outcome measures to assess interventions for spasticity. *Arch Phys Med Rehabil.* 1996;77:1083–1089.
21. Richardson D, Sheean G, Werring D et al. Evaluating the role of botulinum toxin in the management of focal hypertonia in adults. *J Neurol Neurosurg Psychiatry.* 2000;69(4):499–506.
22. Johnson CA, Burridge JH, Strike PW, et al. The effect of combined use of botulinum toxin type A and functional electric stimulation in the treatment of spastic drop foot after stroke: a preliminary investigation. *Arch Phys Med Rehabil* 2004;85:902–9.
23. Caty GD, Detrembleur C, Bleyenheuft C, et al. Effect of simultaneous botulinum toxin injections into several muscles on impairment, activity, participation, and quality of life among stroke patients presenting with a stiff knee gait. *Stroke* 2008;39:2803–08.
24. McHorney CA, Ware JE Jr, Raczek AE. The MOS 36-Item Short-Form health survey (SF-36): II. Psychometric and clinical tests of validity in measuring physical and mental health constructs. *Med Care* 1993;31(3):247–63.
25. Bouffioulx E, Arnould C, Thonnard JL. SATIS-Stroke: A satisfaction measure of activities and participation in the actual environment experienced by patients with chronic stroke. *J Rehabil Med* 2008;40(10):836–43.
26. Turner-Stokes L. Goal Attainment Scaling (GAS) in rehabilitation: a practical guide. *Clin Rehabil* 2009;23(4):362–70.
27. Abu-Shakra S, VanDenburgh A, Zhou J, Charles D, Zafonte RD, Esquenazi A, Beddingield F. Clinically meaningful improvements in the Ashworth Scale for spasticity. In Press.
28. National Institute of Neurological Disorders and Stroke, Stroke: hope through research. NINDS Washington DC 2008.
29. American Heart Association, Heart disease and stroke statistics 2007 update. AHA Dallas TX, 2008.
30. Center for Disease Control, Morbidity and Mortality Weekly report. CDC, Atlanta GA 2005.
31. Spasticity in adults: management using botulinum toxin national guidelines. Royal College of Physicians. London. 2009.
32. Esquenazi A, Mayer N. Instrumented assessment of muscle overactivity andspasticity with dynamic polyelectromyographic and motion analysis for treatment planning. *Am J Phys Med Rehabil.* October 2004;83(10 Suppl):S1–29.
33. Sheean GL. Botulinum treatment of spasticity: why is it so difficult to show a functional benefit? *Curr Opin Neurol* 2001 Dec;14(6):771–6.
34. Mayer NH, Esquenazi, A. Childers, M.K. Common patterns of clinical motor dysfunction. In: *Spasticity and other forms of muscle overactivity in the UMNS.* Brashear and Mayer, editors. We Move 2008.
35. Hyman N, Barnes M, Bhakta B, et al. Botulinum toxin (Dysport) treatment of hip adductor spasticity in multiple sclerosis: a prospective, randomised, double blind, placebo controlled, dose ranging study. *J Neurol Neurosurg Psychiatry* 2000 Jun;68:707–12.
36. Opara J, Hordyńska E, Swoboda A. Effectiveness of botulinum toxin A in the treatment of spasticity of the lower extremities in adults—preliminary report. *Ortop Traumatol Rehabil* 2007;9(3):277–85.
37. Kirazli Y, On AY, Kismali B, Aksit R. Comparison of phenol block and botulinus toxin type A in the treatment of spastic foot after stroke: a randomized, double-blind trial. *Am J Phys Med Rehabil* 1998;77(6):510–5.
38. Bhakta BB, Cozens JA, Chamberlain MA, Bamford JM. Impact of botulinum toxin type A on disability and carer burden due to arm spasticity after stroke: a randomized double blind

placebo controlled trial. *J Neurol Neurosurg Psychiatry* 2000 Aug;69(2):217–21.

39. Mayer N, Esquenazi, A. Muscle overactivity and movement dysfunction in the upper motoneuron syndrome. *Phys Med Rehabil Clin N Am* 2003;14:855–883.

40. Esquenazi A, Mayer N. Laboratory analysis and dynamic polyEMG for assessment and treatment of gait and upper limb dysfunction in upper motoneuron syndrome. *Eura Medicophys.* 2004;40:111–122.

41. Steiner WA, Ryser L, Huber E, Uebelhart D, Aeschlimann A, Stucki G. Use of the ICF model as a clinical problem-solving tool in physical therapy and rehabilitation medicine. *Phys Ther* 2002;82(11):1098–107.

42. Brin MF. Dosing, administration, and a treatment algorithm for use of botulinum toxin A for adult-onset spasticity. The Spasticity Study Group. *Muscle Nerve Suppl.* 1997;20(suppl 6): S208–S220.

43. Sheean G. Botulinum toxin treatment of adult spasticity. *Expert Rev Neurother* 2003;3:773–785.

44. Dietz V, Trippel M, Burger W. Reflex activity and muscle tone during elbow movements in patients with spastic paresis. *Ann Neurol* 1991; 30:767–779.

45. Reiter F, Danni M, Lagalla G, et al.Low-dose botulinum toxin with ankle taping for the treatment of spastic equinovarus foot after stroke. *Arch Phys Med Rehabil* 1998 May;79(5):532–5.

46. Rousseaux M, Compère S, Launay MJ, Kozlowski O. Variability and predictability of functional efficacy of botulinum toxin injection in leg spastic muscles. *J Neurol Sci* 2005 May 15;232(1-2):51–7.

47. Cioni M, Esquenazi A, Hirai B. Effects of botulinum toxin-A on gait velocity, step length, and base of support of patients with dynamic equinovarus foot. *Am J Phys Med Rehabil* 2006 Jul;85(7):600–6.

48. Bayram S, Sivrioglu K, Karli N, Ozcan O. Low-dose botulinum toxin with short-term electrical stimulation in poststroke spastic drop foot: a preliminary study. *Am J Phys Med Rehabil* 2006 Jan;85(1):75–81.

49. Farina S, Migliorini C, Gandolfi M, et al. Combined effects of botulinum toxin and casting treatments on lower limb spasticity after stroke. *Funct Neurol* 2008 Apr-Jun;23(2):87–91.

50. Fock J, Galea MP, Stillman BC, et al. Functional outcome following botulinum toxin A injection to reduce spastic equinus in adults with traumatic brain injury. *Brain Inj* 2004 Jan;18(1):57–63.

51. Stoquart GG, Detrembleur C, Nielens H, Lejeune TM. Efficiency of work production by spastic muscles. *Gait Posture* 2005 Dec;22(4):331–7. Epub 2004 Dec 23.

52. Robertson JV, Pradon D, Bensmail D, et al. Relevance of botulinum toxin injection and nerve block of rectus femoris to kinematic and functional parameters of stiff knee gait in hemiplegic adults. *Gait Posture* 2009 Jan;29(1):108–12. Epub 2008 Sep 3.

53. Esquenazi A, Mayer N, Garreta R. Influence of botulinum toxin type A treatment of elbow flexor spasticity on hemiparetic gait. *Am J Phys Med Rehabil* 2008 Apr;87(4): 305–10.

54. Pittock SJ, Moore AP, Hardiman O, et al. A double-blind randomised placebo-controlled evaluation of three doses of botulinum toxin type A (Dysport) in the treatment of spastic equinovarus deformity after stroke. *Cerebrovasc Dis* 2003;15(4): 289–300.

55. Mayer NH, Esquenazi A, Keenan MA. Assessing and treating muscle overactivity in the upper motor neuron syndrome. In *Brain injury medicine principles and practice.* N. Zasler, D. Katz and R Zafonte (edts). DEMOS, New York, NY., chapter 2006;35:615–653.

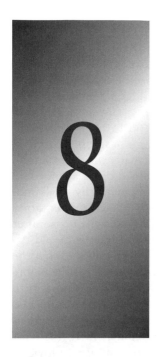

Setting Realistic and Meaningful Goals for Treatment

Elie Elovic

In 1998, O'Brien et al. (1) discussed the importance of goal setting when planning spasticity interventions. Clearly, the setting of proper goals is an important component in the management of this condition. Unfortunately, there is almost no literature that can assist clinicians in this process, forcing clinicians to rely solely on their clinical acumen. Elovic et al. (2) have previously published an extensive discussion and a proposed hierarchy of numerous outcome metrics. However, besides recommending that one should choose functional goals whenever possible, they gave very little guidance regarding the selection of these goals. In the discussion that follows, the author of this chapter will attempt to fill this void and increase the readers' understanding of this critical component in the regimen of spasticity treatment.

Numerous patients, with a variety of neurologic conditions, present for the management of their spasticity or other components of their upper motor neurons syndrome (UMNS). Normally, the person seeking treatment is looking for increased function, a decrease in their pain, improved posture, or easing of their caregiver's burden. Patients do not present to a doctor's office or a therapist's clinic looking for improvement in their range of motion, a higher score on their Fugl-Meyer, a lowering of their Ashworth Scale, or a change in an electophysiologic measure, such as the H/M ratio. Yet, all too often, those are the outcome metrics that clinicians and scientists use

when following up their patients or study participants during the course of treatment. However, patients do not seek treatment just to have changes in physiologic parameter. Instead, they want changes that are meaningful to them. In fact, Taricco et al. (3) suggest that patient-oriented outcomes should not only be important for an individual seeking treatment but should also be the basis for evidence-based clinical practice. Chapter 5 presents an organized and extensive discussion of the numerous parameters that can be used to follow a person's progress while they are undergoing treatment for their spasticity. The importance of choosing outcome measures that stress function and quality of life whenever possible as well as including the patient and family in the decision process cannot be overemphasized. This chapter will help guide clinicians in the process of choosing meaningful and realistic treatment goals.

CHOOSING MEANINGFUL AND REALISTIC TREATMENT GOALS

Patients and their families can be unrealistic and seek functional improvements that are just not likely to be obtainable. This can greatly complicate the efforts of clinicians who are often able to more accurately appraise what can reasonably be accomplished with treatment as compared to the patient or their family members. The challenge is to include the patient, family, and caregivers as members of the goal-setting team while maintaining professional objectivity and knowledge while guiding the treatment team into setting meaningful and obtainable goals. To accomplish this sometimes challenging task, clinicians must communicate with the consumers of health care services while comprehensively evaluating the entire clinical scenario.

So what are the factors that clinicians need to consider when designing treatment goals and programs? These items can be placed into 4 separate categories: (1) the patient, (2) the support system, (3)financial resources, and (4) the skills of the treatment team and availability of different treatment modalities. Each of these items will be discussed in greater detail in the sections that follow. It is critical that the clinicians perform an extensive assessment, including a history and physical evaluation that evaluates the items mentioned above as the first step in the development of an appropriate treatment plan and goals.

The Patient and the Clinical Presentation

The patient's clinical presentation, including the components of UMNS that they are experiencing and its etiology (4), is a critical component of the evaluation process. Other important factors include their prognosis, retained function, and the symptoms that are experiencing. These items along with the other items discussed below are important in the decision process of goal setting for spasticity management.

Spasticity Etiology: Clinical presentations may appear similarly despite having very different etiologies. Spasticity that results from spinal cord injury and multiple sclerosis can respond well to oral antispasticity agents (5–9). As a result, it may be reasonable to set as a goal to control a patient's systemic spasticity and spasms by utilizing oral agents in these populations. This is not the same with spasticity whose etiology is from acquired brain injury. The cognitive side effects and sedation (10), as well as some of the agents' potential for impairing recovery (11) and the limited efficacy (4) of oral systemic antispasticitiy agents, make them relatively poor agents for systemic spasticity, and the goal of reducing tone with them with an acceptable side effect profile with the acute brain injury population is very rarely met (12).

Time Since Onset: The treatment and goals that are pursued early after the onset of the condition often differ from those pursued later in the disease course.

Although clearly there is some overlap, early treatment and goals place a greater emphasis on complication prevention and positioning while allowing and hopefully facilitating the recovery process. Chemodenervation is sometimes performed early on to facility recovery and improve range of motion and positioning but certainly less than later in the tone management program. Early administration of a chemoneurolytic agent could lead to undesirable weakness or potentially block motor recovery because a person's clinical presentation can rapidly change early in the recovery phase after a stroke. As a result, many of the interventional trials with botulinum toxins have as a criterion that the patient is at least 3 months out from the stroke before being eligible for study inclusion (13–17). Studies such as that of Brashear et al. (15) used the Disability Assessment Scale, which evaluated disability in the areas of hygiene, dressing, position, and pain to look for functional changes secondary to treatment. Elovic et al. (16) looked at the effects of repeated open-label injections of botulinum toxin in areas such as quality of life and caregiver burden. These goals are important, but it is the long-term improvement in these areas that is most important clinically. Although there is some overlap in goal setting regarding the use of botulinum toxins, it is a very rare case where definitive procedures (eg, neuro-orthopedic, intrathecal baclofen placement) are performed early in the recovery, as the motor recovery process is nowhere near completion. Often, when clinicians utilize these procedures early on, it is an act of desperation because other more conservative modalities have failed to address the severe tone and significant contractures or other complications are beginning to develop. As a result, when these procedures are introduced early on in the recovery phase, the goals often reflect complication prevention that is commonly seen early in the recovery phase.

Anatomic Distribution: An important consideration when designing both treatment approaches and goals is the distribution of the muscle overactivity. In broad terms, distribution is normally categorized in 3 different groups: focal, regional, or generalized. Focal distribution is the term used to describe when a person's tone-related issues are confined to an area such as the hand or foot (ie, clenched fist or equinus deformity). A regional pattern is seen commonly with hemiplegia when an entire extremity or both on the same side demonstrate sequalae of the UMNS. Finally, the term generalized is used when the increased spasticity is noted through all extremities.

So how will anatomic distribution affect goal setting? When the increased tone is local in nature, then treatment and goals will reflect the area involved. For the hand, this might include decreased discomfort while wearing or greater ease of donning their splint, improved hand hygiene, greater cosmesis, or improved positioning. If there is residual function, then there could also be improved performance on hand and finger tasks, such as object manipulation or a more useful grip. When the foot is the issue, treatment goals could be improved mobility, ease of applying the brace, or an improved weight-bearing surface. When the pattern is more of a regional nature, the treatment and goals should also reflect that; however, there could be some overlap. Intrathecal baclofen is commonly used for regional or generalized spasticity. Goals for its use include improved mobility or easing of perennial hygiene; however, it may also demonstrate an effect on a focal condition and improve the foot's weight-bearing surface. When the muscle overactivity is generalized in nature, functional goals are less likely to be obtainable. Goals that are normally pursued in these cases are more passive in nature and often involve reducing discomfort and easing the caregiver burden; however, mobility can sometimes be addressed with systemic interventions such as intrathecal baclofen.

Functional and Overall Prognosis: The functional prognosis and life expectancy of the person with muscle overactivity need to be considered when making decisions regarding goal setting. If the spasticity that is present is a result of a condition such as a very aggressive lesion with a resultant short life expectancy, then it would be unreasonable to plan complex interventions such as neuro-orthopedic procedures that might theoretically lead to better weight-bearing surfaces and improved mobility. The recuperation time, morbidity, and discomfort that might come from these procedures are likely to outweigh any potential short-lived benefits that might result. Instead goals such as increased comfort, easing of caregiver burden, and the ability to facilitate limited independence of a person are more appropriate. However, if more functional goals can be pursued with less aggressive interventions, such as chemodenervation with toxin, should they be considered.

The issue of functional prognosis can also play an important part in the treatment and goal-setting process. The case of a patient who presents for spasticity management several years after his stroke can serve as a good example of this principal. It may be reasonable to treat with botulinum toxin 1 or 2 times to observe for long-term benefits after the toxin wears off. However, if after several interventions the patient returns to baseline, then the goal should be to effect long-term

change in tone management and a more definitive procedure should be considered. Likewise, in the patient whose prognosis is very guarded, such as permanent vegetative state, the goals should be designed to find long-term, cost-effective solutions to facilitate care, positioning, and complication prevention.

Cognitive Status: It is important to assess a patient's cognitive ability when designing treatment plans and goals. Clinicians must address the person's potential to be compliant and adhere to a prescribed treatment. An issue that must be evaluated is a person's ability to adhere, safely follow, and watch for complications when using a splint or using an oral antispasticity agent. If there are substantial cognitive deficits and a lack of adequate support, much more limited goals must often be the treatment target.

Concurrent Medical Problems: The overall medical condition of the patient being treated must be considered. When designing a treatment plan and setting goals, the medical comorbidities of the person being treated must be taken into account. Although a neuro-orthopedic intervention or placement of an intrathecal baclofen system may be the optimal treatment to achieve the goal of functional mobility and ease of care, sometimes the medical condition may greatly complicate the situation because the general anesthesia that is needed to perform these procedures may not be tolerated because of cardiac risk. An example of this that the author of this chapter was involved in is discussed as Clinical Case V later in this chapter. Other medical issues that may affect treatment and goal setting include impaired cognition, decreased arousal, orthostatic hypotension, problems with skin integrity, or an infected decubitus ulcer that makes the risk of implanting a device far greater.

Residual Function: When discussing problems with the UMNS, the symptoms can be divided into positive symptoms (eg, muscle overactivity, spasticity, clonus, cocontraction, associated reactions) and the negative symptoms (eg, weakness, fatigue, problems with coordination, and lose of motor control). Most of our interventions address the positive symptoms of the syndrome, and our ability to address the problems that result from the negative symptoms is very limited. As an example, when toxin intervention is utilized, although there can be some unmasking of residual function and potential improved motor control, the vast majority of motor movement must already be present before the treatment. When there is none, goals of the treatment must be primarily passive in nature. For there to be active finger extension, the extensor mechanism must be relatively intact before implementation of any treatment intervention. This is less true in the lower extremity, as the use of an orthotic device in combination with toxin treatment may facilitate mobility, even when active ankle dorsiflexion is very limited.

Response to Previous Treatment Efforts: An important component that needs to be assessed is the person's response to past treatment efforts. It would be inadvisable to repeat an effort that has previously failed in other clinicians' hands in the past. The caveat for this rule is to make sure that the past effort gave an adequate trial to assess the potential efficacy of the intervention. Some reasons that may warrant reattempting and intervention include chemodenervation with insufficient doses of botulinum neurotoxin, toxin efforts were not directed at the appropriate muscles, or the dose of the oral antispasticity agents trialed was not titrated to a sufficient level to determine potential benefit. If adequate doses of a particular oral agent did not reduce a person's spasms in the past, it is unlikely to do so in the future. By the same token, if a chemodenervation program with toxin appropriately addressed someone's hand hygiene and pain issues, it is likely to do so in the future. As a general rule, unless there has been a fundamental change in a patient such as developing of resistance to botulinum toxin or there has been a fundamental change in the person's condition (eg, exacerbation of multiple sclerosis), past performance can often guide the decision making and resultant goal-setting process. Therefore, it is extremely important to obtain a history and when possible obtain the records that report the results of previous treatment efforts.

Manifestation of the Upper Motor Neuron Syndrome: There are numerous different positive components of the UMNS. The readers are referred to a different chapter in this text for further discussion of this material. Based on the different presentations of the UMNS, different interventions are required, and the goals that can be achieved must differ. Cocontraction is one such example, and it occurs when a muscle is firing out of its normal phase and often is triggered when the antagonist muscle is firing. One of the most commonly clinical examples of this is when the brachioradialis fires during voluntary elbow extension. The elbow extensors may be weak but may be able to extend the arm if they were not opposed by the brachioradialis firing out of phase. The goal of temporary improvement of elbow extension and reach with the arm can possibly be obtained if a botulinum neurotoxin injection is performed into the cocontracting muscle.

Another example of different goals based on the component of the UMNS is the relationship between equinovarus deformity that is due to spasticity and dystonia. Although both of these conditions may respond to botulinum neurotoxin intervention, the same cannot be said about neuro-orthopedic intervention. Much of the basis of the neuro-orthopedic interventions is the changes that are created in the stretch reflex with tendon lengthening. It is reasonable then to address spastic equinovarus deformity with tendon lengthening. Because dystonia does not involve the velocity-dependent stretch reflex, the goal of improving foot position is obtainable when the deformity is spastic in origin but not when it is secondary to dystonia.

Benefits the Patient Derives From Their Spasticity: An issue that is often spoken about, perhaps more than it should be, is the potential positive effects of spasticity. The classic example that is mentioned is the patient with multiple sclerosis who is standing and using their quadriceps tone to maintain their ability to stand. Although this may be an unusual case, clinicians must consider this issue and be careful with their treatment and goal selection. Building on this issue, the clinicians must be careful that their spasticity intervention of reducing quadriceps tone with the goal of improving the swing phase of the gait cycle is met while there is significant quadriceps weakness and problems with the stance phase.

Available Support System

Support System: People with UMNS often need support from caregivers for their daily function. Caregivers can play an important role in the administration of spasticity treatment. They can offer support in many areas and can actively participate and facilitate the treatment process. One example of the importance of caregivers is their ability to provide supervision to allow for the safe administration of medications. Other examples of the roles they can play include arranging or providing transportation to clinical appointments, follow through with important modalities such as stretching or positioning, or reinforcing of constraint-induced therapy as examples. With the increasing limitations in resources available to support treatment, the role played by caregivers may become even more important in the future. As a result, it is hard to overemphasis the importance of the support system available to the patient. This is especially important when the person being treated has cognitive deficits. An absence of a good support network will often require the treatment team to set more limited goals.

Financial Resources

Financial Issues: As unpleasant as it may be to admit, financial realities can play an important part in the design and implementation of a treatment plan and goal. Botulinum neurotoxin and intrathecal therapy can be quite costly, and the price tag is often out of reach for families with limited means. The 20% copay that is required of Medicare patients without coinsurance can also make procedures too costly to be borne by a patient with very limited income. Geographic location can often play a role in the decision process. In Formosa as an example, the physicians are often limited to 200 U of onabotulinum toxin A. This makes the administration of large doses that are often needed for regions of large spasticity not an option. On the other hand, the patients can receive outpatient therapy for months and sometimes even years after their stroke. Closer to home, there are significant variations in the United States in regards to payment for outpatient therapy services. In New Jersey, as an example, patients with Medicaid as their primary insurance can often receive extensive physical and occupational therapy after toxin administration, which greatly facilitates the ability to effect range of motion and positioning issues in combination with toxin treatment. The state of Utah has a very different approach to reimbursement for therapy from their Medicaid provider. The limited resources that are available to reimburse outpatient services may well limit the goals that can be achieved with treatment. Without appropriate therapy follow-up, it becomes very challenging to develop treatment goals of improved positioning, range of motion, or even active function for patients with long-standing residual tone. This can be true for goals throughout the spectrum, from improved range of motion and positioning all the way to functional mobility.

The Skills of the Treatment Team and Availability of Different Treatment Modalities

I commonly see patients with spasticity secondary to acquired brain injury present to my office on oral baclofen. Because there are only limited data addressing the use of these agents for this condition (18–20) and there are concerns regarding side effects (12) and possible impairing motor recovery (11), one must assume that the clinicians are unable to utilize other treatment modalities that have a more supportive literature base. The use of botulinum toxin for chemodenervation can often not be utilized as a treatment in the inpatient unit because of financial issues. Furthermore, some skill is required, and many clinicians are reluctant to master them. Phenol neurolysis, which was a very common procedure before the introduction of the botulinum toxins, requires even more skills than the use of toxins, and the practitioners who perform this procedure safely and effectively are far fewer than those who treat spasticity. As a result, when there are large areas that require spasticity management, many clinicians are unable to offer the combination treatment approach of toxin and phenol. Finally, there are very few truly skilled surgeons who are experts at performing neuro-orthopedic interventions. Definitive interventions, which may be the only ones that can facilitate the goal of effective lifetime remediation of increased tone, may be unobtainable.

DETERMINING TREATMENT GOALS

So how does the treatment team proceed and develop their treatment approach and the related goals for the patients that present to them? This is a complicated question that involves a complete evaluation that addresses the issues mentioned earlier in this chapter. This needs to be complemented by a discussion with the patient and their family. It is critical that patients and their caregiver be in agreement with the treatment team. It does not mean that there aren't tiers of goals. If the family and/or the patient have goals that are unrealistic to pursue, it is incumbent on the treatment team to address this issue before commencing treatment. Otherwise, there will be great disappointment and potentially the development of an adversarial relationship between the treatment team and the patient and his or her family. The times that the author has gotten himself in trouble is when he has ignored this basic rule. Two things are vital to the development of successful goals. The first is that the patient/family and the remainder of the treatment team come to a general agreement as to what is expected with the planned interventions. The second is that the clinicians are honest and realistic with the family when setting the objectives of treatment. This is not to imply that all hopes of the family must be dashed, but realistic minimal goals are outlined and those potentially more desirable but less likely to be reached are also discussed.

CONCLUSION: SYNTHESIS OF INFORMATION AND CHOOSING TREATMENT GOALS

The treatment team must balance all the factors that have been discussed previously and develop a comprehensive plan. The most important inputs into to the decision process are the residual function, the muscle overactivity, the pathology generated, and the potential changes that can result from the available interventions. Three questions that must be answered to determine if a goal is realistic are the following: (1) Is the inability to reach the goal primarily due to the muscle overactivity or is there some other problem that is a major source of this disability factor that is blocking the desired goal? (2) Is there sufficient residual function present that once an issue is addressed, the function will be performable? and (3) Is there a treatment that can address muscle overactivity without doing serious harm? Integration of all of these materials to choose realistic meaningful goals can be a challenging exercise. The author will present a series of cases to facilitate the reader's understanding of these principals.

CASE DISCUSSIONS

Case I

M.K. is a 42-year-old, right-handed man who has a history of secondary progressive multiple sclerosis who presented to a spasticity clinic with significant hip adductor tone bilaterally. He has been wheelchair-bound for approximately 5 years and is independent at a wheelchair level, including sliding board transfers. His strength is good in the upper extremities, and his tone in the upper extremities is 0 to 1 on the Ashworth Scale. His strength in the lower extremity cannot be assessed secondary to severely increased tone that is a 4 throughout in the bilateral lower extremities. M.K. has previously been performing straight catheterization independently up to 3 months before presentation but has recently become unable to perform these activities secondary to an ability to spread his legs because of the recently increased tone in his legs. His neurologist has placed M.K. on oral baclofen 20 mg, QID; tizanidine 36 mg, per day; and 20 mg valium, q day without improvement in his symptoms. He presents to the clinic for management of his spasticity and particularly his hip adductor tone so he again will be able to perform straight catheterization.

Goal-setting discussion: The goals for this patient's treatment plan are fairly straightforward. Reducing his adductor tone is the primary purpose for the patient presented to your office. Oral medications have been unable to adequately address the severity of his tone. Treatments that could be considered included botulinum toxin injection to the adductor muscles bilaterally, bilateral obturator nerve blocks, or intrathecal baclofen. The tone is regional in nature, and the first two options will only treat the tone at the hip. Utilizing intrathecal baclofen has the potential for treating the

increased muscle activity found throughout both legs. The initial goals will be reducing adductor tone and facilitating M.K.'s ability to perform his self-care activities. There is a remote possibility that there is residual function in the lower extremity that may be unmasked with intrathecal baclofen, and improved mobility may be obtainable. The 5 years of being wheelchair-bound makes this a more remote possibility.

Case II

J.S. is a 66-year-old, right-handed woman who 6 months before presentation to the clinic sustained a right hemispheric middle cerebral artery occlusion with a resultant dense left spastic hemiplegia with her arm more affected more than her leg. She is able to ambulate independently but presents to the clinic requesting evaluation and treatment for her left upper extremity. When she walks she reports that her left elbow flexion increases, which impairs her balance. Her wrist and fingers also get tight, and the overall position is embarrassing to her and a source of pain. On evaluation, the patient has some volitional movement at the elbow wrist and trace finger extension. There is Ashworth 2 tone noted at the elbow wrist and fingers. J.S. is able to extend her elbow slowly with cocontraction appreciated in her elbow flexors that is slowing elbow extension.

Goal-setting discussion: The patient's muscle overactivity is clearly affecting her ability to use her left upper extremity and by her own report impairs her balance. There are numerous levels of potential goals that could be achieved with this patient. At a minimum, botulinum toxin injection would have the potential to lessen the muscle activity and reduce the associated reaction that is causing her elbow to flex when walking. Minimal goals will be to reduce muscle overactivity, reduce J.S.'s pain, and address the associated reaction at the elbow. More advanced goals that are likely to be obtainable would be to improve voluntary elbow extension to facilitate using the left arm as a more effective functional assist to her right arm. A higher-level goal that will depend on the residual function that exists in the finger extensors is the potential to get some functional use from her left hand.

Case III

T.F. is a 75-year-old man who sustained a large intracerebral bleed 9 months before presentation with a dense spastic hemiplegia involving his right upper and lower extremities. He has extremely limited motor function and is wheelchair-bound and only has trace movement in a synergy pattern at his right shoulder. He has significant problems in his right hand and wrist secondary to severe muscle overactivity with an inability to don his hand splint as well as problems with positioning and hygiene.

Goal-setting discussion: This is a very simple case in regard to goal setting because there is no realistic chance of volitional functional recovery. The goals are simply to reduce muscle overactivity, ease donning of T.F.'s hand splint, and the improve passive function of ease of hand hygiene.

Case IV

T.S. is a 25-year-old man who, secondary to a diving accident, sustained a C8 ASIA D injury. He is able to ambulate using Lofstrand crutches. He is totally independent in all areas of activities of daily living but presents to the spasticity clinic with complaints of severe pain and spasms. He has been trialed on Lyrica for pain control, but it has had a negligible effect on T.S.'s symptoms. Secondary to the severe neuropathic pain that he is experiencing, he is requiring substantial doses of opioids by mouth and has also required intravenous narcotics to control his spasms, pain, and tone. On evaluation, he has good strength throughout both lower extremities and is able to ambulate 500 ft without difficulty.

Goal-setting discussion: T.S. is fully independent, but secondary to painful spasticity and spasms that have resulted from his spinal cord injury, he had significant problems with his quality of life. Oral medications have been ineffective in the management of his pain. A reasonable approach at this point is a trial of intrathecal baclofen to evaluate its potential to reduce his painful spasms. Because he is fully independent at this time, it is important to also evaluate T.S.'s function when he is under the influence of intrathecal baclofen. Ideally, intrathecal baclofen can achieve the goal of pain relief while not negatively affecting his motor function.

Case V

B.Z. is a 25-year-old, right-handed man with a ventricular septal defect who sustained an embolic cerebrovascular accident with a spastic left hemiplegia. B.Z. had volitional movement in both his left arm and leg but was severely limited in his ability to move his left side because of significant tone measures (Ashworth 3 to 4) involving his left elbow flexors, left quadriceps, left hip adductors, gastrocsoleus complex, and tibialis posterior. He was able to perform many of his basic self-care activities of daily living with setup and supervision but has his greatest difficulties with mobility. He was able to ambulate with a hemi walker and moderate assistance of 1 for 30 ft, and he could transfer with minimal assistance of 1. When walking or transferring, his elbow went into very significant flexion, which further complicated his ability to walk and transfer. When walking, he demonstrated a narrow base (hip adductors) and stiff knee gait (quadriceps) with initial foot contact on the lateral aspect of the mid foot (equinovarus).

Goal-setting discussion and clinical course: When first evaluated, because of the severity of his tone over large regions of his body, the idea of intrathecal baclofen was introduced to the patient and his family as a means of addressing his significant lower extremity tone, with a plan for chemodenervation for his upper extremity. The goals were to improve his balance and weight-bearing surface to facilitate his transfers and mobility. The family was initially reluctant to have the patient undergo intrathecal baclofen treatment, and they decided to have the patient undergo chemodenervation utilizing onabotulinum toxin A. B.Z. was gradually up to a dose of 800 U of the toxin, but the severity of the tone made addressing all of his areas of muscle overactivity impossible.

Reluctantly, the family agreed to have an intrathecal baclofen system placed, and the initial results were very promising because early titration resulted in improved tone in the lower extremity and ambulation with a hemi walker and minimal assistance of 1. However, 1 month after placement of the pump, it became infected and had to be removed at which time B.Z. reverted back to his previous level of function. The Neurosurgeon was reluctant to replace the pump, and other interventions were planned in efforts to reduce the patient's muscle overactivity. Phenol neurolysis was used to treat the elbow flexor tone, but still, the lower extremity tone could not be managed. Neuro-orthopedic intervention was considered, but because of B.Z.'s cardiac status, clearance for general anesthesia could not be obtained. Finally, after 18 months passed and no other alternative treatment was available, the neurosurgeon replaced the pump without incident.

At the present, B.Z. is ambulating with a hemi walker for 300 ft with contact guard and is transferring with supervision. This case nicely illustrates the challenges faced by clinicians while they are trying to address functional goals with significant medical comorbidities.

References

1. O'Brien CF, Seeberger LC, Smith DB. Spasticity after stroke. Epidemiology and optimal treatment. Drugs Aging 1996;9(5): 332–340.

2. Elovic EP, Simone LK, Zafonte R. Outcome assessment for spasticity management in the patient with traumatic brain injury: the state of the art. J Head Trauma Rehabil 2004;19(2): 155–177.

3. Taricco M, Pagliacci MC, Telaro E, Adone R. Pharmacological interventions for spasticity following spinal cord injury: results of a Cochrane systematic review. Eura Medicophys 2006;42(1):5–15.

4. Elovic E. Principles of pharmaceutical management of spastic hypertonia. Phys Med Rehabil Clin N Am 2001;12(4):793–816, vii.

5. Kirshblum S. Treatment alternatives for spinal cord injury related spasticity. J Spinal Cord Med 1999;22(3):199–217.

6. Duncan GW, Shahani BT, Young RR. An evaluation of baclofen treatment for certain symptoms in patients with spinal cord lesions. A double-blind, cross-over study. Neurology 1976;26(5):441–446.

7. Groves L, Shellenberger MK, Davis CS. Tizanidine treatment of spasticity: a meta-analysis of controlled, double-blind, comparative studies with baclofen and diazepam. Adv Ther 1998;15(4):241–251.

8. Nance PW, Bugaresti J, Shellenberger K, Sheremata W, Martinez-Arizala A. Efficacy and safety of tizanidine in the treatment of spasticity in patients with spinal cord injury. North American Tizanidine Study Group. Neurology 1994;44(11 Suppl 9):S44–S51.

9. Hudson P, Weightman D. Baclofen in the treatment of spasticity. Br Med J 1971;4(778):15–17.

10. Meythaler JM, Guin-Renfroe S, Johnson A, Brunner RM. Prospective assessment of tizanidine for spasticity due to acquired brain injury. Arch Phys Med Rehabil 2001;82(9): 1155–1163.

11. Goldstein LB. Common drugs may influence motor recovery after stroke. The Sygen In Acute Stroke Study Investigators. Neurology 1995;45(5):865–871.

12. Hulme A, MacLennan WJ, Ritchie RT, John VA, Shotton PA. Baclofen in the elderly stroke patient its side-effects and pharmacokinetics. Eur J Clin Pharmacol 1985;29(4):467–469.

13. Bakheit AM, Thilmann AF, Ward AB et al. A randomized, double-blind, placebo-controlled, dose-ranging study to compare the efficacy and safety of three doses of botulinum toxin type A (Dysport) with placebo in upper limb spasticity after stroke [In Process Citation]. Stroke 2000;31(10):2402–2406.

14. Bhakta BB, Cozens JA, Chamberlain MA, Bamford JM. Impact of botulinum toxin type A on disability and carer burden due to arm spasticity after stroke: a randomised double blind placebo controlled trial. J Neurol Neurosurg Psychiatry 2000;69(2):217–221.

15. Brashear A, Gordon MF, Elovic E et al. Intramuscular injection of botulinum toxin for the treatment of wrist and finger spasticity after a stroke. N Engl J Med 2002;347(6): 395–400.

16. Elovic EP, Brashear A, Kaelin D et al. Repeated treatments with botulinum toxin type a produce sustained decreases in the limitations associated with focal upper-limb poststroke spasticity for caregivers and patients. Arch Phys Med Rehabil 2008;89(5):799–806.

17. Gordon MF, Brashear A, Elovic E et al. Repeated dosing of botulinum toxin type A for upper limb spasticity following stroke. Neurology 2004;63(10):1971–1973.

18. Jones RF, Lance JW. Bacloffen (Liorcsal) in the long-term management of spasticity. Med J Aust 1976;1(18):654–657.

19. Pedersen E. Clinical assessment and pharmacologic therapy of spasticity. Arch Phys Med Rehabil 1974;55(8):344–354.

20. Pinto OS, Polikar M, Debono G. Results of international clinical trials with Lioresal. Postgrad Med J 1972;48:Suppl-25.

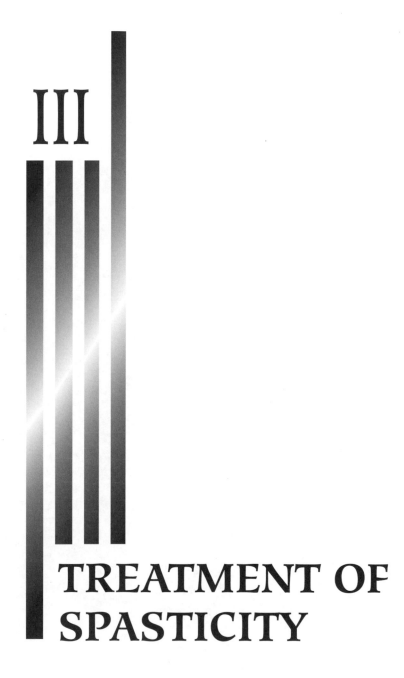

III

TREATMENT OF
SPASTICITY

Chemoneurolysis With Phenol and Alcohol: A "Dying Art" That Merits Revival

9

Lawrence J. Horn
Gurtej Singh
Edward R. Dabrowski

For the 3 decades before the introduction of botulinum toxins (BTs) for the treatment of upper motor neuron syndrome (UMNS) and spasticity, physiatrists were trained in the use of phenol and, less commonly, alcohol for these purposes. In some situations, the technique to apply these agents was considered to be more laborious and requires a modicum of greater skill than is the case with BTs. Given the relative facility of application of BT, its use among physiatrists and other specialists dramatically increased, whereas that of phenol declined. Hence, in the recent past, it was not unusual to refer to those of us using phenol (as well as BT) as practitioners of a "dying art," particularly by those specialists who had never been trained in the application of phenol or alcohol.

The authors' purpose for this chapter is to review the mechanism of action, techniques, proven benefits, and risks associated with phenol neurolysis along with a brief discussion of the use of alcohol. In addition, the authors will provide a comparison between phenol and BT and suggest situations when the practitioner may preferentially select one intervention over another. Given the limitations of BT (expense, the necessity of waiting 3 months between interventions, and the duration of action of BT), it is reasonable to include phenol and alcohol neurolysis, along with BT, in the armamentarium of the less-invasive approaches to the management of the UMNS.

CHEMICAL NEUROLYSIS

Nerve blocks involve the application of substances to a nerve that will interfere with conduction along the nerve on a temporary or permanent basis; local anesthetics, phenol, and alcohol are the most frequently used. Chemical neurolysis involves the application of an agent that will damage a portion of a nerve, impeding conduction. Ultimately, these interventions are intended to treat spasticity, hypertonicity, primitive movement patterns, and possibly other aspects of the UMNS by interfering with the muscle stretch reflex arc. Nerve blocks exhibit their effect primarily through treatment of the efferent component of the arc, but the afferent loop can be involved as well. In essence, the result would be the conversion of a muscle affected by UMNS to one with a partial lower motor neuron syndrome via partial denervation. Neurolysis has been used at every level of the peripheral nerve, from the spinal cord and roots to the motor endplate. The location of intervention will determine the completeness of the block and the number of muscles affected by the treatment.

Phenol and alcohol have been used effectively since the late 1950s. These substances have proven effectiveness in eliminating clonus, improving range of motion (ROM) of joints affected by spastic contracture, reducing scissoring during ambulation, improving seating, improving gait, facilitating the use of orthotics, and ameliorating painful spasms or toe clawing (1–11). In the past, neurolysis has been used effectively to treat spastic external sphincters and reduce urinary retention (4). Several authors have described improved activation, strength, or speed in antagonists of blocked muscles. There is also evidence of a seemingly paradoxical improvement in the strength/control of partially blocked muscles themselves (2–5, 8, 11). Chemical neurolysis has a long history of proven effectiveness and benefits in the management of UMNS.

PHENOL

Phenol is carbolic acid, a derivative of benzene. At room temperature, it is soluble in water at concentrations less than 6.7%. It is also soluble in other commonly used vehicles such as glycerine and is available as colorless hygroscopic crystals. When oxidized, the crystals or phenol solution become pink. Phenol has local anesthetic properties at concentrations of 1% to 2%; it is bacteriostatic at 0.2% concentrations (in water) and bactericidal at 1.0%. In the past, phenol has been the active component in fungicidal skin preparations and was used for embalming by the ancient Egyptians. In the present, it is a component of some over-the-counter throat lozenges. Phenol is considered a chemical, not a drug, by the Food and Drug Administration. As such, it is not technically "approved" for the treatment of spasticity.

When applied to or injected into any tissue at concentrations 5% or greater, phenol denatures protein causing tissue necrosis. This property accounts for both its effectiveness as a neurolytic agent and some of the associated potential side effects. Systemic doses of 8.5 g are considered lethal, principally from cardiovascular failure and severe central nervous system dysfunction including seizures. Doses of phenol injected for neurolysis are a tiny fraction of the lethal dose. Twenty cubic centimeters of a 5% solution contains 1 g. Phenol is easily absorbed through the skin (and dura, for those incorporating it as a component of prolotherapy). After injection, any systemically absorbed phenol is converted by the liver to phenyl compounds and excreted by the kidney as quinols. Chronic exposure can cause renal toxicity, rashes, or gastrointestinal problems.

Phenol Neurolysis: Histologic Changes

Initially, phenol was thought to selectively block small sensory fibers. However, the early electrophysiologic findings after application of phenol to peripheral nerves and nerve roots appear to be more relevant to its anesthetic and not its neurolytic properties (12–15). Subsequent histologic and electron microscopic examinations have demonstrated nonselective destruction of nerve fibers of all sizes (15, 16). These finding may have implications for technique of application and may relate to injection-related complications.

Soon after phenol injection, inflammatory reactions occur followed by patchy areas of complete destruction of nerve fibers in roots and peripheral nerves (17). Burkel and McPhee (16) determined that if phenol is "dropped" onto a nerve, axons in the center of the nerve are spared, but if the chemical is injected into the nerve, all fibers were affected. Wallerian degeneration occurs at the site of injection, followed by subsequent regrowth of most axons. At 14 weeks, the injected/regenerated nerves appeared histologically normal, albeit with increased associated collagen and fibroblasts in the endoneurium. Lower concentrations of aqueous phenol (<1%) were more likely to cause localized demyelination without axon destruction (14–18).

In 1977, Halpern (19) reported his findings from evaluating 144 samples from animals after intramuscular neurolysis with 1% to 7% phenol. Axons of all sizes were destroyed regardless of concentration. Neurogenic atrophy and collateral reinnervation were observed. Muscle recovery varied depending on the concentration of the aqueous phenol: 1% to 3% allowed for near-normal appearance of affected muscle by 3 months, but specimens injected with 5% to 7% continued to show evidence of denervation. The volumes of aqueous phenol used for injected also correlated with the lesion size.

The clinical implications of the above histologic examinations may be summarized as follows:

1. Very low concentrations of phenol (<1%) may only produce local anesthetic effects or mild demyelination with temporary clinical effects.

2. Low concentrations (<3%) may produce a mixture of axonal destruction and demyelination with a possible reduction in the duration of neurolytic block, but with near-normal recovery of nerve and muscle.

3. Concentrations of 5% to 7% are more likely to leave residual evidence for denervation in nerve and muscle at 3 months, a longer duration of clinical effect, but with greater potential for some "permanence" to the block. Most current practitioners use concentrations of 4% or 5%.

4. When phenol is applied to nerves without penetrating the nerve, it essentially affects

what it contacts. Therefore, the practitioner may need to move the needle around the nerve and inject at more than one location in its circumference to reach specific fascicles or nerve bundles to achieve the desired clinical effect (baring in mind that larger volumes will produce larger lesions in nerve and surrounding soft tissue).

5. The development of fibrous tissue in and around the nerve and adjacent soft tissue, coupled with collateral reinnervation and sprouting, may make a desired clinical outcome more challenging with subsequent injections, especially at the site of the original injection.

Technique of Injection for Phenol Neurolysis

Although some clinicians stimulated peripheral nerve and attempted to use electromyographic recording to isolated motor endplates (thus improving localization), this has proven to be a very laborious process and one which offers little advantage in precision when compared to careful clinical observation. The most commonly used technique employs the use of a nerve stimulator capable of delivering pulsed direct current as a square wave of 0.1 to 0.5 millisecond duration once or twice per second. The stimulator should have a rheostat to control the current flow. An ammeter facilitates precise localization. Generally, stimulators attached to electrodiagnostic equipment do not have ammeters, and "guessing" the milliampere flow is not a recommended technique. Localization with this equipment is akin to the use of early electrodiagnostic equipment, the chronaximeter. Essentially, motor points and nerves will respond to much lower amperage of current than surrounding muscle and soft tissue. Because the clinician wishes to preferentially inject proximal to the motor point or nerve, it is desirable to localize a site proximal to these structures, which is identified by obtaining a stimulation with less current. Current flow is between the stimulating electrode and a reference or pad; there is no ground. The needles used with the stimulator are the same as those used for BT injections: Teflon coated, except the bevel, of varying lengths dependent on site and patient morphology, and 22 to 27 gauge often related to the length of the needle. The primary author prefers to connect the needle to the syringe containing the phenol with a short length of intravenous tubing. This allows manipulation of the needle and maintenance of its position when withdrawing before injection and during the injection itself. If possible, a stimulator that allows for superficial, as well as percutaneous, stimulation is preferred. This will allow the clinician to localize nerves, angle of approach, and motor points before the introduction of the needle and facilitate more rapid percutaneous localization with less discomfort for the patient. Of course, superficial stimulation can only be employed for accessible nerves and muscles; deep-muscle motor points (eg, tibialis posterior) may only be reached percutaneously.

The patient should be prepped by having the entire limb being treated exposed. On occasion, special positioning techniques will need to be employed. If accessible nerves or muscles are to be treated, the use of a superficial stimulator to identify points along the course of the peripheral nerve to the motor point will help optimize localization. The current flow is typically between 5 and 30 mA for superficial stimulation. The clinician uses the superficial stimulator to identify the general location of the nerve or motor point by observing for the desired contraction of the muscle or muscle groups to be treated. The current is then reduced while observing for maximal contraction for finer localization (Figures 9.1 and 9.2). The point is then marked, and the skin at the site of injection prepared with alcohol (or povidine and alcohol). The percutaneous electrode (needle) is then introduced. Most stimulators that allow for both percutaneous and superficial stimulation will require a modification of electrode feeds on the stimulator apparatus. A "search" is then undertaken, often in 3 dimensions,

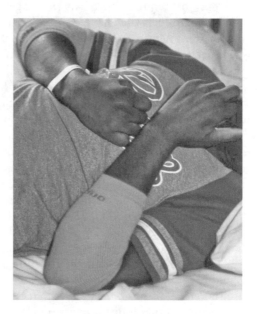

FIGURE 9.1

Early spastic contracture of the left elbow in a patient with traumatic brain injury.

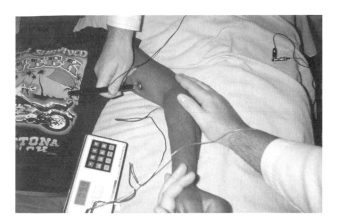

FIGURE 9.2

Superficial identification of left biceps motor point. Notice that the milliamp flow is 9.9.

with the pulsed current typically between 1 and 5 mA. Once maximal desired contraction is obtained, the current is reduced and the localization proceeds as the clinician identifies the site of maximal contraction with the amperage less than 1 mA (optimally closer to 0.5 to 0.7 mA)—the lower the better for precision. This will indicate that the bevel of the needle is optimally positioned. If too much current is used when injection occurs, the "ball of current" at the bevel tip may be stimulating nerve or motor points some distance from the needle; higher volumes than should be necessary of phenol may be required to reach the target area. When the clinician feels they have optimally localized the point for treatment electrically, the phenol should be slowly injected (Figures 9.3 and 9.4). Although as clinicians we are taught to withdraw before injection, this may be even more important with phenol because the potential for toxicity as a result of intravascular injection of the substance is very great. Once the phenol is injected, there should be an almost immediate reduction/cessation of the muscle twitch, with a continued reduction in response to electrical stimulation over 1 to 2 minutes. This occurs for two reasons: the initial local anesthetic effect of the phenol and the fact that the volume of the fluid may impede electrical conduction to some extent. The clinician also needs to consider that the bevel of the needle is directional; there may be a ball of current around the tip, but the injected phenol will be flowing out of the needle in one direction; therefore, if the clinician feels that they have accurately localized the point of injection electrically, yet with injection there is only a minimal reduction in contraction, they may find an improved effectiveness of injection by gently twirling the needle during

slow administration of the phenol. The total volume of phenol injected at one site typically ranges from 0.1 to 1 cc. The total volume of phenol administered to an adult in a given treatment session should not exceed 1 g. We limit our injections to 20 cc of 5% phenol for an adult but typically use less than 10 cc; unlike botulinum, the patient may return in a few days for additional treatments if needed.

Although the above process may sound laborious, normally it actually takes place within a minute or two; of course the speed of the clinician improves with experience. Patient tolerance for the procedure varies considerably; patients may feel some discomfort from the electrical stimulation, from the needle search, and from some burning during the injection of phenol or alcohol. After the treatment session, we typically apply ice or cold packs to the areas of injection to help minimize discomfort from the needle searches. To expedite localization of motor points, various guides for the electromyographer (20) may be used. In addition, there are specific anatomic localization guides for phenol/alcohol neurolysis (21–23).

Site of Injection

As mentioned previously, the lower motor neuron may be, in theory, treated with phenol neurolysis at any point along its course from the spinal cord to the motor point of an individual muscle. If there is a single offending muscle, then one should localize that individual muscle through a motor point injection. However, in some cases, a single injection of a peripheral nerve may treat several muscles contributing to a pattern of spasticity or primitive movement patterns (eg, tibial

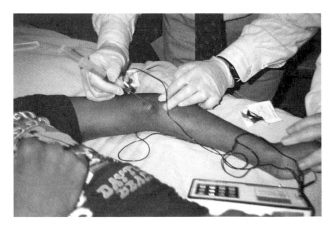

FIGURE 9.3

Percutaneous identification and neurolysis of left brachioradialis motor point.

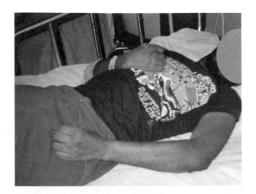

FIGURE 9.4

Result of phenol neurolysis of left biceps and brachioradialis motor points, as compared to untreated right upper limb.

nerve injection in the popliteal space for equinovarus of the foot/ankle with associated toe clawing). Furthermore, given the relative immediacy of the action of phenol, the clinical effect may be titrated during the treatment session: motor points may be injected, and if the effect is insufficient, the clinician may then move proximally to the motor branch or ultimately the peripheral nerve supplying the muscle. This also allows for the patient to "try the block on for size" as to their satisfaction with the result, particularly for gait disorders or orthotic fit, with the potential for the clinician to go back and do additional treatments until the patient is satisfied with the result. Ultimately, the choice of site (motor point, motor nerve, or mixed sensory/motor nerve) will be dictated by the desired clinical effect (including number of muscles being treated in the distribution of a peripheral nerve), the tolerance of the patient for the needle search, the risks of the needle search at different sites, and the risks for other complications such as dysesthesias.

Lumbar and sacral nerve blocks. This procedure is no longer a common technique of treatment. It requires conscious sedation and fluoroscopy to provide optimal localization for the needle. Risks include accidental intrathecal injection and damage to the entire cauda equina with associated sexual, bowel, and bladder dysfunction. Most often, this procedure was undertaken to treat hip flexors. Alternative treatment approaches with BTs have all but eliminated this particular intervention technique.

Mixed motor/sensory peripheral nerve blocks. There are many advantages to this procedure compared with motor point blocks. First, there is a block of sensory fibers, cutaneous and from the muscles themselves, both of which may contribute to the re-

duction of spasticity. Second, it is often possible to identify bundles within the nerve and preferentially block them to target specific muscles with one injection site. Third, most clinicians believe that sensorimotor peripheral nerve blocks produce a more thorough block of longer duration, although this belief does not have more than a teleological basis for support in that it has not been systematically studied. Certainly, a more proximal block will require a longer period of axonal regeneration insofar as this contributes to the recurrence of spasticity. Fourth, this technique is often easier and faster than more peripheral motor branch/point blocks in achieving a desired clinical effect.

The major risk to this type of injection is related to one of its theoretical advantages: the block of sensory (and possibly autonomic) nerve fibers. This can lead to temporary loss of sensation and to the potentially much more bothersome or disabling nerve pain in the distribution of the injected nerve. Identification and management of these problems will be discussed later in the chapter. In addition, the immediate effect of the block can be quite profound and potentially lead to "overcorrection" or overstretching injury if the patient is not properly counseled.

Motor nerve/motor point blocks. There are many points along the peripheral arborization of motor nerves that these blocks can occur. In some cases, the motor branch to a specific muscle can be identified very close to its departure from the mixed sensory/motor nerve from which it originates. More commonly, the motor fascicle is identified near the muscle it innervates. Motor points are the place where this motor branch enters a particular muscle or where there is a cluster of motor endplates. There are usually several motor points for a given muscle. Therefore, as one attempts neurolysis more peripherally along the motor nerve, more injections are necessary. The patient has to endure more needlesticks, and the clinician may become more fatigued over time. The advantage of injecting motor points or motor branches is that they do not contain any cutaneous afferents, and hence, the risk of dysesthesia is greatly reduced compared to mixed sensory motor nerve blocks. Furthermore, it allows the ability to titrate the clinical effect of the block alluded to previously. Certain peripheral nerves (most notably the obturator nerve) contain little to no sensory components and therefore do not have associated dysesthesias with whole nerve blocks.

Open neurolysis. A final technique, also not commonly used, is the open, surgical identification of peripheral and motor nerves followed by the application of phenol. Obviously, this allows for direct visualization of the nerve to be treated and may allow for safer proximal treatment. However, this procedure incorporates the inherent risks of anesthesia and the additional recovery from surgery, along with added costs.

Duration of Action of Phenol Neurolysis

There is an extraordinary wide variability in the literature regarding the duration of effect of phenol. Again, from a teleological perspective, one would assume that the duration of action would be longest for root or peripheral nerve block when compared to intramuscular or motor point block; it takes longer for axons to reinnervate target muscles the more proximal the injection. However, this is not clearly demonstrated in the literature (Table 9.1). Peripheral nerve blocks appear to last from 10 days to as many as 28 months (10). Paravertebral blocks range between 1.5 and 10 months (24) and intramuscular between 1 and 36 months (25, 26). Specific motor point or endplate blocks were reported by DeLateur (8) to last 3 to 6 months and open nerve blocks 6 months to more than 1 year.

The variability in the literature may be explained by several factors. The percent (ranging between 2% and 5%) of aqueous phenol as well as volume (not consistently reported) could account for some discrepancies. The measurement tools used for spasticity and return of spasticity were also quite different and at times extremely subjective. Although it is assumed that all clinicians in the studies were experienced with phenol neurolysis, technique may also influence the outcome/duration. Further, it is not entirely clear from the peripheral nerve studies whether there was evidence for blockade of sensory afferent fibers that might contribute to spasticity.

Other factors might contribute to improving duration of outcome related to postblock interventions. If the injected muscle and associated soft tissue are effectively stretched after the block, this may prolong the clinical effectiveness. If the antagonist is strengthened either by exercise or by electrical stimulation, this may, in theory, produce a clinical improvement in the duration of efficacy through inhibition of the injected muscle.

Repetition of blocks may also improve the duration of effectiveness with the subsequent injections (27). However, most studies (and clinical experiences) that evaluated repetitive blocks seem to indicate that it is somewhat more difficult to perform the subsequent blocks (25). Both the difficulty in achieving the block and the improved duration of effect may be explained by fibrous tissue and sprouting that make localization more difficult but may also impede regrowth of axons.

Side Effects and Complications of Phenol Neurolysis

Side effects of phenol neurolysis may be related to the simple act of placing a needle in the soft tissue (bleeding, compartment syndrome, pain, infection), the effects of the block (overcorrection, strain or sprain from overstretching, temporary loss of useful motor function, atrophy), and specific side effects from phenol (temporary sensory loss, dysesthesias, tender nodules in soft tissue). Venous thromboembolism has been rumored to occur, but the evidence to support that this is an effect of phenol is weak to nonexistent. Patients who were purported to have experienced this problem were few, and evaluations for hypercoaguable states or absence of venous thrombosis before injection were not done. Macek (28) reported (second hand) on 2 cases with purported venous thrombosis related to phenol neurolysis. In neither case was there a specific discussion of the location of the deep vein thrombosis or effectiveness of the blocks. Technologies were limited in the 1980s, but there was no discussion of coagulation disorders. Theoretically, poor technique with intravascular or perivascular injection could cause scar tissue damage or occlude venous structures. A particularly effective block *might* render the "pumping action" of spastic muscle ineffectual, contributing to venous stasis (22). In a similar vein, if the patient was uncomfortable after the block or took a long car or airplane trip, inactivity could lead to stasis as well. Awad (22) has articulated the opinion that when deep vein thrombosis occurs, it is usually in the calf and may be related to the "repeated indiscriminate needle probing and/or the injection of large quantities of phenol solution by the novice."

Side effects from needling. Local bruising, pain, and swelling may occur, as well as infections, if aseptic

---

TABLE 9.1
Expected (Estimated or Projected) Duration of Phenol Neurolysis

ANATOMIC LOCATION	DURATION
Peripheral nerve block	10 days–28 months
Intramuscular block	4 weeks–36 months
Paravertebral block	6 weeks–10 months
Motor point or endplate block	3 months–6 months
Open nerve block	6 months–12 months

technique is not utilized. Aspiration before injection is an obvious precaution. A potential complication relates to bleeding in deeper muscles and the risk of a compartment syndrome. Many patients with stroke are on antiplatelet therapy and may bleed more easily; special care in minimizing needle exploration should be exercised under these circumstances. It is also advisable to stop coumadin or therapeutic anticoagulation in a sufficient time frame before injection to avoid this complication.

Side effects from effective blocks. These include the possibility of atrophy, sprains, and overcorrection, as well the potential loss of useful motor function. There may also be a temporary loss of cutaneous sensation. In terms of atrophy, caution should be observed in exercising the involved musculature to fatigue during the period the block is most "active." Subsequently, after the block has begun to wear off, electrical stimulation and exercise (and the return of spasticity) are usually sufficient to correct what is largely a cosmetic problem.

Peripheral nerve blocks may be very profound in their effect, with clinical changes in several muscles involved in a particular pattern of movement. Most patients will have become accustomed to their spasticity and will have learned compensatory mechanisms for functional activities. The best example would be the use of a tibial nerve block in the popliteal space to treat equinovarus of the foot/ankle as well as toe clawing. In comparison to motor point blocks or BT, there may be a much more complete and immediate abolition of spasticity and possibly motor function in the gastrocnemius, soleus, tibialis posterior, and long and short toe flexors. As a result, the patient does not have the opportunity to acclimate to changes in their spasticity as might be the case with botulinum. Caution should be observed immediately after the block if the patient is accustomed to ambulating. Overstretching of the involved parts should be avoided as well. In this example, there may also be loss of the intrinsic muscle functions of the foot, resulting in sprain from poor dynamic support of the plantar arch; this may be prevented by the use of a foot orthotic or modification of the sole plate of an ankle-foot orthotic. At times, there is overactivity in antagonist muscles that result in "overcorrection" as may be seen in surgical interventions to lengthen or move tendons. In this example, if the tibialis anterior was a powerful contributor to the varus posturing of the foot and ankle, one may see an associated "calcaneal" deformity, at least dynamically, of the foot/ankle complex after tibial nerve block. Appropriate intervention would include motor point blocks or BT injection to the tibialis anterior or peroneal nerve block. Most of the problems of over-correction can be avoided by not being overzealous with injections and titrating the amount and site of injection to patient need.

In evaluating patients before neurolysis, the clinician must be cognizant of the risk of loss of useful motor function, even if it is dominated by spasticity and under poor volitional control. Gait (7, 9) or transfers may be compromised.

Side effects specific to phenol. These side effects are in part related to location of block. Although no longer commonly done, there is the possibility of dural transfer of phenol when done at the level of the nerve roots. The affinity of phenol to cross dura, without the direct penetration thereof, has been confirmed in animal experiments (15). In humans, this may account for case reports of spinal cord injury when the injection was done close to the dura (29, 30). Intrathecal injection of phenol has also been associated with thrombosis of the posterior spinal artery (31).

Dysesthesias. The most worrisome side effect of phenol neurolysis in mixed sensory/motor nerves is that of dysesthetic pain, which occurs in the sensory distribution of the nerve. The pain is of the classical neuropathic type: burning, tingling, electrical feelings, exacerbated by light touch. Onset is not immediate, but delayed by a few days to 2 weeks. The incidence of dysesthetic pain varies widely in the literature (0–32%) and is affected by several variables. There are no reports of dysesthesia with obturator nerve blocks, so in reviewing a series of patients, it is important to identify the percentage of blocks done to this nerve. The skill of the clinician may be relevant, but there is not a clear association with the concentration or volume of phenol. The duration of the discomfort is typically several weeks (21), but may last a few days to as much as a year. Kolaski et al. (32) reported that the use of phenol and botulinum in combination produced a higher rate of complications than botulinum alone, although patients receiving the combined treatment were more likely to have greater severity of spasticity. Most of the complications related to local injection symptoms; the rate of dysesthesias was only 0.4%. However, the mixed sensorimotor nerves injected were the obturator (no reports of dysesthesia) and the musculocutaneous.

The duration and severity may be ameliorated by pharmacologic and other interventions. Classically, the recommended intervention is to repeat the block with the thought that the original intervention was incomplete (10), but it is often difficult to convince patients to repeat the procedure that caused their discomfort in the first place. Modalities for management include compression garments or wraps. Local anesthetic patches may be effective. The primary author would suggest a fairly aggressive pharmacologic approach if it is clear that the pain is neuropathic and not due to overuse or mechanical factors. This includes the use of anti-inflammatories (medrol dose-pack followed by nonsteroidal anti-inflammatories, if symptoms persist), anticonvulsants (pregabalin, gabapentin, carbamazepine), and antidepressants (duloxetine, amitriptyline), and this should be considered in combination and gradually weaned. Finally, an under-recognized complication may relate to the block of autonomic fibers traveling with the sensorimotor nerve. This may result in redness or other discoloration of the skin supplied by said fibers, presumably due to loss of neurogenic vascular control in a paretic limb. There may be associated edema, and the treatment is re-assurance and compressive garments.

Local inflammatory responses. Motor point blocks often involve several injections in a given muscle. As a result, patients may have transient pain or swelling related to both repetitive needling and the inflammatory effects of phenol. This is particularly true in the calf. Tender nodules may develop and may reflect the local damage to muscle with an associated inflammatory reaction described by Halpern (19) in animal studies. These reactions began a few days after injection and began to resolve after 2 weeks. Glenn (21) recommends that the application of icing immediately after the procedure and anti-inflammatory medications can prevent or ameliorate these temporary symptoms.

ALCOHOL

In addition to Phenol, there has been both clinical and literature support for the use of ethyl alcohol (alcohol) in the chemoneurolysis of peripheral nerves as a part of a treatment plan for spasticity (33–37). Although the volume of literature support is limited as compared to phenol and now botulium toxin, there does remain strong efficacy for its use in both achieving desired outcomes (33–37) as well as limiting undesired side effects (34–39).

Jang et al. (34) treated spastic hemiplegia of the ankle using 50% ethyl alcohol in water. They identified the motor branches of the tibial nerve responsible for both the medial and lateral heads of the gastrocnemius muscle. Postinjection and then at 6-month follow-up, there remained a statistically significant decrease in the Modified Ashworth Scale scores, clonus scores, and passive ROM. Although these three measurement tools are scientific in nature, possibly the addition of gait analysis might have further provided added clinical value to their overall outcomes.

Viel et al. (37) used 65% ethyl alcohol for 27 obturator nerve blocks. Radiographic films and stimulator guidance were used to achieve 100% localization. Using their own scales for muscle spasticity, triple flexion, gait, and hygiene, there was significant statistical data to show improvement at the 1, 2, and 4-month follow-up. An interesting aspect to their research was the use of cost analysis. They found a total cost of 10.67 euros for the procedure (8.23 euros for the needle and 2.44 euros for the alcohol solution). The cost for a 4-month supply of dantrolene sodium and oral baclofen was between 500 and 1000 euros and between170 and 134 euros, respectively. One significant cost that was not included in this study was for the use a nonoperative procedure room and conscious sedation or generalized anesthesia used during the ethyl alcohol injection.

Kong and Chua (36) used 100% ethyl alcohol in the treatment of 13 patients with hip adductor spasticity. As with the study of Jang et al, they also found statistical improvement at 6 months for a decreased Modified Ashworth Scale score and an increased passive ROM. Gait analysis was performed in this study, but for only the 3 patients who could ambulate. Even postinjection there was a continued use of assistive devices; however, both patients and authors agreed that there was an improvement in overall balance, decreased scissoring, and increased gait speed. Further studies with a larger ambulatory population may certainly help show the long-term utility and retained functional outcome with the use of ethyl alcohol as an effective chemoneurolytic in patients with spastic gait.

In the early 1960s, Hariga et al. (40), Tardieu et al. (41, 42) proposed injection of a local chemical neurolytic agent directly into muscle. They injected large quantities of 45% alcohol into the limb muscles, at the motor point in children with cerebral palsy. It was reported that spasticity was reduced in most cases, without reducing or affecting voluntary strength. They further reported a duration effect from 6 to 12 months and occasionally as long as 2 to 3 years (40–43). Similar findings were noted by Cockin et al (44) in the United Kingdom in 1976. He injected 45% alcohol into similar muscles, yielding a reduction in spasticity without inducing profound weakness (44).

Other investigators evaluated the Tardieu technique (6, 44–47), which led to modification of the procedure (6, 45, 46). O'Hanlan et al. (6) used the same dilution of alcohol but did not try to target the motor nerves specifically. He injected 45% alcohol in large volumes of 10 to 40 mL into multiple locations within the target muscles of spastic patients. O'Hanlan et al. observed significant reduction in spasticity without loss of motor power in the 10 patients treated. Sensation was also reported to remain intact. He also reported in the *Virginia Medical Monthly* a case of vascular phlebitis when a "poor" so-called state store preparation of alcohol was used. Carpenter (45) and Carpenter and Seitz (46) proposed the concept of "intramuscular" alcohol using 40% to 50% alcohol. This procedure was performed under general anesthesia due to the significant pain caused during the injections. The gastrocnemius demonstrated the best response of those muscles injected. The muscles were divided into quadrants, and each quadrant was injected with 2 to 6 mL of alcohol. Equinus gait was eliminated in 128 of 130 children injected. Duration of effect was shorter than reported by Tardieu et al., with the equinus gait returning 7 to 20 days after injection. Overall, the injections lasted 1 to 6 weeks. Muscle biopsies were also performed 4 to 6 weeks after the procedures, and in 4 to 6 patients revealed a round cell infiltrate without fibrosis.

Intramuscular alcohol has been used to achieve relief of spasticity for a slightly longer duration and is less time-consuming than for motor point blocks (46, 48). In addition, the procedure's duration of effect could be useful for diagnostic purposes when a longer period of evaluation is necessary than can be provided by a local anesthetic agent or for therapeutic purposes when longer-lasting procedures are unnecessary or undesirable. Another advantage of this procedure is that because precise localization of nerves is not necessary, it can be performed quickly in situations where speed is a consideration, for example, in agitated and combative patients and in children (49).

There have been many questions as to the optimal concentration of ethyl alcohol that is to be used in the chemoneurolysis of peripheral nerves. In a classic study of animals, May (50) described how the use of 100% ethyl alcohol causes degeneration and fibrosis with partial regeneration of neurons. It also attempts to link how more dilute solutions do not show an equal correspondence to neuronal destruction and that less concentrated injections may be unpredictable in their overall outcome. Most studies indicate that the concentration of alcohol used is dependent on muscle mass and weight of the patient.

The mechanism of action of alcohol is as a nonselective denaturization of proteins that affect axons, myoneural junctions, muscle fibers, and the interstitial tissue. This may lead to retrograde Wallarian degeneration of the nerve fiber (38, 39). Biopsies from muscles that have undergone intramuscular washing have shown necrosis and inflammatory cells (46).

There is no clear correlation of alcohol concentration to adverse side effects. Most studies have shown limited adverse outcomes with only 1 to 2 patients in each study complaining of local site injection pain or sensory dysesthesias, which lasts for only a few weeks and seem to respond well to select antidepressants (amitriptyline) or antiseizure (carbamazepine) medications (34, 38). Theoretical risks are similar to those seen with the use of phenol and include seizures, central nervous system depression, and cardiovascular collapse (36). A complication unique to the use of ethyl alcohol is inebriation. One study of adults (36) did encounter this side effect but stated that it resolved spontaneously. Critics to the use of ethyl alcohol could theoretically consider its use in the pediatric population unwarranted, because of this, it is our opinion that most children undergoing this procedure are chaperoned by their legal guardians who can help to monitor such a reaction, and we would also advocate for limiting its use in those patients, children, or adults who have any form of liver damage that might inhibit their ability to process its systemic effects.

COMPARISON OF PHENOL NEUROLYSIS AND BT

There are several potential benefits of phenol over BT. Phenol has an immediate onset of action, is much less expensive, and can be titrated in a single visit to optimize dosing/clinical effect. Botulinum dosing may be adjusted but cannot be administered more frequently than every 3 months. Phenol may be repeated in a few days. Indeed, if the patient or clinician is dissatisfied with the results of a botulinum injection (once it has reached full therapeutic effect), "touch-up" blocks could be done with phenol. Phenol can be given anywhere along the motor nerve, from motor point blocks (most akin to botulinum effects) to nerve root. The duration of action of peripheral nerve or motor nerve blocks appears to be longer than those with motor point blocks or botulinum. Furthermore, it may be feasible to inject a single point on a peripheral nerve and treat several muscles simultaneously (tibial nerve block), sparing the patient multiple injections and often getting a more effective block than with botulinum.

On the other hand, there are potential risks to phenol as compared to botulinum. The immediacy of effect, particularly from robust peripheral nerve blocks, may require adjustment by the patient and may transiently interfere with gait or transfers; the more gradual onset of effect from botulinum injection is far less likely to cause this problem. Of course, the major concern from phenol neurolysis compared to botulinum is the potential for sensory disorders. As mentioned above, the exact incidence is not clearly known and varies depending on which sensorimotor nerve is injected. Overall, the incidence appears to be less than 10%; the hyperalgesia/dysesthesia phenomenon is also treatable and typically does not last very long with treatment—of course the presence of this complication may put a bit of a strain on the patient-physician relationship for its duration. Phenol may also produce scars or fibrous depositions in soft tissue. Some of these may be uncomfortable and, more rarely, may affect subsequent surgical releases or other interventions.

Given the wide disparity in cost between phenol and botulinum, it is surprising that there are only a very few studies directly comparing these agents. The studies that do exist have serious flaws, and it is difficult to generalize from them. In 1998, Kirazli et al. (51) reported on what was the "first trial" to directly compare botulinum and phenol for spastic foot after a stroke. Ten patients received 400 U of botulinum, acknowledged by the authors to be a relatively high dose, distributed as 100 U in each of the following muscles under electromyographic guidance: the soleus, medial gastrocnemius, lateral gastrocnemius, and tibialis posterior. Ten patients received 3 cc of 5% phenol injected as a tibial nerve block with percutaneous stimulation, "the primary target being fibers to the gastrocnemius and soleus muscles and the secondary target, the tibialis posterior." The authors were allegedly attempting to do the block just distal to the bifurcation of the sciatic nerve, 7 cm above the popliteal crease. Yet, they also state that the phenol procedure took 1 to 2 hours, and the BT procedure only 15 to 30 minutes. Typically, a phenol block of the tibial nerve should only take 10 minutes.

Follow-up was done using the Ashworth Scale for dorsiflexion and eversion, clonus duration, improvement in active and passive ROM, Brace Wearing Scale, and an ambulation score. This follow-up occurred at 2, 4, 8, and 12 weeks. The authors concluded that the improvement in the eversion Ashworth score improved in the botulinum group but not in the phenol group, and overall, botulinum was more effective at weeks 2 and 4 but that there were no statistically significant differences at weeks 8 and 12. This would contradict the clinical experience that a tibial block would be of longer duration than motor point blocks or botulinum. Furthermore, 2 (20%) of 10 patients developed peroneal nerve palsy and 30% developed dysesthesias lasting 2 to 4 weeks in spite of the authors' seemingly laborious efforts to accurately localize their phenol injections; these complications impacted the results in, at the very least, the Ashworth for eversion and walking capacity that favored BT in the first

2 to 4 weeks after injection. It is not clear whether the 2 patients with inadvertent peroneal palsies also contributed to the 30% of patients that developed dysesthesias. For an experienced clinician, it is not surprising that peroneal palsies developed in 20% of 10 patients and 30% developed dysesthesias given the "localization" of the tibial nerve 7 cm above the popliteal crease. This site is far more rostal than the one used by clinicians with experience performing phenol tibial nerve blocks. Typically, the nerve is identified at the popliteal crease, although additional blocks of the large motor branches to the gastrocnemius bellies may have to be identified just medial and lateral to the nerve at this level or just distally as they enter the bellies of the muscle. Glenn (21) comments on this potential flaw in technique: "When blocking at the apex of the popliteal fossa, the practitioner should be aware of the close proximity of the common peroneal nerve to the tibial nerve and the origin of the sural nerve at this level." Therefore, although this study purports to show a relative advantage of large doses of botulinum for the spastic equinovarus foot compared to phenol, given the small number of patients, the findings and data are severely compromised by the technical inadequacies of the phenol blocks. From a practical perspective, hemiplegic patients may require treatment of additional muscles in other limbs or for spastic toe flexors or striatal toe associated with spastic equinovarus. The use of such large doses of botulinum for the targeted muscles in this study would also have a significant impact on the total dose recommended for the first or subsequent injection; less botulinum would be available to treat other limbs or even muscles involved in the same primitive movement pattern.

A recent retrospective study evaluated 336 children and 764 treatments comparing phenol and BT to botulinum alone for complications (32). Phenol use was confined to the obturator nerve and musculocutaneous nerve blocks. Complications were divided into intraoperative systemic, local, and functional. Patients injected with the combined agents were more likely to have severe impairments with longer treatment sessions and spastic tetraplegia. Systemic complications were more common in the combined group (7.6% vs 2.5%) but were of short duration (3–7 days) and could not be attributed to an effect of phenol versus botulinum by the authors (eg, constipation). Two patients (0.4%) did experience cardiac arrhythmias, which resolved with observation. One of these had mitral valve prolapse, which predisposes to arrhythmia. The authors commented about a previous study with a 19% rate of arrhythmia with phenol, but this study involved intramuscular injection and halothane anesthesia. Local symptoms were more common in the combined group (4.5% vs 1.5%), which included bruising, swelling, and tenderness, but these were not specifically ascribed to the sites of phenol injection, and again, the combined population was subjected to more extensive needling. Dysesthesias were rare (0.4%) and occurred only in the distribution of the musculocutaneous nerve. This is a low incidence compared to other studies and reflects the selection of mixed sensorimotor nerves with little or no significant sensory component. Overall, this study demonstrated the acceptably low risk of combining phenol neurolysis and botulinum injections, especially when treating complex patients where the total safe dose of BT limits the global clinical effect desired by treatment.

Hypothetical Cost Comparisons

Obturator nerve blocks versus botulinum for adducted lower extremities. To optimally treat scissoring gait or severe adductor tone for hygiene, 150 to 200 U of botulinum type A would be required at a cost of $507.42 × 2 = $1014.84 versus 5 cc of 5% phenol ($7.00).

Musculocutaneous nerve block versus botulinum for flexed elbow. Two hundred units of botulinum A for biceps, brachioradialis, and brachialis at a cost of $507.42 × 2.5 = $1268.55 or 3 cc of 5% phenol with low risk for dysesthesias.

Tibial nerve block with dysesthesias. Comparative cost analysis case scenario:

A 48-year-old man with a traumatic brain injury presents to your clinic 6 months postinjury. He has completed both acute inpatient rehabilitation and an outpatient program. A spastic hemiparesis causing plantar-flexion contracture remains as a major barrier in his ability to progress from an assist level to a modified-independent level with activities of daily living (ADLs) and ambulation. Traditional oral antispasticity agents have either failed to resolve his contracture or caused excessive sedation. He is now unable to don an ankle-foot orthosis, even with the assistance of family.

Interventional options are the following:

- Phenol chemodenervation of the tibial nerve at a point in the popliteal fossa. Five milliliters of prepared 5% phenol in sterile water.
- Botulinum treatment to the medial and lateral gastrocnemius muscles, soleus muscle, and posterior tibialis muscle. One hundred units of botox per muscle group for a total of 400 U.

Procedural similarities:

Assuming that the procedure is performed in an outpatient office setting, the basic cost for physician time, injection needle, nerve stimulation needle for phenol or electromyographic needle for BT, syringes, alcohol prep pads, and other miscellaneous items would be equal for either of the procedure using phenol or BT. If this procedure was performed in a hospital setting, the costs for facility fees would be equal.

Procedural differences:

- Cost of 400 U = $507.42 × 4 = $2029.68
- Cost of 5% phenol in 10 mL sterile water = $7.85

Expected complications:

It has been documented that the use of phenol for chemodenervation can lead to dysesthesias in the territory of the sensory components of that given nerve. Although there are certain nerves (musculocutaneous and obturator) that may have a lesser incidence, there have been a few reports of dysesthesias after phenol use in the tibial nerve. Therefore, we propose that to help treat this potential complication, the patient be given a Medrol Dosepak along with a membrane stabilizer, either gabapentin or pregabalin, for 3 months.

Further costs:

- 1 Medrol Dosepak = $24.60
- 3-month supply of pregabalin, taken as 150 mg PO BID = $341.86
- 3-month supply of gabapentin, taken as 300 mg PO TID × 1 week, then 600 mg PO TID × 1 week, then 900 mg PO × 10 weeks = $984.06

Final cost difference:

- Given that procedural costs, physician time, and equipment are equal: the cost of 400 U of botox is $2029.68, whereas the cost of phenol and its potential side effects is $991.91. This is a difference of $1037.77 (source: Amerisource Wholesale, as of August 11, 2008) (see Table 9.2).
- In this scenario, we have deliberately treated dysesthesias for a prolonged period; most reports indicate a shorter duration of the problem. We have deliberately used expensive medications in this treatment. One should also consider that a tibial nerve block should last at least twice as long as (6 months) BT, so that the

TABLE 9.2
*Cost Comparison of Phenol Tibial Neurolysis and
Botulinum for Equinovarus of the Foot/Ankle*

SUBSTANCE USED	WITHOUT COMPLICATION	TREATMENT FOR NEURITIS WITH STEROID DOSE PACK AND PREGABALIN ×3 MONTHS
Botulinum A (400 U)	$2029.68	$2029.68
Phenol	$7.85	$594.31

actual costs for botulinum are $4060 for a 6-month interval compared to $7.85 for phenol. Finally, the intervention described with botulinum was identical to that described by Kirazli and omitted the long toe flexors and the flexor hallucis longus, which are commonly involved in the extensor equinovarus posture of the lower limb. Although these could be treated with the same $7.85 of phenol, it would take at least an additional 150 U of botulinum type A at an additional cost of $761.13 per 3-month session.

PEDIATRIC CONSIDERATIONS

The treatment of spasticity in the pediatric population generally involves patients who have cerebral palsy with spastic hemiplegia, diplegia, or tetraplegia. Among other diagnoses, spasticity also affects those children with strokes and brain injuries. The utility in aggressive treatment allows for the patient to maintain a certain level of independence with self-care, caregivers ease with hygiene care and ADL management, and potentially provide the patient to ambulate with less assistive technologies.

Phenyl alcohol (Phenol), ethyl alcohol (Alcohol), and BT have all been used in the interventional treatment of spasticity in children. In the past, many studies have discussed the use of motor point blocks for the management of spasticity using both Phenol and Alcohol. Increasingly in the literature, more studies have used either the A or B form of BT alone or in combination with Phenol. This section will discuss those applications of either phenyl or ethyl alcohol.

The administration of either alcohol agent does not differ much in the pediatric population when compared to adults. A similar stimulator, Teflon-coated needle, and use of surface anatomy are employed with

the pediatric procedure as it would be with adults. Generally, in children, there is a greater utilization of a procedure room or even an operating room where an anesthesiologist is consulted to administer either general anesthesia or conscious sedation. Although neither approach is without complications, one study did demonstrate a 1.2% rate of anesthesia-related complications (32). Many sources discuss the advantages of anesthesia to allow the physician greater ease with which to perform this procedure. An agitated child would certainly make placement and further localization of the obturator nerve quite difficult given its proximity to other vascular structures in the inner proximal thigh.

Although not reported explicitly in the literature, one distinct advantage to sedation is to allow the child's muscles to relax after induction of an anesthetic. What may be difficult for a clinician to differentiate during an examination in the office would be how much of a child's deficit is related to spasticity and how much is related to contracture. The use of an anesthetic will allow much of the spastic component to relax, and therefore, a more complete clinical examination to be performed. Overall success of treatment may be better appreciated by the clinician who can then better guide therapy after the chemoneurolysis. This will also help to reassure parents in terms of what to expect from this procedure and possibly prepare them for a further discussion on surgical release of a contracted joint. This being said, it remains vitally important for the clinician to weigh the various risks and benefits of sedation with an anesthetic and communicate this with the parents. Some older children or those whose physical impairments do not compromise their cognitive abilities may be better suited for local anesthetic during the chemoneurolysis, as they are better able to relax during a stressful situation (52).

Many case reports and texts have also discussed the particular complications as they pertain to the use of phenol and alcohol. Although the total number of studies that focus on complications are few, Morrison et al. (52) found that there was no correlation between the plasma concentration of phenol and the risk of cardiac arrhythmias. Although their overall rate of arrhythmias was 19%, or 3 of 16, one was attributed to intraprocedural laryngospasm, and of the other 2 who were noted to have an arrhythmia, there were 4 other patients with higher plasma concentrations that did not experience an arrhythmia (53).

The duration of action for phenol alone has not been studied well in recent literature, as much of it is combined with the use of BT. In the 1970s, Spira (7) performed 136 phenol blocks at various locations in children. Of these, 118 involved the tibial and obturator nerves. Within 48 hours, 80 of the 118 blocks demonstrated "good relief." At 3 weeks, this number was reduced to 77, and between 3 and 6 months follow-up, only 41 of the initial 118 had good relief of their spasticity. "Some relief" was found in 40 blocks, and "no relief" was found in 37 of the initial 118 blocks. Although those children with "moderate spasticity" had a higher percentage of "relief" at 3 months follow-up when compared to the percentage of relief in the "severe spasticity" group, the findings from this study do show that clear advantages of phenol block are both immediate and long-term relief of spasticity, especially in the targeting of the tibial and obturator nerves. Both motor and sensory complications were found in this study. Seventeen patients did have difficulty with push-off during ambulation, suggesting damage to the gastrocnemius muscle, whereas 7 patients experienced dysasthetic pain. Other studies have described both motor and sensory complications after the use of phenol; one noted that the use of gabapentin, in those with sensory complaints, helped to relieve symptoms within a few weeks.

A follow-up study in 1994 by Yadav et al. (54) also carried a large number of patients (116) with the diagnosis of spastic cerebral palsy. Unlike the study mentioned above, they found an average 13 months of effective relief and parasthesias in 5 of the 246 peripheral nerve blocks. These enhanced results may be attributed to the larger sample size or refinement in technique. In addition, unlike the first study, further emphasis was placed on functional outcomes and use of assistive devise with ambulation, showing that 70% of their population was able to ambulate with an assistive devise after phenol injection. Finally, an increase in independence in ADLs was also demonstrated.

Although there are limited data on the use of phenol and alcohol in chemoneurolysis for the treatment of spasticity in the pediatric population, the evidence is clear in terms of safety and efficacy. In addition, there is both a demonstration of immediate and long-acting relief of spasticity, generally found greatest in the application of tibial and obturator nerve blocks. The clinical implication is beneficial for both patient and caregiver. In addition, there is increased independence or ease with which to perform ADLs and hygiene care as well as with ambulation in this patient population. Added benefit from the use of phenol can help guide further interventional care, for example, surgery, if so needed. Although there is an argument that the technical aspects of motor point neurolysis as well as time of procedure are greater than that for the administration of BT, given the severity of spasticity with many patients and therefore the need to treat many muscles, the maximum dose of BT is expended rapidly. The ability to selectively treat 2 or 3 nerves to achieve spastic relief of many muscles may still best be used to argue the utility of chemical intervention.

SUGGESTED APPROACHES FOR SPECIFIC UPPER MOTOR NEURON DISORDERS

Even if the clinician prefers BTs for the treatment of upper motor neuron disorders because of its ease of administration and low side effect profile, he or she is still limited by the recommended safe dosing parameters for a given procedure. Hence, the ability to use phenol to treat some muscle groups at low risk for complications allows for optimal dosing or inclusion of important additional muscles for botulinum treatment. Furthermore, awareness of cost-effectiveness, as well as relative safety/ease of administration, mandates an armamentarium beyond BTs alone. For example, administration of botulinum in an inpatient setting will result in delayed results, impeding the course of interdisciplinary rehabilitation, and could easily consume any or all financial benefit to the institution related to the patient's stay. This is not to say it should not be done, but for selected problems, phenol may prove safe while producing immediate benefit and be more cost-effective than botulinum. Finally, if botulinum injections prove inadequate alone, the clinician could use phenol neurolysis to benefit undertreated areas (Table 9.3).

Examples and Recommendations

Torticollis. Although phenol may be used to treat superficial muscles involved in spastic torticollis (such as the upper trapezius or sternocleidomastoid), it is recommended that BT is the preferable alternative. Certain deep muscles may contribute to the pattern that would not be easily identified with cutaneous stimulation. Given the proximity of important neural and vascular structures, it would be advisable to avoid excessive needle searches for motor points or branches.

Upper Body

Adducted, internally rotated shoulder. The major muscles contributing to this pattern include the pectoralis complex, the subscapularis, teres major, and latissimus dorsi. Techniques have been described to approach the motor points of all of these muscles, although typically the latissimus would be treated with a thoracodorsal nerve block. This nerve can be

TABLE 9.3
Suggested Uses of BT and Phenol

Muscle Group	Botulinum	Phenol Motor Point	Phenol Nerve
Latissimus	X		X
Pectoralis	X	X	
Teres major	X	X	
Subscapularis	X (Preferred technique)		
Biceps	X	X	X (musculocutaneous)
Brachialis	X	X	X (musculocutaneous)
Brachioradialis	X	X	
Wrist flexors	X	X	
Finger flexors	X	X (possible)	
Hand/Finger intrinsics	X		
Hip flexors	X		
Hip adductors	X		X (obturator) (Preferred technique)
Flexed knee (hamstrings)	X	X	
Stiff knee (quadriceps)	X	X	
Equinovarus ankle/foot	X	X	X (tibial)
Striatal toe	X	X	

located both with superficial and percutaneous electrical stimulation between the posterior and middle axillary lines anterior to the lateral border of the scapula. The needle should be inserted almost parallel to the sagittal plane to avoid the thoracic wall. Pectoralis motor points can be easily identified with superficial stimulation with an important point being just below the clavicle at approximately its mid point where a major motor branch can be identified. The teres major motor point is also easily identified with superficial stimulation. The subscapularis motor point cannot be identified with superficial stimulation. Approaches to reach the subscapularis motor point or nerve block have been described by Hecht et al. (55, 56). If the scapula can be "winged," one approach involves having the patient side-lying with the involved shoulder up and inserting the needle at the medial border of the scapula at the level of the scapular spine. Again, the needle should be as close to parallel with the chest wall as possible and pointed

away from the chest wall toward the inner aspect of the scapula. A second approach involves having the patient lying supine and approaching the subscapularis fossa from the lateral aspect. These same approaches may be used for subscapularis botulinum injections.

Given the risks associated with blind needle searches in close proximity to the thorax, it is preferable to approach the subscapularis with botulinum. Treatment of the pectoralis complex can be done either with phenol motor point blocks or botulinum, as can the teres major. In an effort to conserve botulinum with reference to a total dose per treatment session in a 3-month period, serious consideration should be given to a phenol thoracodorsal block rather than botulinum for the latissimus.

Flexed elbow. The major muscles contributing to the flexed elbow pattern include the biceps brachii, brachialis, and brachioradialis. All of these muscles can be approached with phenol motor point blocks or motor fascicle blocks. Again, depending on the number of muscles to be treated in a botulinum session, consideration could be given to a musculocutaneous block to treat the biceps and brachialis and thus conserve botulinum for other muscle groups. To identify the nerve, superficial stimulation can be used initially. The primary author prefers the "distal" approach to better avoid other nerves and vascular structures. The nerve is identified 2 to 3 cm distal to the insertion of the pectoralis major in the upper arm. The brachial artery is palpated and the needle inserted anterior to the artery and directed laterally until contraction of the biceps is identified.

Flexed wrist and fingers. Although motor points or motor branches can be identified with superficial stimulation for the major flexors of the wrist and the flexor digitorum superficialis, it is recommended that this primitive movement pattern be treated with BT rather than phenol neurolysis, at least as an initial treatment. Both the median and ulnar nerves are rich in sensory fibers. The risks of dysesthesias due to suboptimal localization or spread of phenol to these nerves or sensory branches is probably too high to use phenol as an initial treatment.

Lower Body

Flexed hip. Recommended techniques to treat the iliopsoas and iliacus have historically focused on a paravertebral approach, for phenol and botulinum. In the case of phenol, this is undertaken in an effort to reach the branches to the offending muscles. However, it is feasible to obtain a relatively good block with botulinum distally near the insertion of the flexors on the lesser trochanter of the femur. The point for injection is approximately 2 fingerbreadths lateral to the femoral artery and 1 fingerbreadth below the inguinal ligament. This may be done using anatomical landmarks as described or with ultrasound or fluoroscopic guidance.

Adducted hip/scissoring. Dysesthesias have never been reported with phenol neurolysis of the obturator nerve. It is recommended that adductor spasticity is most productively treated with phenol neurolysis to the obturator nerves. This limits the amount of needling and is most cost-effective. The obturator nerve is best identified by the anterior approach described by Glenn (21). The nerve can be identified by superficial stimulation first, but the needle is inserted along the lateral border of the adductor longus 2 cm distal to its origin. The anterior branch is approximately 2 cm deep, and by advancing the needle posteriorly and perpendicular to the coronal plane, in the same sagittal plan, another 2 cm of the posterior branch can be

reached. In some cases, with long-standing spasticity, it may be technically difficult to access the nerve. In this situation, BT can be administered, and before the effect wears off, phenol neurolysis can be performed to the obturator nerves.

Flexed knee. The major flexors of the knee are the hamstring muscles: semimembranosis, semitendonosis, and biceps femoris. These are primarily supplied by branches from the sciatic nerve. Of course, injecting the whole sciatic nerve with phenol is to be avoided. The nerve and branches to the hamstrings should be identified with superficial stimulation first. If one bisects a line between the ischial tuberousity and the greater trochanter, it is easy to identify the nerve. Selective motor branch identification can be somewhat cumbersome but involves inching the stimulator medially or laterally away from the nerve. This is best achieved a few centimeters distal to the point identified above. Although the hamstrings require a large amount of BT for treatment, if interruption of severe knee flexion contraction is the major treatment goal, then botulinum may be the preferred intervention.

Stiff knee. Either phenol motor point blocks or low-dose botulinum can be effective. The advantage of phenol is immediate ability to titrate the dose. In either case, caution must be observed against overzealous intervention leading to knee buckling.

Equniovarus of the ankle/foot. Muscles contributing to this deformity include the gastrocnemius, soleus, tibialis posterior, possibly the tibialis anterior, and if toe clawing is problematic, the flexor hallucis longus and flexor digitorum longus. Nearly all of these muscles could be treated by a tibial nerve block. However, even if done correctly, there remains a (treatable) risk for dysesthesias. The clinician must once again weigh the number of muscles being treated, including other limbs, against the total number of units of botulinum needed, notwithstanding the cost of the botulinum. Consideration could be given to treating the gastrocnemius with motor fascicle blocks with phenol and treating the deep muscles, not available to superficial localization, with botulinum, as an example.

Striatal toe. The major contributing muscle to this pattern is the extensor hallucis. It may be treated either with botulinum or phenol motor point block.

CONCLUSION

In summary, phenol and alcohol neurolysis have a long history in the treatment of upper motor neuron disorders. Phenol is inexpensive and immediately titratable for the desired clinical effect. It is likely that proximal nerve blocks produce a much longer-lasting effect than motor point blocks or BT injections. The risk for dysesthesias in mixed sensorimotor nerve blocks is genuine but typically of short duration and treatable—although for the patient who develops this problem, the duration is not short enough and the discomfort may be incapacitating. However, given the comparatively enormous expense of botulinum, limitations imposed by its duration of action, the inability to retreat or titrate sooner than every 3 months, the ability to complement this medication with phenol neurolysis or motor point blocks would provide an advantage to the clinician and to patients requiring these interventions.

References

1. Katz J, Knott LW, and Feldman DJ. Peripheral nerve injections with phenol in the management of spastic patients. *Arch Phys Med Rehabil* 1967;48:97–99.
2. Khalili AA, Harmel MH, Forster S, Benton JG. Management of spasticity by selective peripheral nerve block with dilute phenol solutions in clinical rehabilitation. *Arch Phys Med Rehabil* 1964;45:513–519.
3. Khalili AA, Benton JG. A physiological approach to the evaluation and the management of spasticity with procaine and phenol nerve block. *Clin Orthop* 1966;47:97–104.
4. Khalili AA, Betts HB. Peripheral nerve block with phenol in the management of spasticity: indications and complications. *JAMA* 1967;200:1155–1157.
5. Halpern D, Meelhuysen FE. Phenol motor point block in the management of muscular hypertonia. *Arch Phys Med Rehabil* 1966;47:659–664.
6. O'Hanlan JT, Galford HR, Bosley J. The use of 45% alcohol to control spasticity. *Va Med Mon* 1969;96:429–436.
7. Spira R. Management of spasticity in cerebral palsied children by peripheral nerve block with phenol. *Dev Med Child Neurol* 1971;13:164–173.
8. DeLateur BJ. A new technique of intramuscular phenol neurolysis. *Arch Phys Med Rehabil* 1972;53:179–185.
9. Mortiz U. Phenol block of peripheral nerves. *Scand J Rehabil Med* 1973;5:160–163.
10. Petrillo CR, Chu DS, Davis SW. Phenol block of the tibial nerve in the hemiplegic patient. *Orthopedics* 1980;3:871–874.
11. Garland DE, Lilling M, Keenan MA. Percuataneous phenol blocks to motor points of spastic forearm muscles in head-injured patients. *Arch Phys Med Rehabil* 1984;65:243–245.
12. Maher RM. Neurone selection in relief of pain: further experience with intrathecal injections. *Lancet* 1957;ii:16–19.
13. Nathan PW, Sears TA. Effects of phenol on nervous conduction. *J Physiol* 1960; 50:565–580.
14. Schaumburg HN, Byck R, Weller RO. The effect of phenol on peripheral nerve. A histological and electrophysiological study. *J Neuropathol Exp Neurol* 1970;29:615–630.
15. Nathan PW, Sears TA, Smith MC. Effects of phenol on the nerve roots of the cat: an electrophysiological and histological study. *J Neurol Sci* 1965;2:7–29.
16. Burkel WE, McPhee M. Effect of phenol injection into peripheral nerve of rat: electron microscope studies. *Arch Phys Med Rehabil* 1970;51:391–397.
17. Fischer E, Cress RH, Haines G, Panin N, Paul BJ. Recovery of nerve conduction after nerve block by phenol. *Am J Phys Med Rehabil* 1971;50:230–234.
18. Mooney V, Frykman G, McLamb J. Current status of intraneural phenol injections. *Clin Orthop* 1969;63:122–131.
19. Halpern D. Histological studies in animals after intramuscular neurolysis with phenol. *Arch Phys Med Rehabil* 1977;58:438–443.
20. Perrotto A, Morrison D, Delagi E, Iazzetti J. *Anatomical guide for the electromyographer: the limbs and trunk.* Springfield, Charles C. Thomas, 2005.
21. Glenn MB. Nerve blocks. In: Glenn, MB, Whyte, J, eds. *The practical management of spasticity in children and adults.* Philadelphia, Lea & Febiger, 1990, pp 251–255.
22. Awad EA. *Injection techniques for spasticity: a practical guide to treatment of cerebral palsy, hemiplegia, multiple sclerosis and spinal cord injury.* Awad OE ed. Minneapolis MN. EA Awad publisher, 1993.
23. Walthard KM, Tchicaloff M. Motor points. In: Licht S ed. *Electrodiagnosis and electromyography* 3rd ed. New Haven CN: Licht, 1971.
24. Meelhuysen FE, Halpern D, Quast J. Treatment of flexor spasticity of hip by paravertebral lumbar spinal nerve block. *Arch Phys Med Rehabil* 1968;49:36–41.
25. Halpern D, Meelhuysen FE. Duration of relaxation after intramuscular neurolysis with phenol. *JAMA* 1967;200:1152–1154
26. Easton JK, Ozel T and Helpern D: Intramuscular neurolysis for spasticity in children. *Arch Phys Med Rehabil* 1979;60:155–158
27. Awad EA. Intramuscular neurolysis for stroke. *Minn Med* 1972;8:711–713.
28. Macek C. Venous thrombosis results from some phenol injections. *JAMA* 1983;249:180.
29. Kowalewski R, Schurch B, Hodler J, Borgeat A. Persistent paraplegia after an aqueous 7.5% phenol solution to the anterior motor root for intercostal neurolysis: a case report. *Arch Phys Med Rehabil* 2002;83:283–285.
30. Abou-Chakra I, Horn LJ, Kane J. Brown Sequard Syndrome as a complication of prolotherapy: a single case report. *Am J Phys Med Rehabil* 2002:81:556 (abstract).
31. Huges JT. Thrombosis of the posterior spinal arteries. *Neurology* 1970;20:659–664.
32. Kolaski K, Ajizian SJ, Passmore L, Pasutharnchat N, Koman LA, Smith BP. Safety profile of multilevel chemical denervation procedures using phenol or botulinum toxin or both in a pediatric population. *Am J Phys Med Rehabil* 2008;87:556–566.
33. Singler, RC. Alcohol neurolysis of siatic and femoral nerves. *Anesth Analg* 1981;60(7):532–533.
34. Jang SH, Ahn SH, Park SM, Kim SH, Lee KH, Lee Zi. Alcohol neurolysis of tibial nerve motor branches to the gastrocnemius muscle to treat ankle spasticity in patients with hemiplegic stroke. *Arch Phys Med Rehabil* 2004;85:506–508.
35. Chua KSG, Kong K-H. Alcohol neurolysis of the sciatic nerve in the treatment of hemiplegic knee flexor spasticity: clinical outcomes. *Arch Phys Med Rehabil* 2000;81:1432–1435.
36. Kong K-H, Chua KSG. Outcome of obturator nerve block with alcohol for the treatment of hip adductor spasticity. *Int J Rehabil Res* 1999;22:327–9.
37. Viel EJ, Perennou D, Ripart J, Pelissier J, Eledjam JJ. Neurolytic blocade of the obturator nerve for intractable spasticity of adductor thigh muscles. *Eur J Pain* 2002;6:97–104.
38. Mooney JF, Koman LA, Smith BP. Pharmacologic management of spasticity in cerebral palsy. *J Pediatr Orthop* 2003;23:679–686.
39. Koman LA, Mooney JF, Smith BP. Neuromuscular blockade in the management of cerebral palsy. *J Child Neuro* 1996;11:S23–S28.
40. Hariga J, Tardieu G, Tardieu C, Gagnard L. Effets de l'application de l'alcool dilue' sur le nerf. Confrontation de l'etude dynamographique et de l'etude histologique chez le chat decerebre'. *Rev Neurol* (Paris) 1964;11:472–474.
41. Tardieu G, Hariga J, Tardieu C, Gagnard L, Velin J. Traitement de la spasticite par infiltration d'salcool dilue' aux

points moteurs, ou par injection epidurale. *Rev Neurol* 1964; 110(6);563–566.

42. Tardieu, C Tardieu G, Hariga J, Gagnard L, Velin J. L'Fondement experimental d'une therapeutique des raideurs d'origine cerebrale (effets de l'alcoolisation menagee du nerf moteur sur le re'flexe d'entrement de l'animal decerebre'). *Arch Fr Pediatr* 1964;21:5–23.

43. Tardieu G, Tardieu C, Haiga J, Gagnard I. Treatment of spasticity by injection of dilute alcohol at the motor point or by epidural route. Clinical extension of an experiment on the decerebrate cat. *Dev Med Child Neurol* 1968;10:555–568.

44. Cockin J, Hamilton EA, Nicholds PJr, Price DA. Preliminary report on the treatment of spacticity with 45% ethyl alcohol injection into the muscles. *Br J Clin Pract* 1971;25:73–75.

45. Carpenter EB. Role of nerve blocks in the foot and ankle in cerebral palsy; therapeutic and diagnostic. *Foot Ankle* 1983;4:164–166.

46. Carpenter EB, Seitz DG. Intramuscular alcohol as an aid in the management of spastic cerebral palsy. *Dev Med Child Neurol* 1980;22:497–501.

47. Pelissir J, Viel E, Enjalbert M, Kotzki N, Eledjam JJ. Chemical neurolysis using alcohol (alcoholization) in the treatment of spasticity in the hemiplegia. *Cah Anesthesiol* 1993;41(2):139–43.

48. Block EE. *Orthopedic management in cerebral palsy*. London, MacKeith Press, 1987.

49. Glenn MV. Nerve blocks, In: *The practical management of spasticity in children and adults*, Glenn & Whyte (Eds), Kea & Febiger, Philadelphia-London. 1990, pp 227–258.

50. May O. The functional and histological effects of intraneural and intraganglionic injections of alcohol. *Br Med J* 1912;31: 465–470.

51. Kirazli Y, On AY, Kismali B, Aksit R. Comparison of phenol block and botulinus toxin type A in the treatment of spastic foot after stroke: a randomized, double-blind trial. *Am J Phys Med Rehabil* 1998;77:510–515.

52. Morrison JE, Hertzberg DL, Gourley SM, Matthews DJ. Motor point blocks in children: a technique to relieve spasticity using phenol injections. *AORN J* 1989;49(5):1346–1354.

53. Morrison JE, Matthews D, Washington R, Fennessey PV, Harrison LM. Phenol motor point blocks in children: plasma concentrations and cardiac dysrhythmias. *Anesthesiology* 1991;75:359–362.

54. Yadav SL, Singh U, Dureja GP, Singh KK, Chaturvedi S. Phenol block in the management of spastic cerebral palsy. *Indian J Pediatr* 1994;61:249–255.

55. Chironna RL, Hecht JS. Subscapularis motor point block for the painful hemiplegic shoulder. *Arch Phys Med Rehabil* 1990. 71;(6):428–9.

56. Hecht JS. Suscapular nerve block in the painful hemiplegic shoulder. *Arch Phys Med Rehabil*, 1992;73(11):1036–39.

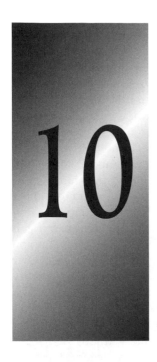

Botulinum Toxin in the Treatment of Lower Limb Spasticity

Alberto Esquenazi

Approximately 700,000 people are affected by a stroke each year in the United States, and there are more than 1,100,000 Americans surviving with residual functional impairment after stroke (1, 2). Traumatic brain injury (TBI) is another form of acquired brain injury and continues to be an enormous public health problem in the 21st century even with modern medicine. Most patients with TBI (75%–80%) have mild head injuries; the remaining injuries are divided equally between moderate and severe categories. The cost to society of TBI is staggering, both from an economic and an emotional standpoint. Almost 100% of persons with severe head injury and as many as two thirds of those with moderate head injury will be permanently disabled in some fashion and will not return to their premorbid level of function. In the United States, the direct cost of care for patients with TBI, excluding inpatient care, is estimated at more than $25 billion annually. The impact is even greater when one considers that most severe head injuries occur in adolescents and young adults with long survival rates.

Acquired brain injury affects a person's cognitive, language, perceptual, sensory, and motor function (3). Recovery is a long process that continues beyond the hospital stay and into the home setting. The rehabilitation process is guided by clinical assessment of motor abilities. Accurate assessment of the motor abilities is important in selecting the different treatment interventions available to a patient.

Spasticity is a term that is often used by clinicians, and although used frequently, it can have different meanings in its interpretation and presentation. Spasticity is just one of the many positive signs of the upper motor neuron (UMN) syndrome, yet, under the heading of "spasticity," clinicians often group all positive signs together and sometimes include negative signs as well. Many of these frequently misidentified phenomena fall under the broader heading of the upper motor neuron syndrome (UMNS)—a condition that has classically been partitioned into a syndrome of positive and negative signs, including weakness, loss of dexterity, increased phasic and tonic stretch reflexes, clonus, cocontraction, released flexor reflexes, spastic dystonia, and associated reactions or synkinesias.

The issue of terminology is more than semantics and of great clinical importance because, for example, treatment of cocontraction, a phenomenon likely to be of supraspinal origin, will differ from treatment of clonus, a phenomenon of the segmental stretch reflex loop. If clinicians desire a concise, descriptive, utilitarian term that captures the essence of positive UMN phenomena, "muscle overactivity" may be a more suitable term than "spasticity," especially since the phrase "muscle overactivity" evokes an image of dynamic muscle contraction, the general hallmark of all positive signs of UMN (4).

Spasticity has classically meant increased excitability of skeletal muscle stretch reflexes, both phasic and tonic, that are typically present in most patients with a UMN lesion. After a UMN lesion, a net loss of inhibition impairs direct descending control over motor neurons. There is also a loss of inhibitory control over interneuronal pathways of the cord that ordinarily regulate segmental spinal reflexes, including stretch reflexes, especially those concerned with antigravity muscles.

Lance characterized spasticity as an increase in velocity dependent tonic stretch reflexes with exaggerated tendon jerks (5). In Lance's consensus definition, tonic stretch reflexes referred to the output response of a muscle group that was stretched at different velocities. "Exaggerated tendon jerks" were examples of "phasic" stretch reflexes. In routine practice at the bedside, the 2 ways of assessing phasic and tonic stretch reflexes are tendon taps and passive stretch of a muscle group at different velocities (6, 7).

Although phenomena of presence are a common source of clinical concern and are frequently treated, phenomena of absence may be at times more functionally disabling and difficult to address. Negative signs signify loss or impairment of voluntary movement assembly and production, a kind of "muscle underactivity" that, in effect, can be described as phenomena of absence (5, 8).

The clinical picture is made more complex by another phenomenon that has not been classically positioned among the positive signs, namely, contracture or better described as the physical changes in the rheologic properties of muscle tissue. Contracture is well recognized by rehabilitation clinicians as a major source of disability for patients with UMNS. Ironically, phenomena of absence and phenomena of presence can both provide a context for the development of contracture (9).

FUNCTIONAL IMPLICATIONS OF SPASTICITY

Fifty years ago, Nikolai A. Bernstein suggested that the basic problem of motor control relates to overcoming redundant degrees of freedom in our multijointed skeletal system, the multijointed limb segments that allow us to interact with the 3-dimensional world we live in. Commonly, there are multiple "agonists" and "antagonists" for virtually any movement direction. To match a required joint torque even across a single joint, the question regarding which muscles should be activated and at what levels of activity is likely to have a very variable answer without a unique solution. For a given patient, however, there may be a "unique" solution in that equinovarus deformity may be solely attributable

to an overactive tibialis anterior in 1 patient, whereas in another, it may be an overactive tibialis posterior (9).

Patterns of limb dysfunction in the UMNS have an impact on the limb utilization for gait or other functional use. A number of muscles typically cross major joints of the extremities, and identifying the actual muscles that contribute dynamically and statically to a UMNS deformity is an important key to clinical management of the resulting gait or upper limb dysfunctions (10, 11). Clinical evaluation is useful to the analysis of movement dysfunction, but gait and motor control assessment laboratory evaluation using dynamic electromyography (EMG) and other assessment techniques is often necessary to identify the particular contributions of offending muscles with confidence. The correct selection of target muscles that contribute to any one pattern of dysfunction may serve as a rational basis for interventions that focus on specific muscles, including chemodenervation with botulinum toxin (BoNT), neurolysis with phenol, and surgical lengthening, transfers, and releases of individual muscles.

This concept, namely, identifying which muscles contribute dynamically and statically to upper motoneuron motor dysfunction, serves as a conceptual basis for this presentation. Simply put, identifying muscles that produce deforming maladaptive joint movements and postures statically and dynamically is an important endeavor in aiding clinical interpretation of gait dysfunction and in rationalizing subsequent treatment interventions (12, 13).

Dynamic EMG, gait, motion analysis, and diagnostic nerve blocks frequently provide the necessary detailed information about specific muscle groups that will guide decision making for treatment. Before selecting treatment interventions, the clinical team and the patient should explicitly develop functional goals. Functional goals may be classified as symptomatic, passive, or active in nature (9). A symptomatic goal refers to clonus, flexor or extensor spasms, and pain among others as some of the targeted goals. Active functions refer to a patient's direct use of the limb to carry out a functional activity. Passive function on the other hand refers to the passive manipulation of limbs to achieve functional ends, typically through patient's passive manipulation of their limb with their noninvolved limbs or their caregivers perform it. Identifying muscles with volitional capacity is important to the achievement of this goal. In broad terms, clinical evaluation focuses on the identification of several factors: Is there selective voluntary control of a given muscle? Is the muscle activated dyssynergically (ie, as an antagonist in movement)? Is the muscle resistive to passive stretch? Does the muscle have fixed shortening (contracture)? In the Gait and Motion Analysis Laboratories, dynamic EMG is acquired and examined in reference to simultaneous measurements of joint motion (kinematics) and ground reaction forces (kinetics) obtained from force platforms. Kinetic, kinematic, and dynamic EMG data augment the clinician's ability to interpret whether voluntary function is present in a given muscle and whether that muscle's behavior is also dyssynergic (Figure 10.1). Combined with clinical information, the laboratory measurements of muscle function often provide the degree of detail and confidence necessary to optimize the rehabilitation interventions. In addition, evaluation under the effect of temporary diagnostic nerve or motor point blocks can help the clinician distinguish between obligatory and compensatory limb postures and gait patterns (14).

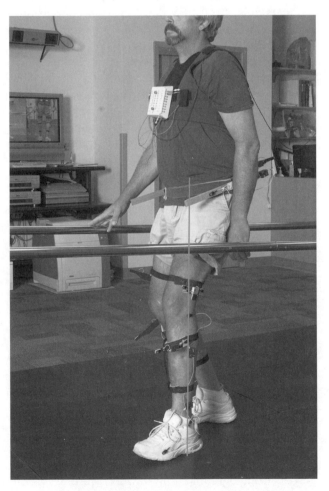

FIGURE 10.1

Subject instrumented for gait analysis data collection including dynamic EMG and CODA 3-D motion sensors. Red vertical line represents the ground reaction force.

CLINICAL ASSESSMENT OF SPASTICITY

There are many assessment techniques used in the routine clinical examination. Motor control, passive range of motion, manual muscle strength, Ashworth, and Tardeau are examples of such techniques that are frequently used.

For more information the reader is encouraged to review chapter 3 of this text. Passive range of motion can be used to determine the available movement for each joint but does not provide information on the cause of limitations if present. Spasticity, muscle overactivity, contracture, or pain can all play a role in limited passive range of motion.

Manual muscle testing allows grading of available strength if normal control is present; the grading is done using a 6-point scale, where 5 is a normal rating with ability to resist significant force and 0 is unable to move. In UMNS, testing of strength may be affected by impaired motor control, the presence of synergistic patterns, and cognitive deficits.

The Ashworth Scale allows assessment of muscle tone; in the modified Ashworth, the rating uses a 5-point scale. The scale has only been validated for the elbow and requires the movement of the joint through its available range in 1 second. Ideally, the test should always be done in the same position and under similar conditions (15). One disadvantage is that this test does not take in consideration the presence of contracture or other factors that may limit joint motion.

The Tardeau test was developed in the pediatric population in the mid 1960. It attempts to assess spasticity by varying the speed of joint motion available from very slow (V1) to as fast as possible (V3). The difference between the parameters permits an estimation of the effect of spasticity (16) (Figure 10.2).

Unfortunately, none of these assessments provides a functional perspective, such as during walking, and cannot precisely determine the source of the problem. Based in our clinical experience, methods based on a functional perspective such as those described below can be more helpful in this regard.

The Impact of Gait

Gait is a functional task performed by most humans. The 3 main functional goals of ambulation are to move from one place to another, to move safely, and to move efficiently. These 3 goals are frequently compromised in the patient with residual UMNS. Most patients will be able to perform limited ambulation, but they will often have problems because of inefficient movement strategies, the presence of instability or pain due to abnormal limb postures, and decreased safety. Some

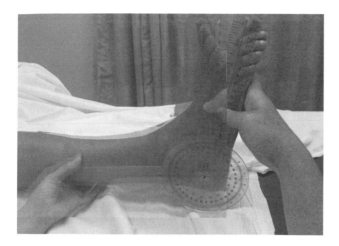

FIGURE 10.2

Demonstrating the Tardeau measurement.

generalizations can be made about the gait of patients with acquired brain injury. These include a decrease in walking velocity with a reduction in the duration of stance phase and impairment of weight-bearing in the affected limb with an increase in the duration of stance time of the less affected limb (17). Ochi et al. (18) reported on differences in temporospatial parameters of locomotion among patients with residual stroke and TBI. From a functional perspective, gait deficiencies can be categorized with respect to the gait cycle. In the stance phase, an abnormal base of support can be caused by equinovarus, toe flexion, or ankle valgus. Limb instability can occur due to knee buckling (sudden flexion) or hyperextension, which may result in knee joint pain or lack of trunk control. This may result in unsafe, inefficient, or painful walking.

During the swing phase, inadequate limb clearance caused, for example, by a stiff knee and inadequate limb advancement caused by limited hip flexion or knee extension may interfere with the safety and energy efficiency of walking. To identify the potential source of the problem and to focus more appropriately on the essence of multifactorial gait dysfunction, formal gait analysis in a laboratory may be required. Combining clinical evaluation with laboratory measurements will increase the degree of resolution needed to understand the common patterns of gait dysfunction in the UMN (17).

Patterns of UMN Dysfunction

Because of scope and space limitations, only the most common patterns of UMN dysfunction in the lower limb that affect walking have been selected for review in this chapter, and they include (1) equinovarus foot, (2) hyperextended great toe, (3) stiff knee, (4) adducted (scissoring) thighs, and (5) flexed hip (9, 12). The first 2 patterns are considered to be problematic throughout the gait cycle. Stiff knee and adducted thigh are predominantly deviations of swing phase, and both can interfere with limb clearance and advancement. The flexed hip is considered a stance phase deviation.

Equinovarus

Equinovarus foot is the most prevalent UMN posture affecting walking and requiring intervention after an acquired brain injury. The foot and ankle are turned down [Figure 10.3(A)], and toe curling or toe clawing may coexist. The lateral border of the foot is the main weight-bearing surface. Skin breakdown over the metatarsal head may develop from concentrated pressure particularly over the fifth metatarsal head; weight-bearing typically occurs when walking but may take place against the footrest of a wheelchair. In walking, equinovarus is frequently maintained throughout stance phase and inversion may increase, causing ankle instability during weight-bearing. Limited ankle dorsiflexion during early and midstance prevents the appropriate forward advancement of the tibia over the stationary foot, promoting knee hyperextension. Impairment in dorsiflexion range of motion in the late stance and preswing phases interferes with push-off and forward propulsion of the center of mass, and combined with reduce walking velocity, it results in marked reduction in joint power generation. During swing phase, equinus posture of the foot may result in limb clearance problem, whereas the lack of appropriate posture of the foot in stance phase may result in instability of the whole body. Under the later presentation, correction of this problem is essential even for limited ambulation.

A number of muscles may generate the abnormal forces with respect to the equinovarus pattern (19). Muscles that can potentially contribute to the equinovarus deformity include the tibialis anterior, tibialis posterior, long toe flexors, gastrocnemius, soleus, extensor hallucis longus (EHL) and the weakness of the peroneus longus, peroneus brevis, and the long toe extensors. As mentioned before, dynamic polyelectromyographic (poly-EMG) recordings of the above-mentioned muscles in combination with clinical examination provide a more detailed understanding of the genesis of this deformity. Dynamic poly-EMG recordings often demonstrate prolonged activation of the gastrocnemius and soleus complex, as well as the long toe flexors as the commonest cause of plantar

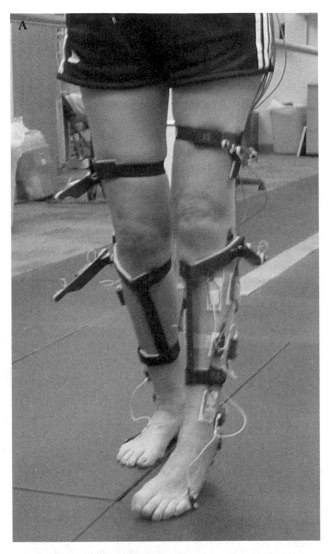

FIGURE 10.3(A)

Equinovarus left foot posture after cerebrovascular accident. Patient has a large bursa under the base of the fifth metatarsal with complaints of pain and instability during the stance phase.

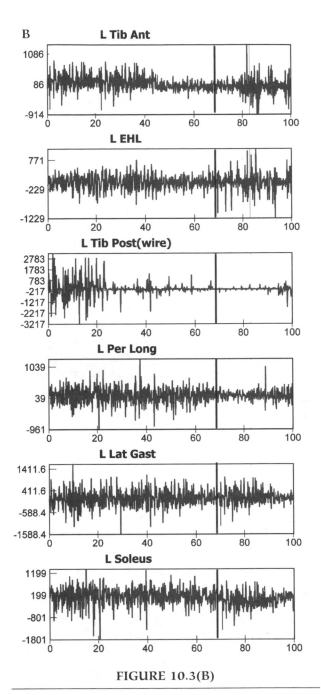

FIGURE 10.3(B)

Dynamic EMG data of the subject seen in panel (A) with equinovarus foot posture after cerebrovascular accident. Data are normalized, and vertical line at 62% indicates the initiation of the swing phase. Note overactive tibialis anterior, EHL, and gastroc soleus complex during swing phase.

flexion. Occasionally, the gastrocnemius and soleus may activate differentially, and treatment interventions must take this into consideration. Ankle inversion is the result of the overactivation of the tibialis posterior and anterior in combination with the gastrocnemius and soleus and, at times, the EHL [Figure 10.3(B)]. If the tibialis posterior and anterior are both apparently contributing to the ankle varus deformity, a decision has to be made about which one of the 2 muscles is the main contributor. Two approaches are possible for this differentiation. The first one is to use the EMG data and the joint powers obtained as part

of the kinematic data in routine gait analysis. The second possibility is a diagnostic tibial nerve block with a short-acting anesthetic. One has to be mindful that reducing the activation of the gastrocnemius-soleus complex will tend to increase ankle dorsiflexion and that tightness of the toe flexors usually becomes more apparent as a result of the toe flexor tenodesis effect brought on by the allowed increased dorsiflexion.

Based on dynamic poly-EMG correlated with clinical findings, the frequent treatment of choice is injection of BoNT into the tibialis posterior, gastrocnemius, soleus, and long toe flexors (19). When a contracture is evident, serial casting may need to be attempted or surgical intervention may need to be considered.

Hyperextended Great Toe

Hyperextended great toe is a deformity that is characterized by toe extension throughout the gait cycle, sometimes referred to as striated toe or "hitchhiker's toe." Ankle equinus and varus may accompany this foot deformity (Figure 10.4). When wearing shoes, the patient may complain of pain at the tip of the big toe, and during stance phase, abnormal concentration of forces under the first metatarsal head can also produce pain. Toe extension during early and midstance affects weight-bearing and can impair gait due to inefficient translation of the center of gravity during late stance phase. It also has an impact on center of gravity stability during stance phase single limb support. Extensor hallucis longus hyperactivity is the main deforming force causing great toe hyperextension. A weak flexor hallucis longus may not be able to compensate and offset the extension force of EHL. When equinovarus is also present, analysis of the contributions of tibialis anterior, tibialis posterior, gastrocnemius, soleus, and

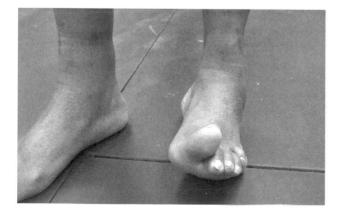

FIGURE 10.4

Hyperextended hallux after cerebrovascular accident. Patient complains of pain at the tip of the big toe and pressure under the first metatarsal base.

the long toe flexors needs to be taken into consideration as well. Chemodenervation with BoNT or motor point injection of EHL with phenol can easily be achieved to alleviate this problems.

Stiff Knee

The stiff knee, as previously mentioned, is a swing phase deformity by definition. The knee is kept extended during preswing and initial swing, resulting in a reduction of the knee arc of motion with its peak less than 40° at mid swing (normal reference approximately 60°) (14). In addition, there may be delay in the timing of flexion and a concomitant reduction in hip flexion [Figure 10.5(A)]. Knee flexion during normal walking is primarily generated by the inertial forces produced by hip flexion. Reduction in swing phase hip flexion may result in decreased knee flexion. The limb appears to be functionally longer because it remains extended at the knee throughout swing phase, resulting in toe drag that may cause tripping and falling. To achieve compensated foot clearance for this relative leg length discrepancy, the patient may attempt contralateral vaulting (early heel rise), ipsilateral circumduction, or hip hiking. All of these compensations increase energy consumption and can result in diminished walking capacity. Electromyographic recordings frequently demonstrate a reduction in the activation of iliopsoas (a hip flexor) along with excessive activation of the rectus femoris, vastus intermedius, vastus medialis, and vastus lateralis. An overactive gluteus maximus in swing phase may act to restrain hip flexion and impair swing limb advancement resulting in an extended knee pattern, and at times, excessive activation or out-of-phase activation of the hamstrings may be seen. If ankle equinus is also present, a reduction in joint power generation and plantar flexion moment may further reduce knee flexion (14, 20).

Based on clinical and laboratory findings, chemodenervation with BoNT to individual heads of the quadriceps may be considered; caution in dosing is suggested to avoid overweakening of the knee extensor mechanism that may result in knee instability. If there is uncertainty of the quadriceps force-generating capacity during walking, it may be advisable to perform a diagnostic block of the motor branch of the femoral nerve to the knee extensors with a short-acting anesthetic to better determine it. If involvement of the gluteus maximus is evident, this can also be treated with chemodenervation with BoNT [Figure 10.5(B)]. Treatment should also incorporate marching exercises, and if the patient exhibits an abnormal ankle posture, appropriate interventions for this problem should be implemented.

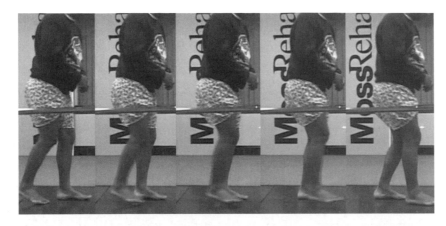

FIGURE 10.5(A)

Stiff knee gait evident in the swing phase in a patient with residual UMNS from TBI. Note lack of knee flexion during swing phase possibly forcing the patient to use compensatory mechanisms for limb clearance, such as circumduction and hip hiking.

Adducted (Scissoring) Thigh

This deformity is characterized by adduction of the hip during the swing phase of locomotion. Hip ad-

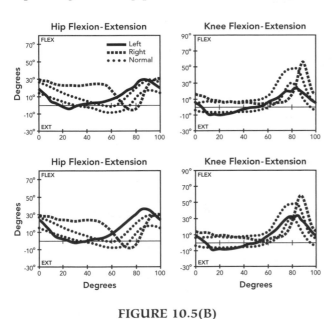

FIGURE 10.5(B)

CODA 3-D kinematic data before (top) and after (bottom) treatment of stiff knee gait in the patient depicted in Figure 10.4. Note marked improvement in left knee (solid line) peck flexion and hip flexion. The dashed line represents right leg and the dotted line represents normative data that are velocity matched. Data are normalized; vertical line at 65% to75% indicates the beginning of the swing phase. Based on dynamic EMG and gait analysis, patient was treated with 200 U of BoNT-A (Botox®) injected to the right rectus femoris (100 U), vastus medialis (50 U), lateralis (50 U), and gluteus maximus (50). See color insert.

duction posturing at the end of swing phase generates a narrow base of support during stance, ultimately making upright balance uncertain. It can also interfere with limb advancement because the adducting swing phase limb may collide with the contralateral stance limb. When adductor spasticity is complicated by hip flexion, other functional activities such as toileting and perineal access can be affected and posture in a chair requires frequent repositioning of the patient (Figure 10.6), Dynamic poly-EMG recordings will

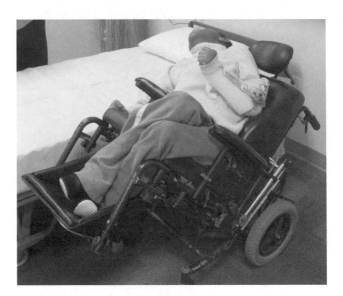

FIGURE 10.6

Adducted hips in a nonambulatory patient with UMNS caused by TBI. Passive function is impaired for dressing and hygiene.

frequently demonstrate overactivation of the hip adductors, medial hamstrings, and pectineus. Weakness of the hip abductors and the iliopsoas may also contribute to this deformity because the patient may be attempting to use the hip adductors during walking in a compensatory manner to advance the limb forward during swing phase.

It is essential to ascertain if the hip adductor deformity is obligatory (the result of adductor overactivity) or compensatory (the result of weak hip flexors) because treatment will differ. If the clinician is uncertain, a diagnostic temporary obturator nerve block can be helpful to differentiate the role of hip adduction in an obligatory-versus-compensatory pattern. Longer-term interventions, such as chemodenervation with botulinum neurotoxin, can be easily carried out. Other treatment options, such as a percutaneous phenol obturator nerve block, exist. After the intervention, aggressive stretching of the hip adductors and exercises to strengthen the hip flexors and abductors should be implemented. Electrical stimulation to the hip abductors may be used to facilitate strengthening (14, 20).

Flexed Hip

The patient with excessive hip flexion potentially experiences difficulty during walking with negative impact during both phases of the gait cycle. In normal gait, the hip is flexed 30° at initial contact but thereafter extends throughout stance phase to about 10°. This deformity can also interfere when standing up from a seated position and during perineal care and sexual intimacy. The UMN pattern of hip flexion is defined as persistent hip flexion throughout stance. Knee flexion deformity may develop as a consequence of severe hip flexion deformity, since in supine position, the knee flexes to allow the heel to touch the bed. During walking, a shortened contralateral step results from stance phase excessive hip flexion. Excessive hip flexion may also affect single limb support stability of the center of gravity. Dynamic poly-EMG recordings during walking may identify overactive iliopsoas, rectus femoris, hip adductors, or lack of activation of the hip extensors and paraspinals. Interventions to reduce overactive hip flexors (iliopsoas and rectus femoris), particularly chemodenervation with botulinum neurotoxin, to these 2 muscles can be easily performed guided by electrical stimulation or ultrasound and followed by appropriate rehabilitation techniques including the implementation of hip stretching and attempting long step walking (14).

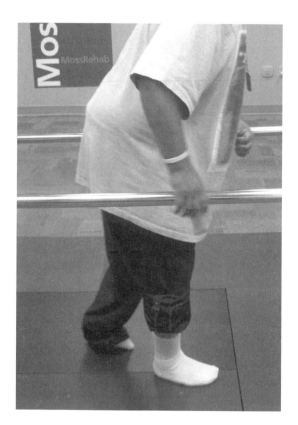

FIGURE 10.7

Flexed hip (right) in a patient with UMNS caused by TBI. Note short left step length caused by limitation in right hip extension.

THE ROLE OF BoNT IN THE TREATMENT OF SPASTICITY

Intramuscular injection of BoNTs inhibit the release of acetylcholine at the neuromuscular junction causing muscle weakness. Three steps are involved in the toxin-mediated paralysis: (1) internalization, (2) disulfide reduction and translocation, and (3) inhibition of neurotransmitter release. The toxin must enter the nerve ending to exert its effect. BoNT-A (formulated as Botox) injection is currently approved by the US Food and Drug Administration for the treatment of blepharospasm, facial spasm, strabismus, cervical dystonia, hyperhidrosis and upper limb spasticity. In Europe, Canada, and several countries in Latin America, BoNT-A (formulated as Botox and Dysport®) is also approved for the management of cerebral palsy and stroke-related spasticity. BoNT-B (formulated as Myo-Bloc® in the United States and NeuroBloc® elsewhere) is approved by the US Food and Drug Administration only for the treatment of cervical dystonia. The reader is encouraged to read other chapters of this text for further information (21, 22).

The purpose of BoNT injections in the management of the UMNS is to reduce force produced by a contracting overactive muscle or muscle group. A reduction in muscle tension can lead to improvement in passive and active range of motion and allows for more successful stretching of tight musculature. More subtly, and more importantly as well, improved motor control and posture may provide the patient with the opportunity to develop compensatory behaviors during functional activities (9). A reduction in muscle overactivity in one muscle or muscle group may have consequences for tone in other muscle groups of the limb through a reduction in the overall effort required to perform movement and/or, through changes in sensory information going to the central nervous system from that limb, may influence more distant muscles or benefit function (21). Finally, the application of external devices such as braces, splints, casts, and even shoes can be facilitated by interventions with chemodenervation.

Botulinum toxin is injected directly into an offending muscle. The major advantages in its use are the ease of application that permits its injection without anesthesia and its predictable effect. The most common adverse effect is excessive weakness of injected muscles, which occasionally spread to nontarget muscles. Given sufficient time, when the patient has a strong response to the paralytic effect of the toxin with excessive weakening, strength will gradually return. No adverse effect on the sensory system is evident with BoNT-A, but pain relieve when present has been reported in some patients (22, 23). In rare cases, nausea, headache, and fatigue have also been reported. No anaphylactic response has ever been reported due to BoNT-A injection. Depending on the size of the muscle being injected, therapeutic doses of Botox® have ranged between 10 and 300 U. In cases of accidental poisoning, an antitoxin is available. Because of the potential risk of migration out of the muscle and the possibility of antibody formation, usually not greater than 600 U of Botox® or 1500 units of Dysport® is administered in a single-treatment session (24). This may be sufficient, however, to treat a number of muscles in that one session (22, 25). Based upon clinical experience and prospective randomize trials, the development of resistance to BoNT-A therapy does not impact the management of patients with muscle overactivity. However, to minimize the risk of immunoresistance, clinicians should use the smallest possible effective dose, extend the interval

---

TABLE 10.1
Suggested Botox Dosing for Adults

CLINICAL PATTERN	POTENTIAL MUSCLE INVOLVED	BOTOX DOSE UNITS/SESSION	NO. OF INJECTION SITES
Equinovarus foot	Gastrocnemius	50–250	2–4
	Soleus	50–200	2–4
	Tibialis posterior	25–150	1–2
	Flexor halucis longus	25–75	1–2
	Flexor digitorum longus	25–100	1–2
	Flexor digitorum brevis	20–40	1
	Tibialis anterior	20–120	1–3
Flexed hip	Iliacus	50–150	2
	Psoas	50–150	2
	Rectus femoris	75–200	2–4
Flexed knee	Medial hamstrings	50–200	2–3
	Lateral hamstrings	50–200	2–3
	Gastrocnemius (as knee flexors)	50–150	2–4
Extended (stiff) knee	Rectus femoris	50–200	2–4
	Vasti	50–150	2–4
Hyperextended toe (striatal)	EHL	20–100	1–2
Adducted thigh	Adductor longus/magnus/brevis	75–300	4–6

Modified from Spasticity and Other Forms of Muscle Overactivity in the UMNS We Move 2008 (20).

between treatments for at least 3 months or longer if possible, and avoid the use of booster injections in between treatment. Careful documentation of muscle selection, dose, and effects is encouraged to allow for dose or muscle selection adjustment in the next treatment cycle if necessary. In our practice, if multiple large muscles are to be injected, we try to concentrate the available dose to a few of them and we may increase dilution and use electrical stimulation before the treatment to enhance the effect and consider using other agents such as phenol injected to other muscles or motor nerves to achieve a complete treatment strategy. With the currently available information, we recommend not injecting BoNT to patients who are pregnant or lactating or have significant medical comorbidities (22, 25, 26).

Before using BoNT in the clinical management of spasticity, the physician should be knowledgeable about the diagnosis and medical management of the condition producing the UMNS. The physician should be proficient in the relevant anatomy and kinesiology and have a clear understanding of the potential benefits of unmasking function and of the limitations of this therapeutic intervention. Unlike the patient with dystonia where voluntary capacity is not an issue, spastic muscles may very well have evidence or potential for voluntary capacity, which the clinician would like to preserve or unmask, and therefore, titration of the paralytic effect of the toxin becomes a much more critical factor in its administration (5). The duration of toxin effectiveness ranges between 10 weeks and 4 months. In our experience, patients have received doses greater than 400 U of Botox® at 3-month intervals for more than 3 years without evidence of loss of effectiveness of the medication. Gordon et al. (26) have reported an increase in duration of effect over time under similar treatment paradigm. The toxin might be an effective tool to "simulate" the effects of surgery to the benefit of the surgeon and patient alike (24).

The strategy of performing a BoNT-A injection is as follows: the skin is prepared by cleaning it with alcohol before insertion of the Teflon-coated, 25-gauge stimulating injecting needle. The electrically conductive inner core of the tip of the needle is used to pass current to the tissues or to record EMG activity. Before or soon after injection, muscle activation should be encouraged to increase the availability of Synaptobrevin 2, a major factor in the uptake and internalization of BoNT-A. As the paralytic effect appears evident, aggressive stretching, muscle reeducation, and functional training are important parts of the treatment protocol (17) (Table 10.1).

CONCLUSION

This chapter reviews the most salient points related to the clinical presentation of UMNS in the lower limb especially during walking. Negative signs of the UMNS include weakness and loss of dexterity. Positive findings such as spasticity, increased phasic and tonic stretch reflexes, clonus, cocontraction, released flexor reflexes, spastic dystonia, and associated reactions or synkinesias can all be summed up in the term muscle overactivity, which produces gait impairment. The clinical picture is made more complex by changes in the viscoelastic properties of muscle and other soft tissues in the form of a contracture. Identifying the specific possible source of the deforming force is of the essence for proper treatment planning and intervention. The combined effects of these phenomena are well recognized by rehabilitation clinicians as a major source of disability for patients with UMNS. This syndrome produces upper and lower limb patterns of dysfunction that commonly affect more than one joint at a time and that need to be correlated with their clinical presentation and resulting impairment. Dynamic poly-EMG and motion analysis can be used to identify the contributors to the specific pattern, and when the technology is not available, thorough careful clinical assessment and selected use of diagnostic nerve blocks can be used to develop a successful BoNT chemodenervation management strategy for this patient population.

References

1. American Heart Association, Heart disease and stroke statistics 2005 update. AHA Dallas TX 2004.
2. Center for Disease Control, Morbidity and Mortality Weekly report. CDC, Atlanta GA, 2001.
3. National Institute of Neurological Disorders and Stroke, Stroke: hope through research. NINDS Washington DC 2004.
4. Mayer N, Esquenazi A, Keenan MAE. Assessing and treating muscle overactivity in the upper motor neuron syndrome. In *Brain injury medicine principles and practice*. N. Zasler, D. Katz and R Zafonte (edts). DEMOS, New York, NY: 2006;35: 615–65.
5. Mayer, N, Esquenazi, A. Muscle overactivity and movement dysfunction in the upper motoneuron syndrome. Phys Med *Rehabil Clin N Am* 2003:14:855–883.
6. Lance JW: Symposium synopsis: In: Feldman RG, Young RR, Koella WP, eds. *Spasticity: disordered motor control*. Chicago: Yearbook Medical: pp 485–494,1980.
7. Okuma Y, Lee RG: Reciprocal inhibition in hemiplegia: correlation with clinical features in recovery. *Can J Neurol Sci* 1996;23:15–23.
8. Dewald JPA, Rymer WZ: Factors underlying abnormal posture and movement in spastic hemiparesis. In AF Thilmann, DJ Burke, WZ Rymer, editors. *Spasticity: mechanisms and management*, Berlin: Springer-Verlag: 1993;123–38.
9. Esquenazi A, Mayer N. Instrumented assessment of muscle overactivity and spasticity with dynamic polyelectromyo-

graphic and motion analysis for treatment planning. Am J Phys Med Rehabil Vol. 83, No. 10 (Suppl). October 2004.

10. O'Dwyer N, Ada L, Neilson PD: Spasticity and muscle contracture following stroke. *Brain* 1996;119:1737–1749.

11. Rosenbaum DA: *Human motor control.* Academic Press, San Diego, CA 1991.

12. Mayer NH, Esquenazi A, Childers MK. Common patterns of clinical motor dysfunction. Muscle Nerve 20:Suppl 6: S21–S23, 1997.

13. Mayer, NH. Esquenazi, A. and Keenan, MAE. Patterns of upper motoneuron dysfunction in the lower limb. *Gait disorders, advances in neurology*, Ruzicka, Hallet and Jankovic (edts). Lippincott Williams & Wilkins, Philadelphia. Vol 87, 311–319, 2001.

14. Esquenazi, A. Talaty, M. Gait analysis: technology and clinical application. In *Physical medicine and rehabilitation*, 3rd ed. R.L. Braddom (edt.) Saunders, Elsevier Inc., Philadelphia, PA. chapter 5. 93–110, 2007.

15. Bohannon RW, Smith MB. Interrater reliability of a modified Ashworth scale of muscle spasticity. *Phys Ther* 1987 Feb;67(2):206–7.

16. Tardieu G, Dalloz J. Principles of examination of stiffness in the cerebral palsied child. *Arch Fr Pediatr* 1963 Dec; 20: 1201–9.

17. Esquenazi Alberto, Mayer Nathaniel and Albanese Alberto. Botulinum toxin for the management of adult spasticity Special Issue Toxins 2008 Highlights Elsevier: 2009 in press.

18. Ochi F, Esquenazi A, Hirai B, Talaty M. Temporal-Spatial features of gait after traumatic brain injury. *J Head Trauma Rehabil* 1999;14(2):105–115.

19. Esquenazi A, Mayer N and Kim S. Patient registry of spasticity care. Archives of PMR. Nov 2008.

20. Mayer NH, Esquenazi, A. Childers, M.K. Common patterns of clinical motor dysfunction. In: *Spasticity and other forms of muscle overactivity in the UMNS.* Brashear and Mayer, editors. We Move 2008.

21. Esquenazi A, Mayer N and Garreta R. Influence of botulinum toxin type A treatment of elbow flexor spasticity on hemiparetic gait. *Am J Phys Med Rehabil* 87:305–311, April 2008.

22. Jankovic, J, Esquenazi, A, Fehlings, D, Freitag, F, Lang, A, Naumann, M. Evidence-based review of patient-reported outcomes with botulinum toxin type A. *Clin Neuropharmacol* Volume 27, Number 5, 234–244. September–October 2004.

23. Childers MK, Brashear A, Jozefczyk P, Reding M, Alexander D, Good D, et al. Dose-dependent response to intramuscular botulinum toxin type A for upper-limb spasticity in patients after a stroke. *Arch Phys Med Rehabil* 2004 Jul;85: 1063–9

24. The upper motor neuron syndrome and muscle overactivity including spasticity and the role of botulinum toxin. Mayer, N, Brashear, A (eds), 2008.

25. Brin MF: Botulinum toxin: chemistry, pharmacology, toxicity, and immunology. *Muscle Nerve* 1997;20(suppl 6) S146–S168.

26. Gordon MF, Brashear A, Elovic E, Kassicieh D, Marciniak C, Gonzaga McGuire JR. Effective use of chemodenervation and chemical neurolysis in the management of poststroke spasticity. *Top Stroke Rehabil* 2001;8:47–55.

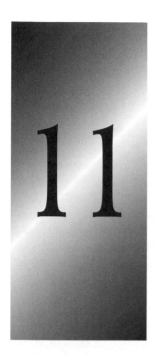

Botulinum Toxin in the Treatment of Upper Limb Spasticity

11

Allison Brashear

The use of botulinum toxin (BoNT) to treat spasticity of the upper extremity has dramatically improved the care of patients with increased tone as part of the upper motor neuron syndrome (UMNS). Before the introduction of BoNT, chemodenervation was only performed by relatively few physicians with injections of phenol and alcohol. The limited access to those performing these injections coupled with concerns about pain and long-term sequlae left many patients without adequate treatment of their UMNS. The introduction of BoNT for the treatment of increased tone has greatly increased the ability of physicians to manage spasticity of the UMNS, focusing on symptoms that interfere with activities of daily living and the ability of the caregiver to care for the patient. Today, the use of BoNT for the treatment of tone in patients with UMNS is one of the most effective and well-tolerated tools physicians use to treat this disabling medical problem.

In 1989, BoNT type A was approved in the United States for injection in the face and eye muscles. Dr Scott and his colleagues developed BoNT as a drug for a temporary treatment of strabismus in children. Dr Scott theorized that small amounts of the potent toxin could temporarily cause relaxation of the injected eye muscle (1, 2). Later, the adaptation of BoNT to treat overactive muscles in the neck, jaw, and limbs was spearheaded by physicians seeking to treat focal medically refractory increases in muscle tone in a variety of movement disorders (3). The ability to select specific muscles, titrate doses for selective relaxation, and avoid systemic side effects allows physicians to treat overactive muscles in many diseases in which there had been no successful treatment before the introduction of BoNT.

Botulinum toxin injections allow the treatment to be focused on a particular muscle or movement. Treatment of upper extremity spasticity with BoNT enables physicians to focus on specific activities and functions important to the patient and/or caregiver. The definition of function varies from patient to patient, and as a result, it is important for clinicians to individualize their treatment approach for each patient. Although all patients with upper extremity spasticity have increased tone, the pattern of presentation may vary by etiology. Likewise, the ability of the patient to participate in adjunct therapy after BoNT treatment may also vary by etiology. For example, central nervous system injury from traumatic brain injury or cerebral palsy may preclude some form of occupational therapy due to cognitive impairment, whereas those with poststroke spasticity may have spatial, language, or speech issues interfering with therapy.

The heterogeneous presentations of upper extremity spasticity have led some investigators to focus on the treatment of spasticity by etiology. As a result, many trials of upper extremity spasticity are limited to common diseases, such as poststroke spasticity. To study a more homogeneous group, many studies have limited enrollment to poststroke spasticity, and further studies may often limit enrollment to those patients requiring sufficient communication skills to complete scales or perform tasks. In clinical practice, the dosing, technique, and benefits noted in the poststroke spasticity trials have been extrapolated to those with traumatic brain injury and cerebral palsy, but trials including adults with spasticity due to traumatic brain injury, adult cerebral palsy, and multiple sclerosis have been small. Therefore, the focus of this chapter will be on poststroke spasticity, but the reader is urged to keep the other causes of the UMNS in mind.

MECHANISM OF ACTION OF BONT

Botulinum toxins are protein neurotoxins produced by several different strains of the *Clostridium botulinum* bacterial species with varying serotype (designated types A through G) (4). Only serotypes A and B have been developed for routine use in health care. Within a serotype, the production varies by manufacturers, and therefore, no generic equivalent is available for these toxins (5). In addition, among serotype A, there are different formulations with different standard doses, and the use of one formulation cannot be easily substituted for another (5). It is important to note that of the commercially available toxin products, the biological activity units are unique to each BoNT preparation and cannot be compared or converted into another.

The mechanism of action of all BoNT serotypes is to inhibit the vesicle-dependent release of acetylcholine and other neurotransmitters from the presynaptic nerve terminal. The binding of the vesicle containing acetylcholine and other transmitters requires a complex set of proteins called "SNARE" proteins (soluble N-ethylmaleimide–sensitive factor attachment protein receptor), which include synaptobrevin (inhibited by serotypes B, D, F, and G); SNAP-25 (inhibited by BoNT-A, -C, and -E); and syntaxin (inhibited by serotype C). The light chain of each serotype acts at a distinct site for one or more of the proteins required for vesicle release. Even when the same protein is affected as in serotypes A, C, and E, the different serotypes affect it at a different site.

In a normally functioning presynaptic nerve terminal, transmitters from the vesicle are released into the synaptic cleft and then bound by receptors on the muscle cell. All of the serotypes of BoNT interfere with this process. The effect of BoNT injection is inhibition of acetylcholine release into the presynaptic cleft. As a result on the postsynaptic membrane, the muscle perceives no input from the nerve terminal and thus becomes "chemically denervated."(3)

CONCERNS ON DOSING

In April 2009, the United States Food and Drug Administration (FDA) mandated a new label warning and risk mitigation strategy for all BoNT sold in the United Sates. A release from the FDA noted that it instigated the labeling change due to reports of systemic spread in some patients and the potential for serious risks associated with the lack of interchangeability among the 3 licensed BoNT products (Botox®, Dysport®, and MyoBloc®). According to the FDA Web site, reports of "spread of toxin has been reported to other areas of the body causing symptoms similar to those of botulism, including unexpected loss of strength or muscle weakness, hoarseness or trouble talking, trouble saying words clearly, loss of bladder control, trouble breathing, trouble swallowing, double vision, blurred vision and drooping eyelids. These symptoms have mostly been reported in children with cerebral palsy being treated with the products for muscle spasticity, an unapproved use of the drugs. Symptoms have also been reported in adults treated both for approved and unapproved uses." The FDA recommended that health care professionals who use BoNTs should do the following: "understand that dosage strength (potency) expressed in 'Units' is different among the botulinum toxin products; clinical doses expressed in units are not interchangeable from one product to another; be alert to and educate patients and caregivers about the potential for effects following administration of botulinum toxins such as unexpected loss of strength or muscle weakness, hoarseness or trouble talking, trouble saying words clearly, loss of bladder control, trouble breathing, trouble swallowing, double vision, blurred vision and drooping eyelids; understand that these effects have been reported as early as several hours and as late as several weeks after treatment; and advise patients to seek immediate medical attention if they develop any of these symptoms." (6)

As part of the new warning, the FDA mandated a risk mitigation strategy on the part of the manufacturers of BoNT in the United States. In the United States, physicians are required to discuss the risk noted above and at each visit give the patient an FDA-approved handout detailing the concerns. This handout is part of the FDA-approved package insert and is included in each package of BoNT. This risk mitigation strategy reminds physicians who use BoNT to be aware of dosing differences between serotypes and between formulations of the same serotypes. The new FDA requirements are a reminder that BoNT is a potent medication that requires skilled use and detailed knowledge of dosing and potential side effects.

WHY DOES BoNT WORK FOR SPASTICITY?

Currently, there are 4 main BoNT products available worldwide for clinical use: BOTOX (Allergan, Inc, Irvine, CA), Dysport (Ipsen Pharmaceuticals, Slough, UK), MyoBloc/Neurobloc® (Solstice Neurosciences, Inc, South San Francisco, CA /Solstice Neurosciences Ltd, Dublin, Ireland), and Xeomin® (Merz Pharmaceuticals GmbH, Frankfurt, Germany). Of the 4 products, 3 are BoNT serotype A (BoNT-A) products (BOTOX, Dysport, and Xeomin), whereas MyoBloc is a BoNT serotype B (BoNT-rim) product. In 2009, the FDA suggested new names to identify the different formulations of BoNT. Botulinum toxin type A (formulated as Botox) is to be referred to as *onabotulinumtoxinA*. Botulinum toxin type A formulated as Dysport is to be referred to as Botulinum toxin type A, formulated as Xeomin, is to be referred to as incobotulinum toxin A. Botulinum toxin type B formulated as MyoBloc is to be referred to as *rimabotulinumtoxinB*. Although no generic forms of BoNT exist, these terms are designed to steer away from brand name terminology in literature and continued medical education (CME) accredited events. The adoption of this new terminology is evolving as physicians and CME providers adjust to FDA recommendations (see Table 11.1) (7).

A majority of the work in the literature in upper extremity spasticity is with either BoNT-ona or BoNT-abo—both type A toxins. BoNT-Inc is the newest type A toxin to appear in the market, and most of the work to date has been limited to studies in blepharospasm and cervical dystonia. Small trials have explored the use of BoNT-rim in spasticity, but large trials with serotype B in spasticity have been lacking (8, 9).

Studies of BoNT-ona in Poststroke Spasticity

In 1996, Simpson et al. (10) published a small double-blind, placebo-controlled, multicenter trial of BoNT-ona in 39 patients with poststroke spasticity. In this dose-finding study, the authors sought to determine the minimally effective dose to treat spasticity at the wrist and elbow in patients with spasticity naive to any BoNT treatment. All patients were at least 9 months poststroke and received treatment of the elbow and wrist flexors only. The finger flexors were not treated. Dosing groups included a total dose of 75, 150, or 300 U of BoNT-ona compared with placebo. The largest dosage group (300 U BoNT-ona) resulted in a statistically and clinically significant mean decrease in wrist flexor tone of 1.2 points ($P = .028$), 1.1 points ($P = .044$), and 1.2 points ($P = .026$) and elbow flexor tone of 1.2 points ($P = .024$), 1.2 points ($P = .028$), and 1.1 points ($P = .199$) at weeks 2, 4, and 6 postinjection. The lower 2 dosage groups of BoNT-ona showed some improvement in tone but did not reach statistical significance. No appreciable changes were noted in the goniometry measurements or functional measures. Adverse effects were limited and well tolerated.

In a multicenter randomized, placebo-controlled study of 3 doses of BoNT-ona across all 3 joints, Childers et al. (11) studied treatment of elbow, wrist, and finger flexors with 3 doses (90, 180, and 360 U) compared to placebo. The primary outcome was the Modified Ashworth (0–4 with half points allowed), a patient and a physicians global rating of change and a frequency of pain rating scale (0–5), and quality of life scales. Patients received up to 2 treatments of either placebo or a total dose of 90, 180, or 360 U. Patients were followed up for a total of 24 weeks. The Modified

---

TABLE 11.1
FDA Terminology for Different Formulations of Botulinum Toxins[a]

Serotype	Brand Name	Manufacturer	FDA Recommended Term	Abbreviation for FDA Recommended Term in This Chapter
A	Botox	Allergan	OnabotulinumtoxinA	BoNT-ona
	Dysport	Ipsen	AbobotulinumtoxinA	BoNT-abo
	Xeomin	Merz	Incobotulinum toxin A	BoNT-inc
B	Myobloc	Solstice	RimabotulinumtoxinB	BoNT-rim

[a]No particular serotype is indicated by BoNT.

Ashworth (0–4 with half point allowed), pain, 36-Item Short Form, and Functional Independence Measure were assessed at 6, 9, 12, and 24 weeks posttreatment. The muscles injection included biceps (50–200 U), flexor digitorium sublimis (7.5–30 U), flexor digitorium profundus (7.5–30 U), flexor carpi radialis (15–60 U), and flexor carpi ulnaris (15–60 U) and were all given with electromyographic guidance. Of the 19 centers involved, a total of 91 subjects enrolled with 77 patients completing the study.

As noted in the earlier Simpson study, the highest total dose of BoNT-ona (360 U) produced the greatest improvement in muscle tone. Those treated with the 180 and 90 U dosages demonstrated less reduction in tone. There were no changes in the 36-Item Short Form, Functional Independence Measure, or life scores. The results of the Simpson and Childers study demonstrated the need for sufficient dosing at multiple joints in the spastic limb. Although a decrease in tone was documented by the Ashworth (see Table 11.2) and Modified Ashworth, neither study demonstrated a functional change.

In 2002, the largest double-blind, placebo-controlled study of toxin-naive patients with spasticity of the wrist and fingers after stroke trial demonstrated sustained improvement over 12 weeks in muscle tone and disability. In addition, Brashear et al. (13) used a novel scale specifically developed for upper extremity BoNT studies, the Disability Assessment Scale (DAS) (see Table 11.3). The DAS was administered with the patient and/or caregiver and physician together rating the impairment of hand hygiene, pain in the hand, look of the hand (cosmesis), or use of the hand in dressing on a simple 0-to-3 scale. The patients selected one (dressing, hygiene, pain, cosmesis) as the most important disability to improve with the treat-

---

TABLE 11.2
Ashworth Scale

0 = no increase in tone (none)
1 = slight increase in tone, giving a catch when the limb is moved in flexion or extension (mild)
2 = more marked increase in tone but limb is easily flexed (moderate)
3 = considerable increase in muscle tone (passive movement difficult, severe)
4 = limb rigid in flexion or extension, (very severe)

Brashear A, Zafonte R, Corcoran M et al. Inter- and intra-rater reliability of the Ashworth Scale and the Disability Assessment Scale in patients with upper-limb poststroke spasticity. Arch Phys Med Rehabil 2002;83(10):1349–1354.

TABLE 11.3
Disability Assessment Scale

Hygiene: Assess the extent of maceration, ulceration, and/or palmar infection; palm and hand cleanliness; ease of cleanliness; ease of nail trimming; and the degree of interference caused by hygiene-related disability in the patient's daily life.
Dressing: Assess the difficulty or ease with which the patient could put on clothing and the degree of interference caused by dressing related disability in the patient's daily life.
Limb Position: Assess the amount of abnormal position of the upper limb.
Pain Assess: the intensity of pain or discomfort related to upper-limb spasticity.

Scoring of DAS

0 = no disability: 1 = mild disability (noticeable but does not interfere significantly with normal activities); 2 = moderate disability (normal activities require increased effort and/or assistance); 3 =severe disability (normal activities limited).

Brashear A, Zafonte R, Corcoran M et al. Inter- and intra-rater reliability of the Ashworth Scale and the Disability Assessment Scale in patients with upper-limb poststroke spasticity. Arch Phys Med Rehabil 2002;83(10):1349–1354.

---

ment. The chosen subscale of the DAS was followed as a secondary outcome measure in the study. As in other large trials with BoNT, the primary outcome measure remained the muscle tone as measured by the Ashworth.

At the end of 12 weeks, subjects treated with BoNT-ona had greater improvement in the wrist and finger flexor tone at each visit than did the placebo group. The maximal difference between the 2 groups in the mean change from baseline occurred at week 4 (wrist: -1.78 active group, -0.42 placebo group [$P < .001$]; finger: -1.59 active , -0.27 placebo group [$P < .001$]). Subjects who received BoNT-ona demonstrated a decrease in muscle tone compared to placebo at all time points in the study ($P < .001$).

The preselected goal of treatment (one subscale of the DAS) demonstrated greater improvement in the treated group than those treated with placebo. At 6 weeks after injection, 40 patients of the active group (62%), as compared to 17 patients in the placebo group (27%), had improvement in their chosen subscale of the DAS. In addition, the treated group demonstrated similar improvement in the DAS subscale at weeks 4 ($P < .001$), 6 ($P < .001$), 8 ($P = .03$), and 12 ($P = .02$). In addition, there was an improvement in all areas measured by the DAS (pain, limb position, hygiene, and dressing) in those treated with drug. Six weeks after injection, 53 (83%) of 64 patients had at east 1-point improvement on the DAS in one or more areas compared with 33 (53%) of 62 patients who received placebo (*P* = .007) (13).

An additional secondary outcome measure, the physicians and patient global assessment also demonstrated improvements in those treated with BoNT-ona. The physicians' assessment was improved in the treated group at all 5 time points in the study (*P* < .001). The patient/caregiver assessment likewise rated more overall improvement in the treated group. (weeks 1, 4, and 6, *P* < .001; weeks 8 and 12, *P* = .002). At week 6, 67% of the patient receiving toxin had a least a 2-point improvement in the physician global rating scale than those receiving placebo (11% with a 2-point improvement). There were no significant differences between the groups of specifically monitored adverse event. The results of this phase III multicenter trial of poststroke spasticity (13) demonstrated that when patients and their physicians jointly select prospectively the goal of treatment, BoNT-ona offers more improvement than placebo.

Sustained Improvement With Repeated Injections

Two clinical trials with repeated use of BoNT-ona in patients with poststroke spasticity in the upper extremity have demonstrated a sustained decrease in muscle tone. In a small study of 28 patients, repeated injections of BoNT-ona in the upper extremity every 3 to 5 months demonstrated continued improvement (14). In a larger study, patients participating in the study by Brashear et al were enrolled in a 42-week open-label study where all were treated with BoNT-ona (15). Over the 42 weeks, the average patient received 2.8 treatments with 61% receiving treatments at 12- to 15-week intervals. The results demonstrate sustained improvement in over the 42-week study with a decrease in the Ashworth and the DAS.

The Ashworth score 6 weeks postinjection at the wrist, finger, and thumb continued to decrease over the course of the study. After the first treatment, 48.2% of patients demonstrated at least a 2-point improvement in their Ashworth 6 weeks after injection, and after the fourth cycle, 61.5% demonstrated at least a 2-point improvement in their Ashworth. Likewise, using the DAS measurement, patients who reported a one or more improvement on the DAS demonstrated the following percent for each subscale: hygiene, 50% to 60%; dressing, 40% to 45%; pain, 25% to 33%; limb position, 46% to 60%.

Like most studies with BoNT-ona, the adverse events were mild or moderate, with 20 (18.2%) of the 110 patients reporting treatment-related adverse events during the entire study. As would be expected with BoNT-ona, injections were well tolerated with the most frequent treatment-associated adverse event of muscle weakness (5.5%, 6/110) and injection site pain (3.6%, 4/110).

Studies of BoNT-abo

BoNT-abo (a different formulation of BoNT-A than discussed above) is approved for use in many countries in Europe for the treatment of spasticity. As of July 2009, BoNT-abo has been approved in the United States for cervical dystonia. The results of several double-blind, placebo-controlled trials demonstrate efficacy in reducing muscle tone of limb spasticity after injection.

In a small 1996 study of 17 subjects, Bhakta treated patients with poststroke spasticity with up to 200 U of BoNT-ona or 1000 U of BoNT-abo. Patients were required to have severe spasticity and "no function" in the arm with no prior benefit from oral medication or physiotherapy. At study enrollment, functional problems reported by the patients before treatment were difficulty with cleaning the palm, cutting fingernails, putting the arm through a sleeve, standing and walking balance, putting on gloves, and rolling over in bed. Treatment consisted of injections to the flexors of the elbow, wrist, and fingers (biceps, flexor digitorum sublimus, flexor digitorum profundus, and flexor carpi ulnaris). Assessment 2 weeks after treatment demonstrated improvement in tone and also improvement in more functional activities. These included improved hand hygiene in 14 of 17 patients, difficulty with sleeves improved in 4 of 16, standing and walking balance improved in 1 of 4, shoulder pain improved in 6 of 9, and wrist pain improved in 5 of 6. Passive range of movement at shoulder, elbow, and wrist also improved after treatment (16).

In a follow-up double-blinded, placebo-controlled 2000 study, Bhakta reported results of 40 patients with poststroke spasticity. Patients were treated with 1000 U of BoNT-abo or placebo. At follow-up, the treatment group demonstrated 22% improvement in disability as compared to a 4.7% improvement in those treated with placebo. Analysis of the individual patients demonstrated improvement in cleaning the palm, putting arms through sleeves, doing physiotherapy at home, and cleaning the armpit of the affected arm. Of 40 patients, 36 had caregivers. The reduction in caregiver burden was reduced compared to those treated with placebo. Of 17 patients who depended on the caregiver to "clean the palm," 8 became independent as compared to no change 17 in the placebo-treated group (17). Bhakta concluded that BoNT-abo is useful for treating patients with stroke who have self-care difficulties due to arm spasticity.

Bakheit et al. (18) reported the results of a double-blind, placebo-controlled trial of 59 patients. Those who received BoNT-abo had a significant reduction in the Modified Ashworth at week 4 compared with the placebo group (P = .004). The magnitude of benefit over the 16-week follow-up period was significantly reduced for the treated group in the wrist (P = .004) and the finger joints (P = .001) when compared with the placebo. The findings of both Bakheit and Bhakta confirm that treatment with BoNT-abo reduced muscle tone in patients with poststroke upper limb spasticity.

Repeated dosing of BoNT-abo in poststroke upper limb spasticity was also reported by Bakheit et al. on 41 subjects who had impairment in a Patient Disability and Caregiver Burden Rating Scale. The Patient Disability Caregiver Burden Rating Scale includes 8 items including cleaning the palm, cutting fingernails, putting the affected arm thru a sleeve, cleaning under the armpit, cleaning around the elbow, standing balance, walking balance, and the ability to perform physiotherapy at home. The caregiver portion included the rating cleaning the palm, cutting fingernails, dressing, and cleaning the armpit (19). In this open-label trial, patients received up to 3 injections of 1000 U of BoNT-abo at least 12 weeks apart. Patients treated with 1000 U of BoNT-abo maintained improvements in muscle tone, patient's perception of disability, and caregiver burden.

Studies of BoNT Type B in Spasticity

BoNT-rim was approved in the United States in 2000 for treatment of cervical dystonia, an involuntary and often painful movement of neck muscles. The literature using BoNT-rim for diseases other than cervical dystonia is limited. Three small pilot studies in the literature discuss the use of BoNT-rim for spasticity (8, 9, 20).

An open-label pilot study suggested that 10,000 U of BoNT-rim in the arm, wrist, and fingers flexors could decrease muscle tone as measured by the Modified Ashworth Scale at weeks 4, 8, and 12 but that dry mouth was reported in 9 of 10 patients (8). A follow-up double-blind, placebo-controlled, 16-week study suggested that 10,000 U is not effective (9). Dry mouth was reported in 8 of the 9 subjects during the double-blind study. A third report combined the treatment of arms and legs with a total fixed dose of 10,000 U (20). Although some benefit was noted, little can be extrapolated from this third small pilot study as the doses varied throughout the study. At this time,

the literature does not suggest that the total BoNT-rim at the dose used for cervical dystonia is effective for spasticity in the upper extremity when used to treat spasticity at the elbow, wrist, and fingers. The use of BoNT-rim to treat spasticity will require further study of dosages before it can be considered an option in the clinical setting.

Defining Clinical Impact

A recent attempt to assess quality of life in 96 patients with upper extremity spasticity treated over 2 cycles with BoNT-abo failed to show changes between the active and placebo group in ratings of quality of life, pain, mood, disability, or care burden. As noted in most prior studies, patients treated with BoNT-abo demonstrated greater reduction in spasticity (Modified Ashworth Scale) (P < .001), which translated into higher Goal Attainment Scales scores (P < .01) and greater global benefit (P < .01). The study reemphasizes the difficulty in capturing quality of life impact when treating a focal body region, even when there is improved ability to achieve personal goals by the participants (21).

Results of a study with 35 sites and 279 patients with upper extremity poststroke spasticity followed up participants for up to 5 serial intramuscular injections of BoNT-ona (200–400 U) divided among the wrist, finger, thumb, and elbow flexors. In addition to muscle tone, each patient's health-related quality of life was assessed by using the Stroke Adapted Sickness Impact Profile and the Visual Analog Scale of the European Quality of Life-5 Dimensions questionnaires. This large, multicenter, open-label study of repeated BoNT-ona treatment in patients with upper-limb poststroke spasticity showed substantial improvements in patients' functional disability, health-related quality of life, and muscle tone (22).

Despite the continued interest in quantifying the clinical impact of BoNT treatment in the upper extremity, physicians continue to increase the use of BoNT. Although there are 2 BoNTs currently available in the United States as of summer 2009, none are FDA-approved for spasticity. Although the lack of FDA approval does not allow marketing for the spasticity indication, the use of BoNT for upper extremity spasticity continues to gain momentum. Injection of BoNT is often the mainstay of therapy of the UMNS, and injections incorporated with an aggressive therapy regimen can often benefit patients and caregivers, improving the use of the arm for activities of daily living and warding off complications such as skin breakdown and contractures. Physicians continue to learn about the injection technique, dosing, and side effects through courses sponsored by leading specialty organizations and CME providers. The interest in BoNT treatment is likely to expand should the FDA approve its use for spasticity. At that time, instruction will become even more important after more physicians, patients, and caregivers become aware of the impact of decreasing tone. Vigilance about dosing, follow-up, and difference between serotypes and formulations will be paramount.

Common Presentations of Upper Extremity Spasticity

Clinical Presentations

The common presentations of spasticity in the upper extremity reflect the pathophysiology of the UMNS. These include flexed elbow, flexed wrist, forearm pronation, clenched hand, and adducted and internally rotated shoulder and any combination of them together. In an individual patient, one part of the limb may be more affected. For example, the patient may retain range of motion at the elbow but have a severely clenched fist, not allowing proper cleaning of the palm (see Figure 11.1).

Treatment of the individual patient must take into account the severity, but also acknowledge the synergy, of the pattern of movement. For example, a clenched hand is often paired with a flexed wrist, but the wrist may be less affected. If the clinician only addresses the finger flexors, there may be cosmetic improvement in the clenched hand, but less functional improvement may be noted if the wrist is not treated because of the synergistic movement of the wrist and fingers. Therefore, treatment of common patterns must

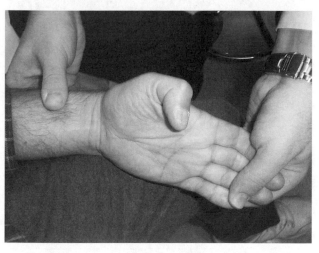

FIGURE 11.1

The thumb in palm deformity seen with hand spasticity.

be taken together as a holistic picture of the impairment of the patient's upper extremity and to what degree spasticity plays a role versus the contribution of the other parts of the UMNS in the overall functional disability of the patient.

The flexed elbow commonly interferes with simple tasks such as reaching, dressing, and eating. Superimposed with difficulty in pronation/supination can further impair the ability to do self-care, feed, and dress. The treatment of the flexed elbow typically involves larger doses than for the finger/wrist flexors. Moreover, treatment of elbow flexors can demonstrate an isolated improvement but may limit an overall improvement in the limb when more complicated movements are required.

The flexed wrist typically presents with some degree of flexion of the fingers and elbow. Isolated treatment of the flexed wrist may be warranted if the wrist flexion is causing pain but the remainder of the hand is loose (see Figure 11.2). However, given the position of an isolated flexed wrist, treatment of the wrist may result in tightening of the fingers secondary to a tenodesis effect and the relationship between the muscles in the hand and wrist. Those treating flexed wrists are encouraged to view it as part of the entire posture of the flexed hand. The muscles involved in a flexed wrist include flexor carpi ulnaris, palmaris longus, and flexor carpi radialis with doses depending on past dosing history and the degree of spasticity.

The clenched hand is by far the best-known presentation of the UMNS in the upper extremity (see Figure 11.3). By virtue of the intricate details of the hand, treatment of the clenched hand with BoNT can improve hand hygiene, allowing the palm to be accessed; can allow participation in occupational therapy and wearing of splints; and can improve self-care such as dressing and feeding.

Injection Technique

Many injectors of BoNT use electromyographic guidance or stimulation to determine the muscles needed for injections. More recently, some physicians are using ultrasound for localization of difficult-to-reach muscles (23). Some physicians may use palpation and/or clinical presentation to determine which muscles require treatment. None of these techniques have been studied in a comparative large trial. A recent American Academy of Neurology (AAN) position paper on BoNT noted that there is insufficient data to support or refute the use of electromyography or stimulation in the treatment of limb spasticity (24). A recent study looked at the utility of finding end plates in injection of the elbow flexors and found benefit to this

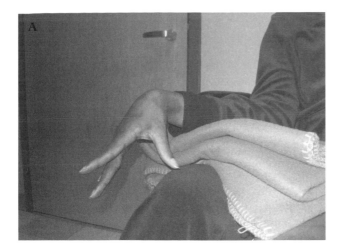
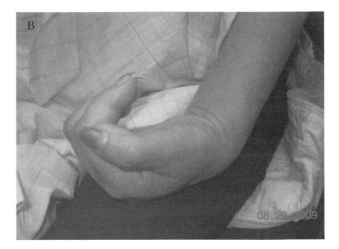

FIGURE 11.2

Flexed wrist. (A) The impact of increase tone at the wrist on function despite good range of motion at the fingers. (B) The flexed wrist as part of the typical flexed elbow, wrist, and fingers seen in poststroke spasticity.

technique (25). However, the time and discomfort of localizing end plates needs to be considered when translating this technique to clinical practice.

Dosing of BoNT is determined by past experiences, size of the muscle, amount of tone, residual function of the spastic muscles, potential of functional loss that may result from decreased tone, and experience of the treating physicians. As an example, a patient who relies on tone to hold a steering wheel to drive may be disappointed to have the tone reduced. Dosage tables recently published in a large monograph of spasticity are based upon feedback of experts in the

field (26). Although dose-finding studies on upper extremity spasticity with 2 of the specific formulations of type A serotypes (BoNT-ona and BoNT-abo) have been performed, the volume delivered and the number of sites per muscle has not been studied.

CASE REPORT 1: TREATMENT TO IMPROVE PASSIVE FUNCTION

A 60-year-old woman presented with spasticity in the arm and wrist after a stroke. The stroke 5 years prior left

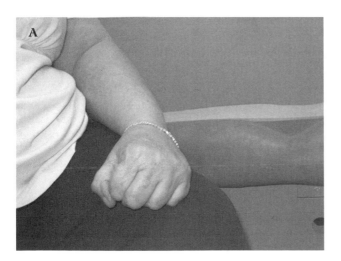
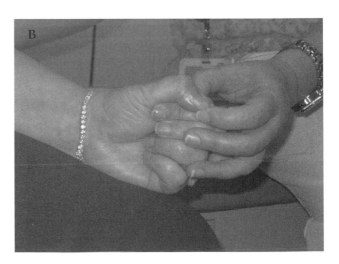

FIGURE 11.3

Clenched fist. (A) Position of the clenched fist interfering with splinting and hand hygiene. (B) An additional view of the clenched fist, note the potential for maceration of the palm by nails and difficulty with hand hygiene and caregiving.

her with a right hemiparesis and some word-findings difficulties. Immediately after the stroke, she had 8 weeks of inpatient therapy and was discharged to a skilled nursing faculty with a splint and with oral medications. Her daughter brought her to a clinic to report excessive sedation and problems with cleaning the hand.

On examination, the patient had a clenched fist with difficulty in opening the fingers and the thumb. The palm was macerated with a foul smell. The wrist was flexed and difficult to move. The elbow had full preserved passive range of motion. The splint the daughter brought to the clinic was impossible to apply and attempts brought complaints of pain from the patient.

The Ashworth scores were the following: the elbow, 1; wrist, 3; and fingers, 4. The DAS scores were the following: hygiene, 3; cosmesis, 2; dressing, 3; and pain, 3.

The patient was treated with BoNT at the elbow (biceps), wrist (flexor carpi ulnaris, flexor carpi radialis), finger flexors (flexor digitorum superficialis, flexor digitorum profundus), and thumb (flexor policis brevis). Follow-up 4 weeks late in the clinic noted improved passive range of motion at the elbow, wrist, and finger with a reported improvement in the ability to clean the palm. The patient's daughter reported that she would now wear her splint at bedtime.

CASE REPORT 2: TREATMENT TO IMPROVE ACTIVE FUNCTION

A 25-year-old man presented to a clinic with increased tone in the fingers and wrist. He is 1 year from a traumatic brain injury and already has had 8 weeks of inpatient therapy. The patient had an intrathecal baclofen pump placed 4 months before presentation to treat excessive tone in the lower extremities with good success. His complaint in coming to the clinic include inability to release his grip on objects like soda cans and that his thumb is always flexed and constantly caught on clothing The occupational therapist notes that his tone in the finger flexes interferes with his ability to have a useful grip and that his thumb is also problematic. She also recommends splinting that allows more active movement and suggests therapy be started after tone is reduced.

Examination reveals an Ashworth score of 2 at the wrist and finger flexors, with a score of 1 at the elbow. He has good active function at the elbow and is able to reach for items with good extension. After consultation with the therapist and counseling the patient about the risk and benefits of BoNT injections,

the patient is treated with injections in the finger flexors and wrist flexors. The dose is much lower than the patient in case 1 because of the desire to improve active function in the hand. The patient started occupational therapy 2 weeks after injections with an intensive program to the upper extremities.

CONSENSUS STATEMENTS AND EVIDENCE REVIEWS

In 2008, the AAN published a position statement on the use of BoNT in the treatment of spasticity (24). The review was focused on BoNT use in general and did not focus on specific serotypes. Authors reviewed, abstracted, and classified articles on BoNT and spasticity using the AAN criteria (class I-IV criteria). Based upon the 14 class I studies in adult spasticity, the experts recommended that BoNT should be offered as a treatment option for the treatment of spasticity in adults. Similarly, in 2009, a European group of clinicians experienced in the use of BoNT for treatment of spasticity after brain injury published a consensus statement of the management of spasticity in adults. Authors noted that BoNT should be provided as part of an integrated program. As noted elsewhere in the literature, the authors noted, "there is not simple or accurate way to converting the unit potency of one preparation to anther, it is important that clinicians are familiar with the characteristics and dosages of each preparation they use and do not try to covert or extrapolate from one preparation to another." (27)

SUMMARY

BoNT is an effective therapy for the increased tone associated with UMNS. Treatment with BoNT should involve appropriate goal selection. Chemodenervation with BoNT should be considered one component of the management of this condition. Dosage selection of BoNT should be individualized to obtain optimal results. Physicians treating patients with BoNT should be aware of the different serotypes, formulations, and literature in spasticity.

References

1. Scott AB, Magoon EH, McNeer KW, Stager DR. Botulinum treatment of strabismus in children. Trans Am Ophthalmol Soc 1989;87:174–180.
2. Scott AB, Rosenbaum A, Collins CC. Pharmacologic weakening of extraocular muscles. Invest Ophthalmol 1973; 12(12):924–927.

3. Jankovic J, Brin MF. Therapeutic uses of botulinum toxin. N Engl J Med 1991;324(17)1186–1194.

4. Hatheway CL. Botulism: the present status of the disease. Curr Top Microbiol Immunol 1995;195:55–75.

5. Brashear A. Clinical comparisons of botulinum neurotoxin formulations. Neurologist 2008;14(5):289–298.

6. http://www.fda.gov/NewsEvents/Newsroom/PressAnnouncements/ucm149574.htm accessed July 19,2009. 7–19–0009. 7–19–0009.

7. http://www.fda.gov/Drugs/DrugSafety/PostmarketDrugSafetyInformationforPatientsandProviders/DrugSafetyInformationforHeathcareProfessionals/ucm174949.htm. 2009. 10–3–0009.

8. Brashear A, McAfee AL, Kuhn ER, Ambrosius WT. Treatment with botulinum toxin type B for upper-limb spasticity. Arch Phys Med Rehabil 2003;84(1)103–107.

9. Brashear A, McAfee AL, Kuhn ER, Fyffe J. Botulinum toxin type B in upper-limb poststroke spasticity: a double-blind, placebo-controlled trial. Arch Phys Med Rehabil 2004;85(5): 705–709.

10. Simpson DM, Alexander DN, O'Brien CF et al. Botulinum toxin type A in the treatment of upper extremity spasticity: a randomized, double-blind, placebo-controlled trial. Neurology 1996;46(5):1306–1310.

11. Childers MK, Brashear A, Jozefczyk P et al. Dose-dependent response to intramuscular botulinum toxin type A for upper-limb spasticity in patients after a stroke. Arch Phys Med Rehabil 2004;85(7):1063–1069.

12. Brashear A, Zafonte R, Corcoran M et al. Inter- and intrarater reliability of the Ashworth Scale and the Disability Assessment Scale in patients with upper-limb poststroke spasticity. Arch Phys Med Rehabil 2002;83(10):1349–1354.

13. Brashear A, Gordon MF, Elovic E et al. Intramuscular injection of botulinum toxin for the treatment of wrist and finger spasticity after a stroke. N Engl J Med 2002;347(6):395–400.

14. Lagalla G, Danni M, Reiter F, Ceravolo MG, Provinciali L. Post-stroke spasticity management with repeated botulinum toxin injections in the upper limb. Am J Phys Med Rehabil 2000;79(4):377–384.

15. Gordon MF, Brashear A, Elovic E et al. Repeated dosing of botulinum toxin type A for upper limb spasticity following stroke. Neurology 2004;63(10):1971–1973.

16. Bhakta BB, Cozens JA, Bamford JM, Chamberlain MA. Use of botulinum toxin in stroke patients with severe upper limb spasticity. J Neurol Neurosurg Psychiatry 1996;61(1): 30–35.

17. Bhakta BB, Cozens JA, Chamberlain MA, Bamford JM. Impact of botulinum toxin type A on disability and carer burden due to arm spasticity after stroke: a randomised double blind placebo controlled trial. J Neurol Neurosurg Psychiatry 2000; 69(2):217–221.

18. Bakheit AM, Pittock S, Moore AP et al. A randomized, double-blind, placebo-controlled study of the efficacy and safety of botulinum toxin type A in upper limb spasticity in patients with stroke. Eur J Neurol 2001;8(6):559–565.

19. Bakheit AM, Fedorova NV, Skoromets AA, Timerbaeva SL, Bhakta BB, Coxon L. The beneficial antispasticity effect of botulinum toxin type A is maintained after repeated treatment cycles. J Neurol Neurosurg Psychiatry 2004;75(11):1558–1561.

20. O'Brien CF. Treatment of spasticity with botulinum toxin. Clin J Pain 2002;18(6 Suppl):S182–S190.

21. McCrory P, Turner-Stokes L, Baguley IJ et al. Botulinum toxin A for treatment of upper limb spasticity following stroke: a multi-centre randomized placebo-controlled study of the effects on quality of life and other person-centred outcomesJ Rehabil Med 2009;41(7):536–544.

22. Elovic EP, Brashear A, Kaelin D et al. Repeated treatments with botulinum toxin type a produce sustained decreases in the limitations associated with focal upper-limb poststroke spasticity for caregivers and patients. Arch Phys Med Rehabil 2008;89(5):799–806.

23. Elovic EP, Esquenazi A, Alter KE, Lin JL, Alfaro A, Kaelin DL. Chemodenervation and nerve blocks in the diagnosis and management of spasticity and muscle overactivity. PM R 2009; 1(9):842–851.

24. Simpson DM, Gracies JM, Graham HK et al. Assessment: botulinum neurotoxin for the treatment of spasticity (an evidence-based review): report of the Therapeutics and Technology Assessment Subcommittee of the American Academy of Neurology4. Neurology 2008;70(19):1691–1698.

25. Gracies JM, Lugassy M, Weisz DJ, Vecchio M, Flanagan S, Simpson DM. Botulinum toxin dilution and endplate targeting in spasticity: a double-blind controlled study Arch Phys Med Rehabil 2009;90(1):9–16.

26. Brashear A. Clinical trials in the treatment of spasticity with botulinum toxin. Brashear A, Mayer NH, (eds.). Spasticity and other forms of muscle overactivity in the upper motor neuron syndrome.NY, 2008:163–170. We move.

27. Wissel J, Ward AB, Erztgaard P. et al. European consensus table on the use of botulinum toxin type A in adult spasticity. J Rehabil Med 2009;41(1):13–25.

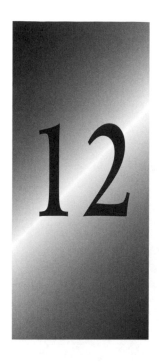

Anatomical Correlation of Common Patterns of Spasticity

Mayank Pathak
Daniel Truong

Spasticity and upper motor neuron syndrome produce abnormal involuntary postures of the affected body parts. The particular posture assumed depends on the size, strength, and relative degree of tone among the various muscles that act across the joint in question. The summation of the various force vectors exerted by these muscles, a complex interaction of agonists, antagonists, and supplementary muscles, along with the viscoelasticity of the muscles involved, determines the particular posture assumed at any joint or set of joints. Thus, it is important to understand not only the structure of a particular joint and the different directions in which it can move but also the location and relative strengths of muscles that cross it. Knowledge of the origins and insertions of these muscles will help the practitioner understand the kinesiology and directions of their pull and thus determine which ones are most active in a particular spastic patient. To facilitate a better understanding of this clinical phenomenon, this chapter will address these anatomical considerations for major joints of the upper and lower limbs.

THE SHOULDER

Anatomy

Joint: To facilitate its function, the shoulder has the most degrees of freedom of movement of any joint in the body. The primary shoulder joint, that is, the glenohumeral articulation, is a multiaxial joint, with the spheroid head of the humerus being held in the shallow concavity of the glenoid fossa of the scapula (1). This nominal ball-and-socket arrangement would fall apart if not strapped together by the muscles and tendons that run across it. As a result of this fact, numerous postural abnormalities may be encountered as a result of upper motor neuron syndrome. The actions of various shoulder muscles are complex and may be different, depending on the starting position, which part of a particular muscle is exerting the most force, and whether their points of origin or insertion are fixed at the start of the motion. In discussing the major shoulder muscles below, they will be arranged according to their major vector of action among patients with spasticity.

Abduction: The deltoid originates along the acromion and adjacent clavicle, running across the shoulder joint to insert on the shaft of the humerus (Figures 12.1 and 12.9). Its action is to abduct the humerus (2). It is generally overpowered by adductors in spasticity.

External Rotation: Underneath the deltoid lies a group of 4 muscles that make up the rotator cuff. Three of these comprise the external rotators: the supraspinatus, infraspinatus, and teres minor, all of which originate on the posterior aspect of the scapula and insert on the posterior surface of the proximal part of the humerus, at and below the greater tubercle (Figure 12.1).

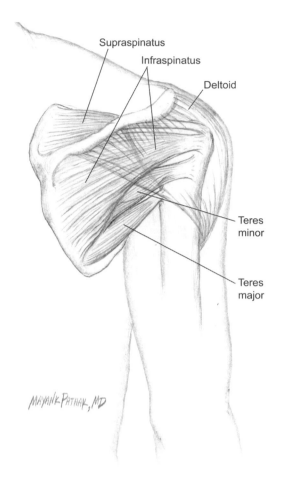

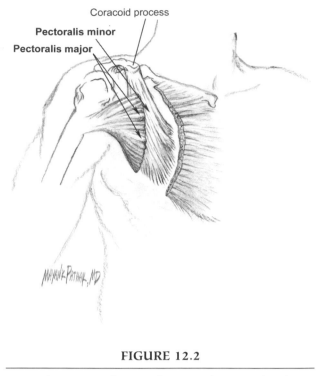

FIGURE 12.2

Pectoralis major and pectoralis minor. (Reprinted with permission from Daniel Truong, Dirk Dressler, Mark Hallett, Eds. *Manual of Botulinum Toxin Therapy*, 2009, © Cambridge University Press.)

FIGURE 12.1

Deltoid, supraspinatus, infraspinatus, teres minor, and teres major. (Reprinted with permission from Daniel Truong, Dirk Dressler, Mark Hallett, Eds. *Manual of Botulinum Toxin Therapy*, 2009, © Cambridge University Press.)

Their action is to externally rotate the humerus, with the supraspinatus also contributing to abduction (3).

Internal Rotation: The fourth rotator cuff muscle, that is, the subscapularis, originates on the anterior surface of the scapula, extending forward to insert on the lesser tubercle on the anterior surface of the humerus, thereby preventing anterior subluxation of the humeral head; its action is to internally rotate the humerus while thrusting the scapula forward (4).

The most powerful internal rotator is the pectoralis major, which has a clavicular head originating from the medial half of the clavicle on its anterior side and a sternocostal head originating from the sternum, the costal cartilage of ribs 1-6, rib 7, and the aponeurosis of the external oblique (Figure 12.2). These fibers all converge to insert on the anterolateral humerus. The

principal action of the pectoralis major is to adduct and medially rotate the humerus, and it also acts as a flexor of the glenohumeral joint for the first 60°(5, 6).

The teres major originates on the posterior surface of the scapula near the inferior angle, inserting medial the anterior midline bicipital ridge of the humerus (Figures 12.1 and 12.3). It is involved in internal rotation and extension of the humerus (5).

Elevation: The next 2 muscles to be discussed are shoulder elevators. The levator scapulae originates from the transverse processes of C1-C4, inserting on the upper medial border of the scapula (Figure 12.4), its actions being to elevate the scapula and rotate the top outward. The trapezius originates from the occiput, nuchal ligament, and spinous processes of the cervical and thoracic vertebrae (Figure 12.4). Its upper fibers insert on the lateral clavicle and acromion, and its middle and lower fibers insert along the scapular spine. The upper fibers elevate the scapula and the entire shoulder joint. Activation of the middle and lower fibers can adduct and depress the scapula (7).

Other Muscles: The latissimus dorsi originates along a wide stretch of medial back structures from

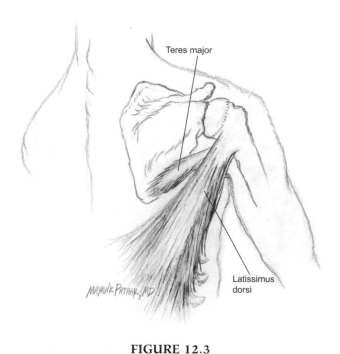

FIGURE 12.3

Latissimus dorsi and teres major. (Reprinted with permission from Daniel Truong, Dirk Dressler, Mark Hallett, Eds. *Manual of Botulinum Toxin Therapy*, 2009, © Cambridge University Press.)

the sacrum to the midthoracic vertebrae, inserting medial to the anterior midline of the proximal humerus (Figure 12.3), its main actions being adduction, internal rotation, and extension (8, 9).

The coracobrachialis originates on the coracoid process and inserts on the medial surface of the humeral shaft, flexing and adducting the humerus (10). The pectoralis minor originates on ribs 3-5 and runs diagonally cephalad and laterally to insert on the coracoid process of the scapula (Figure 12.2). With the ribs fixed, it pulls the scapula downward and forward, moving the shoulder joint anteriorly.

Spastic Postures

Shoulder Adduction and Internal Rotation: Muscles that adduct and internally rotate the humerus at the glenohumeral joint are the strongest; thus, the adducted and internally rotated posture is the most commonly encountered among spastic patients (Figure 12.5). Activities that are impaired by this posture and that can be ameliorated by the application of botulinum toxin include donning and doffing of clothing, caregiver-assisted mobility and transfers, and hygienic care of the axilla (11). The principal muscles involved in this posture include the pectoralis major, latissimus

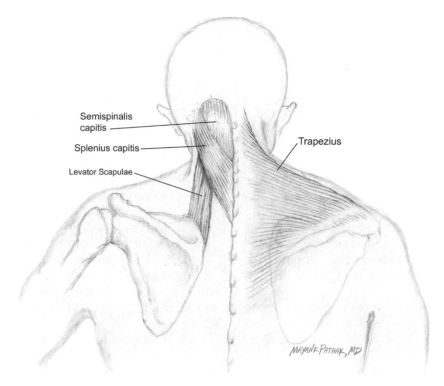

FIGURE 12.4

Semispinalis capitis, splenius capitis, levator scapulae, and trapezius. (Reprinted with permission from Daniel Truong, Dirk Dressler, Mark Hallett, Eds. *Manual of Botulinum Toxin Therapy*, 2009, © Cambridge University Press.)

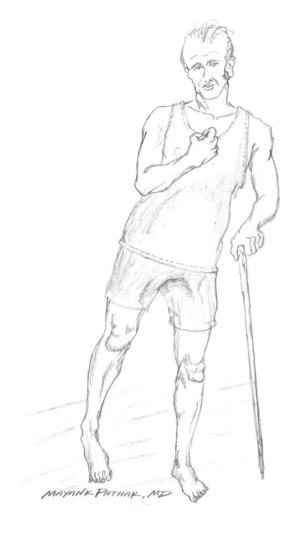

MAYANK PATHAK, MD

FIGURE 12.5

Right-sided spastic hemiplegia. (Reprinted with permission from Daniel Truong, Dirk Dressler, Mark Hallett, Eds. *Manual of Botulinum Toxin Therapy*, 2009, © Cambridge University Press.)

dorsi, teres major, and subscapularis, any or all of which may be targeted for chemodenervation.

Shoulder Hyperextension: Hyperextension is a less common pattern of spastic posture but can occur if the subscapularis and pectoralis muscles are not strongly contractile. This allows the latissimus dorsi and teres major, along with the posterior deltoid and long head of triceps, to pull the humerus in a posterior direction. With spasticity in the shoulder extensor muscles, active shoulder flexion may be slowed.

Shoulder Subluxation: After acute central nervous system injury, there is an initial period of flaccidity before the onset of spasticity. During this flaccid

phase, sufficient laxity may occur in the rotator cuff and other shoulder strap muscles to allow inferior and/or anterior subluxation of the glenohumeral joint, especially when traction is placed on the paretic limb by caregivers attempting to move the patient (12). This subluxation may become a chronic problem, failing to resolve after the onset of spasticity, and can lead to long-term pain and increase in disability (13, 14). In treating shoulder joint spasticity with botulinum toxin, it is important to assess for the presence of subluxation and to avoid exacerbating the problem by chemodenervation of rotator cuff muscles or by excessive dosing of other muscles crossing the humerus. These can include the deltoid and the pectoralis major and minor.

THE ELBOW

Joint Anatomy: The elbow is capable of 4 types of movement: flexion, extension, pronation, and supination. Flexion/Extension movements occur at the humeroulnar joint, a hinge-like complex comprised of the rounded trochlea of the distal humerus resting in the concave trochlear notch of the proximal ulna. Pronation and supination occur at the humeroradial joint, a biaxial joint that can rotate along the long axis of the radius as well as being able to move in a transverse axis during flexion/extension (15). Any combination of these directions of movement can be involved in spastic posturing.

Flexion and Supination: Because the flexors and supinators are more powerful, they generally predominate in spasticity; thus, the flexed elbow with the forearm supinated is most frequently encountered among patients (Figure 12.5).

The principal muscles involved are the biceps, brachialis, brachioradialis, and pronator teres (discussed under pronators). The elbow flexors are strongest in work in different positions. The biceps is strongest in supination, whereas the brachialis is most involved in pronation, and the brachioradialis is strongest in the neutral position The biceps has 2 heads, each originating on different parts of the scapula: a short head originating on the coracoid process and a long head originating on the supraglenoid tubercle (Figure 12.6). The biceps inserts onto the radial tuberosity and also forms the bicipital aponeurosis, which inserts into the fascia of the medial forearm (Figure 12.7). The biceps thus produces both flexion and strong supination of the forearm at the elbow joint (16).

The brachialis originates over a large area of the distal half of the anterior humerus and inserts onto the coronoid process and tuberosity of the proximal

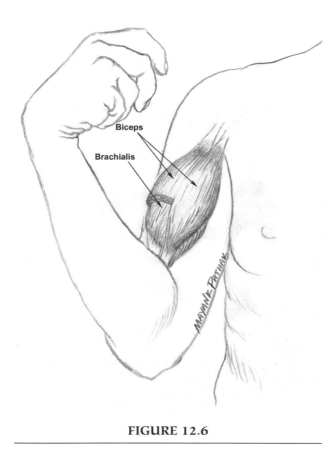

FIGURE 12.6

Biceps and brachialis. (Reprinted with permission from Daniel Truong, Dirk Dressler, Mark Hallett, Eds. *Manual of Botulinum Toxin Therapy*, 2009, © Cambridge University Press.)

ulna (Figure 12.6). It is a pure flexor of the elbow; not inserting on the radius, it has no contribution to the rotation of the radius and therefore does not pronate or supinate the forearm (17). The third elbow flexor, that is, brachioradialis, originates on the distal humerus and inserts distally on the styloid process of the radius (Figure 12.8).

Extension: Extension is a less common spastic posture at this joint and is produced by 2 muscles, that is, the triceps brachii and anconeus. The triceps, forming the bulk of the posterior upper arm, has, as its name indicates, 3 heads (Figure 12.9). Two of these, that is, the medial and lateral heads, originate along the posterior humerus, whereas the third, that is, the long head, originates on the infraglenoid tubercle of the scapula. The triceps crosses the elbow joint to insert on the olecranon process of the ulna. The second elbow extensor muscle is the anconeus. Originating on the lateral epicondyle of the humerus, it inserts distal to the joint on the olecranon and adjacent part of the proximal ulna (18). Its belly can be palpated over the lateral part of the olecranon, and it plays a minor role in extension movements.

Pronation: Pronator teres has a humeral head originating on the medial epicondyle of the humerus and contributing to elbow flexion and an ulnar head originating on the coronoid process of the proximal ulna and producing pronation of the forearm (Figure 12.7). Pronation movement also occurs at the wrist, being produced by the pronator quadratus, which originates

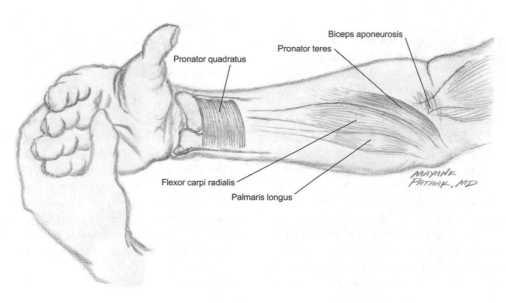

FIGURE 12.7

Flexor carpi radialis, palmaris longus, pronator teres, and pronator quadratus. (Reprinted with permission from Daniel Truong, Dirk Dressler, Mark Hallett, Eds. *Manual of Botulinum Toxin Therapy*, 2009, © Cambridge University Press.)

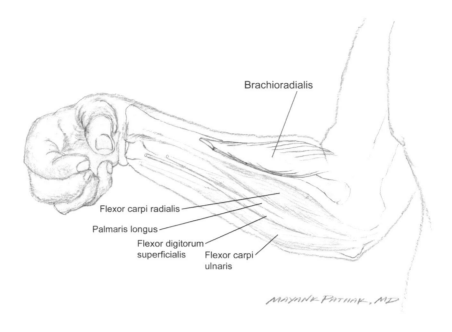

FIGURE 12.8

Flexor digitorum superficialis, FCU, brachioradialis, FCR, and palmaris longus. (Reprinted with permission from Daniel Truong, Dirk Dressler, Mark Hallett, Eds. *Manual of Botulinum Toxin Therapy*, 2009, © Cambridge University Press.)

on the anteromedial surface of the distal ulna and inserts on the anterior surface of the radius (19).

THE WRIST

Joint Anatomy: The wrist joint consists mainly of the distal ends of the radius and ulna against the proximal surfaces of the scaphoid, lunate, and triquetrum (20). The spastic wrist is usually flexed and often accompanies a flexion of the elbow and fingers.

Flexion: Three principal muscles will be discussed. The flexor carpi radialis (FCR) starts at the common flexor tendon, which originates on the medial epicondyle of the humerus, and runs longitudinally along the medial half of the anterior forearm to insert on the second and third metacarpals. It flexes the wrist with slight abduction. Closely related to the FCR, sharing a common origin and running a parallel course adjacent to its medial edge, is the palmaris longus, whose tendon of insertion merges into the palmar aponeurosis (Figures 12.7 and 12.8). This muscle is variable in morphology and may be absent or entirely tendinous in some persons. The flexor carpi ulnaris (FCU) has 2 heads, that is, a humeral head that arises from the common flexor tendon and an ulnar head originating from the medial surface of the olecranon

of the ulna (Figure 12.8). The FCU runs a longitudinal course in the medial forearm, inserting on the pisiform carpal bone (21). Finger flexor muscles, discussed elsewhere, also contribute to wrist flexion.

Extension: Extension is a less frequently encountered posture because the muscles producing this movement are relatively weaker. The extensor carpi radialis longus crosses 2 major joints. Originating on the lateral supracondylar ridge and lateral epicondyle of the humerus, it courses along the posterolateral forearm, its fibers becoming tendinous along the way, and inserts on the base of the second metacarpal. Closely related to the extensor carpi radialis longus is the extensor carpi radialis brevis, which originates at the common extensor tendon from the lateral epicondyle of the humerus and inserts on the base of the third metacarpal. Both of these muscles produce extension at the wrist joint along with abduction of the hand. The third major extensor, that is, the extensor carpi ulnaris, originates at the common extensor tendon of the lateral epicondyle of the humerus and runs longitudinally in the medial half of the dorsal surface of the forearm to insert along the dorsal surface of the fifth metacarpal. It extends and adducts the hand at the wrist (22). It should be noted that spastic activation of the wrist extensors also tends to produce

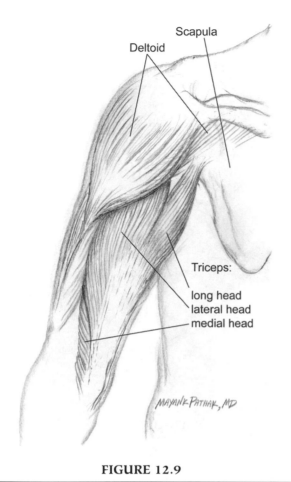

FIGURE 12.9

Triceps and deltoid. (Reprinted with permission from Daniel Truong, Dirk Dressler, Mark Hallett, Eds. *Manual of Botulinum Toxin Therapy*, 2009, © Cambridge University Press.)

secondary flexion at the metacarpophalangeal (MCP) joints as the tendons of the long finger flexors come under tension when the wrist is extended.

THE HAND

Anatomy

Joint: The principal joints to be considered are the 5 MCP joints at which the main directions of movement are flexion and extension, with smaller adduction/abduction movements, and the proximal and distal interphalangeal (IP) joints of the fingers and IP joint of the thumb, at which flexion and extension occur. The stronger muscles are the flexors and adductors; thus, the clenched fist, along with curled thumb, is the most frequently encountered posture in spastic patients; however, other patterns are important to consider as well.

Finger Flexion: Flexion at the proximal IP joint is produced mainly by the flexor digitorum superficialis (FDS). The FDS has one head that originates on the coronoid process of the ulna and the common flexor tendon and another head that originates on the anterior surface of the radius. The fibers of FDS insert on the middle phalanges of the 4 fingers (Figure 12.10). Flexion at the distal IP joints is produced by the flexor digitorum profundus (FDP), which originates on the antereomedial shaft of the ulna and interosseous membrane; it inserts into the ventral side of the bases of the distal phalanges, producing flexion at the distal IP joints (Figure 12.11). Flexion at the MCP joints of the

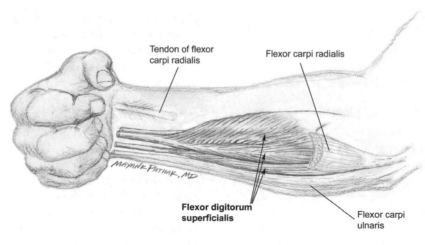

FIGURE 12.10

Flexor digitorum superficialis, FCR, and FCU. (Reprinted with permission from Daniel Truong, Dirk Dressler, Mark Hallett, Eds. *Manual of Botulinum Toxin Therapy*, 2009, © Cambridge University Press.)

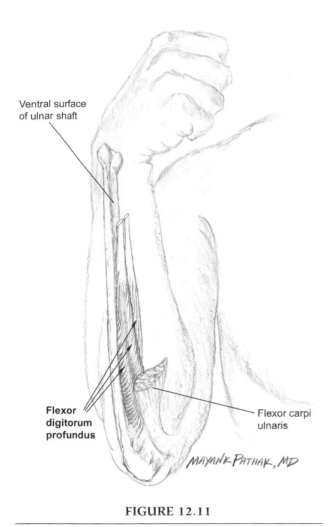

Ventral surface
of ulnar shaft

**Flexor
digitorum
profundus**

Flexor carpi
ulnaris

MAYANK PATHAK, MD

FIGURE 12.11

Flexor digitorum profundus and FCU. (Reprinted with permission from Daniel Truong, Dirk Dressler, Mark Hallett, Eds. *Manual of Botulinum Toxin Therapy*, 2009, © Cambridge University Press.)

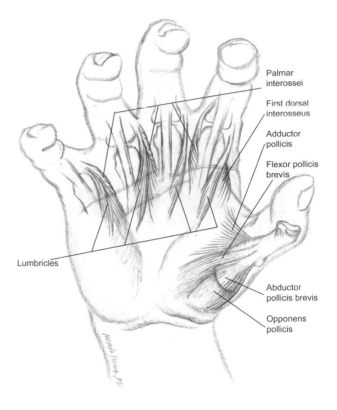

Palmar
interossei

First dorsal
interosseus

Adductor
pollicis

Flexor pollicis
brevis

Lumbricles

Abductor
pollicis brevis

Opponens
pollicis

FIGURE 12.12

Adductor pollicis brevis, flexor pollicis brevis, opponens pollicis, adductor pollicis, palmar interossei, dorsal interossei, and lumbricles. (Reprinted with permission from Daniel Truong, Dirk Dressler, Mark Hallett, Eds. *Manual of Botulinum Toxin Therapy*, 2009, © Cambridge University Press.)

4 fingers is produced by the FDS and FDP because their tendons must cross this joint to insert on the phalanges, as well as by a set of intrinsic hand muscles, that is, the lumbricles, to be discussed later (23).

Abduction and Adduction: Abduction and adduction at the MCP joints are produced by the interossei. Originating from the metacarpals and inserting onto the proximal phalanges, a set of 4 dorsal and 3 palmar interossei occupy the spaces between the metacarpals (Figure 12.12). The palmar group adducts the fingers, drawing them together in the common spastic posture; the dorsal group may sometimes act to spread the fingers (24).

Spastic Postures

The Clenched Fist: Fist clenching is produced by spastic action of the muscles discussed above and may be combined with either a flexed or extended wrist, for which the principal muscles of action have already been reviewed. The clenched fist may impair hygienic care of the hand and lead to maceration or ulceration of the palmar surface.

Flexion Plus Extension: Another posture, which is occasionally encountered, is the combination of flexion at the MCP joints and extension at the IP joints. This posture is produced by the interaction of the extrinsic finger flexors and extensors located in the forearm, as well as by a set of intrinsic hand muscles, that is, the lumbricles (Figure 12.12). Originating from the tendons of FDP, the lumbricles insert on the tendons of the extensor digitorum, producing a hand posture that might be used to hold this book by its edge (25).

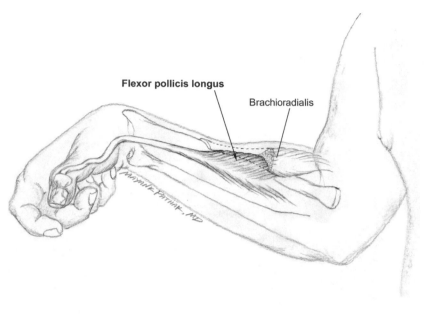

FIGURE 12.13

Flexor pollicis longus and brachioradialis. (Reprinted with permission from Daniel Truong, Dirk Dressler, Mark Hallett, Eds. *Manual of Botulinum Toxin Therapy*, 2009, © Cambridge University Press.)

Thumb Curling: The MCP joint of the thumb is more mobile than those of the other digits, and thus, the thumb can move to oppose any of the other fingers at this joint as well as moving in flexion, extension, adduction, and abduction. In spasticity, the thumb may be curled over the flexed fingers or may be bent into the palm. The muscles of the thenar eminence, that is, the flexor pollicis brevis, abductor pollicis brevis, and opponens pollicis, originate from carpal bones and the flexor retinaculum. The first 2 muscles insert on the proximal phalanx, and the opponens inserts on the first metacarpal (Figure 12.12). Their collective action is to pull their bones of insertion anteriorly and medially, drawing the thumb across the hand and flexing the MCP joint. The adductor pollicis (Figure 12.12), which spans the web between the first 2 metacarpals, draws these 2 bones together as well as flexing the MCP joint. The final muscle to consider for the thumb is the flexor pollicis longus (Figure 12.13), which originates from the anterior radius and inserts on the base of the thumb's distal phalanx, producing flexion at the IP joint (26).

THE HIP

Joint Anatomy: The hip is a multiaxial joint in which the hemispheroid head of the femur rests in the deep socket of the acetabulum. This relatively deep articulation, together with the joint's capsule and ligaments, makes it more stable in comparison with the shoulder and less prone to subluxation at the expense of some reduction in range of mobility. The hip is capable of flexion up to 120° (with the knee flexed) and extension of up to 30° with the knee extended. In addition to these principal motions, the hip can be moved in adduction, abduction, internal rotation, and external rotation (27). The actions of the various hip muscles are complex and vary depending on the starting position, which part of a particular muscle is activated, and whether the pelvis or the femur is fixed at the start of the motion. Muscles will therefore be described in regard to their major contribution to abnormal posture in spastic patients.

Flexion: The 3 strongest contributors to hip flexion are the rectus femoris (described later among the knee extensors), the psoas, and the iliacus (Figure 12.14). The psoas originates along vertebral bodies, transverse processes, and intervertebral discs of the lower spine from T12 to L5. The iliacus originates broadly on the anterior surface of the iliac fossa. Its fibers converge onto the tendon of the psoas. The fibers of these 2 muscles converge onto a common tendon that inserts on the lesser trochanter of the proximal femur (28). Other thigh muscles that cross the hip joint also contribute to hip flexion.

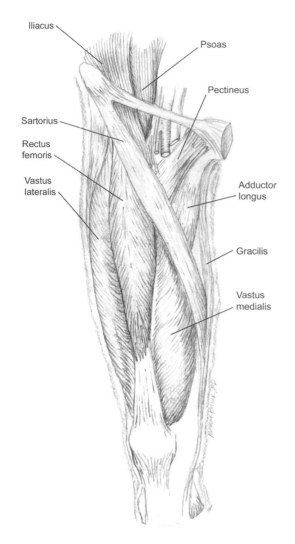

FIGURE 12.14

Rectus femoris, vastus lateralis, vastus medialis, sartorius, iliacus, psoas, pectineus, adductor longus, and gracilis. (Reprinted with permission from Daniel Truong, Dirk Dressler, Mark Hallett, Eds. *Manual of Botulinum Toxin Therapy*, 2009, © Cambridge University Press.)

Extension: Extension of the hip is occasionally a clinically problematic posture among spastic patients. The gluteus maximus (Figure 12.15), originating from the posterior iliac fossa, sacrum, and sacrotuberous ligament, and inserting on the posterior femoral shaft and the fascia latae, is the major contributor among pelvic muscles (29). The hamstring group, discussed below, also contributes.

Internal Rotation: There are 3 principal muscles of internal rotation. The gluteus minimus and the glu-

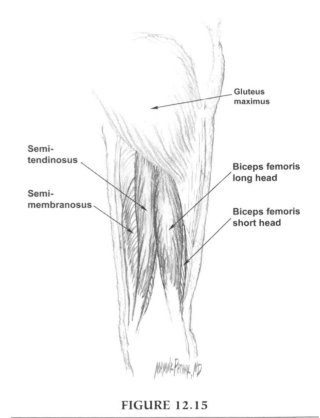

FIGURE 12.15

Gluteus maximus, biceps femoris long head, biceps femoris short head, semitendinosus, semimembranosus. (Reprinted with permission from Daniel Truong, Dirk Dressler, Mark Hallett, Eds. *Manual of Botulinum Toxin Therapy*, 2009, © Cambridge University Press.)

teus medius originate on the external iliac fossa, their fibers converging on the anterolateral aspect of the greater trochanter. Tensor fascia latae originates from the anterior iliac crest and inserts onto the ileotibial tract, a band of fibrous tissue running down the lateral thigh from the lateral tibia and fibula (30).

External Rotation: A group of 6 deep muscles originate on the pelvic bones and insert on or near the greater trochanter of the femur. Among other actions, they produce external rotation of the femur at the hip joint. These muscles include the piriformis, obturator internus, obturator externus, quadratus femoris, gemellus superior, and gemellus inferior. In addition to these, the biceps femoris (long head) and the adductor muscles (see below) assist in external rotation (31).

Adduction: Adduction is produced by 5 principal muscles (Figure 12.16). The anterior portion of the adductor magnus originates from the ischiopubic ramus and inserts along the posteromedial length of the

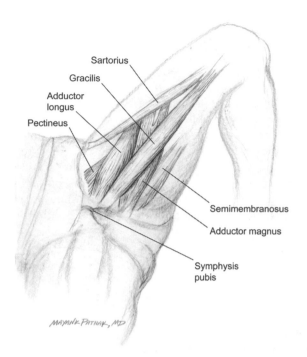

FIGURE 12.16

Adductor magnus, adductor longus, gracilis, pectineus, sartorius, and semimembranosus. (Reprinted with permission from Daniel Truong, Dirk Dressler, Mark Hallett, Eds. *Manual of Botulinum Toxin Therapy*, 2009, © Cambridge University Press.)

femur, and the posterior portion originates from the ischial tuberosity and inserts just proximal to the medial femoral condyle (32). Three other adductors, that is, pectineus, adductor brevis, and adductor longus, originate on the pubis and insert on the posteromedial femur. In addition to adduction, these 4 muscles assist in the external rotation of the femur. The fifth adductor, that is, the gracilis, originates on the inferomedial pubis, crosses both the hip and knee joints, and inserts on the medial side of the proximal tibia. As a polyarticular muscle, it can also flex and medially rotate the knee. Other contributors to adduction include biceps femoris (long head), gluteus maximus (deep part), psoas, and iliacus (33).

Abduction: Abduction at the hip is rarely a clinically significant posture among spastic patients. Four of the principal muscles, that is, gluteus medius, gluteus minimus, and tensor fasciae latae, have already been described. The superficial part of the gluteus maximus, originating on the sacrum and posterior iliac crest and inserting on the fascia latae, extends, externally rotates, and abducts the femur at the hip (34).

THE KNEE

Joint Anatomy: The knee is a complex joint consisting of the hinge-like tibiofemoral joint, in which articulation of the convex femoral condyles against the flat tibial condyles is stabilized by the presence of 2 menisci that conform to their respective surfaces. The joint complex also consists of the patellofemoral joint, that is, a gliding joint. These joints share a common capsule and are stabilized by a number of ligaments (35). Although some rotation can occur at the knee, its

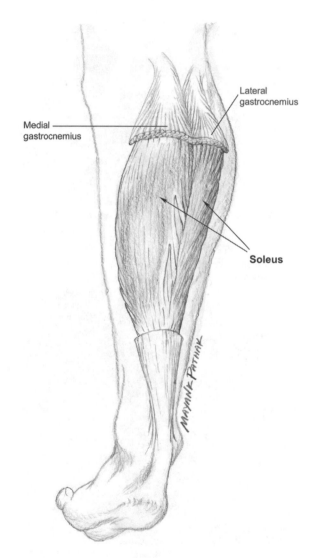

FIGURE 12.17

Gastrocnemius and soleus. (Reprinted with permission from Daniel Truong, Dirk Dressler, Mark Hallett, Eds. *Manual of Botulinum Toxin Therapy*, 2009, © Cambridge University Press.)

2 principal directions of motion, that is, flexion and extension, will be considered here. Spastic patients can present with either a flexed or extended posture at the knee.

Flexion: Flexion is mainly produced by the hamstring muscle group of the posterior thigh. This consists of the semitendinosus, semimembranosus, and the long and short heads of biceps femoris (Figure 12.15). Except for the short head of biceps femoris, all of these component muscles arise on the ischium and insert on the proximal tibia or fibula. Acting thus across 2 joints, they both flex the knee and extend the hip (36). Flexion posture at the knee tends to be more problematic than extension because it precludes erect posture, impedes stride, and may prevent heel strike during gait.

Extension: Extension is mainly produced by the quadriceps femoris group of the anterior thigh. Of these muscles, the vastus lateralis, vastus medialis, and vastus intermedius originate on the femoral shaft, whereas the rectus femoris originates on the anterior inferior iliac spine and crosses the hip joint before merging with the tendons of the other 3 muscles (Figure 12.14). This common tendon inserts on and envelopes the patella, whose tendon continues distally across the tibiofemoral joint to insert on the tibial

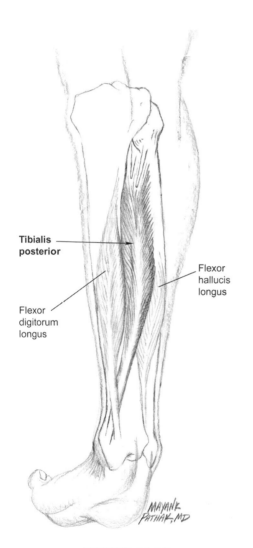

FIGURE 12.18

Tibialis posterior, flexor digitorum longus, and flexor hallucis longus. (Reprinted with permission from Daniel Truong, Dirk Dressler, Mark Hallett, Eds. *Manual of Botulinum Toxin Therapy*, 2009, © Cambridge University Press.)

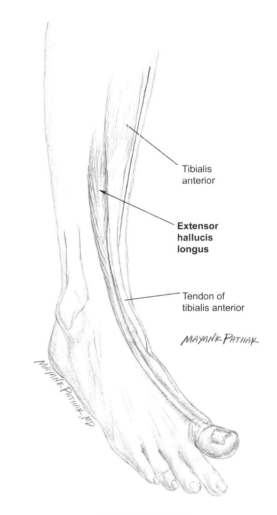

FIGURE 12.19

Tibialis anterior and extensor hallucis longus. (Reprinted with permission from Daniel Truong, Dirk Dressler, Mark Hallett, Eds. *Manual of Botulinum Toxin Therapy*, 2009, © Cambridge University Press.)

tuberosity (37). Rectus femoris, acting across the hip joint, also contributes to hip flexion.

Extension posture, although troublesome, is sometimes utilized by the patient for weight-bearing during stance, transfers, and gait. Excessive reduction of extensor tone by use of botulinum toxin or other means may result in functional loss of these abilities.

THE ANKLE AND FOOT

Joint Anatomy: The ankle complex consists of the talocrural joint, an articulation of the tibia, fibula, and talus, and the subtalar joint between the talus and calcaneus. The principal motions of dorsiflexion, plantar flexion, inversion, and eversion will be considered (38). Because of the relative strengths of the different muscles, plantar flexion and inversion are the common postures among spastic patients.

Plantar Flexion: Plantar flexion is produced chiefly by the triceps surae group of the posterior calf. Most superficial is the gastrocnemius, of which a lateral head and a medial head arise from the respective condyles of the distal femur, running distally across the knee joint. Deep to these is the soleus, originating along the proximal posterior shafts of the tibia and fibula. The fibers of all the triceps surae converge onto the Achilles tendon, which then crosses the talocrural and subtalar joints and inserts on the posterior calcaneus, thus acting to plantar flex the foot (Figure 12.17). The gastrocnemii, by having crossed the knee joint posteriorly, also contribute to knee flexion (39).

Inversion: Inversion is produced by a number of muscles, including the triceps surae, which exerts a slight inversion during plantar flexion. Other than these, the tibialis posterior is the most important. It originates from the proximal posterior shafts of the tibia and fibula as well as from the interosseus membrane between them, its tendon running behind the medial malleolus to insert on the medial and plantar surfaces of several foot bones (Figure 12.18). The tibialis posterior is flanked in the deep calf by 2 other muscles, that is, the flexor digitorum longus medially and the flexor hallucis laterally, both of which also contribute to inversion (40). In addition, the tibialis anterior may also contribute to inversion of the ankle and foot (40).

Dorsiflexion: Dorsiflexion is less of a problem in spastic persons. The strongest dorsiflexor is the tibialis anterior (Figure 12.19), originating from the lateral condyle and anteromedial shaft of the tibia to insert on the inferomedial surface of the cuneiform bone and the base of metatarsal I (41). Deep and adjacent to this muscle are the extensor digitorum longus and the ex-

tensor hallucis longus (described below), which also assist in dorsiflexion.

Great Toe Extension: This posture is encountered frequently among spastic patients and is produced by the extensor hallucis logus (Figure 12.19), which originates from the anteromedial surface of the fibula and inserts on the dorsal surface of the distal phalanx of the great toe (42).

Eversion: Eversion, rarely a clinical problem, is produced chiefly by peroneus longus and peroneus brevis, which arise along the head and shaft of the fibula; longus inserts on the medial cuneiform bone and the base of metatarsal I, whereas brevis inserts on metatarsal V (43).

References

1. Watkins J. Structure and function of the musculoskeletal system. Champaign, Il.: *J Hum Kinet* 1999:131, 181.
2. Dimon, Jr. T. *Anatomy of the moving body.* 2nd ed. Berkley, Ca.: North Atlantic Books, 2008:152.
3. Calais-Germain B. *Anatomy of movement.* Seattle, Wa.: Eastland Press, Inc., 2007:126–127.
4. Dimon, Jr. T. *Anatomy of the moving body.* 2nd ed. Berkley, Ca.: North Atlantic Books, 2008: 149–150.
5. Calais-Germain B. *Anatomy of movement.* Seattle, Wa.: Eastland Press, Inc., 2007:130–131. 135.
6. Dimon, Jr. T. *Anatomy of the moving body.* 2nd ed. Berkley, Ca.: North Atlantic Books, 2008:146.
7. Calais-Germain B. *Anatomy of movement.* Seattle, Wa.: Eastland Press, Inc., 2007:123–124.
8. Dimon, Jr. T. *Anatomy of the moving body.* 2nd ed. Berkley, Ca.: North Atlantic Books, 2008:142.
9. Calais-Germain B. *Anatomy of movement.* Seattle, Wa.: Eastland Press, Inc., 2007:131.
10. Calais-Germain B. *Anatomy of movement.* Seattle, Wa.: Eastland Press, Inc., 2007:129.
11. Braun RM, Botte M. Treatment of shoulder deformity in acquired spasticity. *Clin Orthop Relat Res* 1999;368:54–65.
12. Fitzgerald-Finch OP, Gibson II. Subluxation of the shoulder in hemiplegia. *Age Ageing* 1975; 4(1):16–8.
13. Paci M, Nannetti L, Taiti P, Baccini M, Rinaldi L. Shoulder subluxation after stroke: relationships with pain and motor recovery. *Physiother Res Int* 2007;12(2):95–104.
14. Suethanapornkul S, Kuptniratsaikul PS, Kuptniratsaikul V, Uthensut P, Dajpratha P, Wongwisethkarn J. Post stroke shoulder subluxatin and shoulder pain: a cohort multicenter study. *J Med Assoc Thai* 2008;91(12):1885–92.
15. Watkins J. Structure and function of the musculoskeletal system. Champaign, Il.: *J Hum Kinet*, 1999:131, 186.
16. Strandring, S, ed. *Gray's anatomy: the anatomical basis of clinical practice.* 40th ed. Philadelphia,Pa: Churchill, Livingstone, Elsevier, 2008:825–826.
17. Strandring, S, ed. *Gray's anatomy: the anatomical basis of clinical practice.* 40th ed. Philadelphia,Pa: Churchill, Livingstone, Elsevier, 2008:826.
18. Strandring, S, ed. *Gray's anatomy: the anatomical basis of clinical practice.* 40th ed. Philadelphia,Pa: Churchill, Livingstone, Elsevier, 2008:826–850.
19. Strandring, S, ed. *Gray's anatomy: the anatomical basis of clinical practice.* 40th ed. Philadelphia,Pa: Churchill, Livingstone, Elsevier, 2008:845, 148.
20. Watkins J. Structure and function of the musculoskeletal system. Champaign, Il.: *J Hum Kinet*, 1999:187.

21. Calais-Germain B. *Anatomy of movement*. Seattle, Wa.: Eastland Press, Inc., 2007:172–173.
22. Calais-Germain B. *Anatomy of movement*. Seattle, Wa.: Eastland Press, Inc., 2007:174–175.
23. Calais-Germain B. *Anatomy of movement*. Seattle, Wa.: Eastland Press, Inc., 2007:176–177.
24. Dimon, Jr. T. *Anatomy of the moving body*. 2nd ed. Berkley, Ca.: North Atlantic Books, 2008:177–180.
25. Calais-Germain B. *Anatomy of movement*. Seattle, Wa.: Eastland Press, Inc., 2007:181.
26. Calais-Germain B. *Anatomy of movement*. Seattle, Wa.: Eastland Press, Inc., 2007:186–189.
27. Watkins J. Structure and function of the musculoskeletal system. Champaign, Il.: *J Hum Kinet*, 1999:189–190.
28. Stone RJ, Stone JA. *Atlas of skeletal muscles*. 4th ed. New York, NY.: McGraw Hill Higher Education, 2003:156–157.
29. Stone RJ, Stone JA. *Atlas of skeletal muscles*. 4th ed. New York, NY.: McGraw Hill Higher Education, 2003:164.
30. Stone RJ, Stone JA. *Atlas of skeletal muscles*. 4th ed. New York, NY.: McGraw Hill Higher Education, 2003:165–168.
31. Calais-Germain B. *Anatomy of movement*. Seattle, Wa.: Eastland Press, Inc., 2007:228, 253.
32. Calais-Germain B. *Anatomy of movement*. Seattle, Wa.: Eastland Press, Inc., 2007:246.
33. Calais-Germain B. *Anatomy of movement*. Seattle, Wa.: Eastland Press, Inc., 2007:245–247, 253.
34. Calais-Germain B. *Anatomy of movement*. Seattle, Wa.: Eastland Press, Inc., 2007:250.
35. Watkins J. Structure and function of the musculoskeletal system. Champaign, Il.: *J Hum Kinet*, 1999:191.
36. Strandring, S, ed. *Gray's anatomy: the anatomical basis of clinical practice*. 40th ed. Philadelphia,Pa: Churchill, Livingstone, Elsevier, 2008:1377–1378.
37. Strandring, S, ed. *Gray's anatomy: the anatomical basis of clinical practice*. 40th ed. Philadelphia,Pa: Churchill, Livingstone, Elsevier, 2008:1373–1374.
38. Watkins J. Structure and function of the musculoskeletal system. Champaign, Il.: *J Hum Kinet*, 1999:206.
39. Calais-Germain B. *Anatomy of movement*. Seattle, Wa.: Eastland Press, Inc., 2007:292.
40. Dimon, Jr. T. *Anatomy of the moving body*. 2nd ed. Berkley, Ca.: North Atlantic Books, 2008:230–234.
41. Stone RJ, Stone JA. *Atlas of skeletal muscles*. 4th ed. New York, NY.: McGraw Hill Higher Education, 2003:186.
42. Dimon, Jr. T. *Anatomy of the moving body*. 2nd ed. Berkley, Ca.: North Atlantic Books, 2008:228.
43. Dimon, Jr. T. *Anatomy of the moving body*. 2nd ed. Berkley, Ca.: North Atlantic Books, 2008:230.

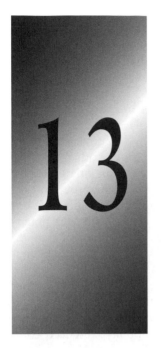

13 The Role of Physical and Occupational Therapy in the Evaluation and Management of Spasticity

Robert Shingleton
Jonathan H. Kinzinger
Elie Elovic

Whereas research efforts have continued to develop novel interventions for the management of spasticity, therapeutic interventions remain a critical component of the overall treatment plan. As a result, physical and occupational therapists continue to be vital members of the treatment team and have and will likely continue to play an important role in the management of a person with spasticity for many years. Over the years, a wide variety of therapeutic modalities and interventions have been developed to treat the upper motor neuron syndrome (UMNS) (1–3). Range of motion (ROM), stretching, positioning, functional electrical stimulation (ES), neuroprosthetics, neurodevelopmental training (NDT), serial casting (SC), dynamic splinting, therapeutic exercise, and constraint-induced therapy are only a handful of the many treatment options available to the therapist. With the current health care climate and focus on evidence-based treatment, however, the efficacy of such interventions needs to be validated with continued research.

This chapter will review the role of physical and occupational therapies in the evaluation and management of spasticity as a component of the UMNS. In addition, the many factors that play a role in determining the course of treatment and the role of therapeutic modalities in the treatment of spasticity will be discussed. Individual and combination therapies will be covered, with issues such as cost, morbidity, and potential efficacy reviewed to facilitate the construc-

tion of a decision-making framework to assist the clinician in determining the best course of treatment for the patient.

FACTORS TO CONSIDER

When determining the optimal course of management for a patient with spasticity, the therapist must weigh the many aspects that can influence the evaluation and treatment decision process. These include, but are not limited to, benefits versus detriments of spasticity, distribution (focal vs generalized), age of the patient, prognosis, time since onset, medical condition, and underlying etiology of the UMNS.

Whereas severe spasticity can be devastating to the overall function of the client, there are several benefits of the condition that should be considered in the treatment decision process (4). Spasticity can help maintain muscle tone and bulk over areas that are prone to pressure and skin breakdown and potentially mitigate the condition. In addition, the muscle pumping action that results from muscle overactivity can potentially aid in overall circulation and reduce the risk of deep vein thrombosis. Increases in spasticity in a person with spinal cord injury (SCI) can serve as a red flag and warn of urinary tract infection, skin breakdown (5), development of heterotopic ossification (1), or syringomyelia (6). Spasticity can also facilitate function because it can assist in the performance of transfers, bed mobility, standing, ambulation, sexual function, and bladder management (7). The clinical team must weigh the loss of the positive effects of UMNS against the benefits of treatment when making their decision. It would be unfortunate, as happens in some cases, if addressing muscle overactivity decreases the person's overall ability to perform functional activities of daily living (ADL).

The deleterious effects of spasticity, especially when it interferes with function, must also be considered. They can interfere with almost all ADL, including bed mobility, transfers, wheelchair mobility, ambulation, eating, toileting, hygiene, sexual function, and dressing (4, 7–9). Not only can spasticity greatly impair the overall functional mobility, but it can also be extremely painful. The pain and spasm cycle can become debilitating to the person emotionally, leading to severe depression and further isolation (10, 11). When left untreated over long periods, it can lead to shortening of the muscles and tendons and ultimately to the development of joint contractures (5, 12, 13). When this occurs in the hips, knees, and/or ankles, transfers, ambulation, positioning in bed, and wheelchair may become impossible even if the person has sufficient underlying strength. This impairs the person's ability to participate in therapeutic exercise or rehabilitation programs, leading to additional functional losses. Based on the problems that can result from spasticity and UMNS, the need to treat moderate to severe spasticity is clear. Therapeutic modalities and interventions can play an important role in mitigating the negative sequelae and minimizing the complications that can occur as a result of UMNS.

When developing a treatment plan, a therapist must take into account several key factors when assessing the patient, for example, the anatomic distribution of spasticity, how dependent it is on positioning, and the UMNS's fluctuation throughout the day, to name a few. If the spasticity is regional or generalized, the person may respond better to a general ROM, stretching, exercise, and positioning program. When the condition is focal, functional ES, bracing, SC, stretching, dynamic splinting, and/or taping may prove more appropriate. Tone that is positional in nature may respond well to an educational program for the patient and/or their caregiver on proper bed and wheelchair positioning as well as transfer training to maximize their ability to assume the best position. When fluctuation occurs throughout the day, scheduling, proper timing of ROM, stretching, and other interventions are important for the proper management of the condition.

Other important issues that the therapist must include in the assessment process are the source of UMNS, spinal versus cerebral, and the age of the person with the condition. When treating children, the fact that significant tone can place stresses on bones and joints, which can in turn lead to deformity, must enter into the decision process. On the other hand, an older adult with osteoporosis could potentially sustain a fracture from an aggressive stretching program.

Choosing appropriate goals is crucial to the development of a treatment plan. Examples of potential targets include, but are certainly not limited to, maintaining or improving the patient's overall functional mobility and independence, alleviating pain, improving balance and gait, preventing or limiting contracture development, maintaining skin integrity, improving positioning and overall functioning with wheelchair management and mobility, and decreasing the level of assistance required by caregivers. The setting of unrealistically high goals can be every bit as much a problem as choosing ones that are too low. It is important to develop a plan of care that is tailored to the individual and has buy in from the patient and caregivers.

EVALUATION

The evaluation of individuals with spasticity requires a multidisciplinary approach, including physicians, physical and occupational therapists, nurses, and most importantly the patient and their caregivers. A thorough assessment incorporating all of the factors discussed above is required for the development of the optimal treatment plan. A standard neuromuscular evaluation including ROM, strength, coordination, balance, transfers, sensation, cranial nerve testing, gait, and reflexes is a vital component of the evaluation process. That being said, the assessment of a patient with UMNS remains a challenge because the understanding of the pathophysiology and subsequent definitions of spasticity remains unclear (5, 14, 15). Spasticity, abnormal reflexes, muscle spasms clonus, and dyssynergic movement patterns have been described as the "positive" features of UMNS. The "negative" features include weakness, loss of dexterity, and fatigability (16). Both positive and negative components of UMNS contribute to the functional deficits that are seen clinically, and evaluation for their presence must be part of the patient assessment. Perhaps the most frequently cited definition comes from Lance (17), who defined spasticity as "a motor disorder characterized by a velocity dependent increase in tonic stretch reflex (muscle tone) with exaggerated tendon jerks, resulting from hyper excitability of the stretch reflex, as one component of the upper motor neuron syndrome." The term *spasticity* has become commonly used almost in a generic sense to include all the other components of the UMNS, including hyperreflexia, clonus, clasp-knife rigidity, exaggerated cutaneous reflexes, cocontractions, dystonia, and associated reactions that occur as a result of positional changes or noxious stimuli (13, 18). Pandyan (14) described spasticity as more than a pure motor disorder that does not result solely from the hyperexcitability of the stretch reflex. Instead, it should be defined as "disordered sensori-motor control, resulting from an upper motor neuron lesion, presenting as intermittent or sustained involuntary activation of muscles"(14). This definition is more broad than Lance's because it includes not only the velocity-dependent spasticity produced as a joint is rapidly flexed or extended at a single point in time but also the increase in tone and muscle spasms witnessed with positional and postural changes during phases of gait and with other nonpassive, functional movements. Spasticity is not just an isolated event to be assessed only at a single point in time but instead is a dynamic event that requires a functional-based assessment to fully appreciate the impact it has on the overall function.

To allow scientists and clinicians to evaluate changes and treatment efficacy, they must use appropriate metrics. Numerous outcome metrics are available for this purpose; however, an extensive discussion of this topic can be found elsewhere in this book. To facilitate a better understanding of the authors' comments, some of the scales most commonly used by the therapist will be briefly discussed to facilitate the readers' understanding. The authors have placed them into 3 categories based on the data collected to obtain the score: physical, self-reported assessments to assist in the overall evaluation, and treatment framework (see Tables 13.1 and 13.2). For the therapist treating the patient, it is important to not only quantify the severity of spasticity but also evaluate its effect on function. If the aim of spasticity management programs is to be patient oriented, then research, clinical trials, and evaluation tools all need to include the patients' self-report and experience to supplement the current battery of measures (19).

Physical Assessments

Physical assessments of spasticity often involve moving the affected joint rapidly through its available ROM and quantifying the severity of the tonal response. Commonly used manual methods for evaluating spasticity include the Ashworth Scale (AS) and the Modified Ashworth Scale (MAS), which are discussed in Table 13.1. There are numerous other measures, including the Tardieu and Modified Tardieu Scales, which are discussed.

Whereas the AS and MAS are easy to perform and require no specialized equipment to complete, the score obtained is subjective. Their validity, interrater reliability, and correlation to other measures of spasticity and function are inconsistent and often questioned as useful tools in the literature, (4, 16, 20–23) particularly when assessing the lower extremity (24).

TABLE 13.1

Ashworth and Modified Ashworth Scale

AS	MAS
0 (1) = no increase in tone	0 = no increase in tone
1 (2) = slight increase in tone, giving a catch when the affected part is moved in flexion or extension	1 = slight increase in tone, manifested by a catch and release, or by minimal resistance at end ROM when the affected limb is flexed or extended
2 (3) = more marked increase in tone but the affected part is easily flexed	(1+) = slight increase in muscle tone, manifested by a catch, followed by minimal resistance throughout the remainder (less than half) of the range of movement
3 (4) = considerable increase in tone, passive movement is difficult	2 = more marked increase in muscle tone through most of the ROM, but the affected part is easily moved
4 (5) = affected part is rigid in flexion or extension	3 = considerable increase in muscle tone, passive movement is difficult
	4 = affected joint is rigid in flexion or extension

TABLE 13.2

Self-reported Assessments of Spasticity

Scale	PSFS	PRISM	SCI-SET	MSSS-88
Attributes	*Part 1*: spasm frequency scale. *Part 2*: spasm severity scale. Easy to administer. No functional component. Validated for MS and spinal cord lesion.	41 items, 7 subscales that can be evaluated independently. Easy to administer. Identifies beneficial and detrimental aspects of spasticity. Validated for SCI.	35 items, targeted mainly at ADLs. Bidirectional response scale. No subscales. Identifies beneficial and detrimental aspects of spasticity. Validated for SCI.	88 items divided into 8 subscales. Subscales can be evaluated independently. Validated for MS.
Scoring	*Part 1*: spasm frequency 0 = no spasms 1 = mild spasms at stimulation 2 = infrequent strong spasms less than 1 time per hour 3 = spasms more often than 1 time per hour 4 = spasms more than 10 times per hour *Part 2*: spasm severity 1 = mild 2 = moderate 3 = severe	0 = never true for me 1 = rarely true for me 2 = sometimes true for me 3 = often true for me 4 = very often true for me	*−3 to +3 bidirectional scale:* −3 = extremely problematic −2 = moderately problematic −1 = somewhat problematic 0 = no effect +1 = somewhat helpful +2 = moderately helpful +3 = extremely helpful	1 = not at all bothered 2 = a little bothered 3 = moderately bothered 4 = extremely bothered

In contrast, Brashear et al. (25) found good interrater and intrarater reliability when assessing the spasticity of the wrist, fingers, and elbow in persons who have had a stroke. Likewise, Skold et al. (26) found significant correlation between the MAS and the patient-reported spasticity using a Visual Analog Scale (VAS) in 45 persons with SCI.

The AS and the MAS are subjective tests in nature in that they do not have standardized procedures for patient positioning, scoring, or overall test implementation (22). Ideally, the clinician should choose a position that is most comfortable for the patient and gives the best picture of the overall spasticity. It is important that the patient be tested in the same position in subsequent sessions to optimize reliability. The affected joint is passively moved through its available ROM at a speed sufficient to induce a spastic response. This presents a major limitation to both scales because the speed of movement has not been well established.

Multiple studies report that 1 second may be the best time to take a joint through its available ROM (11). The resistance to movement, where it occurs in the ROM, and the strength of the resistance are noted and quantified. The AS uses a 5-point 0–4 scale, whereas the MAS adds 1+ to the scale as well. The 1+ grade was added in the MAS to enhance the sensitivity of the test in elbow flexor tone in people with multiple sclerosis (MS) (27) (see Table 13.1).

The AS was originally designed to evaluate the antispasmodic effects of Carisporodol in MS (28). Both scales have subsequently been used with a variety of etiologies including brain injury (22), stroke (25), and SCI (4). The fact that spasticity differs based on etiologies may account for some of the variability in the literature that has examined the MAS and AS. (4, 11) Additional factors to consider when administering either scale include the time of day, emotional status, current health issues, repeated stretching or ROM before the testing period, pain, and fatigue (11). Any of these factors can either lead to an increase or decrease in spasticity, thereby giving the tester a skewed result. In addition, it is important to note that the AS and MAS only evaluate the velocity-dependent nature of spasticity across a single joint (4) at a single point in time. Although both scales have been weakly associated with quality of arm skills, gait velocity, stride length, and gross motor functions (22), there have been limited data that have demonstrated a significant association between the AS and any specific function. Therefore, the clinician must use caution when assessing velocity-induced tone and functional limitations because they may not be directly related. Experienced therapists have witnessed the patient with marked tone as assessed by the AS/MAS at rest, only to see minimal tone and impairment in those same muscle groups during functional activities. The converse can also be true where a patient has minimal tone when evaluated at rest but exhibits increased tone during repositioning, transfers, standing, and other functional tasks.

Hypertonia may also result from muscle hypoextensibility (contracture), which consists of the shortening of the muscle due to a decrease in the number of sarcomeres (29). The precise association between spasticity and contracture remains unclear. The therapist using AS or MAS must not confuse muscle stiffness or contracture with spasticity.

Patient Reported Assessments

A critical component to the overall evaluation and management of spasticity is the feedback from the patient and their caregivers. Because tone can fluctuate based on many factors as described above, a patient's self-assessment can provide therapists with a clearer picture of the overall nature of spasticity and the impairment and functional deficits that it evokes. This can facilitate the development of an appropriate treatment plan. Research has shown that clinical examination does not always elicit spasticity in patients who report it and that examination of one or more symptoms of spasticity does not correlate with the person's self-report of spasticity, with function, or with each other (30, 31). Therefore, it is crucial that the therapist take into account the person's self-report of their symptoms and how it affects their function because the patient and the caregiver are often the best judge of its effects overall (10). The Penn Spasm Frequency Scale (PSFS) (32), the Patient Reported Impact of Spasticity Measure (PRISM) (33), the Spinal Cord Injury Spasticity Evaluation Tool (SCI-SET) (10), and the Multiple

Sclerosis Spasticity Scale (MSSS-88)(19) are 4 self-assessment tools discussed below (see Table 13.2).

Penn created the 5-point spasm frequency scale to follow the effects of intrathecal baclofen in 20 patients with MS and spinal cord lesion (32). The scale was later modified to include a spasm severity component to better capture the true nature of the person's spasticity (4). The first part involves a 5-point scale in which the patient assesses the frequency of their spasms with "0 = no spasms" to "4 = spontaneous spasms greater than 10 times per hour." The second part is a self-report of the severity of spasms with "1 = mild" to "3 = severe." The second part is only completed if the person reports a score greater than 0 in the first part of the battery.

Priebe et al. (30) found a weak relationship between the PSFS and the patient-reported scales of pain and function associated with spasticity in persons with SCI. In addition, the PSFS, AS, and other clinical tests of spasticity, including tendon taps, clonus, and plantar stimulation, demonstrated poor correlation to each other in persons with SCI, suggesting that each test may be evaluating a different component of spasticity as it relates to the UMNS (30), and what is being tested clinically may not correlate to what the person is experiencing throughout the day functionally (4). Whereas the PSFS is a good tool for incorporating the patient's report because it provides the clinician with valuable information regarding the daily fluctuations of the person's spasticity, it is important for the therapist to standardize the time of day and the time frame (e.g. over the last 24 hours or the last 7 days) to capture the most accurate assessment from the patient. Further studies are required to test the reliability of the PSFS in persons with SCI and to establish validity with other clinical measures of spasticity.

The PRISM was developed to measure the impact of spasticity on the quality of life of persons with SCI (33). The PRISM is a 41-item, self-assessment tool rated on a 0–4 scale with "0 = never true for me" and "4 = very often true for me." The 7 subscales within the instrument evaluate the effects of altered motor control with respect to social avoidance and anxiety, psychological agitation, daily activities, need for assistance or positioning, need for interventions, and social embarrassment, as well as the positive impact of altered motor control on function.

The PRISM offers the therapist a clinical tool that is easy to administer and captures a wide span of the impacts of spasticity through its subscales. Each subscale is independently scored, so the therapist may choose to focus evaluation and track treatment efforts on one area of interest (e.g. daily activities), as factor analysis has shown that each domain addresses a unique aspect of spasticity as it relates to the quality of life in persons with SCI (33, 34). Another intriguing feature of the tool is its ability to differentiate the beneficial versus detrimental effects of spasticity on the client's overall functional status. This is an invaluable information for therapists in their efforts to develop a treatment program that maximizes appropriate spasticity reduction while maintaining or improving overall patient function. Whereas the PRISM was designed and validated with a large pool of persons with SCI, the statements are generic enough that it should apply to any population affected by spasticity as a result of UMNS. However, it has not yet been validated in other populations. Further work is needed to validate this relatively new instrument with varying patient populations who have spasticity.

The SCI-SET is a 35-item self-report of the impact of spasticity on the targeted ADL over a 7-day recall period (10). The instrument allows the client to rate both problematic and beneficial aspects of their spasticity on a –3 to a +3 bidirectional scale. Like the PRISM, it was validated among people with SCI, but because its statements are generic, they could potentially be used in other populations with spasticity (e.g. stroke, brain injury, and MS), although it too has not been validated in these groups. It is quick and easy to administer and provides the therapist with valuable information related to the impact of spasticity on functional ADLs. As a tool that allows the therapist and patient to see the helpful and problematic effects of spasticity on specific functional tasks, such as balance, gait, and dressing, the SCI-SET is significant as an aid in treatment decision making, in outcome tracking, and for research purposes.

The MSSS-88 is an 88-item questionnaire that quantifies the impact of spasticity over a 2-week period in 8 areas: spasticity-specific symptoms (muscle stiffness, pain and discomfort, and muscle spasms), functional areas (ADL, walking, and body movements), and 2 areas related to emotional health and social functioning (19). Scoring is based on a 1–4 scale with "1 = not bothered at all" and "4 = extremely bothered." Like the PRISM, the MSSS-88 provides the clinician a picture of the impact of the person's spasticity over a wide range of activities and circumstances. It also allows the therapist to examine each subscale individually, as each is a unique instrument that can be analyzed separately from the whole. This allows the specific tailoring of the evaluation, treatment planning, and goal setting with the patient because each section can independently add to the evaluation and management process. Whereas the instrument has been validated for persons with MS, we believe that many of the items and subscales are generic enough to

be applied to other diagnoses, as with the PRISM and SCI-SET. Validation studies within different diagnostic groups of patients could make the MSSS-88 a powerful tool that could be utilized across the spectrum of spasticity as it relates to the UMNS.

Functional Assessments

Evaluating the effects of spasticity on functional activities and quantifying it should be the primary goal in spasticity evaluation and management. This would allow clinicians to directly measure the results of the treatment program on spasticity during specific functional activities and give additional meaning to traditional outcome measures. As discussed earlier, clinical assessments that primarily analyze velocity-induced spasticity have shown weak correlation to actual patient function(22) and should not be relied upon solely as an indication of the degree of the person's spasticity. Self-reported assessments are an effective tool for gathering the perspective of the patient and caregiver and can provide valuable information as to the nature and overall impact of spasticity on both function and caregiving. However, self-reported assessments are subjective and provide no clinical objective measurement of spasticity. That being said, tests that examine spasticity during functional activities are needed to reliably assess the true nature and impact of spasticity on the patient and their caregiver (35). There are many standardized functional tests available to therapists that effectively analyze gait, coordination, balance, functional independence, ability to perform ADL, and various combinations of upper extremity and lower extremity functions. Unfortunately, there are no tests that specifically address, quantify, and analyze the impact of spasticity on those areas of function. Many tests simply quantify the degree to which a function can or cannot be performed and the level of assist required. Whether the underlying issue causing the limited performance is decreased strength, ROM, impaired motor control, coordination, or spasticity, it is left up to the clinician for further evaluation and testing to determine. Because of this, it is important that the therapist pick the appropriate test to examine spasticity based upon the patient's diagnosis, their current status and ability to perform ADL, and patient/caregiver goals. The clinician can then assess the impact of spasticity on the ability of the patient/caregiver to complete the test. For example, if a patient is performing a 10-meter walk test, then it is not simply the time it takes to walk the distance that should be noted. The affect of spasticity on overall gait mechanics, step and stride lengths, knee stability in midstance, and knee flexion and extension during the swing phase are all potential areas where spasticity can greatly impair the person's ability to walk 10 m in a certain time. When assessing a caregiver's ability to transfer a patient with severe spasticity that has no volitional movement, the degree to which the spasticity increases the caregiver burden should be addressed. The question is how do we measure or quantify the degree to which the observed spasticity affects the function? Ng and Hui-Chan (36) demonstrated poor correlation between ankle plantar flexion spasticity as measured by the Composite Spasticity Scale (CSS) (37) and the Timed Up and Go (TUG) test in 11 patients poststroke. Their results contrasted with others, who found a positive correlation between TUG and ankle plantar flexion spasticity (38, 39), and agreed with other researchers, who also demonstrated poor correlation between the 2 measures (40, 41). A potential limitation found in many of the studies attempting to correlate spasticity to function is that spasticity is often assessed through the use of passive, velocity-dependent, nonfunctional tests that are then compared to the results of dynamic, non–velocity-dependent functional tasks. Spasticity measured passively may be quite different when observed during dynamic activities. For example, knee extensor spasticity, which measures 4/5 on the MAS in supine, may not present as significantly during functional gait analysis as one might expect, whereas the mild 2/5 spasticity may be magnified in standing and interfere greatly with the ability of the knee to flex during gait. The point is that, when attempting to measure the effects of spasticity on function, the test of spasticity should mimic that function as closely as possible. Unfortunately, accurately measuring and quantifying spasticity during functional activities and determining the true impact on function may require the use of expensive motion analysis systems, surface electromyography (EMG), and dynamometers, (21) which are often neither readily available nor practical in the clinical setting. To that end, the therapist is somewhat limited to observational analysis when assessing the impact of spasticity on function. Whether the test is the Dynamic Gait Index, the 6-minute walk test, the 10-meter walk test, the TUG, the Wolf Motor Function Test, or the Fugl-Meyer Upper Limb Test, the therapist assessing spasticity must take into account where the spasticity is occurring, in what muscle group(s), and how it is affecting the overall ability to complete the task. Because video has recently become easily accessible and affordable through smaller handheld units, it offers the therapist a valuable clinical tool for documenting and analyzing spasticity during different positions and function. The therapist can then document changes in spasticity and function throughout the treatment process.

TREATMENT OPTIONS

The primary goal of any spasticity management program should be to maximize function; balance, motor control, gait mechanics, speed, transfers, bed mobility, dressing, hygiene, and reducing caregiver burden are all examples of functional domains that should be addressed. In addition, making a task easier to perform, more energy-efficient, and safer are all reasonable goals for the treatment team. There are numerous treatment options available to therapists to treat spasticity and UMNS. For the purpose of this chapter, we have divided them into the following:

1. Physical treatments (ROM, stretching, SC, dynamic splinting, and constraint induced therapy);
2. Therapeutic exercise (strengthening, cycling, and body weight–supported gait training);
3. Modalities (electrical and thermal);
4. Combination therapies.

Electrical modalities may include functional/neuromuscular ES (FES/NMES), transcutaneous ES (TENS), and neuroprosthetic devices that incorporate NMES into a device that produces functional movements. Thermal modalities may include heat (hot packs, ultrasound [US], fluidotherapy, diathermy, and infrared [IR]). Cryotherapy applications often include cold packs, cold baths, vapocoolants, and ice massage. Although these treatment options have been used for many years, the efficacy of these techniques in the treatment of UMNS needs to be validated. Because clinicians are increasingly expected to offer evidenced-based treatment, it is important that therapists take an active role in guiding this research.

Physical Treatments

Stretching

The exercises and protocols that fall in the category of stretching are some of the primary intervention strategies used by both physical and occupation therapists in the management of patients with spasticity. Stretching is defined as the process of producing elongation. As an intervention, it is commonly used to address numerous other impairments other than spasticity, such as limitations in ROM and functional mobility.

There are numerous methods of applying the modality of stretching to a person, but historically, it is provided by clinicians in a hands-on manual fashion. Manual stretching techniques are heavily utilized as an adjunct to other therapeutic interventions but are very difficult to standardize and objectify. This has complicated efforts to scientifically study and develop evidence-based practice (EBP). The use of a mechanical device to apply a stretch, such as a dynamometer (Cybex), is another method to deliver a stretch to a person. In contrast to manual stretch, the use of these devices increases ones ability to be more objective, allows better standardization for clinical treatment and research protocols, and may better facilitate the creation of guidelines for EBP. On the other hand, these devices can be both extremely expensive and inaccessible to many clinicians, particularly in rural settings. One may be forced to choose between treatments that can be well controlled and objectively measured but functionally irrelevant on the one hand and on the other functionally relevant, practical but with a very limited means of standardizing and measuring the treatment applied (42).

There are many variables that must be considered when applying stretch. These include the characteristics of intensity, duration, dose, frequency, and repetitions (42). The aggressive stretching program that would be administered to a young relatively active and healthy individual with cerebral palsy (CP) would differ dramatically from that prescribed to a 90-year-old, chronic, nonambulatory stroke survivor with bony metastases. To better delineate the differences in the methods of applying stretch, the authors will now define for the readers the different variables used to describe the act of stretching.

When therapists describe the differences used in the application of stretch to a person, these are the common terms used. *Intensity* refers to the amount of tension that is applied to structure(s). *Duration* is the period that the structures are elongated within one repetition. *Dose* is the total end range time. *Frequency* is the periodicity ranging from one session to daily sessions for weeks, months, or even years. *Repetitions* are the number of times stretched in a single session. Although these terms are good in describing the treatment, and the treatment is in wide use, there is scant work and extremely limited EBP guidelines on how to vary these parameters in the treatment of different conditions. To be effective, stretches are typically reported to require at least 30 seconds, but the "longer the better" is often encouraged based on in vitro studies performed by Williams (43). However, based on a detailed review of the literature, Bovend'Eeerdt et al. (42) was unable to demonstrate a relationship between the duration of a stretch and its effectiveness. In their review, the authors noted a wide variance in how stretch was applied. Stretching protocols ranged from single sessions to several months of treatment,

with durations ranging from 1.5 to 45 minutes; the durations of a single stretch vary from 20 seconds to 45 minutes.

As time limitations become progressively more of a barrier, therapists are often looking for more efficient and effective strategies to manage the stretching of individuals. As mentioned above, dynamometers can be used but are often cost prohibitive and not necessarily functional, whereas manual stretching is labor-intensive with limited objectivity. Therapists have looked for other means of applying stretch to a patient and avoid the limitations discussed above. The search to find cost-effective means to apply appropriate stretch that is clinically relevant and cost-effective has lead the clinicians at our institution to seek creative solutions to the complex problem. Because many people have multiple deficits, choosing a treatment that can address more than one problem is a clear advantage to both clinician and patient.

Traditionally, the use of tilt tables has been used widely to manage limitations in joint range and minimize the sequelae of spasticity and deficits in the ROM of the lower extremity joints, particularly the triceps surae. When used effectively, numerous joints, including knee, hip, trunk, and even the upper extremities, can be treated simultaneously. The intensity of the stretch provided can be modulated by controlling the ankle that the tilt table is set at. By increasing the angle and making the patient more upright, there is an increased weight-bearing load borne through the feet. There are also increased physiological benefits when this occurs. This includes postural improvement, decreased orthostatis, better pulmonary toilet, and improved bone mineral density (BMD), to name a few. With respect to BMD, most publications report no improved BMD; however, a recent review article reported some positive effects of standing weight-bearing activities on bone density if the treatment intensity was sufficiently long and high. These benefits were also more pronounced if begun early after SCI and continue over the long term. Otherwise, there appears to be no physiological benefit of weight-bearing on BMD (44).

Early after a neurologic insult, the tilt table can be used to address each of these issues. As individuals stabilize after prolonged immobilization, the continued use of a tilt table should be encouraged. However, the standing frame is another method to achieve the same goals with the same benefits in a more functional position. Both devices should be utilized to address the numerous potential benefits and complications, particularly considering that there is minimal burden on therapists from a time management or physically demanding perspective.

The standing frame often allows for more active participation from individuals and provides a greater sense of security to individuals who use it.

Similar to the tilt table, standing frames are often used to address the same issues as the tilt table with some additional benefits and can be used as a progression from the tilt table. The standing frame often allows for more active participation from individuals and provides a greater sense of security to individuals who use it. The standing frame is used often in our clinic as an adjunctive modality, where therapists will often place individuals upright at the end of a treatment session for subsequent participation in occupational, recreation, and speech therapy sessions. It has been our experience that attention, arousal, and alertness are improved with overall improved functional improvements and participation, particularly in the stroke population. In addition, this device, which is often combined with a mirror, is used for individuals with Pusher syndrome and other midline awareness deficits. Although this is anecdotal, we are presently tracking the data for analysis and publication (Figure 13.1).

Another easily accessible piece of equipment that is useful in the management of decreased ROM and spasticity is the Total Gym. It is frequently used in our clinic to address stretching of the lower extremities, as described above, and to also address the strength and motor control deficits observed in the neurologic population. Active neuro reeducation of the lower extremities can occur in-between passive stretching routines and can be graded in terms of intensity as the tilt table can. Using this piece of equipment allows for the isolation of the impaired Lower Extremity (LE) muscle groups to be facilitated. Strength training was once avoided and criticized as an activity that would increase spasticity. However, resistance training, in general, has been shown to produce increased strength, gait speed, functional outcomes, and improved quality of life without exacerbation of spasticity in the stroke population (Figure 13.2) (45).

Dynamometers such as Cybex, Kin-Com, and Biodex, as well as intelligent feedback-controlled devices, are less commonly used but are being utilized in an increasing manner by clinicians to provide well-controlled and standardized stretching interventions.

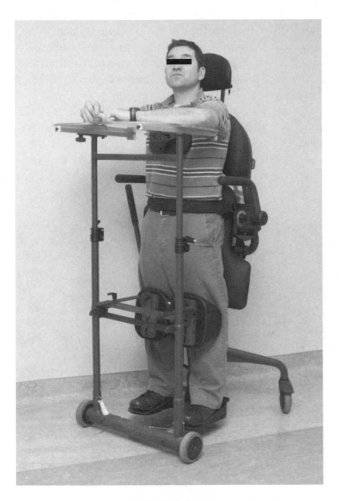

FIGURE 13.1

Utilization of standing frame to promote increased weight-bearing while providing static stretch to the ankle plantar flexors and hip flexors.

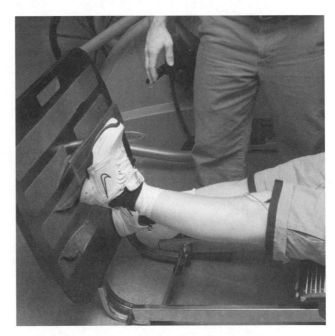

FIGURE 13.2

Provision of static stretch to the ankle plantar flexors using the Total Gym.

Intelligent feedback devices are driven by a motor controlled by a digital signal processor. The stretching velocity was controlled so that the speed is inversely proportional to the resistance torque. Near the end of the ROM, an increased resistance slows the motor in stretching the muscle-tendon complex slowly and safely. Once the specified peak resistance torque is reached, the motor held the joint at the end position for a period to allow "stress relaxation." Chung et al. (46) utilized intelligent feedback to assess the benefits of stretching on several variables, including spasticity. Although the changes in reflex components were not statistically significant, it was observed that the force-generating capacity of hemiparetic muscles was improved after intervention. These effects of intelligent stretching were not seen in the healthy muscle.

The effects of stretching on spasticity are limited, with evidence showing no long-lasting changes on spasticity or the underlying etiology. However, the treatment of spasticity through stretching allows for an opportunity to treat functional impairments and deficits such as gait with greater emphasis on normalizing movement patterns. If used judiciously with education provided to families and caregivers, one can decrease the risk of contracture and permanent muscle shortening over time. This in turn will minimize the secondary complications and the need for other interventions, such as surgical tendon-lengthening procedures. It is important to remember stretching as an intervention that is not without its risks. Patients have experienced numerous problems as a result of aggressive ROM activities. At times, one can create the very problem that they seek to avoid as a result of providing painful and noxious stimuli. Although rare, avulsions and fractures have been reported in the literature (47). These complications arise often in the presence of other chronic impairments associated with the underlying pathology. Overall, evidence is lacking, particularly with respect to spasticity management and stretching. However, it is widely accepted that stretching will aid in maintaining ROM and help prevent secondary complication in the presence of spasticity. This will ultimately improve functional mobility and potential throughout the lives of individuals with neurologic injury.

Serial Casting

The use of SC, also called inhibitory casting, in the management of spasticity has been utilized for decades. It was first described in the 1960s in individuals with CP (48, 49). Since then, casting has evolved to include treatment in multiple central nervous system disorders, including brain injury, SCI, stroke, and MS.

Because spasticity places a muscle into a shortened position for prolonged periods, the resulting contractures are a leading complication. This often leads to limitations and impairments in functional mobility and ADL and in severe pain, among others. Therefore, a primary indication for SC is in minimizing these secondary complications. Typically, the elbow, wrist, finger, and ankle joints are the ones that are most commonly treated with this modality.

Too often, SC is recommended and used once contractures are present and limitations are already present A more proactive approach is ideal, and patients who are deemed at risk should be identified early and treated.

Serial casting involves the stepwise application of a plaster or fiberglass cast applied circumferentially around a spastic and/or contracted joint(s). The repeated application of casts with the joint being stretched further with each application leads to improve ROM, increased function, and/or decreased pain (48). Serial casting is discontinued when no increase ROM is noted in 2 sequential casts or maximal ROM is achieved (50). At this point, the final cast is bivalved to serve as maintenance orthosis (Figures 13.3, 13.4, and 13.5).

The proposed theories suggest that SC reduces spasticity and hypertonia, but the underlying mechanism is largely unknown. However, numerous theories do exist. The neurophysiological theory proposes that casts minimize changes in muscle length, which in

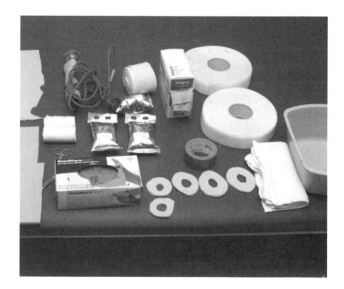

FIGURE 13.3

Material used in SC including cast padding, foam padding, fiberglass casting material and stockinette (cutout foam to protect bony prominences).

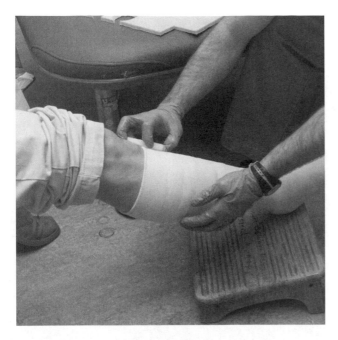

FIGURE 13.4

Application of serial cast to treat ankle plantar flexor contractures and muscle overactivity. The clinician is wrapping high on the calf to maximize the mechanical advantage of the cast to provide optimal stretch.

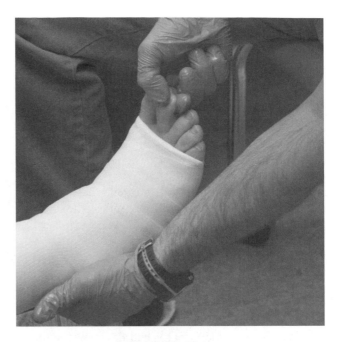

FIGURE 13.5

Clinician performing checking of capillary refill, a critical component of checking the limb after casting.

turn reduces excitatory input through afferent receptors in the muscle spindles, which in turn reduces reflexive alpha motor neuron excitability. The increased tension on the spastic muscle also results in increased stimulation of the golgi tendon organs, which inhibits the alpha motorneurons through type Ib afferent fibers (48). Another proposed mechanism, although the evidence is not strong, is that the neutral warmth provided by the cast may inhibit motor neuron excitability and promote muscle relaxation (51). Another proposed component is that the circumferential pressure around the spastic muscle and joint provided by the cast is thought to reduce cutaneous sensory input (48), which reduces the overall level of interneuron and motor neuron excitability, thus decreasing spasticity (52). A similar effect has been seen with air splints applying circumferential pressure (53).

A mechanical explanation has also been given as an explanation for the efficacy of SC. When a cast is applied, it provides a stretch of load and long duration, which helps to prevent and correct joint contractures (54, 55). Alterations in the mechanical properties of the muscle and tendon itself have been exhibited through casting studies, with animal studies showing an increase in the number of sarcomeres in series in response to casting (56).

Wearing Schedules: As mentioned above, serial casts are applied in a sequential and stepwise manner to progressively increase gains in ROM. Traditionally, casting is a lengthy process, and several cast changes are frequently required to achieve the desired ROM. The standard practice has historically been changes every 5 to 7 days (50). Pohl et al. (50) have been performing cast changes at much shorter intervals ranging from 1 to 4 days. Utilizing this wearing schedule, they have observed equally effective ROM outcomes in shorter periods with fewer complications.

Possible Complications: The patient population that often requires a cast is often as risk of being a poor communicator regarding problems with the cast. This may be due to sensory loss cognitive impairment, decreased arousal, or communication deficits. As a result, the treating clinicians must maintain a vigil to avoid them. Possible problems include a burn either secondary to heat generated from the water used to wet the cast or heat generated from the cast itself (57). Other problems including the development of a compartment syndrome and skin breakdown have been reported. The possibility of a deep vein thrombosis developing increases with the duration of the application of the cast. Osteopenia and osteoporosis with a risk of pathologic facture is also reported with prolonged use.

Dynamic Splinting

Dynamic splinting are devices that incorporate an active, active assistive, or passive component into the device. This typically allows for functional movement patterns out of the spastic pattern. Commonly used dynamic splints include dynasplint, Saeboflex, and other custom fabricated devices often using a combination of springs and pulley systems to provide the dynamic component. They can also be designed and fabricated to allow motion at certain joints without the use of external assistance (58). Most often, these types of splints are utilized in upper extremities, the hand in particular. However, they can be used for lower extremity spasticity and ROM impairments, particularly the dynasplint. Dynasplints are thought to encourage reductions in spasticity through the same principles and rationales described throughout this chapter; however, no evidence exists regarding their efficacy on spasticity management.

Burtner et al. (58) published data on the differences between no splint, dynamic splinting, and static splinting in 10 children with hemiplegic CP. Specifically, they examined EMG muscle activation patterns but not spasticity specifically. They also collected data on grip and pinch strength as well as dexterity through peg board testing. Results revealed improved grip strength and dexterity in children with spasticity when wearing dynamic splints. This suggests improved function with dynamic splinting. Significantly less EMG activity was noted during grip with static splinting with increased compensatory shoulder muscle activation. This suggests both a possible decrease in spastic muscle activity but also may lead to decreased motor control and muscular atrophy.

Saeboflex

The Saebo splints include the Saeboflex, the Saeboreach, and the Saebostretch, with each providing specific effects to specific joints. The SaeboFlex orthosis was designed to allow rapid training of grasp and release activities in hemiplegic hands where there is flexor muscle activity but limited extension or extension that is limited by the flexor hypertonicity (59). It involves the use of repetitive task-specific activities. In a study by Farrell et al. (59) SaeboFlex training occurred in a constraint-induced movement therapy (CIMT) fashion. Thirteen chronic hemiplegic stroke survivors participated in 6 hours per day over a 5-day intervention period. The study lacked a control group and involved other interventions such as neuromuscular stimulation and exercise focused on strength, ROM, and motor control. Therefore, it is difficult to attribute any changes in outcome measures solely to

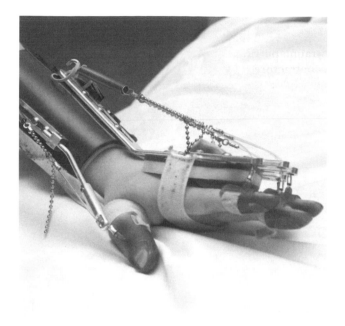

FIGURE 13.6

Dynamic stretching of finger flexors using the Saeboflex dynamic splint.

the SaeboFlex. Results of the study demonstrated reductions in spasticity as measured by the MAS. They also demonstrated improvements in active movement at the shoulder and elbow. Passive ROM in wrist extension improved, but not in wrist flexion or finger flexion or extension. Participants were pain-free throughout the study and demonstrated no negative consequences. No other evidence-based publications are available at the time of this publication that discuss the Saeboflex (Figure 13.6).

Dynasplints

These dynamic splints are made for numerous joints including the shoulder, elbow, wrist, and hand for the upper extremity and knee and ankle for the lower extremity. They provide continuous low load, long-duration stretches to various muscle groups affected by joint contracture, spasticity, and other causes of ROM deficits (60). These devices consist of padded adjustable cuffs with medial and lateral struts that are hinged at the joint axis. Unique to this device is the ability to adjust the tension and force applied across a given joint. This allows for a progressively greater amount of stretch coupled with an increase in duration of the wearing time, which in turn allows for progressive improvement in ROM. Wearing times can progress rapidly with limited risk of skin breakdown and patient discomfort. In a case study, a patient with traumatic brain injury (TBI) used an elbow flexion contracture splint. Wearing time was progressed from 30 minutes to 10 hours per day and an additional 2 hours at night within the first month of use. Ultimately, wearing time ranged between 8 and 12 hours daily. Tension was gradually increased from 2 to 10 by the end of the 2.5-month protocol. Over the course of the case study, elbow extension ROM increased from an initial value of –67° to –15°. No objective measure was used to document spasticity, but the author states "a decrease in tone of the elbow flexion musculature detectable by a gradual lessening in resistance to passive movement." Another study demonstrates improvements in ROM but not spasticity in a randomized control trial comparing the effects of botulinum toxin type A (BTX-A) and manual therapy combined with dynamic splinting with the dynasplint (experimental group). The control group received botulinum toxin and manual therapy alone. Elbow extension improved 33.5% versus 18.7% in the experimental and control groups, respectively. The MAS scores were nonsignificantly reduced 9.3% versus 8.6% in the experimental and control groups, respectively (61). One final study (62) addressed the utility of the dynaplints in the maintenance of increased ROM obtained from injection with botulinum toxin to treat elbow spasticity.

Lycra Garments

Designed to produce continuous stretch of spastic muscles when worn for several hours each day, Lycra garments have demonstrated rapid splinting and antispastic effects on wrist and fingers in patients with hemiplegia (63). These garments are constructed in segments that are stretched in the desired orientation to promote a specific direction of pull and sewn together. The material's elasticity exerts direction stress on the targeted segments to provide continuous stretch. Although not commonly used in the United States, their use is becoming fashionable in some rehabilitation units (64). They have demonstrated effectiveness but require custom fitting and may become hot and uncomfortable for some individuals. Barnes (64) suggested that Lycra garments may be a more comfortable alternative to some cumbersome splints as well as serial casts. Limited evidence exists regarding these garments, particularly as it relates to spasticity. However, Gracies et al. (63) reported on short-term improvements in 16 patients wearing this Lycra garments for 3 hours as splints for the management of their upper extremity spasticity. Results demonstrated significant beneficial effects on wrist and finger spasticity and small improvements in the ROM of the shoulder.

THERAPEUTIC EXERCISE

Exercise is an essential component of the rehabilitation process as it relates to the UMNS (65–67). However, the effects of exercise on spasticity have been less clear however and even considered as contraindicated for persons with MS and stroke as strenuous exercise has been clinically observed to increase spasticity in some patients (66). More recently, new evidence is emerging that advocates for the addition of therapeutic exercise to the rehabilitation program of persons with spasticity as it relates to the UMNS (45, 68, 69).

Unloaded Cycling

A study by Motl et al. (70) evaluated the effects of unloaded leg cycling on spasticity as measured by both the H reflex and MAS in 27 person's with MS. Individuals with relapsing-remitting primary or secondary progressive MS who were not on any antispasticity medications performed exercise on a cycle ergometer for a single session of 20 minutes at an unloaded resistance. Measurements were taken before and at 10, 30, and 60 minutes after exercise. Results demonstrated significant reductions in both MAS and Hmax/Mmax ratios at each experimental time frame. These changes were not noted in the control condition, which consisted of resting comfortably for the same period in the same environment. The authors concluded that unloaded cycling was beneficial in decreasing spasticity in patients with MS. In a follow-up study (71), the effects of a 4-week program of unloaded cycling in 22 persons with MS were examined. The exercise participants cycled 3 times per week for 30 minutes over the 4-week period. Metrics gathered at 1 day after, and 1 and 4 weeks after the 4-week period included the H reflex, (MAS), and the MSSS-88. The researchers found no significant changes in the objective measures of spasticity, H reflex, or MAS spasticity scores. However, there was a reduction in a subjective assessment of spasticity, the MSSS-88.

In a small study of 9 patients poststroke (average of 22 months), Diserens et al. (72) studied the impact of upper extremity ergometry on spasticity and motor performance. After cycling 5 days per week for 3 weeks, there was a reduction in spasticity as measured by the AS of the elbow flexors and extensors.

There was also a significant increase in active elbow ROM and in the force production of the affected upper extremity.

The studies examining the effects of cycling on spasticity are limited and often involve small subject samples as described above. From the limited research available however, it appears that unloaded cycling can have a positive impact on spasticity and does not appear to increase spasticity as once thought. Larger well-controlled studies are needed to examine the effects of resistance cycling on spasticity and to determine optimal treatment parameters for varying UMNS etiologies.

Body Weight–Supported Ambulation

Body weight–supported ambulation has been proposed as a means for improving mobility skill after stroke (73). There are many theories as to its mechanism of action, but Hesse (74) suggests that body weight–supported ambulation is an example of translation work and task-specific repetitive training. There are literally thousands of papers in the literature extolling its potential utility to improve gait more efficiently than the more classically used modalities. It has been used in various populations including CP (75), stroke (76–79), SCI, and MS. It is uncertain if this modality is actually more effective than standard gait training regarding improved gait parameters, and no study has yet demonstrated noted significant improvement in spasticity using this modality.

Strength Training

In a review of 7 randomized controlled trials (RCTs) examining the effects of strength training in persons poststroke with hemiplegia, it was found that neither effortful activities or high-intensity strength training has an excitatory effect on spasticity and that progressive resistive training has a positive impact on overall function (66). A meta-analysis of 15 RCTs that examined the effects of strength training in persons with acute (2 weeks to 4.5 months) and in persons with chronic (2 to 8 years) poststroke concluded that strength training can improve strength, improve activity, and does not increase spasticity (80). These results are further supported by a more recent evidenced-based review of 11 studies performed by Pak and Patten (45), which looked at the effects of high-intensity resistance training on spasticity and function in persons poststroke. The authors found substantial evidence that resistance training increases gait speed and strength with no increase in spasticity.

The reviews above clearly show that strength training in persons poststroke should not be excluded from the rehabilitation program due to a concern for increased spasticity as a result. Although spasticity reduction does not appear to be a benefit of strength training, the positive effects of increased strength and improved function should outweigh any concerns of spasticity exacerbation. Additional research examining strength training and its effect on spasticity in persons with MS, SCI, TBI, and CP are needed to add further clarification to this issue.

MODALITIES

Electrical Stimulation

Electrical stimulation is a commonly used modality for reducing spasticity, improving muscle tone, improving sensation, reducing pain, and facilitating function. The FES and TENS are the 2 most commonly applied forms of ES in current practice and are discussed below. Care must be taken to ensure that the patients and their caregivers understand the nature of ES and its risks and contraindications. Proper electrode placement, care of electrodes, and potential skin irritation/breakdown should be a critical part of the educational component when prescribing these modalities for home and clinic use. Electrical stimulation should not be applied in people with an active implant, for example, pacemaker, in persons who are pregnant, directly over a known tumor or active malignancy, in persons with seizure disorders, over active sites of bleeding, or over growing epiphysis (81, 82).

Functional ES

Functional ES has become a widely accepted form of treatment for paralysis after SCI, stroke, brain injury, and other upper motor neuron disorders (83). Functional ES uses the effects of NMES on intact lower motor neurons and incorporates the movement produced into a functional task (84). Functional ES has historically been used to supplement paralyzed or weakened muscles with functional tasks including standing, gait, and upper extremity function utilizing neuroprosthetic (84) devices (see Figures 13.1, 13.2, and 13.3/insert PT shot 5, 4, 3) Controlled studies that have examined the effectiveness of FES/NMES treatment in the management of spasticity are discussed below (85–89). The FES/NMES look to be promising interventions for the short-term reduction in spasticity, as a tool to facilitate functional movement, and as an adjunct to medical management.

Popovic et al. (87) examined the effects of functional electrical therapy (FET) using an upper extremity neuroprosthesis over a 3-week study period on the paretic arm of 28 persons with acute hemiplegia in a randomized, single-blinded control study. Subjects were randomly assigned to 2 control and 2 FET groups. Each group consisted of a higher functioning group (HFG) and a lower functioning group (LFG) based on the person's ability to move their Upper Extremity (UE) and hand through specified ranges of movement. The 2 control groups received the same physical therapy interventions as the study groups without the FET. The FET groups participated in 30-minute sessions per day over a 3-week period. During the FET sessions, participants were asked to perform a variety of functional UE tasks including brushing the teeth and hair, using a telephone, and manipulating various cans and juices aided by a neuroprosthetic device. Both study groups received daily conventional Bobath therapy during the 3-week study period as well. Outcomes were measured using the Upper Extremity Function test, Drawing Test, MAS of key hand and UE muscles, and the Reduced Upper Extremity Motor Activity Log (MAL). Evaluations were performed both before and after the 3-week program. In addition, follow-up was performed at 6, 13, and 26 weeks after the treatment was completed. The MAS was assessed only at the start of the study and at the 26-week follow-up. At the 26-week follow-up evaluation, the higher functioning FET group demonstrated a statistically significant reduction in UE spasticity when compared to the lower functioning FET group and to the LFG/HFG control groups. The other groups did show reduction in spasticity, albeit nonsignificantly. In addition, all groups demonstrated improvements in the functional outcome measures; however, the gains in the FET groups were significantly larger as compared to the control groups. No adverse events or reactions to the described treatments were noted by the authors. The results from this study outline the importance of adding a FET component to the treatment plan. The combination of FET and functional-based therapies proved to be a beneficial one as the results show. Although therapy alone exhibited good results, the addition of FET improved the outcomes in all metrics studied.

Ring and Rosenthal (86) evaluated the potential effectiveness of home usage of the upper extremity (NESS H200) neuroprosthesis (see Figure 13.2/insert PT shot 4) on upper limb spasticity and active hand function over a 6-week study in 22 patients with moderate to severe upper limb paresis, 3 to 6 months poststroke.

Treatment was initiated at 10 minutes, 2 times per day, and was increased to 50 minutes, 3 times per day, over the first 2 weeks and remained at that level for the remainder of the study. Two modes of stimulation were used: intermittent finger extension and alternating finger flexion and extension. Both the control group and the study group also attended outpatient therapy 3 times per week for a minimum of 3 hours per day for traditional stroke rehabilitation therapies that did not include the NESS H200. Other, nonspecified treatment modalities were available for use to both the control and treatment groups. At the conclusion of the 6-week program, a significantly greater improvement in spasticity and active hand function was noted in the treatment group as compared to the control group as assessed by the MAS, the Box and Blocks, and 3 Jebsen-Taylor hand function tests. It is of interest to note that in the muscle groups with spasticity grades of moderate to severe (3 to 4), 64% of those in the study group improved to grade 2 or less, whereas only 9% of the control group improved to a MAS grade of 2 or less. The authors reported no adverse events or reactions from the treatment in either group.

Yan and Hui-Chan (85) investigated the effects of FES on lower extremity spasticity. Spasticity, motor control, and the ability to walk were assessed, with the TUG test utilized to evaluate walking and motor control. Forty-six patients with an acute stroke within 2 weeks of onset were assigned to 1 of 3 groups: an active FES group that received FES 30 minutes per day, 5 days per week to the ankle dorsiflexors; a sham stimulation group that received 30 minutes of nonfunctioning FES stimulation; and a control group. All 3 groups received standard stroke rehabilitation therapy 5 days per week for 3 weeks. After 3 weeks of the protocol, the treatment group demonstrated a significant improvement in the CSS and ankle dorsiflexion (DF) torque as compared to the sham FES and control groups. In addition, 85% of the FES group was able to ambulate with an assistive device after the 3 weeks of treatment as compared to 60% of the placebo and 46% of the control group; 84.6% of the FES group returned home, which was significantly greater than the other 2 groups. The authors reported that no reactions or adverse events occurred during the study.

Bakhtiary and Fatemy (89) evaluated the effects of NMES combined with inhibitory Bobath techniques on ankle plantar flexor tone, passive ankle DF, and DF strength in an RCT of 40 patients with stroke. Subjects were randomly assigned to a NMES group or to a NMES plus Bobath treatment group. The Bobath plus NMES group underwent 20 daily sessions of

15 minutes of Bobath inhibitory techniques for the LE followed by 9 minutes of NMES applied to the anterior tibialis (cathode) and to the fibular head (anode) over the peroneal nerve. Neuromuscular ES was set at 100 Hz with a 4-second surge on and a 6-second surge off. Outcomes were assessed after each session and included the MAS for spasticity, ankle DF ROM, ankle DF strength, and the soleus H reflex amplitude. The investigators found a significant improvement in ankle plantar flexion spasticity, DF muscle strength, and ROM in both the NMES control group and in the Bobath plus NMES group. In addition, a significant improvement in muscle tone, ankle DF ROM, and DF strength was observed when comparing the NMES plus Bobath group to the NMES only group. The authors concluded that a combination of Bobath techniques plus NMES may be an effective tool for the treatment of spasticity. No adverse events or reactions were noted as a result of the treatment.

Mesci et al. (88) studied the effects of NMES in combination with a traditional rehabilitation program on ankle DF ROM and spasticity in 40 patients with chronic stroke. Forty patients were assigned to equal groups of treatment and control. Both groups received poststroke physical therapy over the 4-week study period. In addition, the treatment group received NMES to the hemiplegic ankle dorsiflexors 5 day per week for the 4-week period. After the study period, the researchers found significant reduction in spasticity and improved ankle ROM when comparing pretreatment and posttreatment measurements over the 4-week study in the treatment group ($P < .05$). Functional ambulation also improved significantly in both groups; however, the difference between the two was not significant. No adverse events or reactions occurred during the study.

All 5 studies discussed demonstrate significant short-term reduction in spasticity using various combinations of FES/NMES. The study by Popovic et al. (87) also showed a sustained reduction in spasticity 26 weeks after the study period, indicating that FES/NMES may potentially play a role in the longer-term management of spasticity. It is important to note that most randomized controlled studies involving FES/NMES examine its effects on poststroke patients. There are numerous, nonrandomized studies with small subject sizes that also demonstrate significant reduction in spasticity in patients with SCI (90, 91), and in persons with MS (92) that were not included in the discussion. Additional well-controlled studies with larger study populations are needed to evaluate its effect on spasticity as a result of SCI, brain injury, and other diagnoses related to the UMNS. The studies reviewed suggest that FES/NMES may provide the

therapist and patient a tool that can be used both clinically and at home to provide short-term relief in spasticity, as well as assistance in performing functional tasks and therapeutic activities. The associated costs, daily treatment time requirements, contraindications, and the ability of the patient and caregivers to carry out a home schedule effectively and safely must all be considered when offering FES/NMES as a home treatment option. Further studies are also needed to determine standardized treatment parameters, patient and caregiver effectiveness in providing treatment, and what, if any, carryover effect FES has on longer-term spasticity management.

Transcutaneous Electrical Nerve Stimulation

Transcutaneous ES is a treatment modality that delivers ES using a current intensity and frequency that are below the motor threshold but above the sensory threshold. It is commonly used as a pain-alleviating modality by physical therapists, and it has also been shown to reduce spasticity in the patient with hemiplegia (93, 94) and in those with SCI (95). More recently, studies have been performed that evaluated the effectiveness of TENS in the management of spasticity in patients with SCI (1), CP (96), MS (97), and stroke (36). Transcutaneous ES is either applied directly to the spastic muscle group, to the antagonistic group, or to both. The exact mechanism of TENS in reducing spasticity remains unclear but has been attributed to the stimulation of cutaneous afferent fibers that would suppress motoneuronal excitability (13). This could occur through a depression of propriospinal interneurons or through synaptic changes in the primary efferent fibers in the dorsal (sensory) horn when applied to the spastic muscle group (98) or through stimulation of the Ia-reciprocal inhibition pathway and subsequent reduction of motoneuronal excitability (99).

Aydin et al. (1) compared the effect of TENS to oral baclofen in a sample of 21 patients with SCI-related spasticity. Eleven patients were treated with TENS, and 10 with oral baclofen. Transcutaneous ES was applied to the bilateral tibial nerves to incorporate the gastrocnemius muscle at a frequency of 100 Hz at an intensity of 50 mA for 15 minutes for 15 days. Clinical spasticity scores including the lower extremity AS, spasm frequency scale, painful spasm scale, clonus, deep tendon reflex, plantar stimulation response scores, and electrophysiological variables consisting of various H reflex responses were measured 15 minutes after the first TENS application and 15 minutes after the 15th application. The patients in the oral baclofen group received 5-mg increases every 3 or 5 days, taking into account the patient's tolerance until a sufficient clinical response was reached, or a maximum dosage of 80 mg/d. Posttreatment evaluation was made after 8 weeks on the therapeutic dose. Significant improvement ($P < .05$) was found in the lower extremity Ashworth score, spasm frequency scale, deep tendon reflex score, functional disability score, and Functional Independence Measure (FIM) scores in both the TENS and oral baclofen groups after treatment. The most noted improvement in the TENS group was 15 minutes after the 15th treatment session in the lower limb Ashworth score. The percentage of change in the clinical, electrophysiological, and functional measurements due to baclofen did not differ significantly ($P > .05$) from the changes due to repeated TENS treatments. The authors concluded that TENS may be recommended as a supplement to medical management of spasticity and as a clinical tool to be used before stretching and ROM. No adverse events or reactions to the treatments were noted by the authors (Figure 13.7).

Another group (96) examined the effects of TENS and exercise on spasticity and function in ambulatory children with CP as measured by the CSS, D and E portions of the Gross Motor Function Measure (GMFM), and walking speed. Thirty-eight control and 40 study group participants all received a standard exercise program over the initial 6-week period that was continued at home by the caregivers for the remainder of the 24-week period. The treatment group received TENS to the spastic agonist and antagonist muscles of the affected leg for 20 minutes per session, 5 days per week for 6 weeks. Both control and study group

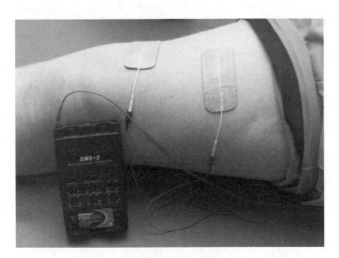

FIGURE 13.7

Demonstration of TENS lead placement to address quadriceps tone.

participants demonstrated a decrease in spasticity and improvements in motor function and ambulation at 6, 12, and 24 weeks of therapy ($P < .05$). In addition, the TENS group showed a statistically significant decrease in the CSS and GMFM and an increase in walking speed when compared to the control group after 6, 12, and 24 weeks of treatment. The study demonstrated that TENS combined with exercise was more effective in reducing spasticity and improving function than exercise alone. This study also demonstrated that TENS may offer an adjunctive form of longer-term management as the decrease in spasticity was maintained 18 weeks after the TENS treatments had ended. No reactions or adverse events were noted by the researchers.

Miller et al. (97) evaluated the potential benefit of TENS on spasticity in 32 patients with MS in a single, blind repeated crossover study. Two groups were evaluated over a 2-week period in which they either received TENS for 8 hours throughout the day or for 60 minutes per day. The TENS was applied at 100 Hz per 0.125 millisecond pulse width per continuous mode. After the initial 2-week period, each group took 2 weeks off and then switched treatments for another 2-week period. A repeated measures analysis of variance of the Global Spasticity Scale was performed before and after the TENS treatments to ensure the order of the treatment did not affect the results. Because there were no significant differences between the 2 groups or in the order in which they received treatment, the results from both groups were combined before and after outcome comparisons. Although their results did not show statistical significance between the 2 treatment interventions as measured by the Global Spasticity Scale on the quadriceps of the most affected limb, there was a significant reduction in spasm frequency per the PSFS and in pain reduction per a 10-point VAS in the 8-hour treatment session. The overall reduction in spasticity, albeit nonsignificant, remains clinically important as therapists can utilize the short-term reduction in spasticity achieved after TENS application before therapy into therapeutic activities that incorporate strengthening, ROM, and functional exercises. It is also worthy to note that the authors reported a significant reduction in the Penn Spasm Scale after the 2 week, 8 hour/day TENS intervention. Although it would not be feasible or pragmatic to apply TENS for 8 hours per day over multiple muscle groups to a person with generalized spasticity, it might be applicable for focal spasticity treatment. The authors reported one dropout due to failure to adhere to the protocol. Two others dropped out due to health and scheduling issues. Otherwise, there were no adverse events or reactions as a result of the treatment.

Ng and Hui-Chan (36) studied the effects of TENS and a TENS plus task-related training (TRT) program on spasticity and gait velocity in 88 patients with stroke in a randomized control study. The participants were assigned to 1 of 4 groups: a control group that received no treatment; a (TENS) group which received TENS at 100 Hz per 0.2 millisecond pulse width over 4 acupuncture points of the affected lower extremity for 60 minutes per day, 5 days per week for 4 weeks; a placebo plus TRT group (placebo + TRT) group that received sham TENS for 60 minutes per day plus a home task training session of 60 minutes per day that consisted of 4 weight-bearing and stepping exercises; and a TENS + TRT group that received both TENS and a TRT home program. Ankle plantar flexion spasticity was measured by the CSS before and after 2 and 4 weeks of treatment and at follow-up 4 weeks after treatment had ended. All 3 treatment groups demonstrated a significant reduction in spasticity when compared to the control group at the 2 and 4 week mark. The TENS and the TENS +TRT groups demonstrated significantly more reduction in spasticity than the placebo + TRT group at the 2-week assessment. The combined TENS + TRT group showed significantly greater improvement in gait velocity when compared TENS alone or with placebo + TRT. This study is important for the therapist because it demonstrates the effectiveness of combining treatment interventions and shows the positive affect of TENS alone as an intervention. It should also be pointed out that the positive results of this study were maintained at the 4-week follow up after the final treatment session, again demonstrating the potential of TENS as a an adjunct therapy for longer-term spasticity management. No adverse events or reactions to the treatment were reported by the authors.

The studies suggest that TENS has the potential to be an effective adjunct to the medical management of spasticity. The short-term reduction in spasticity obtained can provide a window of opportunity for the patient and therapist to address the underlying features of weakness, coordination, balance, and impaired function so often seen as a result of the UMNS. Although TENS may not be appropriate for the patient with generalized spasticity due to the complexity of application to multiple sites, it should be considered as a focal treatment. Furthermore, TENS may have a place in long-term spasticity management as described above. As with any piece of equipment prescribed for home use, the therapist must take into account cost-effectiveness, the ability of the patient and/or their caregivers to effectively and safely carry out

the home program, and how the device fits into the overall goals of the patient and the therapy program. A critical component to the success of any home program involves a detailed discussion with the patient and caregiver(s) regarding proper setup and safety.

Thermal Modalities

Heat and cold (Cryotherapy) applications have been used for decades in the treatment of pain, inflammation, muscle spasms, and spasticity as a result of the UMNS (2, 100). Cold is typically applied through ice packs, ice massage, or cold baths but can also be applied through cold air circulation and vapocoolants. Heat modalities include hot packs, warm baths, US, diathermy, and IR. Although these modalities are commonly used, their efficacy in the treatment of spasticity remains inconclusive and in need of further validation through rigorous, well-controlled studies.

Cold

Although the underlying physiology of cold in reducing spasticity remains clearly undefined, there are several proposed mechanisms for its effectiveness. Cold may cause a slowing of nerve conduction, a decrease in muscle spindle activity, desensitization of cutaneous receptors, and changes in central nervous system excitability (100–103). All of these mechanisms could lead to an overall reduction in the monosynaptic stretch reflex activity, thereby reducing spasticity (2). Cold should not be applied to known areas of circulatory insufficiency and over known malignancy or tumor and should be used with caution in person's who are pregnant or over areas of insensate skin, as prolonged cold application at lower temperatures could lead to tissue damage (81, 82).

Chiara et al. (104) examined the effects of a 24°C (75.1°F) cold bath on oxygen consumption, perceived exertion, and spasticity as measured by the MAS in 14 patients with minimal to moderate lower extremity spasticity (MAS 1–3) with MS. Each subject was given 2 treatments in random order: (1) rest at ambient room temperature (approximately 24°C) × 20 minutes (AT group) and (2) immersion in a cold bath at 24°C × 20 minutes (CT group). After 20 minutes, subjects in both groups walked on a treadmill for 10 minutes, rested for 30 minutes, and then walked an additional 10 minutes. This was performed on 2 separate days in random order. Spasticity was measured before treatment, immediately after the 20 minutes of AT or CT, and again just before the second trial of walking. Spasticity was significantly higher in the CT group immediately after the 20 minutes of treatment

(1.6 vs 1.4). It should be noted that baseline mean spasticity measurements for both groups was 1.4, which remained constant throughout the AT group sessions, and spiked to 1.6 in the CT group, but returned to the 1.4 mean at the 30-minute testing mark. The authors reported 50% of the CT group subjects were visibly shaking after the cold bath immersion, which could easily explain the increase in spasticity at the second assessment.

Another group of investigators (100) studied the effects of a hydrotherapy exercise program on spasticity, spasm severity, FIM scores, and oral baclofen intake on 20 patients with SCI. The subjects were divided into 2 groups: (1) the control group received passive ROM exercises twice per day and their prestudy oral baclofen as prescribed for 10 weeks; (2) the study group received the same treatment as the control group and an additional 20 minutes of full immersion hydrotherapy exercises in a 71°F pool 3 times per week. Outcome metrics were taken before and after the 10-week study period. Both groups demonstrated a statistical improvement in spasticity per the AS scale (4.1 to 1.7) in the study group as compared to (3.9 to 2.1) in the control group, although the difference between the 2 groups was not significant. There was a significant decrease in the spasm severity scores of the hydrotherapy group when compared to the control. Both groups significantly improved with FIM scores, with the hydrotherapy group demonstrating a larger change. When looking at baclofen intake, the hydrotherapy group significantly decreased its use of oral baclofen from 100 to 45 mg/d over the 10-week period, whereas the control group remained unchanged at 96 mg/d. Their results contradict the previous study in which no change in spasticity was seen. There are several plausible explanations for the difference. First, the prior study examined and found that patients with MS with spasticity of cerebral origin which may respond differently to cooler water than patients with spasticity of spinal origin. Second, the baseline spasticity scores in the previous study were relatively low to begin with (1.4) for both groups on the MAS as compared to (3.9) the control and (4.1) the study groups using the AS of the present study. Finally, it is possible that the combination of baclofen and hydrotherapy produced a larger treatment effect in the present study. There was no mention of baclofen intake in the prior study, only that the patients stayed on their current medication schedule throughout the study (104).

Other researchers (105) studied the influence of cold air therapy on 46 paraplegic rabbits with spasticity. Cold air was applied for 60 minutes to the triceps surae group at a distance of 10 cm to elicit intramuscular temperatures of 25°C, 30°C, and 32.5°C in the 3 study groups, respectively. Clinical spasticity measurements (muscle tone per the MAS, stretch reflex, Babinski sign, and ankle clonus) were taken immediately after intramuscular temperatures were achieved and at 30 and 60 minutes after. Spasticity was also measured electrophysiologically through the H/M and F/M ratios. Although significant reductions in spasticity were found in all 3 groups, the reduction lasted up to 30 minutes in the 30°C and 25°C groups, respectively, and less than 30 minutes in the 32.5°C group per clinical measurements. At 60 minutes, the mean value of spasticity in the 25°C and 30°C groups was still lower than pretreatment values, although nonsignificantly. When measured electrophysiologically, the reduction in spasticity was observed immediately and not at all after 30 and 60 minutes postcooling. This study supports the limited research on the effects of cold in that it offers a short-term reduction in spasticity of approximately 20 to 30 minutes. (106) Although this is a relatively short amount of time, it does provide a window of opportunity for the patient and therapist to focus on the negative aspects of the UMNS with a reduction in the debilitating effects of spasticity.

Bell and Lehmann (107) investigated the effects of cooling on the Hoffmann (H) reflex and the tendon tap (T) reflex through surface EMG recordings in 16 healthy subjects before and after cooling of the triceps surae muscle group. They found no significant change in the H reflex amplitude precooling and postcooling but did find a nonsignificant decrease in the height of compound action potentials when observing T waveforms. Their findings dispute earlier claims that cooling can facilitate the excitatory alpha motoneuron as measured by the H reflex and increase spasticity, and reinforce claims that cooling decreases muscle spindle activity as measured by the T reflex. Price et al. (108) also studied the influence of cryotherapy on spasticity of the triceps surae in 25 participants with TBI, stroke, and SCI. Spasticity was measured precooling, during cooling, and 1 hour postcooling using the viscoelastic properties of the muscle as a baseline. The researchers found a statistically significant reduction in spasticity during cryotherapy, but only a mild trend toward a decrease postcooling. Of interest to note is 2 of the participants had a clear increase in spasticity postcooling, which reinforces some claims that cooling may increase spasticity initially due to an increase in alpha motoneuron excitability (2).

The effectiveness of cold application in the treatment of spasticity remains questionable. The mixed results discussed leave questions as to the temperatures being studied and the methods of application. There is no clearly defined definition as to the temperature range that constitutes "cold." Further, well-controlled human studies looking at different temperature applications through cooling garments, moist ice packs, or colder air/bath immersion would be of interest, as would research examining what effect antispasmodic medications in combination with various cold therapies has on spasticity. From the limited research available, cold application may be useful as a short-term intervention to allow therapists and patients a small window of up to 30 minutes to address areas such as weakness, balance, and impaired functional mobility. The time needed to produce an effect is also unclear and would largely depend upon the treatment modality utilized. In the studies above, cold was applied between 20 and 60 minutes at temperatures ranging from 24°C to 32.5°C to achieve the desired effect. When using ice massage or vapocoolants, the application time would need to be decreased because these modalities cool the skin rapidly and could lead to skin injury if applied too long. In addition, studies where participants exhibit moderate to severe spasticity at baseline may elicit different results, as studies with low baseline means have less room for a treatment effect. Finally, we could not find any studies that examined the effects of cold therapy on functional improvements in subjects with spasticity. Research in this area would be highly beneficial when making clinical decisions as to the optimum course of treatment. As a long-term solution to spasticity management, cold applications do not appear to represent a viable solution at this time based upon the absence of well-controlled, randomized studies.

Heat

Heat has also been used in the management of spasticity as a component of the UMNS. The exact mechanism of heat in affecting spasticity is undefined. As heat is capable of reducing pain, this may be a plausible explanation for its reported effectiveness (2), as pain is known to increase spasticity. The majority of the limited research examining heat as a treatment modality revolves around the use of US. This is probably due to the inherent nature of US to penetrate deeper than superficial hot packs, hot baths, fluidotherapy, and paraffin. Diathermy and IR modalities are also capable of deeper heat production (2). However, there is little research into their effectiveness in the treatment of spasticity as a component of the UMNS and are not discussed in detail in this chapter.

Researchers (109) compared the effects of US and IR therapies on ROM and spasticity of the ankle plantar flexors in 21 patients with stroke. Subjects were randomly assigned to either the US or the IR groups.

Ultrasound was applied for 10 minutes and IR for 20 minutes to the ankle plantar flexors. Clinical measures including the H reflex, AS, and ROM were evaluated before treatment, immediately after, and again 15 minutes after treatment. The researchers found no significant reduction in spasticity immediately after treatment or 15 minutes later in either the US or the IR groups per the H reflex and AS scores. This study contradicts an earlier study by Ansari et al. (110) in which 12 patients with stroke were divided into a US group and a sham US group to determine the effects of US on ankle plantar spasticity. Outcome measures included the AS and the H reflex. Continuous US was applied for 15 minutes, 3 days per week, and every other day for 15 sessions. The authors found a significant reduction in the AS and in the H reflex ratios of the study group. However, the reduction in the AS was not significant when compared to the sham US group. The reduction in the H reflex ratio was significant between the 2 groups, and the H reflex actually increased in the placebo group. The researchers concluded that US can reduce Hmax/Mmax ratio measure as a measure of alpha motoneuron excitability and spasticity as measured by the AS in ankle plantar flexor spasticity in patients with stroke.

As with cold applications, the use of heat as a therapeutic modality in the management of spasticity remains unclear and anecdotal due to the limited research available. The 2 studies above using US found different results with similar populations, similar interventions, and using the same outcome measures. We could find only one relevant study examining IR as discussed above and no randomized controlled studies looking at diathermy, paraffin, hot packs, warm bath immersion, or fluidotherapy, although many of these modalities are commonly listed as treatment options for spasticity (2). Because varying forms of heat have been utilized for years for differing pathologies, studies examining its effectiveness in reducing spasticity as a component of the UMNS with diverse modalities, different temperatures, and applications would be beneficial to the patient and therapist in the overall management and treatment of this condition.

COMBINATION THERAPIES

To this point, this chapter has focused largely on individual forms of treatment for spasticity. It is clinically intuitive, however, to hypothesize that a combination of therapeutic interventions would have a cumulative effect and offer a wider range of management options. Experienced therapists rarely utilize one form of treatment in isolation. Rather, they combine various interventions based on clinical experience, research, and judgment to affect the desired outcome. Of the literature discussed to this point, many of the researchers utilized a combination of modalities plus therapeutic exercise/activities in the treatment groups that demonstrated statistically significant spasticity effect: TENS + TRT (36), neuroprosthetic FES program in combination with outpatient therapy, (86) Bobath techniques plus NMES (89), TENS combined with home exercise (96), and NMES in combination with a traditional rehabilitation (88). To allow patients with moderate to severe spasticity to more effectively take part in functional-based therapy programs however, other interventions should be included to achieve the maximal effect on spasticity (111).

Botulinum toxin type A injection and baclofen (oral and intrathecal) are mainstays in the medical management of spasticity. There is a growing body of research (111–114) and systematic reviews (115) examining the effects of BTX-A in combination with therapeutic exercise, constraint-induced therapy (116–118), SC (119–122), or ES (123–125) on spasticity intervention that is worthy of discussion, as these combinations represent the importance of the multidisciplinary approach to the management of the patient with spasticity and ultimately to improve function.

Botulinum Toxin Type A Injection and Electrical Modalities

Chang et al. (111) looked at the effects of BTX-A injection in combination with 6 weeks of postinjection (FES) and repetitive hand task therapy on hand spasticity and function in 14 patients with hemiplegia due to stroke or TBI. The participants were divided into 2 groups: 5 patients in the Chedoke-McMaster Assessment HFG and 9 patients in the Chedoke-McMaster Assessment LFG. Both groups received BTX-A injection within 7 days of the initial study assessment in combination with six 1-hour therapy follow-up visits. They also received 12 weeks of 60 minutes per day of home-based FES-assisted repetitive hand tasks, such as dealing cards, stacking canned goods, placing pennies into coin sleeves, and washing mirrors and countertops. Outcome measures were recorded at baseline, 6, 9, and 12 weeks postinjection. Outcome measures including the MAS, MALs, and the Action Research Arm Test (ARAT) improved significantly for both groups over the 12-week study period, although the change was not significant between the groups when looking at the ARAT or the MAS. No adverse events or reactions to the treatment protocol were noted. The results of this study indicate that BTX-A injections combined with postinjection therapy and FES

can improve hand function and decrease spasticity in persons with stroke or TBI who present with either high or low baseline functional deficits.

Baricich et al. (125) studied the combined effects of BTX-A with taping, ES, or stretching on ankle plantar flexor spasticity in 23 chronic (a minimum of 6 months poststroke) hemiplegic persons with spastic equinus foot. Subjects were randomly assigned to each of the 3 treatment groups. Outcome measures including the MAS, ankle PROM, gastrocnemius medialis motor action potential, and maximum ankle DF in stance phase were taken before injection and at 10, 20, and 90 days postinjection. Both heads of the gastrocnemius on the affected side were injected. The ES group received stimulation at 5 Hz to the injected muscles for two 30-minute sessions daily for 5 consecutive days. Stretching of the ankle plantar flexors with the knee straight for 20 minutes followed each ES session. Participants in the taping group had the thigh and ankle taped into ankle DF. Taping was checked daily for 5 days and reapplied to maintain maximal stretch of the affected muscles. Subjects in the stretching group received two 30-minute sessions of stretching to the affected muscle for 7 days. At 10 days postinjection, spasticity had significantly improved in the ES group only, although all groups demonstrated a decrease. All 3 groups improved significantly in the other outcome measures. Twenty days postinjection, all 3 groups continued to show a significant decline in spasticity as compared to baseline with the ES and taping groups improving significantly more than the stretching group. At 90 days postinjection, the ES and taping groups remained significantly lower in MAS scores than at baseline, although scores were higher than at the 20-day mark, indicating that the treatment effect had reached its ceiling and was in decline. Overall, the groups receiving BTX-A injection combined with ES and stretching or with taping and stretching performed significantly better than the group that received injection and stretching only in all metrics collected. There was no report of any adverse events or reactions to the treatments performed. The results of this study demonstrate that combining BTX-A injection with ES and taping could be beneficial in the treatment of persons with spastic equinovarus foot. Although the results from the combination BTX-A injection and stretching group were not significant when compared with the other groups, stretching and BTX-A combined exhibited reduced spasticity significantly as compared to baseline 20 days postinjection.

Another group (123) examined the combined effects of BTX-A and NMES on ankle plantar flexor spasticity and DF ROM in 18 children with CP. In the 7 treatment group participants, NMES was applied to the motor points of the gastrocnemius muscle at 40 Hz to a visible muscle contraction for 30 minutes, twice per week for the 2-week study period. The 11 control group subjects received BTX-A only. Both groups also continued with their prestudy physical therapy sessions twice per week for the 2-week period. At the 2-week and 3-month follow-ups, both the control and treatment groups demonstrated significant reductions in ankle plantar flexor spasticity per the MAS when compared to baseline. Although the combined effect of NMES was not significant versus the control group, it is important to note that ankle DF ROM was significantly improved at 2 weeks and 3 months in the treatment group when compared to the control group and significantly in gait per the Physician Rating Scale at the 3-month mark. No adverse reactions or events were noted as result of the treatments in this study. This study demonstrates that although BTX-A combined with NMES has no greater affect on spasticity than BTX-A alone after 3 months of treatment, the combination of the 2 interventions does provide a significant effect on ankle ROM and in gait mechanics per the Physician Rating Scale. These 2 improvements alone would enable the patient and therapist to continue to work on functional-based interventions such as gait and ankle balance strategies. No adverse reactions or events were noted as result of the treatments in this study.

Botulinum Toxin Type A Injection and CIMT

Page et al. (116) introduced the concept of spasticity reduction through a combination of BTX-A chemodenervation injections with modified constraint-induced therapy (mCIMT). Their results were presented through a case study of a 44-year-old man who had experienced a stroke 14 months before beginning treatment. The patient participated in a 10-week combination of Physical Therapy (PT) and Occupational Therapy (OT), which consisted of ½ hour each, 3 times per week. The majority of OT (24 minutes) concentrated on the affected UE with functional-based tasks and the remainder on compensatory strategies. PT focused mainly on UE stretching, gait, and balance with approximately 5 minutes dedicated to compensatory strategies for the unaffected side. In addition, the patient's unaffected UE was restrained through the use of a mesh mitt and hemisling secured by Velcro straps for 5 hours, every weekday for the 10-week period. After 10 weeks of mCIMT, the patient demonstrated marked improvement in UE function per the Fugl-Meyer Assessment of Motor Recovery After Stroke (Fugl) and ARAT. The subject still exhibited stiffness in his fingers and the inability to extend his Proximal Inter Phalangeal

(PIP) joints in the ring and middle fingers. The patient received a BTX-A injection 2 weeks after the end of the mCIMT therapy to the affected muscle groups. Four weeks after injection, the patient continued to demonstrate improvements in the Fugl and ARAT. Spasticity in the affected finger flexors decreased from a 2 on the MAS to a 1+. The patient also reported good improvement in his ability to manipulate a larger variety of objects versus before injection. Although the results are from a single case study, they remain clinically relevant in that they demonstrate the promising affect this combination could have on spasticity and UE function in persons who have sustained a stroke and opened the door for a larger controlled trials (117, 118).

Sun et al. (117) followed the above case study with a randomized controlled study that examined the combined effects of BTX-A injection with mCIMT on UE spasticity and function in 32 patients with chronic stroke (≥1 year poststroke). All participants began the treatment protocols 1 day after BTX-A injection into the affected muscle groups of the hemiplegic UE. The 14 subjects in the control group attended traditional rehabilitation 3 times per day for 3 months. Treatment consisted of 1 hour each of PT and OT. Therapy focused on neurodevelopmental training techniques, balance, gait, UE function, and endurance. The 15 study group participants received shaping exercises and intensive massed practice of the affected UE for 2 hours per day, 3 days per week for the 3-month period. In addition, the nonaffected UE was restrained for 5 hours per day during the patient's awake hours with a soft mitt. A behavioral contract and patient diary dictated what exercises could be performed at home with and without the restraint. The primary outcome measure was the MAS of the affected UE. Secondary measures included the MAL and the ARAT. Outcome assessments were measured before BTX-A injection, at 4 weeks, 3 months, and 6 months after injection. All participants demonstrated significant reductions in UE spasticity at 4 weeks and 3 months postinjection without differences between the groups. At the 6-month follow-up, the study group sustained a significant difference from baseline in the elbow, wrist, and finger flexors, which was also significant as compared to the control group, which maintained significant reduction in spasticity in the wrist flexors only. Both groups demonstrated improvement in the ARAT scores 4 weeks postinjection without differences between the 2 groups. The study group continued to improve in ARAT scores with significant differences at 3 and 6 months versus the control group. The study group also exhibited significantly greater improvement in both subscales of the MAL at 3 and 6 months compared to the control group. Two adverse events in both groups were noted due to mild injection site pain, which was transient. No adverse reactions were noted with either treatment group. Although the results of this study are highly promising, it was the only controlled study we could find that examined the combined effects of BTX-A and mCIMT on spasticity management. Additional research examining this combination on spasticity and improved function would be welcomed and likely very beneficial to the treatment of the patient with spasticity.

Botulinum Toxin Type A Injection and Therapeutic Exercise

In an RCT of 38 patients with MS and severe focal spasticity per the MAS (grades >3–4), (114) the combined effects of BTX-A injection with exercise therapy consisting of stretching and active movement over a 12-week study period were examined. The control ($n = 18$) received BTX-A injections to the affected muscle groups of both the UEs and LEs. The study group ($n = 20$) received similar BTX-A injections and physical therapy 7 days per week for a total of 15 consecutive days. Therapy sessions consisted of a combination of active and passive movements designed to maintain muscle length, including injection site–specific stretching and reciprocal movement techniques for a total of 40 minutes per session. Outcome data included the MAS and a 0-10 VAS patient rating of spasticity relief. Data were collected preinjection and at 2, 4, and 12 weeks postinjection. The researchers found a significant decrease in spasticity at 2, 4, and 12 weeks postinjection as compared to the control group ($P < .01$). The study group also demonstrated significant improvement over the control group per the VAS at weeks 4 and 12, but not at week 2. This could be attributed to the relatively short amount of time after the BTX-A injection and the differences between patient report of spasticity versus clinical measures, which may or may not correlate with each other as discussed earlier in this chapter. This study supports the use of stretching in combination with BTX-A injection as a strategy for spasticity management in persons with MS and for persons poststroke as discussed earlier in this chapter (125). The reduction in spasticity obtained through BTX-A injection can allow the therapist and patient to effectively work on functional-based therapies including gait, balance, and ADL. No adverse events or reactions to the treatment protocols were noted by the authors.

Another study (113) evaluated the effects of BTX-A plus OT versus injection alone, OT alone, or a control group in 80 patients with spastic quadriplegia, triplegia, or hemiplegic CP. Main outcome measures included the Canadian Outcome Performance Measure (COPM) and the Global Attainment Scale (GAS). Secondary outcomes included the Melbourne Assessment of Unilateral Upper Limb Function, the Australian Authorized Adaptation of the Child Health Questionnaire, the Quality of Upper Extremity Skills Test, the Pediatric Evaluation of Disability Inventory, and the Tardieu Scale for spasticity assessment. Metrics were collected at baseline, 2 weeks, 3 months, and 6 months after baseline evaluation. One week before beginning the OT protocols, participants in the BTX-A injection groups received an injection to the affected muscle groups. The OT protocol consisted of 1 hour a week of therapy for 12 weeks. Therapists were free to use treatments deemed appropriate for this population and included, stretching, casting, splinting, motor training, environmental modification, and practice of specific goal-related activities. Subjects in the OT groups and control group were also allowed to continue their pretrial OT sessions throughout the 6-month study period, which presents a major limitation to this study, as these sessions were not controlled in any way. No adverse events were reported in the control group. The study groups reported a total of 9 adverse events that comprised nausea, vomiting, flu-like symptoms, fever, and upper respiratory tract infection. The BTX-A plus OT group demonstrated significantly greater gains on the COPM and GAS at 3 and 6 months as compared to the others. There was no difference noted between the BTX-A only and the OT only groups. These are important findings because both measures are patient/caregiver reports indicating that the BTX-A plus OT group attained both functional performance and lifestyle goals as a result of the treatment protocol. No difference between any of the groups was observed in the Quality of Upper Extremity Skills Test metrics. Spasticity decreased significantly in both groups that received BTX-A injections up to the 3-month mark with no significant difference between the 2 groups. The effect began to wear off at 3 months, and spasticity returned to baseline by 6 months. However, the results of the COPM and GAS remained throughout the 6-month period reinforcing the argument that what is reported functionally by the patient and/or their caregiver may not correlate to what is observed clinically, especially when it comes to spasticity and the effect it has on function be it positive or negative.

Botulinum Toxin Type A Injection and SC

Farina et al. (119) examined the combined effects of BTX-A injection plus casting in 13 subjects poststroke with equinovarus foot. Control subjects and

6 treatment participants received BTX-A injections to the tibialis posterior and gastroc-soleus muscles of the affected LE. The treatment group was casted with a removable cast that was worn at night for 4 months. Outcome measures including static and dynamic baropodometric tests, the MAS, and the 10-meter walk test were taken before injection and at 2 and 4 months postinjection. Two months after injection, both groups demonstrated therapeutic effects, although not significantly between the two. At 4 months, the treatment group demonstrated continued clinical improvements in all outcome measures, whereas the control group had returned to baseline measures. Although the study was based on a small sample size, the results reinforce the concept of combining casting with BTX-A for persons poststroke who demonstrate equinovarus deformities. No adverse reactions in either group were reported by the researchers.

Newman et al. (120) evaluated the effects of delayed SC in contrast to immediate casting after BTX-A injection in 12 children with CP and partially reducible spastic equinus foot. All children received BTX-A injections to the gastroc-soleus complex of the affected LE. Participants were randomized into 2 groups. The first group (n = 6) received immediate casting. The second group (n = 6) was casted 4 weeks after injection. Casts were replaced every week for 3 weeks. Three children in the immediate casting group complained of pain and had to be recasted before the prescribed recasting. None of the delayed group required recasting. Outcome was measured by the fast DF angle of the Tardieu Scale (R1). Results were measured at 3 and 6 months postinjection. After 3 months, the delayed casting group demonstrated a 27°improvement in the DF angle vs a 17° improvement in the immediate casting group. At 6 months postinjection, the delayed casting group had maintained a 19° improvement, whereas the immediate casting group had decreased to 11°. Although the within- and between-group differences were not significant and the sample size was small, the results demonstrate that delayed SC of up to 4 weeks after BTX-A injection can reduce ankle plantar flexor spasticity greater than with immediate casting in children with spastic ankle equinus foot. A larger study with the same parameters and metrics would be welcomed, as the questions of casting, not casting, and when are often asked with this patient population.

In a similar study (126) of 10 children with CP with equinus foot, the control group was placed in an ankle foot orthosis immediately after injection, whereas the study group was casted. Outcome measures were measured before injection and at 1, 4, and 12 months and included the MAS, GMFM, ROM, and gait analysis. The researchers found significant reduction in spasticity after 1 month in both groups and after 4 and 12 months in the group that was casted. In addition, walking speed and GMFM were significantly improved in the casted group at 4 months. No change was noted in ankle kinematics during the gait cycle in either group throughout the study.

Ackman et al. (127) compared the cumulative effects of 3 treatment sessions of BTX-A injection only, placebo injection and SC, and the combination of BTX-A injection and SC in the management of dynamic equinus deformity in ambulatory children with spastic CP. Thirty-nine children were enrolled in the randomized, double blind, placebo-controlled prospective study. Children were randomly assigned to 1 of 3 treatment groups: BTX-A only (B), placebo injection plus casting (C), or BTX-A plus casting (B + C). Three treatments including injection and casting were administered at baseline, 3 months, and 6 months. Evaluations were performed at baseline, 3, 6, 7.5, and 12 months after initial treatment. Primary outcome measures included ankle kinematics, gait velocity, and stride length. Secondary outcome measures included ankle spasticity as measured by the AS and Tardieu Scale, ankle plantar flexion strength, ROM, and ankle kinematics during initial contact, stance, and swing phases of gait. The BTX-A injection only group (B) demonstrated no significant change in any metric throughout the study period. In addition, ankle spasticity was not significantly decreased in group B at any time throughout the study period. The placebo injection plus casting (group C) demonstrated a significant decrease in spasticity on both the Ashworth and the Tardieu Scales ($P \leq .02$) from baseline to each follow-up assessment. The BTX-A plus casting (group B + C) did not demonstrate significant reduction in spasticity on the AS at any assessment interval but did demonstrate a significant reduction in spasticity on the Tardieu Scale ($P \leq .05$) from baseline to 6, 7.5, and 12 months. Of interest is the significant increase in spasticity in the placebo injection plus casting and BTX-A injection plus casting groups on the Tardieu Scale ($P \leq .05$) and in group C on the AS between 7.5 months and 1 year. The degree of spasticity, however, remained below the baseline values at 1 year follow-up. There was no skin breakdown resulting from the casts, no injuries during cast removal, nor any early removal of the cast for any of the participants. Noted adverse events included 2 children falling more often than usual immediately after treatment, which resolved within 1 to 2 weeks. Results of this study indicate that BTX-A injection alone demonstrated no improvement in the outcomes measured, whereas casting alone and BTX-A plus casting were effective in the short-term and long-term management of dynamic equinus in children with spastic CP.

Many of the above results are contrasted in a systematic review of the effects of casting, casting plus BTX-A injection, or BTX-A injection only on foot equinus in children with CP (<20 years old). In addition, the timing and sequencing of casting with BTX-A injection was also examined (122). Twenty-two articles were reviewed including 7 RCTs. The authors concluded that there is little evidence that casting is superior to no casting, but the protocols of casting in current use have not been compared with any treatment in a control group in any of the reviewed RCT. This makes sense in that the population being studied is children with CP. We suggest it would be difficult for any parent to withhold treatment that could provide benefit to their child, regardless of the study. It was also concluded that there is no strong and consistent evidence that combining SC and BTX-A injections provides any greater benefit than using each intervention alone. Finally, it was determined that there was no evidence that the order or timing of treatment (casting before BTX-A versus BTX-A before casting) affects outcome. In the review, the authors pointed out that much of the evidence reviewed both positive and negative is weak and that the results could be explained by limitations found within the various studies. It should also be mentioned that most studies examining SC and BTX-A injections focus on children with CP. Studies examining the effects of these treatments in other etiologies including MS, stroke, TBI, and SCI are needed because these populations also demonstrate significant contractures related to spasticity as a component of the UMNS.

SUMMARY

Pharmacology, surgical options, intrathecal medications, and chemodenervation are what many commonly think of when considering interventions for spasticity management. However, as the authors have discussed in this chapter, there are many therapeutic treatments that can play an important role in the treatment of patients who have sequelae from the UMNS. Although commonly prescribed and performed, there are significant deficiencies in the literature in regards to large double-blinded trials proving that fully supports their use. However, progress has been made, and studies like the EXCITE trial have given strong scientific evidence to support their use. The authors have reviewed many of the commonly used therapeutic interventions, the indications for their use, and the

decision process used by skilled clinicians to design the most appropriate treatment approach. Therapy can be an extremely useful tool in the management of spasticity, either as a single treatment or as a part of a multifaceted approach to maximize a person's overall function. The authors hope that the information provided will be useful to both clinicians planning treatments and rehabilitation scientists as they develop novel interventions to further improve treatment options. Finally, the safety and risks of treatment options is discussed to further assist the reader in their treatment choices.

References

1. Aydin G, Tomruk S, Keles I, Demir SO, Orkun S. Transcutaneous electrical nerve stimulation versus baclofen in spasticity: clinical and electrophysiologic comparison. *Am J Phys Med Rehabil* 2005;84(8):584–592.
2. Watanabe T. The role of therapy in spasticity management. *Am J Phys Med Rehabil* 2004;83(10 Suppl):S45–S49.
3. Woldag H, Hummelsheim H. Evidence-based physiotherapeutic concepts for improving arm and hand function in stroke patients: a review. *J Neurol* 2002;249(5):518–528.
4. Hsieh JT, Wolfe DL, Miller WC, Curt A. Spasticity outcome measures in spinal cord injury: psychometric properties and clinical utility. *Spinal Cord* 2008;46(2):86–95.
5. Adams MM, Hicks AL. Spasticity after spinal cord injury. *Spinal Cord* 2005;43(10):577–586.
6. Kramer KM, Levine AM. Posttraumatic syringomyelia: a review of 21 cases. *Clin Orthop Relat Res* 1997;(334):190–199.
7. Adams MM, Ginis KA, Hicks AL. The Spinal Cord Injury Spasticity Evaluation Tool: development and evaluation. *Arch Phys Med Rehabil* 2007;88(9):1185–1192.
8. Armutlu K, Meric A, Kirdi N, Yakut E, Karabudak R. The effect of transcutaneous electrical nerve stimulation on spasticity in multiple sclerosis patients: a pilot study. *Neurorehabil Neural Repair* 2003;17(2):79–82.
9. Ashworth NL, Satkunam LE, Deforge D. Treatment for spasticity in amyotrophic lateral sclerosis/motor neuron disease. *Cochrane Database Syst Rev* 2004;(1):CD004156.
10. Adams MM, Ginis KA, Hicks AL. The Spinal Cord Injury Spasticity Evaluation Tool: development and evaluation. *Arch Phys Med Rehabil* 2007;88(9):1185–1192.
11. Biering-Sorensen F, Nielsen JB, Klinge K. Spasticity-assessment: a review. *Spinal Cord* 2006;44(12):708–722.
12. Ashworth NL, Satkunam LE, Deforge D. Treatment for spasticity in amyotrophic lateral sclerosis/motor neuron disease. *Cochrane Database Syst Rev* 2006;(1):CD004156.
13. Elbasiouny SM, Moroz D, Bakr MM, Mushahwar VK. Management of spasticity after spinal cord injury: current techniques and future directions. *Neurorehabil Neural Repair* 2010;24(1):23–33.
14. Pandyan AD, Gregoric M, Barnes MP et al. Spasticity: clinical perceptions, neurological realities and meaningful measurement. *Disabil Rehabil* 2005;27(1-2):2–6.
15. Wood DE, Burridge JH, van Wijck FM et al. Biomechanical approaches applied to the lower and upper limb for the measurement of spasticity: a systematic review of the literature. *Disabil Rehabil* 2005;27(1-2):19–32.
16. Malhotra S, Pandyan AD, Day CR, Jones PW, Hermens H. Spasticity, an impairment that is poorly defined and poorly measured. *Clin Rehabil* 2009;23(7):651–658.

17. Lance JW. The control of muscle tone, reflexes, and movement: Robert Wartenberg Lecture. *Neurology* 1980;30(12): 1303–1313.

18. Young RR. Spasticity: a review. *Neurology* 1994;44(11 Suppl 9):S12–S20.

19. Hobart JC, Riazi A, Thompson AJ et al. Getting the measure of spasticity in multiple sclerosis: the Multiple Sclerosis Spasticity Scale (MSSS-88). *Brain* 2006;129(Pt 1):224–234.

20. Ansari NN, Adelmanesh F, Naghdi S, Tabtabaei A. The effect of physiotherapeutic ultrasound on muscle spasticity in patients with hemiplegia: a pilot study. *Electromyogr Clin Neurophysiol* 2006;46(4):247–252.

21. Burridge JH, Wood DE, Hermens HJ et al. Theoretical and methodological considerations in the measurement of spasticity. *Disabil Rehabil* 2005;27(1-2):69–80.

22. Platz T, Eickhof C, Nuyens G, Vuadens P. Clinical scales for the assessment of spasticity, associated phenomena, and function: a systematic review of the literature. *Disabil Rehabil* 2005;27(1-2):7–18.

23. Fleuren JF, Voerman GE, Erren-Wolters CV et al. Stop using the Ashworth Scale for the assessment of spasticity. *J Neurol Neurosurg Psychiatry* 2010;81(1):46–52.

24. Allison SC, Abraham LD, Petersen CL. Reliability of the Modified Ashworth Scale in the assessment of plantarflexor muscle spasticity in patients with traumatic brain injury. *Int J Rehabil Res* 1996;19(1):67–78.

25. Brashear A, Zafonte R, Corcoran M et al. Inter- and intrarater reliability of the Ashworth Scale and the disability assessment scale in patients with upper-limb poststroke spasticity. *Arch Phys Med Rehabil* 2002;83(10):1349–1354.

26. Skold C, Lonn L, Harms-Ringdahl K et al. Effects of functional electrical stimulation training for six months on body composition and spasticity in motor complete tetraplegic spinal cord-injured individuals. *J Rehabil Med* 2002;34(1): 25–32.

27. Bohannon RW. Variability and reliability of the pendulum test for spasticity using a Cybex II isokinetic dynamometer. *Phys Ther* 1987;67(5):659–661.

28. Ashworth B. Preliminary trial of carisoprodol in multiple sclerosis. *Practitioner* 1964;192:540–542.

29. Yelnik A, Albert T, Bonan I, Laffont I. A clinical guide to assess the role of lower limb extensor overactivity in hemiplegic gait disorders. *Stroke* 1999;30(3):580–585.

30. Priebe MM, Sherwood AM, Thornby JI, Kharas NF, Markowski J. Clinical assessment of spasticity in spinal cord injury: a multidimensional problem. *Arch Phys Med Rehabil* 1996;77(7):713–716.

31. Lechner HE, Frotzler A, Eser P. Relationship between self- and clinically rated spasticity in spinal cord injury. *Arch Phys Med Rehabil* 2006;87(1):15–19.

32. Penn RD, Savoy SM, Corcos D et al. Intrathecal baclofen for severe spinal spasticity. *N Engl J Med* 1989;320(23): 1517–1521.

33. Cook KF, Teal CR, Engebretson JC et al. Development and validation of Patient Reported Impact of Spasticity Measure (PRISM). *J Rehabil Res Dev* 2007;44(3):363–371.

34. Hill MR, Noonan VK, Sakakibara BM, Miller WC. Quality of life instruments and definitions in individuals with spinal cord injury: a systematic review. *Spinal Cord* 2009.

35. Crenna P. Spasticity and 'spastic' gait in children with cerebral palsy. *Neurosci Biobehav Rev* 1998;22(4):571–578.

36. Ng SS, Hui-Chan CW. Transcutaneous electrical nerve stimulation combined with task-related training improves lower limb functions in subjects with chronic stroke. *Stroke* 2007;38(11):2953–2959.

37. Yan TB, Hui-Chan CW, Li LS. [Effects of functional electrical stimulation on the improvement of motor function of patients with acute stroke: a randomized controlled trial]. *Zhonghua Yi Xue Za Zhi* 2006;86(37):2627–2631.

38. Hsu AL, Tang PF, Jan MH. Analysis of impairments influencing gait velocity and asymmetry of hemiplegic patients

after mild to moderate stroke. *Arch Phys Med Rehabil* 2003;84(8):1185–1193.

39. Eng JJ, Kim CM, Macintyre DL. Reliability of lower extremity strength measures in persons with chronic stroke. *Arch Phys Med Rehabil* 2002;83(3):322–328.

40. Nadeau S, Arsenault AB, Gravel D, Bourbonnais D. Analysis of the clinical factors determining natural and maximal gait speeds in adults with a stroke. *Am J Phys Med Rehabil* 1999;78(2):123–130.

41. De BE, Nadeau S, Bourbonnais D, Dickstein R. Associations between lower limb impairments, locomotor capacities and kinematic variables in the frontal plane during walking in adults with chronic stroke. *J Rehabil Med* 2003;35(6): 259–264.

42. Bovend'Eerdt TJ, Newman M, Barker K, Dawes H, Minelli C, Wade DT. The effects of stretching in spasticity: a systematic review. *Arch Phys Med Rehabil* 2008;89(7):1395–1406.

43. Williams PE. Use of intermittent stretch in the prevention of serial sarcomere loss in immobilised muscle. *Ann Rheum Dis* 1990;49(5):316–317.

44. Biering-Sorensen F, Hansen B, Lee BS. Non-pharmacological treatment and prevention of bone loss after spinal cord injury: a systematic review. *Spinal Cord* 2009;47(7):508–518.

45. Pak S, Patten C. Strengthening to promote functional recovery poststroke: an evidence-based review. *Top Stroke Rehabil* 2008;15(3):177–199.

46. Chung S, Bai Z, Rymer WZ, Zhang LQ. Changes of reflex, non-reflex and torque generation properties of spastic ankle plantar flexors induced by intelligent stretching. *Conf Proc IEEE Eng Med Biol Soc* 2005;4:3672–3675.

47. Chua SG, Kong KH. Complete semimembranosus rupture following therapeutic stretching after a traumatic brain injury. *Brain Inj* 2006;20(6):669–672.

48. Mortenson PA, Eng JJ. The use of casts in the management of joint mobility and hypertonia following brain injury in adults: a systematic review. *Phys Ther* 2003;83(7): 648–658.

49. Lannin NA, Novak I, Cusick A. A systematic review of upper extremity casting for children and adults with central nervous system motor disorders. *Clin Rehabil* 2007;21(11): 963–976.

50. Pohl M, Ruckriem S, Mehrholz J, Ritschel C, Strik H, Pause MR. Effectiveness of serial casting in patients with severe cerebral spasticity: a comparison study. *Arch Phys Med Rehabil* 2002;83(6):784–790.

51. King TI. Plaster splinting as a means of reducing elbow flexor spasticity: a case study. *Am J Occup Ther* 1982;36(10): 671–673.

52. Lehmkuhl LD, Thoi LL, Blaize C, Kelley CJ, Krawczyk L, Bonte CF. Multimodality treatment of joint contractures in patients with severe brain injury: cost, effectiveness, and integration of therapies in the application of serial/inhibitive casts. *J Head Trauma Rehabil* 1990;5(4):23–42.

53. Robichaud JA, Agostinucci J. Air-splint pressure effect on soleus muscle alpha motoneuron reflex excitability in subjects with spinal cord injury. *Arch Phys Med Rehabil* 1996;77(8):778–782.

54. Gossman MR, Sahrmann SA, Rose SJ. Review of length-associated changes in muscle. Experimental evidence and clinical implications. *Phys Ther* 1982;62(12):1799–1808.

55. Kottke FJ, Pauley DL, Ptak RA. The rationale for prolonged stretching for correction of shortening of connective tissue. *Arch Phys Med Rehabil* 1966;47(6):345–352.

56. Shah SB, Lieber RL. Simultaneous imaging and functional assessment of cytoskeletal protein connections in passively loaded single muscle cells. *J Histochem Cytochem* 2003; 51(1):19–29.

57. Halanski M, Noonan KJ. Cast and splint immobilization: complications. *J Am Acad Orthop Surg* 2008;16(1):30–40.

58. Burtner PA, Poole JL, Torres T et al. Effect of wrist hand splints on grip, pinch, manual dexterity, and muscle activa-

tion in children with spastic hemiplegia: a preliminary study. *J Hand Ther* 2008;21(1):36–42.

59. Farrell JF, Hoffman HB, Snyder JL, Giuliani CA, Bohannon RW. Orthotic aided training of the paretic upper limb in chronic stroke: results of a phase 1 trial. *NeuroRehabilitation* 2007;22(2):99–103.

60. MacKay-Lyons M. Low-load, prolonged stretch in treatment of elbow flexion contractures secondary to head trauma: a case report. *Phys Ther* 1989;69(4):292–296.

61. Lai JM, Francisco GE, Willis FB. Dynamic splinting after treatment with botulinum toxin type-A: a randomized controlled pilot study. *Adv Ther* 2009;26(2):241–248.

62. Lai JM, Francisco GE, Willis FB. Dynamic splinting after treatment with botulinum toxin type-A: a randomized controlled pilot study. *Adv Ther* 2009;26(2):241–248.

63. Gracies JM, Marosszeky JE, Renton R, Sandanam J, Gandevia SC, Burke D. Short-term effects of dynamic lycra splints on upper limb in hemiplegic patients. *Arch Phys Med Rehabil* 2000;81(12):1547–1555.

64. Barnes MP. Spasticity: a rehabilitation challenge in the elderly. *Gerontology* 2001;47(6):295–299.

65. Reid S, Hamer P, Alderson J, Lloyd D. Neuromuscular adaptations to eccentric strength training in children and adolescents with cerebral palsy. *Dev Med Child Neurol* 2009; 52(4):358–363.

66. Patten C, Lexell J, Brown HE. Weakness and strength training in persons with poststroke hemiplegia: rationale, method, and efficacy. *J Rehabil Res Dev* 2004;41(3A):293–312.

67. Dalgas U, Stenager E, Jakobsen J et al. Resistance training improves muscle strength and functional capacity in multiple sclerosis. *Neurology* 2009;73(18):1478–1484.

68. Teixeira-Salmela LF, Olney SJ, Nadeau S, Brouwer B. Muscle strengthening and physical conditioning to reduce impairment and disability in chronic stroke survivors. *Arch Phys Med Rehabil* 1999;80(10):1211–1218.

69. Rimmer JH, Chen MD, McCubbin JA, Drum C, Peterson J. Exercise intervention research on persons with disabilities: what we know and where we need to go. *Am J Phys Med Rehabil* 2010;89(3):249–263.

70. Motl RW, Snook EM, Hinkle ML, McAuley E. Effect of acute leg cycling on the soleus H-reflex and Modified Ashworth Scale scores in individuals with multiple sclerosis. *Neurosci Lett* 2006;406(3):289–292.

71. Sosnoff J, Motl RW, Snook EM, Wynn D. Effect of a 4-week period of unloaded leg cycling exercise on spasticity in multiple sclerosis. *NeuroRehabilitation* 2009;24(4):327–331.

72. Diserens K, Perret N, Chatelain S et al. The effect of repetitive arm cycling on post stroke spasticity and motor control: repetitive arm cycling and spasticity. *J Neurol Sci* 2007;253(1–2): 18–24.

73. Hesse S, Bertelt C, Schaffrin A, Malezic M, Mauritz KH. Restoration of gait in nonambulatory hemiparetic patients by treadmill training with partial body-weight support. *Arch Phys Med Rehabil* 1994;75(10):1087–1093.

74. Hesse S, Bertelt C, Jahnke MT et al. Treadmill training with partial body weight support compared with physiotherapy in nonambulatory hemiparetic patients. *Stroke* 1995;26(6): 976–981.

75. Mutlu A, Krosschell K, Spira DG. Treadmill training with partial body-weight support in children with cerebral palsy: a systematic review. *Dev Med Child Neurol* 2009;51(4): 268–275.

76. McCain KJ, Pollo FE, Baum BS, Coleman SC, Baker S, Smith PS. Locomotor treadmill training with partial body-weight support before overground gait in adults with acute stroke: a pilot study. *Arch Phys Med Rehabil* 2008;89(4):684–691.

77. Hesse S. Treadmill training with partial body weight support after stroke: a review. *NeuroRehabilitation* 2008;23(1): 55–65.

78. Franceschini M, Carda S, Agosti M, Antenucci R, Malgrati D, Cisari C. Walking after stroke: what does treadmill training with body weight support add to overground gait training in patients early after stroke: a single-blind, randomized, controlled trial. *Stroke* 2009;40(9):3079–3085.

79. Miyai I, Suzuki M, Hatakenaka M, Kubota K. Effect of body weight support on cortical activation during gait in patients with stroke. *Exp Brain Res* 2006;169(1):85–91.

80. Ada L, Dorsch S, Canning CG. Strengthening interventions increase strength and improve activity after stroke: a systematic review. *Aust J Physiother* 2006;52(4):241–248.

81. Perret DM, Rim J, Cristian A. A geriatrician's guide to the use of the physical modalities in the treatment of pain and dysfunction. *Clin Geriatr Med* 2006;22(2):331–354.

82. Allen RJ. Physical agents used in the management of chronic pain by physical therapists. *Phys Med Rehabil Clin N Am* 2006;17(2):315–345.

83. Dimitrijevic MR. Clinical practice of functional electrical stimulation: from "yesterday" to "today". *Artif Organs* 2008;32(8):577–580.

84. Sheffler LR, Chae J. Neuromuscular electrical stimulation in neurorehabilitation. *Muscle Nerve* 2007;35(5):562–590.

85. Yan T, Hui-Chan CW. Transcutaneous electrical stimulation on acupuncture points improves muscle function in subjects after acute stroke: a randomized controlled trial. *J Rehabil Med* 2009;41(5):312–316.

86. Ring H, Rosenthal N. Controlled study of neuroprosthetic functional electrical stimulation in sub-acute post-stroke rehabilitation. *J Rehabil Med* 2005;37(1):32–36.

87. Popovic MB, Popovic DB, Sinkjaer T, Stefanovic A, Schwirtlich L. Clinical evaluation of functional electrical therapy in acute hemiplegic subjects. *J Rehabil Res Dev* 2003;40(5):443–453.

88. Mesci N, Ozdemir F, Kabayel DD, Tokuc B. The effects of neuromuscular electrical stimulation on clinical improvement in hemiplegic lower extremity rehabilitation in chronic stroke: a single-blind, randomised, controlled trial. *Disabil Rehabil* 2009;31(24):2047–2054.

89. Bakhtiary AH, Fatemy E. Does electrical stimulation reduce spasticity after stroke? A randomized controlled study. *Clin Rehabil* 2008;22(5):418–425.

90. Szecsi J, Schiller M. FES-propelled cycling of SCI subjects with highly spastic leg musculature. *NeuroRehabilitation* 2009;24(3):243–253.

91. Krause P, Szecsi J, Straube A. Changes in spastic muscle tone increase in patients with spinal cord injury using functional electrical stimulation and passive leg movements. *Clin Rehabil* 2008;22(7):627–634.

92. Szecsi J, Schlick C, Schiller M, Pollmann W, Koenig N, Straube A. Functional electrical stimulation-assisted cycling of patients with multiple sclerosis: biomechanical and functional outcome–a pilot study. *J Rehabil Med* 2009;41(8):674–680.

93. Tekeoglu Y, Adak B, Goksoy T. Effect of transcutaneous electrical nerve stimulation (TENS) on Barthel Activities of Daily Living (ADL) index score following stroke. *Clin Rehabil* 1998;12(4):277–280.

94. Potisk KP, Gregoric M, Vodovnik L. Effects of transcutaneous electrical nerve stimulation (TENS) on spasticity in patients with hemiplegia. *Scand J Rehabil Med* 1995;27(3):169–174.

95. Goulet C, Arsenault AB, Bourbonnais D, Laramee MT, Lepage Y. Effects of transcutaneous electrical nerve stimulation on H-reflex and spinal spasticity. *Scand J Rehabil Med* 1996;28(3):169–176.

96. Xu KS, He L, Li JL, Mai JN. [Effects of transcutaneous electrical nerve stimulation on motor function in ambulant children with spastic cerebral palsy: a randomized trial]. *Zhonghua Er Ke Za Zhi* 2007;45(8):564–567.

97. Miller L, Mattison P, Paul L, Wood L. The effects of transcutaneous electrical nerve stimulation (TENS) on spasticity in multiple sclerosis. *Mult Scler* 2007;13(4):527–533.

98. Dewald JP, Given JD, Rymer WZ. Long-lasting reductions of spasticity induced by skin electrical stimulation. *IEEE Trans Rehabil Eng* 1996;4(4):231–242.

99. Kuo JJ, Lee RH, Johnson MD, Heckman HM, Heckman CJ. Active dendritic integration of inhibitory synaptic inputs in vivo. *J Neurophysiol* 2003;90(6):3617–3624.

100. Kesiktas N, Paker N, Erdogan N, Gulsen G, Bicki D, Yilmaz H. The use of hydrotherapy for the management of spasticity. *Neurorehabil Neural Repair* 2004;18(4):268–273.

101. Jozefczyk PB. The management of focal spasticity. *Clin Neuropharmacol* 2002;25(3):158–173.

102. Kirshblum S. Treatment alternatives for spinal cord injury related spasticity. *J Spinal Cord Med* 1999;22(3):199–217.

103. Parziale JR, Akelman E, Herz DA. Spasticity: pathophysiology and management. *Orthopedics* 1993;16(7):801–811.

104. Chiara T, Carlos J, Jr., Martin D, Miller R, Nadeau S. Cold effect on oxygen uptake, perceived exertion, and spasticity in patients with multiple sclerosis. *Arch Phys Med Rehabil* 1998;79(5):523–528.

105. Lee SU, Bang MS, Han TR. Effect of cold air therapy in relieving spasticity: applied to spinalized rabbits. *Spinal Cord* 2002;40(4):167–173.

106. Elovic E, Zafonte RD. Spasticity management in traumatic brain injury. *State of the Art Review of Rehabilitation* 2001;15(2):327–348.

107. Bell KR, Lehmann JF. Effect of cooling on H- and T-reflexes in normal subjects. *Arch Phys Med Rehabil* 1987;68(8):490–493.

108. Price R, Lehmann JF, Boswell-Bessette S, Burleigh A, deLateur BJ. Influence of cryotherapy on spasticity at the human ankle. *Arch Phys Med Rehabil* 1993;74(3):300–304.

109. Nakhostin AN, Naghdi S, Hasson S, Rastgoo M. Efficacy of therapeutic ultrasound and infrared in the management of muscle spasticity. *Brain Inj* 2009;23(7):632–638.

110. Ansari NN, Naghdi S, Bagheri H, Ghassabi H. Therapeutic ultrasound in the treatment of ankle plantarflexor spasticity in a unilateral stroke population: a randomized, single-blind, placebo-controlled trial. *Electromyogr Clin Neurophysiol* 2007;47(3):137–143.

111. Chang CL, Munin MC, Skidmore ER, Niyonkuru C, Huber LM, Weber DJ. Effect of baseline spastic hemiparesis on recovery of upper-limb function following botulinum toxin type A injections and postinjection therapy. *Arch Phys Med Rehabil* 2009;90(9):1462–1468.

112. Meythaler JM, Vogtle L, Brunner RC. A preliminary assessment of the benefits of the addition of botulinum toxin a to a conventional therapy program on the function of people with longstanding stroke. *Arch Phys Med Rehabil* 2009;90(9):1453–1461.

113. Wallen M, O'Flaherty SJ, Waugh MC. Functional outcomes of intramuscular botulinum toxin type a and occupational therapy in the upper limbs of children with cerebral palsy: a randomized controlled trial. *Arch Phys Med Rehabil* 2007;88(1):1–10.

114. Giovannelli M, Borriello G, Castri P, Prosperini L, Pozzilli C. Early physiotherapy after injection of botulinum toxin increases the beneficial effects on spasticity in patients with multiple sclerosis. *Clin Rehabil* 2007;21(4):331–337.

115. Hoare BJ, Wallen MA, Imms C, Villanueva E, Rawicki HB, Carey L. Botulinum toxin A as an adjunct to treatment in the management of the upper limb in children with spastic cerebral palsy (UPDATE). *Cochrane Database Syst Rev* 2010;(1): CD003469.

116. Page SJ, Elovic E, Levine P, Sisto SA. Modified constraint-induced therapy and botulinum toxin A: a promising combination. *Am J Phys Med Rehabil* 2003;82(1):76–80.

117. Sun SF, Hsu CW, Sun HP, Hwang CW, Yang CL, Wang JL. Combined botulinum toxin type a with modified constraint-induced movement therapy for chronic stroke patients with upper extremity spasticity: a randomized controlled study. *Neurorehabil Neural Repair* 2010;24(1):34–41.

118. Levy CE, Giuffrida C, Richards L, Wu S, Davis S, Nadeau SE. Botulinum toxin a, evidence-based exercise therapy, and constraint-induced movement therapy for upper-limb hemiparesis attributable to stroke: a preliminary study. *Am J Phys Med Rehabil* 2007;86(9):696–706.

119. Farina S, Migliorini C, Gandolfi M et al. Combined effects of botulinum toxin and casting treatments on lower limb spasticity after stroke. *Funct Neurol* 2008;23(2):87–91.

120. Newman CJ, Kennedy A, Walsh M, O'Brien T, Lynch B, Hensey O. A pilot study of delayed versus immediate serial casting after botulinum toxin injection for partially reducible spastic equinus. *J Pediatr Orthop* 2007;27(8):882–885.

121. Kay RM, Rethlefsen SA, Fern-Buneo A, Wren TA, Skaggs DL. Botulinum toxin as an adjunct to serial casting treatment in children with cerebral palsy. *J Bone Joint Surg Am* 2004;86-A(11):2377–2384.

122. Blackmore AM, Boettcher-Hunt E, Jordan M, Chan MD. A systematic review of the effects of casting on equinus in children with cerebral palsy: an evidence report of the AACPDM. *Dev Med Child Neurol* 2007;49(10):781–790.

123. Kang BS, Bang MS, Jung SH. Effects of botulinum toxin A therapy with electrical stimulation on spastic calf muscles in children with cerebral palsy. *Am J Phys Med Rehabil* 2007; 86(11):901–906.

124. Hesse S, Jahnke MT, Luecke D, Mauritz KH. Short-term electrical stimulation enhances the effectiveness of Botulinum toxin in the treatment of lower limb spasticity in hemiparetic patients. *Neurosci Lett* 1995;201(1):37–40.

125. Baricich A, Carda S, Bertoni M, Maderna L, Cisari C. A single-blinded, randomized pilot study of botulinum toxin type A combined with non-pharmacological treatment for spastic foot. *J Rehabil Med* 2008;40(10):870–872.

126. Bottos M, Benedetti MG, Salucci P, Gasparroni V, Giannini S. Botulinum toxin with and without casting in ambulant children with spastic diplegia: a clinical and functional assessment. *Dev Med Child Neurol* 2003;45(11):758–762.

127. Ackman JD, Russman BS, Thomas SS et al. Comparing botulinum toxin A with casting for treatment of dynamic equinus in children with cerebral palsy. *Dev Med Child Neurol* 2005;47(9):620–627.

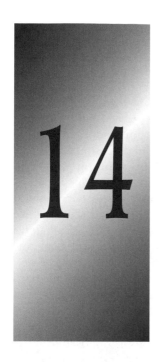

Emerging Technologies in the Management of Upper Motor Neuron Syndromes

14

Ira Rashbaum
Steven R. Flanagan

Diseases and trauma of the central nervous system (CNS) afflict a staggering number of individuals of all ages and often result in lifelong disabilities. To comprehend the scope of the problem, one need only to examine the incidence of a single condition such as stroke, which afflicts 780,000 individuals each year in the United States and is the single most common cause of disability (1). Add to that the incidence of all other conditions affecting the CNS, including both traumatic brain and spinal cord injuries that occur at alarmingly high rates in younger individuals, it becomes clear that efforts to better delineate CNS pathology and reduce its morbidity must be a priority for researchers and clinicians.

In the past, computed tomography (CT) and conventional MR technology permitted imaging of only macrostructural details of the living brain and spinal cord. Methods to examine their in vivo microscopic architecture and physiology were extremely limited, hindering researchers in their attempt to better delineate the complexity of both normal and pathological functioning. Consequently, the development of more effective treatment modalities was hampered. However, recent advances in imaging technologies have substantially increased our knowledge and understanding of both normal and pathological CNS functioning. This enhanced knowledge will be used to better delineate the pathology that results from injury as well as the recuperative responses that ensue, providing clinicians with the clues needed to develop more effective treatments. These advances also offer researchers the opportunity to further assess the changes in the maturing brain that account for developing skills occurring throughout early childhood, adolescence, and adulthood; the adaptive responses to disease and trauma; and the physical interactions between various cerebral regions that underlie normal human function.

New treatment modalities, such as transcranial magnetic stimulation (TMS), virtual reality (VR), electrical stimulation (ES), robotic therapy, constraint-induced movement therapy (CIMT), and body weight–supported treadmill training, are currently being investigated as means to enhance recovery. They incorporate knowledge gained from research and advancements in neuroimaging that have enhanced our understating of neural plasticity and the role it plays in recovery. Advances in technology will demonstrate changes in the management of muscle overactivity in 2 separate yet complementary manners. The first is in the area of improved methods of diagnostic evaluations, whereas the second will address changes in the treatment modalities available for the clinicians in their clinical efforts. This chapter will address advancements in both of these areas as advances in technologies that will likely lead to a more fundamental understanding of the CNS, and amelioration of morbidity caused by disease and trauma will be mentioned in the discussion that follows.

Although many of the technologies that will be discussed are currently used for research purposes, they hold the possibility of providing clinicians valuable information regarding disease processes and outcomes. First, it provides in vivo information pertaining to pathology and physiology that impacts function. Enhanced understanding will help researchers develop new means to treat impairments associated with upper motor neuron disorders. This new knowledge can also be used in conjunction with traditional therapies and to aid in developing new technologies to improve rehabilitation outcomes. Last, it will help guide treatment and predict outcomes that will likely be useful to provide care that is both effective and efficient.

NEUROIMAGING TECHNOLOGIES

Standard CT and T1/T2-weighted MR images of the CNS provide valuable information regarding macrostructural abnormalities arising from trauma and disease. Unquestionably, these technologies have enhanced our ability to treat people in more efficient and definitive ways not feasible before their clinical implementation. However, in the adult human brain, white matter on both CT scans and T1/T2-weighted MR images appear homogeneous despite its inherent complexity. They also cannot adequately assess microscopic lesions such as those associated with diffuse axonal injury or changes in either metabolism or the concentration of biological molecules occurring in specific disease states. Recent advances in imaging technologies are enabling researchers and health care providers to noninvasively peer into the living brain, enhancing our knowledge of the structure and function of the CNS that will ultimately improve our ability to diagnose and treat people with neurologic disabilities.

Diffusion Imaging

Diffusion imaging uses MR technology to detect the movement of water molecules, providing a means to visualize cerebral tissue based on both the speed and direction of its movement. The manner in which water diffuses in biological tissue is impacted in specific ways, such as by the presence and chronicity of particular disease states. For example, restricted diffusion occurs in acutely infarcted cerebral tissue but later increases as the stroke becomes chronic, offering a sensitive means to differentiate acute from chronic stroke. This can be used clinically when combined with findings from cerebral perfusion studies. After

very acute stroke, diffusion images rapidly indicate the area of infarct and theoretically nonsalvageable tissue. Perfusion images identify regions of impaired blood flow, which after very acute stroke is often larger than the region of diffusion abnormality. This difference between diffusion and perfusion abnormalities, referred to as the diffusion-perfusion mismatch, is thought to represent the penumbra, the region of the brain susceptible to infarct if restricted blood flow is not restored. Results of several studies have indicated that thrombolytic therapy may be helpful in reducing stroke volume and improving clinical outcomes when given up to 6 hours after stroke onset, rather than just the currently approved 3-hour window when there is a significant diffusion-perfusion mismatch (2, 3). Improved clinical outcome appears to be more likely in those with mismatch and isolated middle cerebral artery occlusions as opposed to those with concomitant middle cerebral and internal artery occlusions (4).

Diffusion tensor imaging (DTI) takes advantage of the fact that water diffuses faster along the orientation of axons and that fiber bundles as opposed to across them, properties referred to as anisotropy and isotropy respectively. Water diffusion is restricted perpendicular to fiber tracts because of restrictions imposed by the axolemma, myelin, and neurofilaments. However, it is relatively unrestricted along the path parallel to the orientation of the tract. Therefore, the degree of anisotropy, typically referred to as fractional anisotropy (FA), is high in well-organized white matter tracts where water moves rapidly parallel along the orientation of the bundle. Images are derived on the basis of the magnitude of FA as well as the orientation of the fibers within a tract, providing structural information pertaining to the integrity of white matter. For example, in cases of traumatic axonal injury where standard neuroimages are often unremarkable, DTI can image disruption of white matter tracts. Diffusion tensor imaging also provide a means to image the direction of fiber tracts by color coding them according to their orientation: typically red for left-right, green for anterior-posterior, and blue for cranial-caudal directions (5). Although color coding is useful, it is 2-dimensional, which limits its ability to assess integrity along an entire fiber tract. Three-dimensional tractography overcomes this by assessing a tract along its entire length. This offers a means to better assess both the function and integrity of individual fiber tracts that can be used to better understand the function and connectivity of cerebral structures, to examine the impact specific lesions have on motor function, and image damage to white matter not feasible with standard imaging.

Diffusion tensor imaging is becoming more widely accepted as a means to best assess the degree of axonal injury after traumatic brain injury (TBI). It is effective in imaging axonal disruption in the presence of normal-appearing standard MR images (6), the extent and quantity of white matter injury (7), and the location of white matter tract injury associated with motor impairment (8). Diffusion tensor imaging data have also been correlated with both TBI severity and outcomes (9–11) and is becoming a useful tool to predict motor outcomes poststroke. After stroke, FA decreases as the time from the infarct increases. As Wallerian degeneration progresses after stroke in long white matter tracts, DTI detects decreased FA in sites distal but previously connected to the site of injury. The magnitude of FA reduction in the pyramidal tracts has also been correlated with motor outcomes poststroke, providing a potential means to predict outcomes (12).

Magnetic Resonance Spectroscopy

Magnetic resonance spectroscopy (MRS) determines the relative concentrations of various molecules in specific cerebral regions, which provides information regarding the chemical makeup of the brain in both healthy and disease states. Data are presented as a graph depicting the concentrations of various compounds, which are then typically presented as a ratio of one compound to another. Information can be obtained from either a single volume of brain, known as single voxel spectroscopy, or as a 2-dimensional or 3-dimensional analysis obtained simultaneously over wider regions, referred to as MRS imaging. Several compounds of interest measured by MRS include *N*-acetylaspartic acid (NAA), creatine, choline, myo-inositol, glutamate, and lactate. *N*-acetylaspartic acid is located only in the neuronal tissue, with relative decreases in its concentration suggesting neuronal injury. Magnetic resonance spectroscopy has detected reduced levels of NAA after TBI even in the presence of normal-appearing standard imaging (13), with evidence indicating it correlates with outcomes (14–16). Determining the relative concentrations of other compounds provides additional information, as detailed in Table 14.1, which can be used clinically in a number of ways. For example, MRS has been found to be a sensitive means of differentiating neoplastic from nonneoplastic lesions by determining the ration of NAA to choline, which is typically reduced in neoplastic as compared to nonneoplastic lesions (17–22). Magnetic resonance spectroscopy data have also been found to correlate with several poststroke outcomes, including motor recovery (23), apathy (24), and de-

TABLE 14.1
Compounds Detected by MRS and Their Markers

NAA	Neuronal marker
Creatine	Energy metabolism marker
Choline	Cell membrane disruption, inflammation, and changes in myelination
Myo-inositol	Astrocyte marker
Lactate	Metabolism

pression (25). For example, during the first several months after acute stroke, increasing NAA/Cr in the contralesional hemisphere has been found to be associated with improved neurologic status (23).

Functional Magnetic Resonance Imaging

Functional MRI (fMRI) is a technique that images cerebral regions that are activated during specific motor, sensory, or cognitive activities. It generates images by assessing the combination of physiological changes associated with metabolic activity, including localized alterations in blood flow and the levels of various forms of hemoglobin. In a technique known as blood oxygen level difference fMRI, the difference in magnetic properties of oxygenated and deoxygenated hemoglobin is used to study the combination of metabolic activity and changes in local blood flow that result from regional activation. The blood oxygen level difference response is represented as a bright signal on fMRI, indicating a region that is more metabolically active than surrounding tissue. Its temporal and spatial resolutions are good, both of which are better than those obtained by either single photon emission computed tomography or traditional positron emission tomography scans. An additional advantage over positron emission tomography and single photon emission computed tomography is the lack of radiation exposure associated with fMRI that permits for multiple imaging. Like all functional imaging studies, several factors must be considered when interpreting fMRI data. These include a subject's ability to cooperate in a tightly confined MR scanner, medication effects on cerebral activation, adequacy of cerebral blood flow, and inadvertent subject movement during image acquisition. Data interpretation is complex in that it is important to consider the multitude of possible reasons accounting for specific activation patterns. For instance, does an activation pattern in a subject with brain injury differ from a normal control because of the establishment of alternative pathways, practice effects, or differences in performance difficulty that exist between injured subjects and normal controls. Other important issues to consider during interpretation include lesion location and size, time postinjury, subject age, the time postinjury the data are obtained, the subject's cerebral dominance, previous injury, presence of cerebral vascular disease, and type of study design (eg, cross-sectional versus longitudinal). Functional MRI has provided valuable insights into both normal and pathological cerebral physiology, although there are limitations to its use. The type of activity performed in MR imaging (MRI) scanners is restricted, which prevents it from studying many complex real-world activities and limits its ecological validity. It is also subject to the same contraindications as standard MRI. At the present time, it is used as a research tool, although it has potential as a means to guide treatment and assess treatment effects.

Functional Near Infrared Spectroscopy

Functional near infrared spectroscopy (fNIRS) is a technology that, like fMRI, determines the presence of cerebral activity by assessing the different concentrations of oxygenated and deoxygenated hemoglobin associated with metabolic activity. However, rather than assessing the magnetic differences of the 2 compounds, fNIRS assesses the differences in their optical properties. The system uses light sources placed on the scalp using a wearable device. The light passes relatively easily through the scalp and skull and into the top few millimeters of the brain. Light sensors on the scalp detect wavelengths of light that are reflected back to the surface. These sensors can detect the differences in near infrared wavelength absorption of oxygenated and deoxygenated hemoglobin reflective of local metabolic activity. It has demonstrated ability to assess cerebral activity in the human cortex associated with both motor and cognitive tasks (26). It has been used to study various changes in metabolic patterns in subjects with dementia (27–29), schizophrenia, (30), and stroke (31–35). It has several advantages over fMRI in that it is less susceptible to motion artifact as the sensors move with the subject, and it is considerably less expensive. It is also not limited by the same contraindications of fMRI, such as the presence of metal plates and subject claustrophobia. Perhaps most importantly, it is a portable system that can assess changes in cerebral activation during tasks performed in settings more ecologically valid for a particular function. This is not feasible in an MR scanner. For the same reasons, it can also as-

sess activation patterns occurring during specific rehabilitation interventions. It therefore offers excellent temporal resolution that may provide opportunities to better develop and assess specific treatment interventions. It is becoming a more accepted technology now that it has been correlated with fMRI (32, 36, 37). Despite its utility, it is limited by its inability to image beyond the top 2 to 3 mm of cerebral cortex and 1 cm lateral to the topical sensors. As a result, it may be efficacious in evaluating the motor system of the upper extremity but cannot be used to evaluate the lower extremity. In addition, unlike fMRI, cranial reference points are used to correlate activity with specific cerebral regions, decreasing its spatial specificity. Other problems include difficulties regarding the reduction of optical signals by the noncerebral tissue, the impact of pigmentation on signal detection, and the limited spatial resolution (38).

EMERGING TREATMENTS

Constraint-Induced Movement Therapy

Constraint-induced movement therapy has emerged as an exciting therapeutic approach for selected stroke survivors with plegic upper limbs. It is an intensive therapeutic regimen provided over the course of 12 days that restricts the use of the uninvolved upper limb, forcing individuals with stroke to use their plegic limb to perform activities of daily living (ADL). It is based on the theory of learned nonuse, which states a limb weakened by stroke will not improve if it is not actively rehabilitated. For example, during the course of rehabilitation, individuals are taught to walk using their unimpaired and plegic legs, as ambulation requires the use of both lower limbs. However, because many ADL can be performed using only the uninvolved upper limb, there may be reduced rehabilitation efforts directed at improving the use of the plegic arm and hand because the primary focus is often to quickly return an individual to independent function. In this scenario, individuals with stroke are taught not to use their plegic upper limb, a process referred to as learned nonuse. Although compensatory one-handed strategies are useful to quickly improve the performance of specific activities, it does not result in cortical reorganization that leads to enhanced use of the plegic limb. However, CIMT has been shown to improve the use of stroke-weakened limbs in association with cortical changes (39).

There are several critical factors involved in CIMT, including intense, repetitive practice using the plegic limb for common functional tasks. This is accomplished in conjunction with physical restriction of the unimpaired arm and hand for up to 90% of waking hours through the use of a mitt, sling, and/or splint. A therapeutic technique, known as shaping, that trains the plegic limb to move through successive approximations of a desired task is performed. Traditional CIMT is extremely intensive and involves at least 6 hours of daily therapy for 2 weeks. The most comprehensive study examining its effectiveness compared to usual rehabilitation care is the EXCITE trial. It included 222 patients with a single stroke sustained 3 to 9 months before the time of enrollment. Compared to the usual treatment group, those receiving CIMT had less self-perceptions of hand function difficulty and performed better on several tests of upper limb function (40). An interpretation of the EXCITE trial by Dobkin (41) noted that a formalized care strategy for the usual treatment group would have helped clinicians critically interpret the value of CIMT, as the CIMT group may have been biased in its self-appraisal. In addition, a short phase-in of therapy for all subjects could have established whether the subjects were reasonably stable in their affected arm function before randomization, and an interim measure would have partially addressed whether less-intensive CIMT could work as well as traditional CIMT (41). Challenges imposed by the intensity and time commitments of CIMT have led the evaluation of several modifications in the way it is delivered. For example, modified constraint-induced therapy provides treatment 5 hours daily for 5 days followed by 3 hours a day, 3 times weekly over approximately 10 additional weeks. Results using this approach were comparable to traditional CIMT, indicating that alternative methods can be successfully used (42). Other modifications have used online computer sessions or combined CIMT with robotic therapy (43). In one pilot study, subjects with chronic stroke utilized online therapy sessions with computer-based cameras as they restrained their less impaired upper limb resulting in functional improvement after 10 weeks of treatment (43).

There are other factors that limit the effectiveness and application of CIMT. It requires considerable effort and motivation on the part of those receiving it, with some evidence indicating that compliance with the mitt restriction to be as low as 32% (44). Ideally, subjects should not be at risk for falls because restraint of the more functional upper limb may prevent the effective use of walking aids, thus predisposing some individuals to injury. Another important factor restricting its use is the relatively small percentage of individuals with stroke for whom it has shown to benefit. Most trials have included only those individuals with active extension of at least 10° at the fingers and

20° at the wrist, markedly limiting the number of individuals who can benefit from its use.

Challenges ahead for CIMT include clarification of how much of the motor and functional gains are derived from the intervention versus the intensity of treatment and whether modifications in dose intensity impact outcomes. This is an important factor when considering if it is financially feasible in current and future economic environments.

Virtual Reality

Development of computer technology have led to the creation of enhanced VR programs that permit individuals to interact in computer-generated environments that simulate real-world settings (45, 46) for both clinical and research purposes. It is a modality that uses technology to create virtual environments where feedback, intensity, and duration can be modified and used in settings that are more controllable than natural environments. In this scenario, specific therapies can be safely provided that may otherwise be too dangerous or complex in actual settings. Virtual reality environments can therefore reduce concerns over the consequences of allowing a person with physical or cognitive impairments to perform potentially dangerous activities on their own. The technology is extremely flexibility, capable of remaining completely consistent over infinite repetitions or altering the type and pattern of sensory inputs and task complexity that can meet a multitude of clinical, research, and assessment needs. Not surprisingly, it has been gaining wider use in rehabilitation settings for both assessments and treatments.

Virtual reality has been shown to be a useful modality to improve functional skills after stroke. Jaffe et al. (47) developed a head-mounted device worn like a hat displaying virtual objects. Patients wear it while walking on a treadmill, with a harness attached. Movement of lower extremities is promoted by negotiating virtual objects obstructing the path. When a virtual object is not successfully avoided, a virtual collision occurs that results in feedback to the patient. Performance has been shown to improve with additional VR training sessions, resulting in fewer "collisions." This form of VR rehabilitation resulted in improved performance on an actual obstacle course compared to conventional ambulation training (47). Fung et al. (48) applied a treadmill mounted on a platform that interfaced with a rear projector. The projector simulated a walking environment while the subject received auditory, sensory, and visual feedback. Subjects with stroke who were trained on this system were noted to have increased walking velocity (48). Improvement in ambulation has also been demonstrated by combining VR with robotic therapy. Deutsch et al. (49) used a desktop computer combined with a seated system that allowed a subject to use their own ankle movements to operate a foot pedal. The subjects were instructed to use the foot pedal to "navigate" a virtual boat or plane while they received visual, auditory, and sensory feedback. Improvements were noted in gait velocity and endurance after 12 hours of training provided over 4 weeks (49).

Jang et al. (50) investigated cortical reorganization and associated functional recovery using VR in patients with chronic stroke. Virtual reality was used to simulate tasks such as lifting crates and making saves as a soccer goalie. Cortical activation and associated motor recovery were measured before and after the intervention with fMRI and clinical tests assessing motor function. Before the intervention, bilateral primary sensorimotor cortices, contralesional premotor cortex, and ipsilesional supplementary motor areas were activated. After training, the activations in the contralesional hemisphere diminished while ipsilesional senosrimotor activation predominated in association with improved motor function (50). Similar findings of enhancing activation in the lesioned hemisphere after the use of various VR-related therapies suggest it may be a useful modality to induce cerebral plasticity and improve motor skills after stroke (51).

Virtual-reality–based rehabilitation for motor, ADL, and cognitive training show promise, yet additional research is necessary to verify and refine preliminary study findings. For example, only limited studies have compared its effectiveness to therapy provided in a real environment (52). In addition, the potentially synergistic effect of combining different technologies, such as robotic therapy and VR, has received only limited attention (53).

Transcranial Magnetic Stimulation

Transcranial magnetic stimulation is a relatively new rehabilitation modality that has been studied for several decades. It is a noninvasive technology that can both enhance and inhibit focal brain activity, potentially inducing cerebral plasticity and enhancing recovery after injury. Transcranial magnetic stimulation uses short magnetic pulses that are generated by passing a very brief electric current through a stimulating coil, typically made of copper encased in plastic that is held to the scalp's surface. The magnetic pulse enters the brain after passing through the scalp and skull, where depending on the pattern of pulse pro-

vided results in either an increase or decrease in cortical excitability. Therefore, unlike electric stimulation, which excites neurons directly, TMS stimulates neural tissue indirectly by inducing electrical activity via magnetism. The size and extent of the magnetic pulse depend on the spatial configuration of the stimulating coil and the position in which it is held. Current applications of TMS after brain injury include measuring the excitability of central motor pathways, mapping cortical representations, and predicting motor recovery (54–56), whereas other potential uses include enhancing cognitive and motor function resulting from brain injury.

Transcranial magnetic stimulation can be delivered via several patterns, including single-pulse, paired-pulse, and repetitive stimulation (rTMS). Transcranial magnetic stimulation delivered in the form of single-pulse stimulation over the motor cortex provides information pertaining to corticospinal tract excitability by measuring the motor response in the muscle corresponding to area of brain being activated. Paired-pulse stimulation can elicit measurable cortical inhibition or facilitation. These paired pulses are delivered through 1 or 2 magnetic coils at varying intervals to elicit either inhibition or facilitation. Repetitive TMS applies a repeated train of magnetic pulses at either low (1 Hz) or high frequencies (5–20 Hz) that cause suppression or enhancement of cortical excitability, respectively (57–59). Repetitive TMS can induce changes in excitability that last beyond the application of the magnetic pulses (60), suggesting it has the capacity to induce long-term potentiation (61) that may be conducive to cerebral plasticity.

Repetitive TMS alters cortical excitability noninvasively and can be used in distinct ways to better understand cerebral physiology and function. For example, activation in a focal brain region can be inhibited, thereby inducing a temporary "virtual lesion" in an otherwise healthy tissue, resulting in the altered performance of a specific task. This provides information regarding the role of that particular cerebral region in the performance of that skill. Alternatively, activation can be enhanced, which again may impact the performance of a motor or cognitive task. This can potentially lead to a more thorough understanding of both cerebral physiology and the neuroanatomical correlates of impaired function resulting from disease or trauma (62, 63).

Several studies have demonstrated the potential use of TMS as a means to enhance motor recovery after a stroke. For example, high-frequency repetitive TMS applied over the lesioned hemisphere, which enhances excitability, resulted in improved hand function of the impaired limb in subjects with acute stroke

(64). Interestingly, many studies have examined the functional impact of inhibiting the uninjured hemisphere by applying low-frequency rTMS, which is typically overactive after stroke (65, 66). The overactivity of the contralesional hemisphere that is observed during movement of the paretic limb (67, 68) is felt to inhibit activation of the lesioned hemisphere, a process referred to as interhemispheric inhibition. Low-frequency rTMS applied over the primary motor cortex of the contralesional hemisphere, resulting in its inhibition, has been shown to improve the function of the affected hand after acute and chronic stroke in subjects of various ages through the process of transcallosal inhibition (69–73), that is, decreasing the activation of the contralesional motor cortex impairs its ability to inhibit the lesioned cortex, resulting in improved motor skills of the hemiparetic limb. Functional MRI data revealed that overall changes in cerebral activation patterns associated with rTMS-induced inhibition of the contralesional motor cortex appeared similar to normal patterns (74). Transcranial magnetic stimulation may become a practical means to enhance recovery after brain injury because it is portable and can be used during rehabilitation interventions.

The changes in cortical excitability induced by TMS has also been studied as a means to manage spasticity in several upper motor neuron conditions, including stroke (75, 76), multiple sclerosis (77, 78), and cerebral palsy (79). Corticospinal neurons are known to modulate α and γ motoneurons, Ia afferent sensory fibers, and spinal interneurons, all of which are involved in the generation of spasticity. In general, increasing corticospinal tract excitability by using rTMS is theorized to inhibit overexcitability of α and γ motoneurons, thereby reducing spasticity. Various rTMS paradigms have been tested with results indicating that it has considerable potential to either reduce spasticity (76–78) and/or increase passive range of motion (75, 79), thereby an improve functional use of affected limbs caused by CNS lesions.

The primary risk of rTMS is inducing seizures, which can be minimized by adhering to recommendations that limit stimulation parameters, advise monitoring guidelines, and detail contraindications (80). An additional risk may be hearing loss, particularly when sessions are provided regularly over several weeks. Potential uses of TMS after neurologic injury in the future will include enhancing our understanding of the physiology underlying the behavior by better delineating the mechanisms, locations, interactions, and adaptability of neuronal networks (81) and exploiting the effects of stimulation on cerebral plasticity to enhance functional recovery. Limitations of TMS include its inability to stimulate subcortical structures that restricts its impact to only those brain regions close to the scalp. The precise timing of when brain plasticity might best occur with TMS has not yet been determined, although as previously mentioned, it has shown promise at various periods poststroke.

Electric Stimulation

Electrical stimulation can be provided in several ways to improve both motor and functional skills after injury to the CNS. It can be applied to muscles or nerves in the form of neuromuscular electric stimulation (NMES) or to the brain via epidurally placed electrodes. Neural plasticity occurs when motor learning is achieved by the performance of goal-oriented, highly repetitive active movement training, aimed at the improved use of a paretic limb. Electrical stimulation, either applied to muscles involved in a specific goal-oriented activity or to the motor cortex associated with the movement of paretic limbs being trained, provides a means to enhance motor relearning and theoretically improve the functional use of the paretic limb. Neuromuscular electric stimulation has also been studied as a means to reduce shoulder subluxation and its associated pain after stroke, as well as to reduce spasticity. Electrical stimulation enhances movement of paretic muscles incapable of sufficiently contracting on their own power, which when applied during highly repetitive training activities theoretically enhances motor relearning.

Clinical use of NMES can be provided in several ways. Cyclic NMES provides simulation at a set rate for a predetermined period of time. Electromyography (EMG)-mediated NMES detects electrical activity in a muscle that is generated by the intent to move it but is insufficient to contract it for functional activities. Once the device detects inherent muscle activity above a set threshold, it provides an externally generated electrical stimulus that causes the muscle to contract. It has a theoretical advantage over cyclic NMES in that it requires cognitive effort to move a limb, providing a biofeedback component that enhances its impact on neural plasticity. However, it is useful only in those muscles that an individual can at least partially activate on their own. Neuromuscular electric stimulation can also be provided to specific muscles in an appropriate time sequence to complete mobility or ADL tasks, such as to the ankle dorsiflexors during the swing phase of gait. This can be achieved by delivering stimulation by using either single-channel or multichannel units. However, as more muscles are stimulated for complex tasks, such as walking, which require the contraction of multiple muscle groups in a very specific pattern using multiple channels, the system becomes cumbersome and impractical. This is partially being addressed by developing percutaneous systems that will be detailed later.

Neuromuscular electric stimulation has been shown to fairly consistently improve motor function (82–91), strength (85, 88, 90, 91), and use of paretic limbs for specific tasks (eg, lifting and moving objects) (88, 90–94) for individuals with stroke at various times postinjury. When used on paretic lower limbs, it has been found to be an effective means to improve gait speed (94–96), an important predictor of successful community ambulation. It has also been shown to be a more effective means to promote motor recovery than conventional rehabilitation techniques alone (82, 85, 86, 88, 89, 91, 93, 94). However, the stability of results over time remains uncertain, as some studies documented sustained improvements for up to 9 months posttreatment (84, 87), whereas others demonstrated that the benefits diminished as the time postinterventions passed (83, 85). It also remains unclear which forms of ES are most useful, as different applications of NMES have not been directly compared to each other. It has been suggested that EMG-mediated devices have a theoretical advantage over cyclic systems, particularly when they are used to assist in completing functional tasks (97), which was supported by the results of a metanalysis (98). Despite improvements in motor skill and strength, these devices have not yet been sufficiently studied to determine whether they are capable of improving quality of life or enhancing independent function after neurologic injury.

Other studies have focused on novel neuroprostheses, which are used in ways to complete mobility and ADL tasks. For example, NMES incorporated into orthotic devices have been shown to improve both upper and lower limb function (92–94, 99), with early use after stroke appearing to result in better outcomes as compared to using them at later times (99). One study investigated contralaterally controlled functional electrical stimulation, which uses an individual's unimpaired hand to control movement of the impaired hand during functional tasks. An instrumented glove that is worn on the uninvolved hand guides ES provided to the paretic hand during repetitive training activities. This provides people with stroke greater control because it permits them to use their unimpaired hand to guide the motion of the hand being trained. Results of 1 pilot study indicated that intensive training with this system improved use of the paretic hand that may last up to 3 months posttreatment (100). A technological advance in ES has included the development and implementation of mi-

crostimultors that have been successfully implanted into muscles and used to improve the use of paretic upper limbs without adverse effects (101).

Shoulder subluxation occurs in the presence of hemiplegia when there is increased humeral head translation relative to the glenoid fossa. It frequently occurs as a result of hemiplegia and is often accompanied with pain. Reduction in both the degree of subluxation and pain has been achieved in selected individuals undergoing NMES to various muscles supporting the shoulder. Neuromuscular electric stimulation delivery to reduce subluxation has traditionally been provided via skin electrodes overlying the deltoid, supraspinatus, and trapezius muscles. However, surface NMES may cause discomfort given the magnitude of stimulation required to pass through skin sufficient enough to cause muscle contraction. Furthermore, selective muscle stimulation is challenging using surface electrodes, as unintended muscles are likely to be activated. This has been addressed by placing electrodes directly into selective muscles using a percutaneous system. This system, which permits many hours of stimulation daily over a period of many weeks, has been shown to be well tolerated and effective in reducing poststroke shoulder pain associated with subluxation (102), particularly when used early poststroke (103). It avoids the discomfort associated with surface stimulation (102) and has been shown to maintain pain reduction for at least 1 year after discontinuation of treatment (104).

Peripheral nerve ES, delivered by cutaneous electrodes, implanted electrodes, or implanted neural prosthetic systems, can reduce spasticity (105). Improvements in wrist flexor spasticity have been demonstrated (106), as well as for distal lower extremity spasticity (107). Electrical stimulation has also been demonstrated to enhance the effect of botulinum toxin A therapy in treating upper limb spasticity poststroke (108).

Robot Therapy

Clinicians and engineers have worked together to develop various robotic devices with the goal of improving both motor and functional recovery after CNS injury (109). As with ES, it takes advantage of evidence suggesting that intensive, highly repetitive, functionally relevant, and challenging therapies are critical factors contributing to motor recovery (110–112). Rehabilitation robots have been designed to provide intensive and highly repetitive therapies that provide a means to improve motor and functional recovery in ways not feasible or practical using traditional rehabilitation approaches. Robots use computer programs that constrain inaccurate limb movement during specific tasks that can be modified as patients progress in their recovery, promoting more functionally appropriate motor skills. The intensity and automated components of robotic therapies specifically address the time and labor constraints associated with traditional therapies, as it can be used with less involvement of trained professionals. It can also enhance patient compliance by combining games with treatment, which provide immediate feedback on performance that serve to increase motivation. Changes in motor skills can be easily tracked and documented, which can help guide therapy, evaluate the efficacy of treatment interventions, and provide an additional means to monitor progress. Potential drawbacks of robotic therapy include being labor-intensive, the start-up costs, and the current lack of validation from clinical trials. However, the initial labor-intensiveness arising from staff training plus the cost of the equipment may be offset by the long-term cost-effectiveness derived from decreasing the amount of direct contact time therapists must spend with patients.

Several robotic devices have been developed, but none have yet been widely used in rehabilitation settings. The first robot used for rehabilitation of hemiparetic upper limbs was the MIT-MANUS. It has a 2 degree-of-freedom, back-drivable device allowing planar pointing and drawing movements of the shoulder and elbow (113). It uses an impedance controller with a programmable maintenance between the arm location and the desired position (62). It has been shown to improve motor recovery after acute and chronic stroke by providing repetitive massed practice of reaching toward a defined end point. The Mirror Image Motion Enabler is an industrial robot coupled to the arm. It moves the arm in 3 dimensions while the force feedback assists or resists the patient's movement. It can incorporate use of the uninvolved limb by measuring its position and then provide assistance to the weaker limb to mirror its movement. It can also be used unilaterally and work in active, passive, and resistive modes. It should be noted, however, that it was not shown to be significantly better than neurodevelopmental training using Bobath therapy 6 months after treatment cessation (114, 115). The Bi-Manu Track is a bilateral training device focusing on the forearm and wrist, which appears to have an advantage in improving motor skills compared with practice assisted with electric stimulation (116).

The Assisted Rehabilitation and Measurement robot is used to guide the paretic upper limb during linear reaching activities by applying forces that improve accuracy. Variable resistance provides force along a desired trajectory then unexpectedly removes resistance such that patients move along the desired path. It has 4 degrees of freedom and requires subjects to apply specific force patterns before providing external assistance. However, similar to some other devices, it has not been shown to be more beneficial than conventional training (117). The GENTLE/s RT system moves the arm passively (118). The Haptic-MASTER, part of the GENTLE/s RT system, suspends the upper limb from a sling to reduce the impact of gravity. It guides the limb along a smooth predefined trajectory and can operate in assistive and resistive modes. A study showed improved upper limb function as measured by the Fugl-Meyer Scale using the GENTLE/s (119). When compared with task practice with the arm suspended in the sling, the GENTLE/s robot seems to yield a greater rate of improvement for shoulder range of motion and the ability to perform certain arm movements (118). The Activities of Daily Living Exercise Robot provides active assistance as patients reach toward real objects. This system aims to deliver poststroke motor rehabilitation paradigms within an ADL-specific context (120).

Other robotic systems have used an exoskeletal design, such as the Myomo e100. This robot is worn on a paretic arm as an elbow orthosis and permits patients to interact naturally with objects while giving force feedback. It detects surface EMG signals from selected muscles, which are used to provide ES to assist with active elbow extension. It has been shown to improve motor skills and reduce spasticity in a group of patients with chronic stroke (121).

The previously described robots were designed primarily to improve proximal arm function. To improve the functional use of upper limbs, it is also necessary to focus on hand function. Several such systems have been developed and are being investigated. The Cyberglove and Rutgers Master II-ND glove are designed to increase range of motion and finger force via repetitive, stereotyped movements. Evidence suggests that although they can improve upper limb motor control after acute stroke (122, 123), there were no consistent improvements in functional abilities (124). Takahashi et al. (125) studied robot-based hand motor therapy after chronic stroke. Subjects with chronic stroke and moderate weakness of the arm and/or hand received 3 weeks of therapy emphasizing intense active repetitive movements involving attention, speed, timing, force, and precision. Significant gains were noted in the Action Research Arm Test and the arm motor Fugl-Meyer score. This was associated with significantly increased activation within the lesioned hemispherere on fMRI, suggesting the ability of this system to induce neural plasticity (125). Taub et al. (126) examined a more automated version of CIMT using AutoCITE. The system is composed of a computer that interfaces with several workstations where patients are trained to perform specific tasks. The computer provides a series of motor instructions to the patient that mimic the therapeutic interventions of CIMT and provides feedback on their performance as well as encouragement in a manner similar to a therapist. It reduces the amount of time needed by the therapist to supervise treatment and has been shown to be as effective as traditional CIMT (126).

Robotic therapy offers a promising venue for improved motor skills in people with hemiplegia. They are capable of providing repetitive, high-intensity, task-specific, and interactive treatments for the impaired limb. The devices can provide force feedback for sensorimotor-type training; measure the speed, direction, and strength of residual voluntary activity; and evaluate patients' movements interactively to assist them in limb movement through a predetermined trajectory during a given motor task. However, they have not gained widespread use for several reasons. Although most studies examining their use have demonstrated significantly improved motor skills, even in those with chronic stroke, they have not consistently been shown to improve ADL performance (127). This may be because most studies used insensitive measures of function that were not capable of detecting changes in ability to perform ADLs. A seemingly important advantage of robots over conventional rehabilitation is its ability to provide highly repetitive treatments over longer periods. However, it has been shown that equally intensive therapies provided by either robots or conventional means confer similar results (128). Future studies will need to address the functional implications of these devices as well as their economic feasibility and advantage over conventional treatments.

Body Weight–Supported Treadmill Training

Body weight–supported treadmill training (BWSTT), first described by Finch et al. (129), provides a strategy to assist some individuals with neurologic impairments to stand and ambulate. It uses a harness system that supports a percentage of a patient's body weight that unloads the lower extremities while training to walk on a treadmill. Evidence suggests that this may be an effective method of improving gait quality, walking speed, and trunk stability after stroke (130). It may also be an effective means to encourage a symmetrical gait pattern early in the rehabilitation process, as well

as a more appropriate method to facilitate sensory input and maximize much-needed repetition during the critical recovery period (131, 132).

The BWSTT is thought to work on various components of locomotion including posture, balance, weight shifting, and coordination. One means by which it may work is through activation of central pattern generators (CPGs) that are located in the spinal cord. Central pattern generators were initially described in invertebrates where it was demonstrated that neuronal networks interacted with specific sensory inputs resulting in locomotion (133). Although the presence of CPGs has not been definitively confirmed in vertebrates, there is evidence suggesting they exist in mammals. Studies examining cats with induced thoracic spinal cord lesions revealed that BWSTT resulted in an improvement in various aspects of gait, including an increase in both gait speed and number of steps taken compared to control animals (134, 135). This supports the theory that the mammalian spinal cord is capable of producing reciprocal gait patterns by means of these activated CPGs in the absence of supraspinal inputs. The improvements in gait in these animals also support the notion that neural plasticity is possible within the spinal cord. Supraspinal mechanism may also contribute to improved ambulation skills via BWSTT in ways similar to forced-use therapy, as it uses mass practice (the need for multiple repetitions) and shaping (performing sequentially greater approximations of a task) through progressive weight-bearing and forced use of impaired lower limbs (136).

The BWSTT attempts to facilitate automatic walking movements within the context of task-specific training. The patient is placed on a treadmill moving at the maximal comfortable walking speed with a portion of their weight-being supported at the trunk by an overhead harness. The combination of therapists and the physical apparatus of the system controls leg movement, patient posture, and balance that aids in mimicking the normal rhythmic nature of gait. The system offers patients the support to maintain the standing position, which is useful for those who do not have the muscle strength or postural control to begin overground gait training. Furthermore, it may decrease the fear of falling, which combined with its other attributes makes gait training feasible early after CNS injury (137). Early training postinjury theoretically enhances more normal-appearing ambulation, as the pattern associated with BWSTT resembles normal gait better than traditional overground training. Therefore, it may avoid the development of gait deviations such as knee hyperextension during stance phase, poor pelvic and trunk motion, gait asymmetry, and decreased step length often associated with tra-

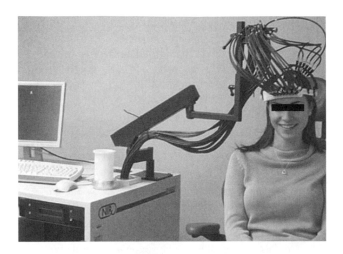

FIGURE 14.1

Functional near infrared spectroscopy. This figure demonstrates the equipment used and the setup for obtaining fNIRS. As noted in the figure, fNIRS is portable, which permits imaging of activated cortical regions during functional tasks in an ecologically valid setting. (Reproduced with permission from Kessler Foundation. Photographer, Richard Titus.)

ditional ambulation training as the patient attempts full weight-bearing. Furthermore, improvements in gait after BWSTT have been associated with changes in cerebral activation patterns in the cerebellum and midbrain, suggesting its ability to enhance cerebral plasticity (138–143).

Studies have largely supported the beneficial effects of BWSTT in term of improvements in the ability to ambulate, posture control, endurance, balance, rate of recovery, and gait velocity predominantly in patients with stroke-related hemiplegia (139, 140), with fewer demonstrating improvements after spinal cord injury (141, 142). Many studies have demonstrated the benefits of BWSTT in improving gait, although a metanalysis of several studies failed to reveal a definitive advantage over traditional therapeutic techniques (143). Possible reasons accounting for this include the heterogenicity in the nature and severity of stroke, the demographic distributions of the patients, variations in the intensity and frequency of training, the methods for assistance, and the placebo effect. However, a recent study demonstrated that BWSTT provided no additional benefit to an equal amount of traditional gait training in subjects with hemiplegia (144). Despite this, there are benefits to ambulation training using BWSTT, including improved cardiovascular fitness (145) and improved upper limb function (146). Hypotheses explaining the later observation include the positive effect of exercise on cerebral blood flow and

angiogenesis, facilitation of information processing caused by release of dopamine and/or norepinephrine, up-regulation of neurotrophins, and improvement in mood with decreased depression (146).

Despite promising results, BWSTT has not received widespread clinical acceptance. A primary drawback has been the time and physical demands placed on therapists to operate the system properly. Several therapists may be required to move the patient's limbs and to operate the machinery while trying to ensure appropriate kinematics of the trunk, pelvis, and lower limb. The BWSTT may also be fatiguing for both patients and therapists, thereby limiting the duration of the therapy sessions (147). Furthermore, it has been suggested that each therapist provide sensory information to the patient on a stride-by-stride basis to achieve maximal benefit. Robotic devices have been developed to address this factor, although these devices are very expensive and recent evidence suggests that their use is no more effective in improving ambulatory skills than

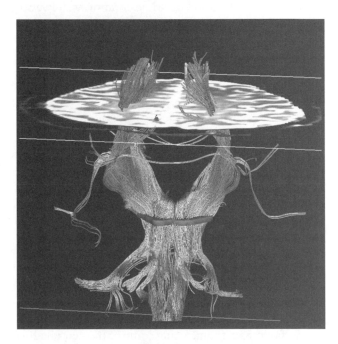

FIGURE 14.2

The DTI image. White matter fiber tracts in the living human brain, visualized noninvasively using DTI, a new and evolving MR technique. Images of this sort are used for basic neuroanatomical research, for clinical diagnosis of subtle neurologic disorders, and for guidance of neurosurgery. Data for this image were acquired using a 1.5-T Siemens Avanto MR scanner in the New York University Langone Medical Center Department of Radiology. (Image courtesy of Dr. Yulin Ge and Dr. Daniel K. Sodickson, Center for Biomedical Imaging, Department of Radiology, New York University Langone Medical Center.) See color insert.

equally intensive conventional therapy (144). Additional studies are needed to address dosing questions, optimal time to initiate treatment, time to progress to overground training, impact of upper extremity support, and most appropriate treadmill speed (41).

Barbeau and Visintin (140) found that both pretraining and posttraining walking speeds were greater on the treadmill than they were in overground walking and that the transfer of training from treadmill walking speed to overground walking speed was greater in the body weight–supported group than in the group without this technique. They also observed that partially unloading the lower limbs during training and progressively increasing the load as the gait pattern improved enhanced the recovery of posture and locomotion (140). Sullivan et al. (148) found that training at fast speeds was more effective in improving speeds of overground walking than training at slow or variable speeds.

In summary, BWSTT has been shown in some studies to be a promising technology in the treatment of patients with neurologic conditions; however, given the cost of the equipment, the labor-intensive nature of BWSTT, and its uncertain clinical efficacy compared to traditional rehabilitation, the clinical viability of BWSTT remains unclear. More studies are required to address these questions adequately.

CONCLUSIONS

Technological advances in the assessment of individuals with neurologic disabilities have led to a greater understanding of both normal and pathological physiological process of the CNS. They have given researchers the ability to explore the in vivo environment of the brain and spinal cord by imaging its microscopic structure, metabolic activity, and molecular makeup. This has provided both researchers and clinicians the knowledge base to better comprehend the complexity of normal human behavior and the pathological conditions that impact them. Using some of the new imaging technologies has the potential to predict prognosis and outcome that may aid one's clinical decision-making process. This knowledge combined with information garnered through other realms of research has been used to develop new treatment modalities that have the potential to enhance recovery caused by diseases or trauma in ways not feasible or poorly understood just a short time ago. However, despite what has been learned in the past few decades, much more remain unknown because these assessment tools have not explained all we need to know about upper motor neuron function and have raised additional questions that

remain unanswered. Accordingly, recovery of function is all too frequently incomplete. Therefore, existing technologies must be refined and new modalities developed to further our ability to effectively ameliorate the physical and cognitive sequelae of neurologic injury. Improved outcomes will only be achieved through greater understanding and dedicated efforts to refine existing treatments and develop new modalities (Figures 14.1 and 14.2).

References

1. Rosamond W, Flegal K, Furie K, et al. Heart disease and stroke statistics—2008 update: a report from the American Heart Association Statistics Committee and Stroke Statistics Subcommittee. *Circulation* 2008;117:e25–146.
2. Parsons MW, Barber PA, Chalk J, et al. Diffusion- and perfusion-weighted MRI response to thrombolysis in stroke. *Ann Neurol* 2002;51:28–37.
3. Albers GW, Thijs VN, Wechsler L, et al. Magnetic resonance imaging profiles predict clinical response to early reperfusion: the diffusion and perfusion imaging evaluation for understanding stroke evolution (DEFUSE) study. *Ann Neurol* 2006;60:508–17.
4. Marks MP, Olivot JM, Kemp S, et al. Patients with acute stroke treated with intravenous tPA 3-6 hours after stroke onset: correlations between MR angiography findings and perfusion- and diffusion-weighted imaging in the DEFUSE study. *Radiology* 2008;249:614–23.
5. Pajevic S, Pierpaoli C. Color schemes to represent the orientation of anisotropic tissues from diffusion tensor data: application to white matter fiber tract mapping in the human brain. *Magn Reson Med* 1999;42:526–40.
6. Nakayama N, Okumura A, Shinoda J, et al. Evidence for white matter disruption in traumatic brain injury without macroscopic lesions. *J Neurol Neurosurg Psychiatry* 2006;77:850–5.
7. Xu J, Rasmussen IA, Lagopoulos J, Haberg A. Diffuse axonal injury in severe traumatic brain injury visualized using high-resolution diffusion tensor imaging. *J Neurotrauma* 2007;24:753–65.
8. Yasokawa YT, Shinoda J, Okumura A, Nakayama N, Miwa K, Iwama T. Correlation between diffusion-tensor magnetic resonance imaging and motor-evoked potential in chronic severe diffuse axonal injury. *J Neurotrauma* 2007;24:163–73.
9. Benson RR, Meda SA, Vasudevan S, et al. Global white matter analysis of diffusion tensor images is predictive of injury severity in traumatic brain injury. *J Neurotrauma* 2007;24:446–59.
10. Huisman TA, Schwamm LH, Schaefer PW, et al. Diffusion tensor imaging as potential biomarker of white matter injury in diffuse axonal injury. *AJNR Am J Neuroradiol* 2004; 25:370–6.
11. Wozniak JR, Krach L, Ward E, et al. Neurocognitive and neuroimaging correlates of pediatric traumatic brain injury: a diffusion tensor imaging (DTI) study. *Arch Clin Neuropsychol* 2007;22:555–68.
12. Thomalla G, Glauche V, Koch MA, Beaulieu C, Weiller C, Rother J. Diffusion tensor imaging detects early Wallerian degeneration of the pyramidal tract after ischemic stroke. *Neuroimage* 2004;22:1767–74.
13. Garnett MR, Blamire AM, Corkill RG, Cadoux-Hudson TA, Rajagopalan B, Styles P. Early proton magnetic resonance spectroscopy in normal-appearing brain correlates with

outcome in patients following traumatic brain injury. *Brain* 2000;123 (Pt 10):2046–54.

14. Marino S, Zei E, Battaglini M, et al. Acute metabolic brain changes following traumatic brain injury and their relevance to clinical severity and outcome. *J Neurol Neurosurg Psychiatry* 2007;78:501–7.

15. Shutter L, Tong KA, Holshouser BA. Proton MRS in acute traumatic brain injury: role for glutamate/glutamine and choline for outcome prediction. *J Neurotrauma* 2004;21:1693–705.

16. Signoretti S, Marmarou A, Fatouros P, et al. Application of chemical shift imaging for measurement of NAA in head injured patients. *Acta Neurochir Suppl* 2002;81:373–5.

17. Butzen J, Prost R, Chetty V, et al. Discrimination between neoplastic and nonneoplastic brain lesions by use of proton MR spectroscopy: the limits of accuracy with a logistic regression model. *AJNR Am J Neuroradiol* 2000;21:1213–9.

18. Hourani R, Brant LJ, Rizk T, Weingart JD, Barker PB, Horska A. Can proton MR spectroscopic and perfusion imaging differentiate between neoplastic and nonneoplastic brain lesions in adults? *AJNR Am J Neuroradiol* 2008;29:366–72.

19. Moller-Hartmann W, Herminghaus S, Krings T, et al. Clinical application of proton magnetic resonance spectroscopy in the diagnosis of intracranial mass lesions. *Neuroradiology* 2002;44:371–81.

20. Poptani H, Gupta RK, Jain VK, Roy R, Pandey R. Cystic intracranial mass lesions: possible role of in vivo MR spectroscopy in its differential diagnosis. *Magn Reson Imaging* 1995;13:1019–29.

21. Poptani H, Kaartinen J, Gupta RK, Niemitz M, Hiltunen Y, Kauppinen RA. Diagnostic assessment of brain tumours and non-neoplastic brain disorders in vivo using proton nuclear magnetic resonance spectroscopy and artificial neural networks. *J Cancer Res Clin Oncol* 1999;125:343–9.

22. Rand SD, Prost R, Haughton V, et al. Accuracy of single-voxel proton MR spectroscopy in distinguishing neoplastic from nonneoplastic brain lesions. *AJNR Am J Neuroradiol* 1997;18:1695–704.

23. Glodzik-Sobanska L, Li J, Mosconi L, et al. Prefrontal N-acetylaspartate and poststroke recovery: a longitudinal proton spectroscopy study. *AJNR Am J Neuroradiol* 2007;28:470–4.

24. Glodzik-Sobanska L, Slowik A, Kieltyka A, et al. Reduced prefrontal N-acetylaspartate in stroke patients with apathy. *J Neurol Sci* 2005;238:19–24.

25. Glodzik-Sobanska L, Slowik A, McHugh P, et al. Single voxel proton magnetic resonance spectroscopy in post-stroke depression. *Psychiatry Res* 2006;148:111–20.

26. Villringer A, Chance B. Non-invasive optical spectroscopy and imaging of human brain function. *Trends Neurosci* 1997;20:435–42.

27. Fallgatter AJ, Roesler M, Sitzmann L, Heidrich A, Mueller TJ, Strik WK. Loss of functional hemispheric asymmetry in Alzheimer's dementia assessed with near-infrared spectroscopy. *Brain Res Cogn Brain Res* 1997;6:67–72.

28. Hock C, Villringer K, Muller-Spahn F, et al. Near infrared spectroscopy in the diagnosis of Alzheimer's disease. *Ann N Y Acad Sci* 1996;777:22–9.

29. Hock C, Villringer K, Muller-Spahn F, et al. Decrease in parietal cerebral hemoglobin oxygenation during performance of a verbal fluency task in patients with Alzheimer's disease monitored by means of near-infrared spectroscopy (NIRS)—correlation with simultaneous rCBF-PET measurements. *Brain Res* 1997;755:293–303.

30. Fallgatter AJ, Strik WK. Reduced frontal functional asymmetry in schizophrenia during a cued continuous performance test assessed with near-infrared spectroscopy. *Schizophr Bull* 2000;26:913–9.

31. Miyai I, Yagura H, Hatakenaka M, Oda I, Konishi I, Kubota K. Longitudinal optical imaging study for locomotor recovery after stroke. *Stroke* 2003;34:2866–70.

32. Kato H, Izumiyama M, Koizumi H, Takahashi A, Itoyama Y. Near-infrared spectroscopic topography as a tool to monitor motor reorganization after hemiparetic stroke: a comparison with functional MRI. *Stroke* 2002;33:2032–6.

33. Sakatani K, Xie Y, Lichty W, Li S, Zuo H. Language-activated cerebral blood oxygenation and hemodynamic changes of the left prefrontal cortex in poststroke aphasic patients: a near-infrared spectroscopy study. *Stroke* 1998;29:1299–304.

34. Takeda K, Gomi Y, Imai I, Shimoda N, Hiwatari M, Kato H. Shift of motor activation areas during recovery from hemiparesis after cerebral infarction: a longitudinal study with near-infrared spectroscopy. *Neurosci Res* 2007;59:136–44.

35. Mihara M, Miyai I, Hatakenaka M, Kubota K, Sakoda S. Sustained prefrontal activation during ataxic gait: a compensatory mechanism for ataxic stroke? *Neuroimage* 2007;37:1338–45.

36. Obrig H, Wenzel R, Kohl M, et al. Near-infrared spectroscopy: does it function in functional activation studies of the adult brain? *Int J Psychophysiol* 2000;35:125–42.

37. Okamoto M, Dan H, Shimizu K, et al. Multimodal assessment of cortical activation during apple peeling by NIRS and fMRI. *Neuroimage* 2004;21:1275–88.

38. Irani F, Platek SM, Bunce S, Ruocco AC, Chute D. Functional near infrared spectroscopy (fNIRS): an emerging neuroimaging technology with important applications for the study of brain disorders. *Clin Neuropsychol* 2007;21:9–37.

39. Liepert J, Bauder H, Wolfgang HR, Miltner WH, Taub E, Weiller C. Treatment-induced cortical reorganization after stroke in humans. *Stroke* 2000;31:1210–6.

40. Wolf SL, Winstein CJ, Miller JP, et al. Effect of constraint-induced movement therapy on upper extremity function 3 to 9 months after stroke: the EXCITE randomized clinical trial. *JAMA* 2006;296:2095–104.

41. Dobkin BH. Confounders in rehabilitation trials of task-oriented training: lessons from the designs of the EXCITE and SCILT multicenter trials. *Neurorehabil Neural Repair* 2007;21:3–13.

42. Page SJ, Sisto S, Levine P, McGrath RE. Efficacy of modified constraint-induced movement therapy in chronic stroke: a single-blinded randomized controlled trial. *Arch Phys Med Rehabil* 2004;85:14–8.

43. Page SJ, Levine P. Modified constraint-induced therapy extension: using remote technologies to improve function. *Arch Phys Med Rehabil* 2007;88:922–7.

44. Kelly BM, Pangilinan PHJ, Rodriguez GM. The stroke paradigm. *Phys Med Rehabil Clin N Am* 2007;18:631–50.

45. Chute DL. Neuropsychological technologies in rehabilitation. *J Head Trauma Rehabil* 2002;17:369–77.

46. Rizzo AA, Buckwalter JG. Virtual reality and cognitive assessment and rehabilitation: the state of the art. *Stud Health Technol Inform* 1997;44:123–45.

47. Jaffe DL, Brown DA, Pierson-Carey C, Buckley E, Lew HL. Stepping over obstacles to improve walking in individuals with poststroke hemiplegia. *J Rehabil Res Dev* 2004;41:283–92.

48. Fung J, Richards CL, Malouin F, McFadyen BJ, Lamontagne A. A treadmill and motion coupled virtual reality system for gait training post-stroke. *Cyberpsychol Behav* 2006;9:157–62.

49. Deutsch JE, Latonio J, Burdea G, Boian R. Post-stroke rehabilitation with the Rutgers ankle system—a case study. *Presence* 2001;10(4):416–30.

50. Jang SH, You SH, Hallett M, et al. Cortical reorganization and associated functional motor recovery after virtual reality in patients with chronic stroke: an experimenter-blind preliminary study. *Arch Phys Med Rehabil* 2005;86:2218–23.

51. You SH, Jang SH, Kim YH, et al. Virtual reality-induced cortical reorganization and associated locomotor recovery in chronic stroke: an experimenter-blind randomized study. *Stroke* 2005;36:1166–71.

52. Fischer HC, Stubblefield K, Kline T, Luo X, Kenyon RV, Kamper DG. Hand rehabilitation following stroke: a pilot study of assisted finger extension training in a virtual environment. *Top Stroke Rehabil* 2007;14:1–12.

53. Mirelman A, Bonato P, Deutsch JE. Effects of training with a robot-virtual reality system compared with a robot alone on the gait of individuals after stroke. *Stroke* 2009;40:169–74.

54. Turton A, Wroe S, Trepte N, Fraser C, Lemon RN. Contralateral and ipsilateral EMG responses to transcranial magnetic stimulation during recovery of arm and hand function afterstroke. *Electroencephalogr Clin Neurophysiol* 1996;101:316–28.

55. Netz J, Lammers T, Homberg V. Reorganization of motor output in the non-affected hemisphere after stroke. *Brain* 1997;120(Pt 9):1579–86.

56. Caramia MD, Iani C, Bernardi G. Cerebral plasticity after stroke as revealed by ipsilateral responses to magnetic stimulation. *Neuroreport* 1996;7:1756–60.

57. Berardelli A, Inghilleri M, Rothwell JC, et al. Facilitation of muscle evoked responses after repetitive cortical stimulation in man. *Exp Brain Res* 1998;122:79–84.

58. Muellbacher W, Ziemann U, Boroojerdi B, Hallett M. Effects of low-frequency transcranial magnetic stimulation on motor excitability and basic motor behavior. *Clin Neurophysiol* 2000;111:1002–7.

59. Chen R, Classen J, Gerloff C, et al. Depression of motor cortex excitability by low-frequency transcranial magnetic stimulation. *Neurology* 1997;48:1398–403.

60. Peinemann A, Reimer B, Loer C, et al. Long-lasting increase in corticospinal excitability after 1800 pulses of subthreshold 5 Hz repetitive TMS to the primary motor cortex. *Clin Neurophysiol* 2004;115:1519–26.

61. Siebner HR, Rothwell J. Transcranial magnetic stimulation: new insights into representational cortical plasticity. *Exp Brain Res* 2003;148:1–16.

62. O'Malley MK, Ro T, Levin HS. Assessing and inducing neuroplasticity with transcranial magnetic stimulation and robotics for motor function. *Arch Phys Med Rehabil* 2006;87:S59–66.

63. Harris-Love ML, Cohen LG. Noninvasive cortical stimulation in neurorehabilitation: a review. *Arch Phys Med Rehabil* 2006;87:S84–93.

64. Khedr EM, Ahmed MA, Fathy N, Rothwell JC. Therapeutic trial of repetitive transcranial magnetic stimulation after acute ischemic stroke. *Neurology* 2005;65:466–8.

65. Shimizu T, Hosaki A, Hino T, et al. Motor cortical disinhibition in the unaffected hemisphere after unilateral cortical stroke. *Brain* 2002;125:1896–907.

66. Murase N, Duque J, Mazzocchio R, Cohen LG. Influence of interhemispheric interactions on motor function in chronic stroke. *Ann Neurol* 2004;55:400–9.

67. Marshall RS, Perera GM, Lazar RM, Krakauer JW, Constantine RC, DeLaPaz RL. Evolution of cortical activation during recovery from corticospinal tract infarction. *Stroke* 2000;31:656–61.

68. Ward NS, Brown MM, Thompson AJ, Frackowiak RS. The influence of time after stroke on brain activations during a motor task. *Ann Neurol* 2004;55:829–34.

69. Mansur CG, Fregni F, Boggio PS, et al. A sham stimulation-controlled trial of rTMS of the unaffected hemisphere in stroke patients. *Neurology* 2005;64:1802–4.

70. Kirton A, Chen R, Friefeld S, Gunraj C, Pontigon AM, Deveber G. Contralesional repetitive transcranial magnetic stimulation for chronic hemiparesis in subcortical paediatric stroke: a randomised trial. *Lancet Neurol* 2008;7:507–13.

71. Liepert J, Zittel S, Weiller C. Improvement of dexterity by single session low-frequency repetitive transcranial magnetic stimulation over the contralesional motor cortex in acute stroke: a double-blind placebo-controlled crossover trial. *Restor Neurol Neurosci* 2007;25:461–5.

72. Takeuchi N, Chuma T, Matsuo Y, Watanabe I, Ikoma K. Repetitive transcranial magnetic stimulation of contralesional primary motor cortex improves hand function after stroke. *Stroke* 2005;36:2681–6.

73. Takeuchi N, Tada T, Toshima M, Chuma T, Matsuo Y, Ikoma K. Inhibition of the unaffected motor cortex by 1 Hz repetitive transcranial magnetic stimulation enhances motor performance and training effect of the paretic hand in patients with chronic stroke. *J Rehabil Med* 2008;40:298–303.

74. Nowak DA, Grefkes C, Dafotakis M, et al. Effects of low-frequency repetitive transcranial magnetic stimulation of the contralesional primary motor cortex on movement kinematics and neural activity in subcortical stroke. *Arch Neurol* 2008;65:741–7.

75. Mally J, Dinya E. Recovery of motor disability and spasticity in post-stroke after repetitive transcranial magnetic stimulation (rTMS). *Brain Res Bull* 2008;76:388–95.

76. Izumi S, Kondo T, Shindo K. Transcranial magnetic stimulation synchronized with maximal movement effort of the hemiplegic hand after stroke: a double-blinded controlled pilot study. *J Rehabil Med* 2008;40:49–54.

77. Centonze D, Koch G, Versace V, et al. Repetitive transcranial magnetic stimulation of the motor cortex ameliorates spasticity in multiple sclerosis. *Neurology* 2007;68:1045–50.

78. Nielsen JF, Sinkjaer T, Jacobsen J. Treatment of spasticity with repetitive magnetic stimulation: a double-blind placebo-controlled study. *Mult Scler* 1996;2:227–32.

79. Valle AC, Dionisio K, Pitskel NB, et al. Low and high frequency repetitive transcranial magnetic stimulation for the treatment of spasticity. *Dev Med Child Neurol* 2007;49:534–8.

80. Wassemann EM. Safety and side-effects of transcranial magnetic stimulation and repetitive transcranial magnetic stimulation. In: Pascual Leone A, Davey NJ, Rothwell J, Wassemann EM, Puri BK, ed. *Handbook of transcranial magnetic stimulation.* New York: Arnold, 2002:39–49.

81. Floel A, Cohen LG. Contribution of noninvasive cortical stimulation to the study of memory functions. *Brain Res Rev* 2007;53:250–9.

82. Sonde L, Gip C, Fernaeus SE, Nilsson CG, Viitanen M. Stimulation with low frequency (1.7 Hz) transcutaneous electric nerve stimulation (low-tens) increases motor function of the post-stroke paretic arm. *Scand J Rehabil Med* 1998;30:95–9.

83. Sonde L, Kalimo H, Fernaeus SE, Viitanen M. Low TENS treatment on post-stroke paretic arm: a three-year follow-up. *Clin Rehabil* 2000;14:14–9.

84. Chae J, Bethoux F, Bohine T, Dobos L, Davis T, Friedl A. Neuromuscular stimulation for upper extremity motor and functional recovery in acute hemiplegia. *Stroke* 1998;29:975–9.

85. Powell J, Pandyan AD, Granat M, Cameron M, Stott DJ. Electrical stimulation of wrist extensors in poststroke hemiplegia. *Stroke* 1999;30:1384–9.

86. Wong AM, Su TY, Tang FT, Cheng PT, Liaw MY. Clinical trial of electrical acupuncture on hemiplegic stroke patients. *Am J Phys Med Rehabil* 1999;78:117–22.

87. Kraft GH, Fitts SS, Hammond MC. Techniques to improve function of the arm and hand in chronic hemiplegia. *Arch Phys Med Rehabil* 1992;73:220–7.

88. Kimberley TJ, Lewis SM, Auerbach EJ, Dorsey LL, Lojovich JM, Carey JR. Electrical stimulation driving functional improvements and cortical changes in subjects with stroke. *Exp Brain Res* 2004;154:450–60.

89. Francisco G, Chae J, Chawla H, et al. Electromyogram-triggered neuromuscular stimulation for improving the arm function of acute stroke survivors: a randomized pilot study. *Arch Phys Med Rehabil* 1998;79:570–5.

90. Cauraugh J, Light K, Kim S, Thigpen M, Behrman A. Chronic motor dysfunction after stroke: recovering wrist and finger extension by electromyography-triggered neuromuscular stimulation. *Stroke* 2000;31:1360–4.

91. Cauraugh JH, Kim S. Two coupled motor recovery protocols are better than one: electromyogram-triggered neuromuscular stimulation and bilateral movements. *Stroke* 2002; 33:1589–94.

92. Kowalczewski J, Gritsenko V, Ashworth N, Ellaway P, Prochazka A. Upper-extremity functional electric stimulation-assisted exercises on a workstation in the subacute phase of stroke recovery. *Arch Phys Med Rehabil* 2007;88:833–9.

93. Alon G, Levitt AF, McCarthy PA. Functional electrical stimulation enhancement of upper extremity functional recovery during stroke rehabilitation: a pilot study. *Neurorehabil Neural Repair* 2007;21:207–15.

94. Alon G, Ring H. Gait and hand function enhancement following training with a multi-segment hybrid-orthosis stimulation system in stroke patients. *J Stroke Cerebrovasc Dis* 2003;12:209–16.

95. Robbins SM, Houghton PE, Woodbury MG, Brown JL. The therapeutic effect of functional and transcutaneous electric stimulation on improving gait speed in stroke patients: a meta-analysis. *Arch Phys Med Rehabil* 2006;87: 853–9.

96. Burridge JH, Haugland M, Larsen B, et al. Phase II trial to evaluate the ActiGait implanted drop-foot stimulator in established hemiplegia. *J Rehabil Med* 2007;39:212–8.

97. Chae J, Sheffler L, Knutson J. Neuromuscular electrical stimulation for motor restoration in hemiplegia. *Top Stroke Rehabil* 2008;15:412–26.

98. de Kroon JR, Ijzerman MJ, Chae J, Lankhorst GJ, Zilvold G. Relation between stimulation characteristics and clinical outcome in studies using electrical stimulation to improve motor control of the upper extremity in stroke. *J Rehabil Med* 2005;37:65–74.

99. Popovic DB, Popovic MB, Sinkjaer T, Stefanovic A, Schwirtlich L. Therapy of paretic arm in hemiplegic subjects augmented with a neural prosthesis: a cross-over study. *Can J Physiol Pharmacol* 2004;82:749–56.

100. Knutson JS, Hisel TZ, Harley MY, Chae J. A novel functional electrical stimulation treatment for recovery of hand function in hemiplegia: 12-week pilot study. *Neurorehabil Neural Repair* 2009;23:17–25.

101. Turk R, Burridge JH, Davis R, et al. Therapeutic effectiveness of electric stimulation of the upper-limb poststroke using implanted microstimulators. *Arch Phys Med Rehabil* 2008;89:1913–22.

102. Yu DT, Chae J, Walker ME, et al. Intramuscular neuromuscular electric stimulation for poststroke shoulder pain: a multicenter randomized clinical trial. *Arch Phys Med Rehabil* 2004;85:695–704.

103. Chae J, Ng A, Yu DT, et al. Intramuscular electrical stimulation for shoulder pain in hemiplegia: does time from stroke onset predict treatment success? *Neurorehabil Neural Repair* 2007;21:561–7.

104. Chae J, Yu DT, Walker ME, et al. Intramuscular electrical stimulation for hemiplegic shoulder pain: a 12-month follow-up of a multiple-center, randomized clinical trial. *Am J Phys Med Rehabil* 2005;84:832–42.

105. Campbell JM, Meadows PM. Therapeutic FES: from rehabilitation to neural prosthetics. *Assist Technol* 1992;4: 4–18.

106. Baker LL, Yeh C, Wilson D, Waters RL. Electrical stimulation of wrist and fingers for hemiplegic patients. *Phys Ther* 1979;59:1495–9.

107. Stefanovska A, Gros N, Vodovnik L, Rebersek S, Acimovic-Janezic R. Chronic electrical stimulation for the modification of spasticity in hemiplegic patients. *Scand J Rehabil Med Suppl* 1988;17:115–21.

108. Hesse S, Reiter F, Konrad M, Jahnke MT. Botulinum toxin type A and short-term electrical stimulation in the treatment of upper limb flexor spasticity after stroke: a randomized, double-blind, placebo-controlled trial. *Clin Rehabil* 1998;12:381–8.

109. Volpe BT, Krebs HI, Hogan N. Is robot-aided sensorimotor training in stroke rehabilitation a realistic option? *Curr Opin Neurol* 2001;14:745–52.

110. Vernon MW, Sorkin EM. Piracetam. An overview of its pharmacological properties and a review of its therapeuticuse in senile cognitive disorders. *Drugs Aging* 1991;1:17–35.

111. Kwakkel G, Kollen B, Lindeman E. Understanding the pattern of functional recovery after stroke: facts and theories. *Restor Neurol Neurosci* 2004;22:281–99.

112. Butefisch C, Hummelsheim H, Denzler P, Mauritz KH. Repetitive training of isolated movements improves the outcome of motor rehabilitation of the centrally paretic hand. *J Neurol Sci* 1995;130:59–68.

113. Krebs HI, Hogan N, Aisen ML, Volpe BT. Robot-aided neurorehabilitation. *IEEE Trans Rehabil Eng* 1998;6:75–87.

114. Lum PS, Burgar CG, Shor PC, Majmundar M, Van der Loos M. Robot-assisted movement training compared with conventional therapy techniques for the rehabilitation of upper-limb motor function after stroke. *Arch Phys Med Rehabil* 2002;83:952–9.

115. Lum PS, Burgar CG, Van der Loos M, Shor PC, Majmundar M, Yap R. MIME robotic device for upper-limb neurorehabilitation in subacute stroke subjects: a follow-up study. *J Rehabil Res Dev* 2006;43:631–42.

116. Hesse S, Werner C, Pohl M, Rueckriem S, Mehrholz J, Lingnau ML. Computerized arm training improves the motor control of the severely affected arm after stroke: a single-blinded randomized trial in two centers. *Stroke* 2005;36: 1960–6.

117. Kahn LE, Lum PS, Rymer WZ, Reinkensmeyer DJ. Robot-assisted movement training for the stroke-impaired arm: does it matter what the robot does? *J Rehabil Res Dev* 2006; 43:619–30.

118. Brewer BR, McDowell SK, Worthen-Chaudhari LC. Post-stroke upper extremity rehabilitation: a review of robotic systems and clinical results. *Top Stroke Rehabil* 2007;14: 22–44.

119. Amirabdollahian F, Loureiro R, Gradwell E, Collin C, Harwin W, Johnson G. Multivariate analysis of the Fugl-Meyer outcome measures assessing the effectiveness of GENTLE/S robot-mediated stroke therapy. *J Neuroeng Rehabil* 2007; 4:4.

120. Wisneski KJ, Johnson MJ. Quantifying kinematics of purposeful movements to real, imagined, or absent functional objects: implications for modelling trajectories for robot-assisted ADL tasks. *J Neuroeng Rehabil* 2007;4:7.

121. Stein J, Narendran K, McBean J, Krebs K, Hughes R. Electromyography-controlled exoskeletal upper-limb-powered orthosis for exercise training after stroke. *Am J Phys Med Rehabil* 2007;86:255–61.

122. Feys HM, De Weerdt WJ, Selz BE, et al. Effect of a therapeutic intervention for the hemiplegic upper limb in the acute phase after stroke: a single-blind, randomized, controlled multicenter trial. *Stroke* 1998;29:785–92.

123. Merians AS, Poizner H, Boian R, Burdea G, Adamovich S. Sensorimotor training in a virtual reality environment: does it improve functional recovery poststroke? *Neurorehabil Neural Repair* 2006;20:252–67.

124. Prange GB, Jannink MJ, Groothuis-Oudshoorn CG, Hermens HJ, Ijzerman MJ. Systematic review of the effect of robot-aided therapy on recovery of the hemiparetic arm after stroke. *J Rehabil Res Dev* 2006;43:171–84.

125. Takahashi CD, Der-Yeghiaian L, Le V, Motiwala RR, Cramer SC. Robot-based hand motor therapy after stroke. *Brain* 2008;131:425–37.

126. Taub E, Lum PS, Hardin P, Mark VW, Uswatte G. AutoCITE: automated delivery of CI therapy with reduced effort by therapists. *Stroke* 2005;36:1301–4.

127. Kwakkel G, Kollen BJ, Krebs HI. Effects of robot-assisted therapy on upper limb recovery after stroke: a systematic review. *Neurorehabil Neural Repair* 2008;22:111–21.

128. Volpe BT, Lynch D, Rykman-Berland A, et al. Intensive sensorimotor arm training mediated by therapist or robot improves hemiparesis in patients with chronic stroke. *Neurorehabil Neural Repair* 2008;22:305–10.

129. Finch L, Barbeau H, Arsenault B. Influence of body weight support on normal human gait: development of a gait retraining strategy. *Phys Ther* 1991;71:842,55; discussion 855–6.

130. Hesse S, Bertelt C, Schaffrin A, Malezic M, Mauritz KH. Restoration of gait in nonambulatory hemiparetic patients by treadmill training with partial body-weight support. *Arch Phys Med Rehabil* 1994;75:1087–93.

131. Visintin M, Barbeau H, Korner-Bitensky N, Mayo NE. A new approach to retrain gait in stroke patients through body weight support and treadmill stimulation. *Stroke* 1998;29:1122–8.

132. Shepherd R, Carr J. Weight supported treadmill training. *Neurorehabil Neural Repair* 1999;13:171–3.

133. Pinsker HK. Integration of reflex activity and central pattern generation in intact aplysia. *J Physiol* 1982;78:775–85.

134. de Leon RD, Hodgson JA, Roy RR, Edgerton VR. Locomotor capacity attributable to step training versus spontaneous recovery after spinalization in adult cats. *J Neurophysiol* 1998;79:1329–40.

135. Barbeau H, Rossignol S. Recovery of locomotion after chronic spinalization in the adult cat. *Brain Res* 1987;412:84–95.

136. Harvey R, Roth EJ, Yu D. Rehabilitation in stroke syndromes. In: Braddom R, Buschbacher RM, Chan L, ed. *Physical medicine and rehabilitation.* 3rd ed. Philadelphia: Saunders Elsevier, 2007:1175–1212.

137. da Cunha IT,Jr, Lim PA, Qureshy H, Henson H, Monga T, Protas EJ. Gait outcomes after acute stroke rehabilitation with supported treadmill ambulation training: a randomized controlled pilot study. *Arch Phys Med Rehabil* 2002;83: 1258–65.

138. Luft AR, Macko RF, Forrester LW, et al. Treadmill exercise activates subcortical neural networks and improves walking after stroke: a randomized controlled trial. *Stroke* 2008;39: 3341–50.

139. McCain KJ, Pollo FE, Baum BS, Coleman SC, Baker S, Smith PS. Locomotor treadmill training with partial body-weight support before overground gait in adults with acute stroke: a pilot study. *Arch Phys Med Rehabil* 2008;89: 684–91.

140. Barbeau H, Visintin M. Optimal outcomes obtained with body-weight support combined with treadmill training in stroke subjects. *Arch Phys Med Rehabil* 2003;84:1458–65.

141. Dietz V, Wirz M, Colombo G, Curt A. Locomotor capacity and recovery of spinal cord function in paraplegic patients: a clinical and electrophysiological evaluation. *Electroencephalogr Clin Neurophysiol* 1998;109:140–53.

142. Wernig A, Muller S, Nanassy A, Cagol E. Laufband therapy based on 'rules of spinal locomotion' is effective in spinal cord injured persons. *Eur J Neurosci* 1995;7:823–9.

143. Moseley AM, Stark A, Cameron ID, Pollock A. Treadmill training and body weight support for walking after stroke. *Cochrane Database Syst Rev* 2005;(4):CD002840.

144. Husemann B, Muller F, Krewer C, Heller S, Koenig E. Effects of locomotion training with assistance of a robot-driven gait orthosis in hemiparetic patients after stroke: a randomized controlled pilot study. *Stroke* 2007;38:349–54.

145. Macko RF, Smith GV, Dobrovolny CL, Sorkin JD, Goldberg AP, Silver KH. Treadmill training improves fitness reserve in chronic stroke patients. *Arch Phys Med Rehabil* 2001;82:879–84.

146. Ploughman M, McCarthy J, Bosse M, Sullivan HJ, Corbett D. Does treadmill exercise improve performance of cognitive or upper-extremity tasks in people with chronic stroke? A randomized cross-over trial. *Arch Phys Med Rehabil* 2008;89:2041–7.

147. Bogey R, Hornby GT. Gait training strategies utilized in poststroke rehabilitation: are we really making a difference? *Top Stroke Rehabil* 2007;14:1–8.

148. Sullivan KJ, Knowlton BJ, Dobkin BH. Step training with body weight support: effect of treadmill speed and practice paradigms on poststroke locomotor recovery. *Arch Phys Med Rehabil* 2002;83:683–91.

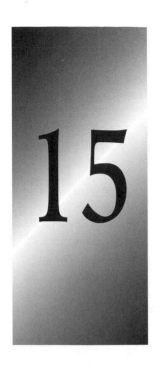

15 Pharmacologic Management of Spasticity: Oral Medications

Jay M. Meythaler
Scott Kowalski

Spastic hypertonia encompasses a variety of conditions that may contribute to increased tone or involuntary movement, including dystonia, rigidity, myoclonus, muscle spasm, posturing, and/or spasticity (1). The neurologic localization of the lesion that is the cause of spastic hypertonia may result in the different clinical manifestations noted. The other conditions associated with spastic hypertonia, such as the "clasp knife phenomenon," Babinsky or Hoffman reflexes, rigidity, and particularly acquired dystonia, may be more disabling than spasticity in acquired brain injury (2, 3), some cases of cerebral palsy (CP) (4), and multiple sclerosis (MS) (5). For this reason, they are often considered to be part of the broader "upper motor syndrome," of which spasticity is a part (6).

One of the hallmarks of upper motor neuron injury or illness above the conus medularis is the development of spastic hypertonia. It is one of the most disabling aspects of central nervous system (CNS) injury or illness. Spastic hypertonia can interfere with the functional use of remaining motor function, limit the range of motion of a joint, or cause pain. This can be very disabling with regard to mobility, transfers, activities of daily living, sitting, or sleep (7–10).

However, there are positive aspects of spastic hypertonia. Spasticity can aid in maintaining muscle tone and mass, resulting in increased blood return in the venous system, decreases the incidence of osteoporosis in paralyzed extremities, and aiding in reflexive

bladder and bowel emptying (11, 12). The increased muscle tone can also provide a fulcrum at various joints to improve posture, aid in sitting, or aid with transfers. The increased muscle mass over bony prominences can help prevent decubitis ulcers. Hence, spastic hypertonia is not an entity we wish to completely eliminate, just modulate.

In general, oral medication has been less successful in managing spastic hypertonia after acquired cerebral injury than in spinally related causes of spastic hypertonia (8, 13). Furthermore, all the potentially useful drugs for spasticity have associated central side effects that need to be carefully weighed when considering their use. The pharmaceutical management of spastic hypertonia after CNS injury or illness has generally been confined to the use of 5 primary medications: baclofen, diazepam, dantrolene sodium, clonidine, and tizanidine (1, 6, 8, 14–17). There is limited evidence that other medications may be useful as well.

Spastic hypertonia clinically presents differently when the lesions are in the spine, brainstem, or cerebral cortex (3, 10). The precise neurologic localization of the lesion can result in different clinical manifestations of spasticity (10). However, one does not treat spastic hypertonia based upon the anatomic location of the lesion. Rather, treatment is focused on the clinical presentation of the patient. Furthermore, it is clear that some medications may be preferred for upper limb spasticity, whereas others may be preferred for lower limb spasticity (5, 17). When one considers the cognitive and other side effects of medications, one needs to customize the treatment of medications quite precisely.

Determining the benefit of oral medications for the treatment of spastic hypertonia must focus on evaluating the patient with physiologic and functional outcome measures (18). The scales listed in Tables 15.1 and 15.2 are the most commonly used clinical methods for assessing the clinical treatment of spastic hypertonia. These scales have been those that have been most often accepted by the Food and Drug Administration (FDA) for pharmaceutical and investigational trials to obtain a clinical indication for use in "spasticity." They are also easily administered and relatively reliable methods for the clinician to utilize in a clinical setting. In addition, the physician should carefully monitor other medications, including "over-the-counter medications" due to potential interactions and the effects these medications may have on spastic hypertonia. We will present in detail the most frequently utilized oral medications and outline briefly the variations in their recommended uses in cerebral disorders versus spinal disorders and when attempting to treat upper extremity spastic hypertonia versus lower extremity spastic hypertonia.

A wide range of potential treatments have been investigated. The *clinical* pharmaceutical management of spastic hypertonia after CNS injury or illness has generally been confined to the use of centrally acting drugs mediated through γ- (19, 20) and peripherally acting drugs that inhibit the release of calcium from the sarcoplasmic reticulum (dantrolene) (15) as well as those that inhibit excitatory neurotransmitter release. We will organize the discussion of these medications by the neurotransmitter, through which they mediate their effect.

TABLE 15.1	
Definition of Ashworth, Spasm Frequency, and Reflex Scores	
Ashworth score	
1	No increase in tone
2	Slight increase in tone, giving a "catch" when affected part is moved in flexion or extension
3	More marked increase in tone, but affected part easily flexed
4	Considerable increase in tone; passive movement difficult
5	Affected part rigid in flexion or extension Spasm frequency score
0	No spasms
1	Mild spasms induced by stimulation
2	Infrequent full spasms occurring less than once per hour
3	Spasms occurring more than once per hour
4	Spasms occurring more than 10 times per hour
Reflex score	
0	Reflexes absent
1	Hyporeflexia
2	Normal
3	Mild hyperreflexia
4	3 or 4 beats clonus only
5	Clonus

Definitions and rating scales used to evaluate muscle tone (1), spasm frequency (2), and deep tendon reflexes (2, 3).

GAMMA-AMINOBUTYRIC ACID AGONISTS

Gamma-aminobutyric acid (GABA) receptor sites are widely present in the CNS, and GABA is the third most prevalent neurotransmitter in the CNS. GABA is present in an estimated 60% to 70% of all synapses in the brain and is inhibitory on a variety of neural pathways associated with spasticity (10, 19, 21). GABA is always an inhibitory neurotransmitter, affecting both presynaptic and postsynaptic inhibitions. GABA is a completely hydrophilic neurotransmitter and therefore is infinitely lipophobic with a complete inability to cross the blood brain barrier (22–24).

GABA receptors are distributed in 3 main receptor subtypes A, B, and C, with GABA-A and GABA-B most clearly involved in the treatment of spastic hypertonia. GABA-A receptors are a heteropentameric molecule that has at least 3 distinct subunits (25). The GABA-A receptor is a ligand-gated chloride ion channel that when activated allows increased chloride ion influx, causing membrane hyperpolarization (26, 27). GABA-B receptors are G-protein coupled and act on voltage-gated calcium channels, including N-methyl-

---

TABLE 15.2A
Spasticity Clinic Initial Evaluation

Name: _____ **MR #:** _____ **Date:** _____

Diagnosis: /_/ Spinal Cord Injury /_/ Multiple Sclerosis /_/ Cerebral Palsy /_/ CVA /_/ TBI /_/

Other _____

Date of Onset: _____ **History:** _____ _____

_____ _____

Surgical Procedures for Spasticity: /_/ None /_/ Rhizotomy /_/ Myelotomy /_/ Neurectomy /_/

Nerve Blocks /_/ Intrathecal Neurolysis /_/ Tendon Lengthening

Other _____

History of Seizures: /_/ Yes /_/ No   **Medication:** _____

_____

Prior/Current Anti-spastic Drug Use:

DRUG	DAILY DOSE	EFFECTIVENESS	SIDE EFFECTS

Neurologic Assessment:

SPASTICITY	LEFT	RIGHT		LEFT	RIGHT
Hip Abduction			Shoulder Abduction		
Hip Adduction			Elbow Extension		
Hip Flexion			Elbow Flexion		
Knee Extension			Wrist Extension		
Knee Flexion			Wrist Flexion		
Ankle Dorsiflexion					
Plantar Flexion					
Spasms: LE			Spasms: UE		
Reflexes: Knee ankle			Reflexes: Biceps		

Functional Assessment:
Mobility: /_/ wheelchair   /_/ ambulatory   /_/ ambulatory with assistive device /_/ bedridden
Urinary Management: /_/ normal   /_/ catheter   /_/ type _____ other: _____
Bowel Management: /_/ normal   /_/ suppository   /_/ digital stim   /_/ other: _____

Additional Findings: _____

_____

_____

_____

Plan: _____

_____

_____

Physician's signature:

_____

Outpatient evaluation sheets for spasticity clinic. (Forms used with permission from Jay Meythaler, MD, University of Alabama at Birmingham. Copyright Jay Meythaler.)

TABLE 15.2B
Baclofen/Clonidine Pump Clinic Follow-Up Evaluation

Name: _____   MR #: _____   Date: _____

Pump Refill: /_/ Yes   /_/ No

Programmer residual volume: _____cc   Actual residual volume: ____cc   Refill volume: _____cc

Concentration: _____ mcg/ml   Lot Number: _____

Program Change: /_/ Yes   /_/ No

Dose: _____ mcg/day   Single bolus given: _____ mcg

Infusion mode: /_/ simple   /_/ complex continuous   /_/ periodic bolus /_/ stopped

Neurologic Assessment:

TONE	LEFT	RIGHT		LEFT	RIGHT
Hip Abduction			Shoulder Abduction		
Hip Adduction			Elbow Extension		
Hip Flexion			Elbow Flexion		
Knee Extension			Wrist Extension		
Knee Flexion			Wrist Flexion		
Ankle Dorsiflexion					
Plantar Flexion					
Spasms: LE			Spasms: UE		
Reflexes: Knee ankle			Reflexes: Biceps		

Functional Assessment:

Mobility: /_/ wheelchair /_/ ambulatory /_/ ambulatory with assistive device /_/ bedridden

Urinary Management: /_/ normal /_/ catheter   /_/ other: _____

Bowel Management: /_/ normal /_/ suppository   /_/ digital stim   /_/ other: _____

Concomitant Medical Problems: /_/ none /_/ UTI /_/ Pressure sore /_/ other: _____

Adverse Effect or System Complication: /_/ Yes   /_/ No

Description: _____

Refill Alarm Date: _____

Other Comments: _____

Physician's signature: _____

Outpatient evaluation sheets for spasticity clinic. (Forms used with permission from Jay Meythaler, MD, University of Alabama at Birmingham. Copyright Jay Meythaler.)

D-aspartate (NMDA) channels (19, 28, 29). G-proteins also increase receptor-operated potassium channel conductance (20). Both mechanisms cause hyperpolarization of the motor horn cells, which is often cited as the predominant mechanism for the antispasticity effects associated with GABA-B agonists (6, 19).

The GABA-B receptors definitely are involved in spasticity treatment (3, 6, 13, 22, 23), whereas the A receptors have some effects on spasticity modulation and have an additional role in seizures management (3, 6). Because GABA crosses poorly into the CNS across any membrane (23, 24), drugs have been developed to either indirectly facilitate the release of GABA or substitute for GABA in CNS as analogs. It has been established that GABA inhibits the release of dopamine, norepinephrine (NE), acetylcholine, and serotonin (5).

Baclofen

Baclofen, 4-amino-3(p-chlorophenyl) butyric acid, is structurally similar to GABA and binds to presynaptic GABA-B receptors within the brainstem, dorsal horn of the spinal cord, and other CNS sites (30–34). Baclofen is a small molecule with a formula weight of 213.67 and the chemical name 4-amino-3(p-chlorophenyl) butyric acid ($C_{10}H_{12}ClNO_2$—see chemical structure above). It is a white to off-white, virtually odorless, crystalline powder with a slightly bitter taste. Structurally, it is very similar to GABA. It is stable as a solid and in solution at room temperatures and decomposes into a lactam at temperatures above 50°C. It was developed in the 1970s and has been a mainstay in the treatment of spastic hypertonia.

Baclofen depresses both monosynaptic and polysynaptic reflexes by blocking the release of neurotransmitters (32, 35). This results in inhibition of gamma motor neuron activity to the muscle spindle intrafusal fibers (19). Hence, baclofen inhibits monosynaptic and polysynaptic reflexes (31, 36). Because these reflexes can facilitate spastic hypertonia, inhibition of these reflex pathways reduces the overactive reflex response to muscle stretching or cutaneous stimulation. Some cases of dystonia also appear to respond to GABA agonists (2, 4, 5). Baclofen has some supraspinal activity that may contribute to clinical side effects.

Orally delivered baclofen reaches relatively low concentrations in the spinal cerebrospinal fluid, even after large oral doses (37). Thus, many patients experience central side effects, such as drowsiness, confusion, or attentional disturbances at the dosages required to reduce spasticity (6, 30, 38, 39). Other central effects of the drug include hallucinations, ataxia, lethargy, sedation, and memory impairment (30, 38–41). Furthermore, those patients with cerebral lesions are felt to be more prone to the centrally mediated side effects of medication (1). There is a significant reduction in attention span in some traumatic brain injury (TBI) patients who have been placed on oral baclofen, even when testing was done after several months on the medication (42). These effects have been reversible with a withdrawal of baclofen. Because cognitive function is critical for survival and adaptation after CNS injury or illness, any impairment of cognition due to medication may significantly adversely effect the severely brain injured patient. The sudden withdrawal of baclofen, including baclofen delivered intrathecally, may lead to seizures and hallucinations (12, 32).

Pharmacokinetics

Oral baclofen is relatively well absorbed with the peak effect within 2 hours of ingestion (42, 43) and a half-life of between 2.5 to 4 hours (6, 43), but it has a tissue half-life in the CNS estimated to be 3 to 5 hours (43). The drug is excreted unchanged by the kidney, and only 6% to 15% is metabolized by the liver (19, 43).

Treatment

The initial dosage of baclofen for spastic hypertonia should be started at 15 mg/d and increased every 3 days by 15 to 20 mg/d in at least 3 times per day due to the relatively short half-life (19, 44). Baclofen is often the first drug of choice in spinal causes of spastic hypertonia of spinal origin (6, 42). It has been utilized predominately for lower limb spastic hypertonia in spinal cord injury (SCI) (27, 45–50) and MS (51–63). Most of these studies on the oral use of the medication have been open-label studies predominately focused on its effects on the lower extremities. The use of baclofen in the upper extremities is based mostly on individual physician experience.

In spasticity due to cerebral origin, the use of baclofen is less well established. There are a few small randomized studies on the use of oral baclofen in CP (47, 48). In stroke and TBI, there is a single open-label trial (5). This 1 trial established that baclofen was effective physiologically in improving spastic hypertonia as measured by the Ashworth score in the lower limbs (5). Based upon the observed decrease in tone, the authors hypothesize that there was a reduced receptor density for GABA-B receptors in the cervical and brainstem regions than the thoracic region (5). Further investigation may delineate if there is a difference of baclofen's effectiveness on the upper extremities versus the lower extremities.

Seizures are a serious side effect of the use of baclofen and appear to lower the seizure threshold, regardless if the dose of baclofen is increased or decreased (64–68). Other complications of oral baclofen include euphoria, hallucinations, ataxia, memory impairment, lassitude, urinary problems, muscle weakness, dizziness, hypotension, sedation, memory problems, and blurred vision (3, 19). Motor weakness is usually the result of those who are overdosed on the medication or were utilizing their reflexive spastic hypertonia for functional status. The most serious side effects involve abrupt withdrawal, which is characterized by increased spastic hypertonia, increased deep tendon reflexes, pruritic symptoms, autonomic instability, hallucinations, central fevers, seizures, and death (19). These side effects are most likely related to a serotonin syndrome and usually develop within 2 and 6 days after abrupt withdrawal regardless of the delivery method of baclofen (12, 32, 65–69).

Surprisingly, there are no pharmacokinetic studies or effectiveness studies on the use of oral baclofen in pediatric patients. This is something that is being addressed currently in a large National Institutes of Health (NIH)-funded clinical trial.

BENZODIAZEPINE DERIVATIVES

Diazepam

Clonazepam

Benzodiazepines were first developed in the 1930s, although clinical usage did not begin until the 1960s

(70, 71). Diazepam is the prototypical benzodiazepine of this class of compounds characteristic of the 1, 4-nitrogenous ring structures most commonly utilized in the United States (70). Diazepam and clonazepam are both documented to be an effective treatment for the initial treatment of spastic hypertonia, but all benzodiazepines (eg, ketazolam, tetraepam,) have been useful in the treatment of spastic hypertonia (19, 70). They differ primarily with regard to the half-life and the cognitive side effects because some are more sedative, whereas others have a more profound hypnotic effect, and this has been the primary differentiation of these medications.

Benzodiazepines do not directly bind to GABA receptors but instead promote the release of GABA from GABA-A neurons by facilitating sodium conductance (19, 72–74). This results in enhanced presynaptic inhibition and is likely why they are useful in epilepsy (70).

These drugs are all CNS depressant medications and are noted for their antianxiety, hypnotic, antispasticity, and antiepileptic properties. The CNS effects are attributed to their ability to enhance GABA-mediated presynaptic inhibition in the CNS and to depress neuronal activity in the descending lateral and ascending reticular system. This also results in their prominent side effects of sedation and lethargy (70, 72, 73). These drugs also impair coordination, and prolonged use can lead to physical and psychological dependence and/or abuse. Effective dosages vary considerably, and upper level doses are primarily limited by tolerance to side effects. Because clonazepam and diazepam are the prototypical medications, they are the focus of this review.

Pharmacokinetics

Diazepam is quickly absorbed, reaches peak serum levels within 1 hour, and has a half-life approaching 60 hours (75, 76). A slow-release preparation does not reach peak serum levels until 3.6 hours after oral delivery (77). Clonazepam reaches peak serum levels in 1 to 4 hours (78, 79) and a 30- to 40-hour serum half-life in adults (80), but only 22- to 33-hour serum half-life in children (81). Clonazepam is primarily metabolized in the liver to glucoronides (79), as is diazepam (70, 75, 76).

Treatment

Diazepam is the prototypical medication utilized in adult spastic hypertonia, and clonazepam, by tradition, is utilized more frequently in pediatric patients.

However, there are many who use clonazepam in adults and vice versa. There are many clinicians who employ other benzodiazepines.

Diazepam is well established in the treatment of spastic hypertonia in MS with several clinical trails in the literature (46, 59–57, 82–84). Diazepam has been traditionally utilized for years in SCI even though the data are less well established, with only a few small studies (46, 85) also in mixed populations of patients with SCI, MS, and stroke. Benzodiazepines have more studies establishing their efficacy in cerebral disorders. In stroke patients, diazepam has been reported to be useful (84-88), but the studies have only small numbers of patients and are likely underpowered. There are only a couple of studies documenting the effectiveness of clonazepam in spastic hypertonia: one in a predominately MS population (89) and another small study in pediatric CP patients (90). Considering its widespread use, it is rather quite remarkable that there are so little data. There is relatively more data on the use of ketazolam, which is not available in the United States. However, in these head-to-head studies with diazepam, there was relatively no advantage except less frequent dosing (84, 91).

Benzodiazepines are sedative hypnotics and as such tend to exacerbate the complications of memory and alertness in patients with cerebral disorders. Hence, lately, they have not been recommended for use at least in the early stages of recovery. Benzodiazepines such as diazepam and lorazepam also have numerous adverse effects, including generalized CNS sedation with fatigue, drowsiness, and dizziness; paradoxical agitation; confusion; and disorientation with periods of blackouts or amnesia (19, 70, 72, 88). Rapid withdrawal has been associated with irritability, tremors, nausea, and seizures (19, 70).

OTHER GABA DERIVATIVES

Gabapentin

Gabapentin is an analogue of GABA. The mechanism of action of gabapentin continues to be a subject of debate. In the past, it was believed that gabapentin's effect was not mediated through interaction with the GABA receptor. However, more recently, it has been thought to interact at the GABA receptor. It is known for certain that gabapentin is not converted metabolically into GABA or GABA agonist, and it is not an inhibitor of GABA uptake or degradation (92). Regardless of the mechanism of action, gabapentin does increase GABA turnover, and no general statements can be made on the effect of gabapentin on NMDA receptors. The mechanism by which gabapentin exerts its anticonvulsant effect is not known. However, it appears now to interact with a unique receptor effecting voltage-gated N-type calcium ion channels (93). It is generally utilized as an adjunctive medication for the treatment of partial seizures (94).

Pharmacokinetics

Gabapentin is predominately renally cleared, leading to its linear pharmacokinetics (93, 95, 96). The bioavailability of gabapentin is not dose proportional (97). As the dose is increased, the bioavailability is decreased. Gabapentin is eliminated unchanged from the systemic circulation by renal excretion, and maximum plasma concentration occurs within 2 to 3 hours (98, 99) of dosing. Unlike other anticonvulsants, gabapentin apparently does not interfere with the elimination of phenytoin, valproic acid, carbamazepine, and phenobarbital (95).

Treatment

Gabapentin was initially designed as a pharmaceutical agent to treat spasticity but was found to be a more potent anticonvulsant for which it is approved for marketing in the United States (98, 100). Nevertheless, there have been small reports of its effectiveness for spasticity of spinal origin (101–104). However, close analysis of these studies indicates that its effectiveness has been marginal, particularly in terms of a reduction in the Ashworth score. However, some physicians continue to note that some patients with spastic hypertonia have a clinically meaningful response to the medication.

The most frequently noted side effects of gabapentin are somnolence (25%), dizziness (23%), ataxia (20%), nystagmus (15%), headache (14%), tremor (13%), fatigue (12%), and nausea/vomiting (9%), although the frequency is claimed to be less frequent than that noted with most other anticonvulsants (19, 95, 98). The usage in children has had mixed results, so it is generally only indicated for those over 12 years of age in children (94, 105). When dosing younger children, there are some pediatric epilepsy dosing guidelines that may be useful that indicate dosing for those 2 years or younger using gabapentin syrup 10 mg/kg (106). Dosing for subjects over 2 years received oral capsules based on weight: 200 mg for 16 to 25 kg; 300 mg for 26 to 36 kg; and

400 mg for 37 to 50 kg (106). There are no studies on the effectiveness of gabapentin on spasticity in children.

Tiagabine

Tiagabine is an anticonvulsant drug that was designed to prevent GABA reuptake into neurons (70). First utilized as an add-on therapy for partial epilepsy (107), more recently, it has been utilized as both an adjunctive medication and a monotherapy for complex-partial seizures and generalized tonic-clonic seizures (105, 108).

Pharmacokinetics

Tiagabine is 96% absorbed orally in most patients reaching peak serum concentration in 45 minutes in most patients although a delay of up to 3 hours has been reported in those with taking other medications that are hepatic metabolized (109). Tiagabine is its spectrum of activity and toxicities have been described as similar to those of vigabatrin and gabapentin (94, 95, 109). Tiagabine is rapidly metabolized via cytochrome P450 enzyme, and drugs that induce this enzyme will increase its metabolism, including carbamazepine and phenytoin (109–111). However, it has a half-life of only 7 to 9 hours (109, 112).

Treatment

Tiagabine is usually initiated at a dose of 4 mg once daily. The dose may be increased by 4 mg at the beginning of the second week and then at weekly intervals by 4 to 8 mg/d, divided in 2 to 4 doses, until a clinical response is achieved (113). The maximum dose is 32 mg/d.

Interestingly, there are no studies on the use of tiagabine in adults with spasticity. However, there are 2 small open-label trials in the use of tiagabine in spastic hypertonia in children (107,114). One small study in 10 subjects indicated an improvement in the Ashworth scores of the children (114). Another study in 14 children who had epilepsy and spastic hypertonia noted an improvement in voluntary motor scores as well (107).

The most frequent adverse effects of tiagabine are dizziness (30%), asthenia (24%), nervousness (12%), tremor (9%), diarrhea (7%), depression (5%), and

emotional labiality (4%) (4). In one large study, serious adverse effects were described in more than 15% of those exposed to the medication (115). Dosage is usually limited to 6 to 36 mg/d (105). Dosages in the 48 to 60 mg/d were linked to paradoxical nonconvulsive status epilepticus, and hence, excessive dosages should be used with caution in those patients with spastic hypertonia with a documented seizure disorder (116).

Vigabatrin

Vigabatrin was another attempt to "tailor make" an irreversible inhibitor of GABA-transaminase predominately as an antiepileptic agent (94). By inhibiting the neurotransporters of GABA and increasing the extracellular GABA, it has been demonstrated that this suppresses seizures (94, 117). Vigabatrin is broadly licensed in Europe and Latin America. Vigabatirn was approved by the FDA in January of 2009, but its release in the United States had been inhibited by its association to vision loss. The drug has generally been utilized for and now is the only FDA-approved medication as an adjuvant therapy for refractory partial seizures in both adults and children (94, 118). Use for spasticity is off-label, and there are no large studies on the use of this drug for spasticity.

Pharmacokinetics

Vigabatrin reaches peak serum concentration within 0.5 to 2 hours (119, 120). It is predominately renally cleared (119) and has a plasma half-life of 5 to 8 hours in adults and 12 to 13 hours in elderly persons (4, 119). Vigabatrin is not metabolized or significantly protein bound (119, 121). The serum levels of liver transaminases are reported to be reduced with vigabatrin, but this has not been associated with hepatic or renal dysfunction (95, 119, 122). It has been noted to decrease the serum level of phenytoin by 20% to 30% (95, 121). The most commonly noted side effects are somnolence/drowsiness (28%), fatigue (28%), dizziness (21%), nystagmus (15%), abnormal vision (11%), agitation (11%), amnesia (10%), depression (10%), and paresthesia (9%) (4, 120). Doses usually start at 25 mg/kg per day and increased up to 125 mg/kg per day as needed. One author generally starts most patients on 1000 mg once a day (118), and the drug is generally increased to a maximum of 4 g a day in 2 divided doses (4, 120).

Treatment

Dosing in adults with spastic hypertonia has been in the range of 2 to 3 g/d in 2 divided doses (121). However, vigabatrin has been of therapeutic value in the treatment of refractory infantile spasms, although these spasms have been linked to seizure activity (123). In 43% of the children there was complete spasm suppression and 95% of the children had a greater than 50% reduction of spasms with initial treatment (123). However, a long-term response was noted in only 75% of children with symptomatic infantile spasms (123).

Vigabatrin can cause psychiatric disturbances, including aggression and psychosis (95, 121, 124). About half of all the patients experience some adverse effects with vigabatrin. The most common are drowsiness and fatigue, although in children, excitation and agitation occur more frequently. Other CNS-related adverse effects include dizziness, nervousness, irritability, headache, nystagmus, ataxia, paraesthesia, tremor, and impaired concentration. Generally, it is felt that patients with significant psychiatric history should be treated with caution with regard to the use of vigabatrin (108). Toxicology studies have associated vigabatrin with intramyelinic vacuolization or edema in the brains of rodents and dogs (94, 95, 118). Vigabatrin may need to be withdrawn if visual symptoms develop. Visual field testing should be performed at baseline and during routine follow up, particularly in children who have visual field deficits or at risk to develop visual field deficits (125–127).

Topiramate

Topiramate is another Anti epileptic drug (AED) for tonic-clonic seizures by blockage of voltage-dependent sodium channels (128), an augmentation of gamma-aminobutyrate acid activity at some subtypes of the GABA-A receptors (4, 129, 130), and antagonism of AMPA/kainite subtype of the glutamate receptor affecting Ca channels (130).

Pharmacokinetics

After oral administration, topiramate reaches peak serum concentration in 1 to 4 hours, averaging 2 hours in most patients (131, 132), and has an elimination half-life of 21 hours (131). Topiramate is only slightly metabolized, and none of the metabolites are felt to be clinically active (133). It is predominately renally cleared (128, 131).

Treatment

Topiramate is usually initiated at doses of 25 to 50 mg/d and increased in increments of 25 to 50 mg per week (131). It has had limited use in spasticity that has been primarily confined to open-label case series of children with spasticity from Canavan disease, which causes early onset leukoencephalopathy and megalencephaly as well as the infantile spasms of West syndrome, when combined with vigabatrin (4, 133, 134). It has been reported to be useful in chorea and hemiballismsus after stroke in 1 case report (135). Topiramate's most significant side effects are somnolence and weight loss (4, 131).

CENTRAL ALPHA-ADRENERGIC AGENTS

The monoamines are widely distributed within the CNS. In spastic hypertonia, they appear to modulate sensory, autonomic, and motor functions through facilitation of presynaptic inhibition of spinal afferent inputs (20). The monoamines have an important role as modulators of spinal neuron excitability (136). Norepinephrine for the spinal pathways is produced in the neurons residing in the brain in the area called the locus ceruleus (20). The mechanism by which noradrenergic pathways modulate spastic hypertonia is predominately by modulating the sensory inputs via presynaptic inhibition of the spinal afferent inputs (20, 137). Norepinephrine also modulates polysynaptic segmental reflexes where NE agonists may restore the vibratory inhibition of spinal reflexes (20, 138). Norepinephrine also has a direct inhibitory effect on interneurons and polysynaptic segmental reflexes (20, 139, 140). In essence, the central NE modulates spastic hypertonia via central alpha-2 and imidazol type-I adrenergic receptor agonist activity by both reducing the stimulating effect of noxious stimulation (20, 141) and modulating the spindle activity directly related to spastic hypertonia (20, 142). When the descending pathways from the brainstem to the spinal cord are disrupted, there is a reduction in the NE in the spinal pathways leading to increased spastic hypertonia.

Clonidine

Clonidine was one of the first central acting central alpha-2 and imidazol type-I adrenergic receptor agonists to be utilized in spasticity (20). Clonidine is also an alpha-1 central adrenergic agonist. This effect is what is felt to be attributable to its effects as an antihypertensive medication, which is antagonized by yohimbine (20, 143–145). Its effects on spasticity are predominately attributed to its alpha-2 adrenergic receptor effects by presynaptic inhibition of sensory afferents (137, 138, 145). This is why it is also attributed to be a profound nocioceptive pain reliever (20). Clonidine's effects on blood pressure appear to be due to the central sympatholytic effect of clonidine. As a result, clonidine has little effect on the blood pressure of people who have complete SCI, but it can lower the blood pressure for normals and those with incomplete injuries (146–148).

Pharmacokinetics

Clonidine is an extremely lipophilic medication with almost uniform distribution whether the medication is delivered via oral (149, 150), transdermal (151–153), intravenous (154, 155), epidural (156), or rectal delivery (157, 158). All reach relatively similar systemic serum levels. Oral clonidine delivered orally reaches peak serum levels in 1 to 1.5 hours and has a scrum half-life of 12 to 16 hours (159). Clonidine is 50% metabolized by the liver with the rest renally cleared largely unchanged (159).

Treatment

Clonidine in the oral form has been utilized quite successfully for spastic hypertonia in SCI (20, 137, 138, 146, 160). However, all the studies were open-label A-B trials. In patients with stroke, there is 1 case report (161). Transdermally, clonidine appears to have had a similar effect as orally (162, 163). It should be pointed out that oral clonidine may have profound effects in patients with SCI on autonomic dysreflexia (164) as well as on bladder reflexes, potentially changing the voiding patterns of the patients (147). There are limited pediatric trials using clonidine for spasticity. The predominant side effects are related to its effects on blood pressure. Other side effects include bradycardia, dry moth ankle edema, and depression (20, 159). Those with a complete high-level SCI may be less likely to have a significant effect on blood pressure (147, 148, 159).

Tizanidine

Tizanidine is a centrally acting, selective alpha-2 adrenergic and imidazole agonist that is structurally related to the antihypertensive drug clonidine (20). However, tizanidine has only one-tenth to one-fiftieth the potency of clonidine in lowering blood pressure or slowing heart rate (165). This is due to the differences in preferential receptor selectivity for alpha-2 receptors rather than alpha-1 adrenergic receptors. Similar to clonidine, tizanidine also has effects on imidazol type I receptors. Tizanidine is active at both segmental spinal and supraspinal levels in both motor and sensory pathways (20). At the spinal segmental level, tizanidine is a presynaptic inhibitor of excitatory amino acid release and also acts to inhibit

---

TABLE 15.3
Table of Most Common Adverse Drug Reactions for Antispasticity Medications

ADR	INCIDENCE	DOSE RELATED	CLINICAL MANAGEMENT	
Sedation	30%–50%	Yes	Reduce dose	Titrate slowly
Dry mouth	30%–50%	Yes	Reduce dose	Titrate slowly
Asthenia	25%–45%	Yes	Reduce dose	Titrate slowly
Dizziness	10%–30%	Yes	Reduce dose	Titrate slowly
Elevated hepatic transaminases	5%	No	Monitor at 0,1-3, and 6 months	Discontinue drug
Hallucinations	0%–3%	No	Ask if present	Discontinue drug
GI effects	4%	No	Monitor symptom	
Hypotension	2%	Yes	Reduce dose	Titrate slowly

Most common side effects with the use of oral tizanidine.

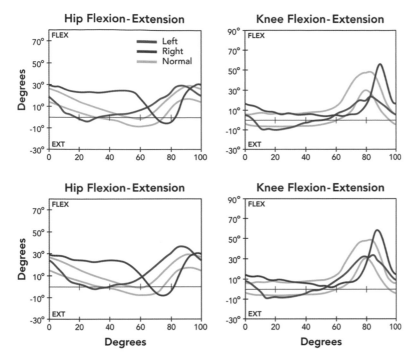

FIGURE 10.5(B) CODA 3-D kinematic data before (top) and after (bottom) treatment of stiff knee gait in the patient depicted in Figure 10.4. Note marked improvement in left knee (blue) peck flexion and hip flexion. Red represents right leg and gray band normative data that are velocity matched. Data are normalized; vertical line at 65% to75% indicates the beginning of the swing phase. Based on dynamic EMG and gait analysis, patient was treated with 200 U of BoNT-A (Botox®) injected to the right rectus femoris (100 U), vastus medialis (50 U), lateralis (50 U), and gluteus maximus (50).

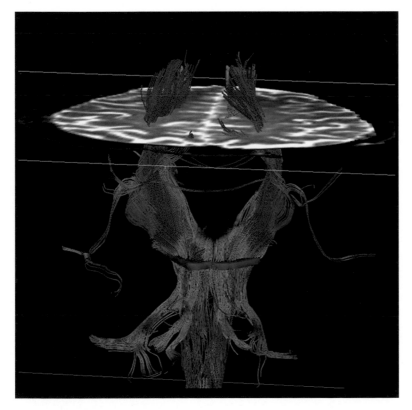

FIGURE 14.2 The DTI image. White matter fiber tracts in the living human brain, visualized noninvasively using DTI, a new and evolving MR technique. Images of this sort are used for basic neuroanatomical research, for clinical diagnosis of subtle neurologic disorders, and for guidance of neurosurgery. Colors assigned to individual nerve fibers represent principal fiber directions (blue: head-to-foot; red: left-to-right; green: front-to-back). Data for this image were acquired using a 1.5-T Siemens Avanto MR scanner in the New York University Langone Medical Center Department of Radiology. (Image courtesy of Dr. Yulin Ge and Dr. Daniel K. Sodickson, Center for Biomedical Imaging, Department of Radiology, New York University Langone Medical Center.)

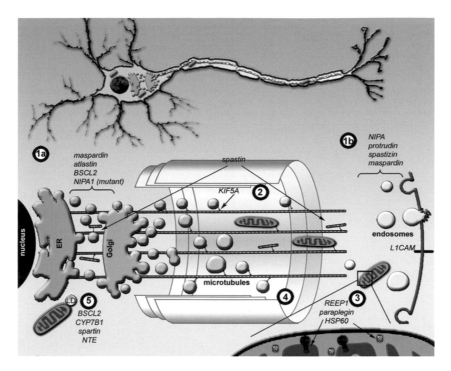

FIGURE 19.1   Model of HSP.

polysynaptic reflexes (166). In the brain, tizanidine inhibits firing of the locus ceruleus, thereby inhibiting the normally facilitatory influence of the descending cerebrospinal pathway. Tizanidine has no effect on monosynaptic reflexes, such as the standard deep tendon reflex (165). More importantly, tizanidine has no activity at the neuromuscular junction and has no direct effect on skeletal muscle fibers, so it does not cause any muscle weakness (167–169). In some reports, patients actually show apparent increases in muscle strength due to central relaxation of the antagonist muscles (167).

Pharmacokinetics

Tizanidine is well absorbed with 50% to 65% absorption from oral doses and undergoes extensive first-pass metabolism (20). None of the metabolites are pharmacologically active. The half-life of tizanidine is 2.1 to 4.2 hours, with peak plasma concentration reached at 1 hour (170, 171). Modified release capsules have a peak serum level of 5.7 hours (172) with 60% of the drug excreted in the urine and 20% recovered in feces (170). Tizanidine is moderately protein bound (about 30%) and exhibits linear kinetics across the range of usual doses. It has no effect on the hepatic P450 enzyme system (20, 170). There is a paradoxical "food effect" that alters the pharmacokinetics of tizanidine. If taken with a meal, the peak plasma concentration is *increased* by 33%, and the time to reach this peak concentration is reduced by 40 minutes (170). The new modified release capsules somewhat temper this "food effect" (170). The overall absorption of the drug remains unchanged (170). There are drug interactions; particularly with the concomitant use of ciprofloxacin, the tizanidine exposure is increased with risks of excessive sedation and hypotension (173, 174).

Treatment

Tizanidine has been effectively utilized in randomized clinical trials for spastic hypertonia in SCI, MS, TBI, and stroke utilizing the Ashworth score as one of the outcome measures (167–169, 175). In stroke, there is another prominent open-label study also demonstrating significant effectiveness utilizing the Ashworth score as one of its outcome measures (173). There are no pediatric studies although it is evident that the medication is utilized off label (176). Dosing should be started at 2 mg at night and increased slowly by 2 mg/d every 2 days to a maximum dosage of 36 mg/d. The effect of tizanidine is clearly dose-related (167, 177).

The most common side effects of tizanidine are sedation, asthenia, dizziness, and dry mouth (167–171) (see Table 15.3). Sedation appears to be the most serious side effect in spasticity trials with an incidence of 41% to 46% (167–169). Despite its similarity to clonidine, there is very little hypotension or bradycardia experienced at clinically relevant doses and virtually none in the lower half of the dose range (177). Rebound hypertension can occur with abrupt cessation from higher does (170). Hallucinations and nightmares have been reported, and some Gastro intestinal (GI) side effects, notably constipation, can occur in up to 5% of Gastro intestinal patients (170). There is excellent agreement between researchers and clinicians with regard to the type and frequency of adverse drug reactions. Perhaps the most significant issue with the chronic use of tizanidine has been its potential for hepatotoxicity, so liver enzymes should periodically be checked as the dosage is increased (20, 170).

SEROTONERGIC AGENTS

The mechanisms by which serotonin affects spastic hypertonia are not clearly understood. It is quite clear that in SCI the presence of serotonin-containing neurons, which originate in the brainstem, is an indication of an incomplete lesion (20). However, it is also clear that in serotonin syndrome there is an increase in tone and spasticity (73, 178, 179). Furthermore, it has been speculated for some time that drugs that can block serotonergic transmission may improve spastic hypertonia (20).

Cyproheptadine

The most profound serotonin blocker utilized to block serotonin is cyproheptadine, which has been studied in spasticity (180–182) as well as to treat the symptoms of the serotonin syndrome associated with baclofen withdrawal (69). It was initially approved for vascular headaches, anorexia, and hives (4).

Pharmacokinetics

Besides its profound effects on blocking serotonin, cyproheptadine has profound anticholinergic and antihistaminic effects as well (4, 69, 183). Dosing is usually at 12 to 20 mg/d in 3 to 4 divided doses with dose increases every 3 to 4 days (4, 69, 182, 183). Cyproheptadine reaches peak serum concentration in 6 to 9 hours after oral ingestion and has a serum half-life of 16 hours (184). The drug is 57% conjugated in the liver, and the rest is renally cleared (184, 185).

Treatment

Clinical data supporting the use of cyproheptadine are quite sketchy. It was first reported to decrease ankle clonus in 6 MS and SCI patients in an open-label study over 25 years ago (180) and later to improve walking speeds in an open-label study of 6 SCI patients (181). A larger 3-armed open-label trial on 25 SCI patients comparing baclofen, clonidine, and cyproheptadine indicated that on the Ashworth Scale and the pendulum test, cyproheptadine was superior to clonidine and equivalent to baclofen. These data are limited because there was no randomization and no placebo group. More recently, there is a report that cyproheptadine may alleviate some of the effects of intrathecal baclofen withdrawal, indicating that GABA-B receptors do inhibit the release of serotonin and that serotonin is involved in movement disorders (69). The most frequent side effects are somnolence and weight gain with the use of cyproheptadine (20, 185).

CANNABINOIDS

Dronabinol

Nabilone

Cannabis, cannabis extracts, and various synthetic cannabinoids have been touted for years as agents to treat spastic hypertonia. It has been the impetus in the United States for various states to legalize the medicinal use of marijuana (4, 186). Tetrahydrocanibinoid (THC) is the active ingredient of cannabis. Synthetic versions such as dronabinol and/or nabilone, developed for nausea, are versions of delta-9-tetrahydrocannabinol (4). Both of these drugs and the cannabis extract have profound antinausea and antianxiety effects. There has been considerable interest in the use of cannabis, particularly in patients with MS (186). The mechanism of action, other than a reduction in anxiety or pain, that may cause spastic hypertonia is not clear.

Pharmacokinetics

Dronabinal reaches peak serum concentration in 1 to 2.5 hours after ingestion and has a biphasic half-life for the active compounds of 19 to 36 hours (187). The drug is rapidly metabolized into the active compound 11-hydroxy-delta-9- tetrahydrocannabinol and is 10% to 15% renally cleared with the rest cleared in the feces (187, 188). Dizziness and somnolence are the most common side effects, although ataxia and memory issues have been reported (187).

Nabilone reaches peak serum concentration in 2 hours and has a half-life of only 2 hours (189). It is extensively metabolized by the liver via the P450 enzyme and predominately excreted in the feces with 20% to 24% renal clearance (189–191).

Treatment

The recommended initial dose for dronabinol in patients is 2.5 mg orally twice daily and slowly increased over and may be gradually increased to a maximum of 20 mg/d (187). Nabilone is started at a dosage of 1 mg/d and increased slowly to a maximum dosage of 6 mg/d in 3 divided dosages (189). There have been several suggestions on the effectiveness of cannabis-related compounds on spasticity for years. These studies were either open-label subjective studies (192–194) or small blinded studies utilizing electromyographic (EMG) analyses (195). Only 2 of the studies were outside of MS, with one having a mixed population of stroke, MS, and SCI (195), and another subjective study in patients with SCI (194).

In a recent large placebo-controlled study, 630 participants were treated with oral cannabis extract (n = 211), delta9-tetrahydrocannabinol (delta9-THC; n = 206), or placebo (n = 213). The trial duration was 15 weeks (196). The primary outcome measure was change in overall spasticity scores using the Ashworth Scale. There was no treatment effect of cannabinoids, either cannabis extract or delta9-THC, on the primary outcome measure (196). However, there was a trend toward improvement that was superior with delta9-THC (196). Interestingly, the placebo group improved significantly, and it is not clear as to whether therapies were controlled for in the study population.

There was some objective improvement in mobility and patients' opinion of an improvement in pain, although there were also some difficulties in the blinding of the study (196).

A 12-month open-label study on these same patients who continued in the trial for 12 months indicated that patients felt that both cannabis extract and delta9-THC helped their spasticity (197). This was confirmed objectively only in the delta19-THC group by an improvement of approximately 2 points on the Ashworth Scale from the baseline. There was suggestive evidence for treatment effects of delta9-THC on some aspects of disability at 12 months as there was in the shorter 15-week study (196, 197). Interestingly, despite the movement for medicinal marijuana, pure cannabis extract was not effective in this extended study (197). There were no major safety concerns. However, memory issues were not addressed, and this appears to be a significant problem even in those who are normal and use cannabis (198). Another more recent randomized trial on 189 patients did not reach statistical significance on the Ashworth Scale but did have an improvement in functional status (190).

Overall, patients felt that these drugs were helpful in treating their disease in the larger trials (196, 197, 199). Others have reported improvement in upper motor neuron-related bladder issues in MS (199). There are those who feel that the side effects of cannabis extract can be alleviated by the use of synthetic cannabinoids (200), and clearly, the dosing is more predictable than the organic version.

OTHER AGENTS

Dantrolene Sodium

Dantrolene, (1-((5-p-nitrophenyl)furfurylidene)amino) hydantoin)sodium hydrate or dantrolene sodium, is the only FDA-approved oral antispasticity medication that is classed as a direct acting skeletal muscle relaxant. Dantrolene does not exert its effect centrally. Rather, it acts in the periphery by decreasing the release of calcium from the sarcoplasmic reticulum of the skeletal muscle cell, thus uncoupling electrical excitation from contraction and decreasing the force of contraction (201–205). This in turn affects intrafusal as well as extrafusal fibers, reducing spindle sensitivity (206, 207). Dantrolene's action is specific for skeletal muscle and affects reflex contractions or spasticity more than voluntary contraction (208). However, its effect is still significant enough that twice the voluntary effort is required to maintain a desired muscle tension (209).

Pharmacokinetics

Dantrolene is well absorbed, approximately 70% (210, 211), and has a half-life of 15 hours after oral administration in adults (212). Peak blood levels are achieved within 3 to 6 hours, and its active metabolite peaks within 4 to 8 hours (42). It is metabolized by the liver via hydroxylation, N-reduction, and acetylation to form 5-hydroxydantrolene and acetylated dantrolene (213). Five-hydroxydantrolene is an active metabolite, albeit less potent and acetylated dantrolene is inactive (212–214). Approximately 20% of an orally administered dose, or 80% of an absorbed dose is eliminated by the kidney in the urine as 5-hydroxydantrolene (79%), acetylated dantrolene (17%), and unchanged parent drug (1%-4%) (212, 215).

Treatment

Dantrolene has been found superior to placebo for the treatment of spasticity secondary to stroke, TBI, SCI, CP, and MS (216–220). However, because of its propensity to cause weakness, several reports advocate limiting its use in CP, spasticity of spinal origin, and MS patient populations, as it may hinder function (15, 85, 217). Correspondingly, in 1980, the American Medical Association released the statement, "Dantrolene should be used primarily in nonambulatory patients and only if the resultant decrease in spasticity will not prevent the patient from functioning" (221). A recent report has recommended dantrolene as a first line agent in the treatment of spasticity after TBI, especially in the acute setting, as it exhibits minimal cognitive effects and may not interfere with neural recovery (217).

The recommended initial dosing for adults is 25 mg daily for 7 days. This may then be increased to 3 times daily dosing for 1 week, then to 50 mg 3 times daily for 7 days, and then to 100 mg 3 times daily if further dose increase is required (212). The maximum daily adult dose is 400 mg (212).

Pediatric dosing is similar to most other medications in that it is weight based. Dosing begins with 0.5 mg/kg daily for 7 days (212). The dose may then be increased as necessary to 0.5 mg/kg 3 times daily for 1 week, then to 1 mg/kg 3 times a day for 1 week, and then to 2 mg/kg 3 times daily to achieve the desired effect (212). Again, a maximum dose of 12 mg/kg per day or 400 mg daily should not be exceeded (212, 205).

Dantrolene use is associated with a significantly increased risk of hepatotoxicity, 1% overall, especially with doses higher than 400 mg a day (212). Not surprisingly, active hepatic disease is a contraindication to its use. Female gender, age more than 35 years, and polypharmacy are additional risk factors for hepatotoxicity (222, 223). In one study of 122 cases of dantrolene-induced adverse hepatic effects, 47 patients (the majority) had asymptomatic elevation of transaminases (224, 225). It is suggested that liver function tests be monitored during dantrolene therapy, and in accordance with good medical practice, the lowest optimally effective dose should be prescribed.

TABLE 15.4
Cerebral Disorders Spastic Hypertonia Treatment Paradigm for the First 6 Months After Brain Injury

---

- Rehabilitation therapies and modalities
  - o Reduce noxious stimulation
  - o Prevent contractures
  - o Reduce exposure to superficial cold
- Splinting and ROM
- Modalities and/or casting
- Systemic medications
  - o Dantrolene sodium
  - o Baclofen* (Meythaler et al. JHTR 2004)
    - Predominate lower limb spastic hypertonia
  - o Tizanidine
    - Predominate upper limb spastic hypertonia
- Neurolytics
  - o Botulinum toxin
  - o Phenol and alcohol
    - Can be irreversable
- Intrathecal baclofen
  - o Controversy over use in the first 6 months after CNS injury

---

Note: This paradigm was first suggested by the NIH TBI clinical trials centers to control confounding variables potentially impacting recovery after injury during the first 6 months after injury. No such paradigms have been established for spinal causes of spastic hypertonia, although most clinicians start with baclofen or benzodiazepines.

Cyclobenzaprine

Cyclobenzaprine is a centrally acting muscle relaxant that has been utilized primarily for muscle spasms. The mechanism of action is felt to be primarily at the brainstem within the CNS as opposed to the spinal cord. It influences both gamma and alpha motor systems by reducing tonic somatic motor activity (226). Cyclobenzaprine is structurally related to and may have actions similar to tricyclic antidepressants and as such has profound anticholinergic effects as well (227). Some of its mechanism of action may be an effect on pain.

Pharmacokinetics

Cylobenzaprine is started at a dosage of 2.5 mg 3 times per day and increased up to 10 mg/d (228). The medication has a peak serum concentration within 4 hours with a half-life of 8 hours for immediate release and longer for various extended release versions (229). It is predominately renally cleared with some hepatic conversion to glucuronides (228, 229).

Treatment

There are no specific studies with this medication, but many physicians use it anecdotally for the treatment of spastic hypertonia and the pain noted with spasticity. One small study on 15 brain injury and SCI patients did not note much of a change in the EMG effect of the patellar deep tendon reflexes (230), but this is not a commonly utilized outcome measure. Dosing starts slowly as above and is titrated up slowly. Somnolence is noted to occur in 39% to 100% of patients taking the medication (226).

Orphenadrine

Orphenadrine citrate is another commonly utilized muscle relaxant (231). It is felt to also work as a

TABLE 15.5
Oral Antispasticity Medications

	Trial	Population, N	Trial Type	Outcome Measure	Result/Comments
Spinal Cord Injury					
Baclofen	Duncan 1976 (50)	25	Double-blind, placebo-controlled, crossover	5-point scale	Baclofen superior ($p < .01$)
	Hinderer 1990 (235)	5	Placebo-controlled	Unspecified	No improvement on baclofen
	Jones 1983 (236)	6	Double-blind, placebo-controlled	5-point scale for spasms	Baclofen favored
Alpha adrenergics	Nance 1994 (182)	124	Placebo-controlled	Ashworth Scale, Pendulum test	Tizanidine superior Ashworth ($p < .0001$), Pendulum ($p = .004$), no difference in daily frequency
	Taricco 2000 (237)	218	Systematic review	Ashworth Scale	Tizanidine superior to placebo, (gabapentin, clonidine, diazepam amytal, oral baclofen) no evidence for significant clinical effectiveness
	Rinne 1980 (57)	32	Head-to-head (tizanidine vs baclofen)	Ashworth Scale	No significant difference
	Nance 1985 (137)	4	Case report	Not specified	Clonidine effective
	Maynard 1986 (160)	12	Open-label	Clinical spasticity	"may benefit from clonidine"
	Nance 1989 (138)	6	Placebo-controlled	Vibratory inhibition Index, H reflex	"Clonidine has an antispasticity effect in SCI patients"
	Donovan 1988 (146)	55	Open-label clinical trial	Observation by patient, therapist, and physician	"56% benefitted"
Benzodiazepines	Corbett 1972 (238)	22	Double-blind, randomized, placebo-controlled, crossover	Clinical improvement as determined by examiner	Valium significantly more effective than placebo
	Roussan 1985 (46)	6	Double-blind, crossover, head to head (baclofen vs diazepam	Frequency of flexor spasms, resistance to passive stretch, ROM, DTR, clonus	No significant difference

(Continued)

TABLE 15.5
(Continued)

	TRIAL	POPULATION, N	TRIAL TYPE	OUTCOME MEASURE	RESULT/COMMENTS
Dantrolene sodium	Gambi 1983 (220)	24	Double-blind, crossover, placebo-controlled	6-point scale	Dantrolene superior ($p < .05$)
	Glass 1974 (85)	16	Placebo-controlled, head-to-head (dantrolene vs diazepam)	6-point scale	Dantrolene favored
	Weiser 1978 (218)	35	Placebo-controlled	4-point scale	Dantrolene superior ($p = .002$)
Cannabinoids	Hagenbach 2007 (239)	25	Open-label, placebo-controlled	Spasticity Sum Score, Modified Ashworth Scale	THC is effective
Other drugs	Gruenthal 1997 (103)	25	Randomized, double-blind, placebo-controlled, crossover	Ashworth Scale	Gabapentin improved spasticity ($p = .04$)
	Priebe 1997 (104)	7	Multicenter, placebo-controlled, cross-over, clinical trial	EMG, Brain Motor Control Assessment	Gabapentin may be effective
	Segal 1999 (240)	21	Randomized, open-label, active-treatment control, dosage-blinded	Modified Ashworth Scale	"Diminished" spasticity with 4-aminopyridine
	Cardenas 2007 (80)	91	Randomized, placebo-controlled	Ashworth Scale	Significant improvement over placebo ($p = .02$)
TRAUMATIC BRAIN INJURY					
Baclofen	Meythaler 2004 (5)	22	Retrospective	Penn Spasm Frequency Scale, Ashworth Scale	Baclofen decreases Ashworth score from 3.5 to 3.2 ($p=.0044$), no significant change in spasm frequency
Alpha adrenergics	Meythaler 2001 (9)	17	Placebo-controlled, prospective	Penn spasm frequency scale, Ashworth Scale	No significant difference Penn Scale, Tizanidine favored Ashworth ($p = .006$)
	Harmon 1996 (241)	2	Prospective, double-blind, placebo-controlled, cross-over, pilot	Modified Ashworth Scale	"Clonidine may be superior to placebo"

Category	Reference	N	Study design	Assessment scale	Outcome
Benzodiazepines Dantrolene sodium Cannabinoids Other drugs	Zafonte 2004 (217)	1	Case report		Tone improved
STROKE					
Baclofen	Hulme 1985 (242)	12	Placebo-controlled	Unspecified	Study stopped due to somnolence as excessive adverse event
	Medaer 1991 (243)	20	Double-blind, crossover, placebo-controlled	Ashworth Scale	Baclofen superior
Alpha adrenergics	Medici 1989 (175)	30	Head-to-head, double-blind, long-term (tizanidine vs baclofen)	Ashworth Scale, 4-point patient self report scale, 5-point muscle strength scale, 3-point clonus scale, Kurtzke Expanded Disability Status Scale	No significant differences
	Maupas 2004 (244)	14	Randomized, placebo-controlled	Modified Ashworth Scale, H reflex	Tizanidine superior
	Groves 1998 (245)	270	Meta-analysis of double-blind, randomized studies	Ashworth Scale	Tizanidine, baclofen, diazepam equally effective
	Gelber 2001 (173)	47	Open-label	Modified Ashworth Scale	Spasticity significantly improved with tizanidine
Benzodiazepines	Bes 1988 (246)	104	Double-blind, head-to-head (diazepam vs tizanidine)	5-point scales for spasticity and spasm severity	No significant differences
	Kendall 1964 (247)	12	Double-blind, crossover	Measurement of PROM and angle of catch	Diazepam reduces spasticity
	Cocchiarella 1967 (87)	19	Randomized, double-blind, placebo-controlled	Objective measures of spasticity	No specific spasmolytic effect observed
Dantrolene sodium	Katrak 1992 (248)	38	Randomized, double-blind, placebo-controlled	0–6 motor assessment scale	No measurable difference
	Ketel 1984 (210)	18	Placebo-controlled	Unspecified	Dantrolene favored
	Chyatte 1971 (249)	9	Double-blind	Methods-Time-Measurement, DTR, Clonus, Resistance to passive movement	Dantrolene effective

(Continued)

TABLE 15.5
(Continued)

	Trial	Population, N	Trial Type	Outcome Measure	Result/Comments
Cannabinoids Other drugs	Stamenova 2005 (250)	120	Randomized, double-blind, placebo-controlled, multicenter, parallel	Ashworth Scale	Tolperisone superior
	Ashby 1972 (230)	15	Double-blind, crossover	5-point scale of muscle tone	No significant difference from placebo
Cerebral Palsy					
Baclofen	Milla 1977 (48)	20	Placebo-controlled	Ashworth Scale	Baclofen superior ($p < .001$)
	Scheinberg 2006 (251)	15	Double-blind, crossover pilot	Goal Attainment Scale, Pediatric Evaluation of Disability Inventory, Modified Tardieu Scale	Baclofen superior to placebo on Goal Attainment Scale
	Lopez 1996 (252)	20	Prospective, placebo-controlled, crossover	Ashworth Scale	"Significant reduction of spasticity"
Alpha adrenergics	Vasquez-Briceno 2006 (253)	40	Randomized, double-blind, placebo-controlled	Ashworth Scale, Posture tone scale	Tizanidine significantly superior
Benzodiazepines	Nogen 1976 (254)	22	Head-to-head (diazepam vs dantrolene)	Unspecified	No significant differences
	Dahlin 1993 (90)	12	Double-blind, placebo-controlled, crossover	Restraint of passive knee movements determined by dynamic dynamometer	Clonazepam significantly reduced spastic restraint ($p < .001$)
	Mathew 2005 (255)	180	Double-blind, parallel, placebo-controlled, randomized	Modified Ashworth Scale	Diazepam significantly reduced tone ($p < .001$)
Dantrolene sodium	Chyatte 1973 (256)	18	Placebo-controlled	4-point scale	No measurable difference
	Denhoff 1975 (219)	18	Placebo-controlled	Unspecified	Dantrolene superior ($p < .04$)
	Haslam 1974 (257)	26	Placebo-controlled	5-point scale	No statistical difference
	Joynt 1980 (258)	21	Placebo-controlled	4-point scale	No statistical difference

Cannabinoids				
Other drugs				
Chlorzoxazone, methocarbamol	Losin 1966 (259)	30	Placebo-controlled	5-point scale	Outcomes not clear
	Bjerre 1971 (260)	44	Placebo-controlled	3-point scale, Johnson Scale	No significant difference
	Hurst 2002 (261)	9	Open-label pilot study	Modified Ashworth Scale	Statistically significant improvement with modafinil
	Maritz 1978 (262)	16	Double-blind, crossover with placebo	Holt's Criteria, 3-point scale	Slight to moderate improvement with piracetam
	Chu 2006 (263)	9	Open label	Modified Ashworth Scale	Tigabine ineffective

MULTIPLE SCLEROSIS

Baclofen	Brar 1991 (264)	38	Placebo-controlled	Ashworth Scale	Baclofen favored
	Duncan 1976 (50)	25	Double-blind, placebo-controlled, crossover	5-point scale	Baclofen superior ($p < .01$)
	Feldman 1978 (51)	33	Double-blind, crossover, placebo-controlled	Unspecified	Baclofen superior
	Orsnes 2000 (265)	14	Placebo-controlled	Ashworth Scale	No significant difference
	Sachais 1977 (29)	166	Placebo-controlled, multicenter	Unspecified	Baclofen superior ($p < .01$)
	Sawa 1979 (58)	21	Placebo-controlled	6-point scale	Baclofen superior ($p < .001$)
	Basmajian 1975 (266)	14	Placebo-controlled	Unspecified	Baclofen favored
	Newman 1982 (60)	36	Head-to-head (tizandidine vs baclofen)	Ashworth Scale, Kurtzke and Pedersen Scales	No significant differences
	Smolenski 1981 (59)	21	Head-to-head, double-blind (tizanidine vs baclofen)	Ashworth Scale, 5-point spasticity scale, 6-point muscle strength scale	No significant differences
Alpha adrenergics	Lapierre 1987 (267)	66	Placebo-controlled	Unspecified	No significant difference
	Smith 1994 (155)	220	Double-blind, placebo-controlled	Ashworth Scale, 4-point Scale, daily counts	No significant difference
	UK Tizanidine Trial Group 1994 (268)	187	Double-blind, placebo-controlled	Ashworth Scale	Tizanidine superior ($p = .004$)
	Bass 1988 (53)	66	Head-to-head (tizanidine vs baclofen)	6-point scale, Kurtzke functional scale, Pedersen functional disability scale	No significant differences
	Eyssette 1988 (52)	100	Multicenter, placebo-controlled, head-to-head (tizanidine vs baclofen)	5-point scale, stretch reflex 1-5 scale	No significant differences

(Continued)

TABLE 15.5
(Continued)

Class	Trial	Population, N	Trial Type	Outcome Measure	Result/Comments
Alpha adrenergics	Hoogstraten 1988 (62)	16	Head-to-head (tizanidine vs baclofen)	Ashworth Scale, 5-point patient self-report, Kurtzke Expanded Disability Status Scale, Kurtzke Functional Systems Incapacity Status, Ambulation index	No significant differences
	Stein 1987 (61)	40	Double-blind, head-to-head (tizanidine vs baclofen)	Ashworth Scale, Kurtzke Expanded Disability, Status Scale, Pedersen Scale	No significant differences
Benzodiazepines	Cartlidge 1974 (55)	40	Head-to-head (diazepam vs baclofen)	Ashworth Scale	No significant differences
	From 1975 (56)	16	Head-to-head, double-blind (diazepam vs baclofen)	Ashworth Scale	No significant differences
	Schmidt 1976 (83)	46	Head-to-head (diazepam vs danrolene)	6-point scales for spasticity, clonus, reflexes	No significant differences
	Cendrowski 1977 (89)	68	Placebo-controlled	Modified Ashworth	Clonazepam and baclofen significantly superior to placebo, No significant difference between clonazepam and baclofen
	Wilson 1966 (269)	21	Double-blind, triple crossover	4-Point Scale	Diazepam significantly superior to placebo
	Basmajian 1986 (91)	14	Double-blind, crossover	EMG	"Ketazolam more effective than placebo"
Dantrolene sodium	Gambi 1983 (220)	24	Double-blind, crossover, placebo-controlled	6-point scale	Dantrolene superior ($p < .05$)
	Gelenberg 1973 (270)	20	Placebo-controlled	Unspecified	Not reported
	Tolosa 1975 (271)	23	Placebo-controlled	7-point scale	Dantrolene favored

Category	Study	N	Study type	Measures	Results
Cannabinoids	Killstein 2002 (272)	16	Randomized, double-blind, placebo-controlled, crossover	Ashworth Scale, Expanded Disability Status Scale	No significant differences
	Vaney 2004 (273)	57	Prospective, randomized, double-blind, placebo-controlled, crossover	Ashworth Scale, self-report of spasm frequency, Rivermead Mobility Index	No statistically significant difference compared to placebo
	Wade 2003 (274)	18	Double-blind, randomized, placebo-controlled, crossover	Patient Reported VAS	Spasticity improved by cannabis medicinal extracts
	Collin 2007 (199)	189	Randomized, double-blind, placebo-controlled	Patient reported spasticity numerical rating,	May be useful
	Zajicek 2003 (196)	667	Randomized, placebo-controlled	Ashworth Scale	No beneficial effect
	Ungerleider 1987 (275)	13	Double-blind, placebo-controlled, crossover	Ashworth Scale, subjective ratings	Significant improvement
Other drugs	Shakespeare 2003 (276)		Cochrane review, double-blind, randomized, placebo-controlled (baclofen, dantrolene, tizanidine, botulinum toxin, vigabatrin, prazepam, threonine, cannabinoids)	Ashworth Scale	No statistically significant differences, No recommendations made, more research needed
	Paisley 2002 (277)	1,200	Systematic review of randomized, controlled trials (baclofen, dantrolene, tizanidine, diazepam, gabapentin, threonine)	Ashworth Scale, "other clinical measures"	Baclofen, diazepam, tizanidine effective, "no evidence to suggest any difference between the drugs"

(Continued)

TABLE 15.5
(Continued)

Trial	Population, N	Trial Type	Outcome Measure	Result/Comments
Other drugs				
Mueller 1997 (101)	15	Double-blind, placebo-controlled, crossover	VAS, Kurtrzke Disability Scale, Ashworth Scale	Statistically significant improvements with gabapentin
Cutter 2000 (102)	22	Prospective, double-masked, placebo-controlled, crossover	Modified Ashworth Scale, Kurtzke Disability Status Scale, Subject self-report	Statistically significant reduction in spasticity with gabapentin
Dunevsky 1998(278)	2	Open-label	Modified Ashworth Scale, Expanded Disability Status Scale	"Satisfactory release of spasticity, significant improvement of functional outcome" with gabapentin
Mondrup 1984 (279)	16	Double-blind, crossover	Measurement of angle at which stretch reflex appeared by mobilisation of limb	Progabide produced medium improvement
Rudick 1987 (280)	32	Double-blind, placebo-controlled, crossover	Ashworth Scale, Kurtzke Expanded Disability Status Scale, Houser Ambulation Index	Progabide effective
Barbeau 1982 (281)	6	Placebo-controlled	Patient report of clonus, EMG activity	"Cyproheptadine substantially reduced the signs associated with spasticity"

centrally acting muscle relaxant. Receptor studies revealed that orphenadrine is an uncompetitive NMDA type glutamate antagonist (4). It is structurally similar to diphenhydramine but does not directly relax muscles (231). It may work by reducing the noxious stimulation of pain (231).

Pharmacokinetics

Orphenadrine is usually started at a dosage of 100 mg orally or 60 mg intravenously once a day as it has a half-life of 13 to 20 hours (231, 232). The medication is predominately renally excreted (231).

Treatment

In one significant study in SCI patients in a double-blind randomized trial, 60 mg of orphenadrine citrate significantly reduced spastic hypertonia by 1 point on the Ashworth score in 11 subjects (233). The predominant side effects of orphenadrine are lightheadedness, syncope, dizziness, drowsiness, dyskinesia, and tremor (231, 234).

TREATMENT PARADIGMS SPINAL DISORDERS VERSUS CEREBRAL DISORDERS

Most clinicians have concluded that one size does not fit all. Although most oral medications except for dantrolene sodium were initially developed for spinal causes of spastic hypertonia, it has become clear that cerebral disorders present their own set of complications. First, there are the cognitive implications, with many of the centrally acting medications having a more profound effect on cerebrally mediated CNS side effects in cerebral causes of spastic hypertonia than in spinal disorders. It has become clear that most clinicians do not readily utilize medications such as benzodiazepines early on in cerebral disorders (Table 15.5).

Furthermore, it is quite clear that in the first few months of recovery, one needs to be careful about inhibiting neurologic recovery. In cerebral disorders, there developed an informal paradigm for the treatment of spastic hypertonia for the first 6 months after injury (see Table 15.4; treatment of spasticity in cerebral disorders). This paradigm was first suggested by the NIH TBI clinical trial centers to control confounding variables potentially impacting recovery after injury in the first 6 months after injury. No such paradigms have been established for spinal causes of spastic hypertonia, although most clinicians start with baclofen or benzodiazepines.

References

1. Mann NH. Functional management of spasticity after head injury. *J Neuro Rehab* 1991;5:51–54.
2. Meythaler JM, DeVivo MJ, Hadley M. Prospective study on the use of bolus intrathecal baclofen for spastic hypertonia due to acquired brain injury. *Arch Phys Med Rehabil* 1996;77:461–466.
3. Meythaler JM. Use of intrathecally delivered medications for spasticity and dystonia in acquired brain injury. Yaksh, editor. *Spinal drug delivery.* Elsevier, New York. 1999, pp. 513–554.
4. Nance PW, Meythaler J. Spasticity management. *Physical medicine and rehabilitation.* Editor Braddom, 2006, pp. 651–662.
5. Meythaler JM, Clayton W, Davis LK, Renfroe SG, Brunner RC. Orally delivered baclofen to control spastic hypertonia in acquired brain injury. *J Head Trauma Rehabil* 2004;19:101–8.
6. Young RR, Delwaide PJ. Spasticity (part one of two parts). *New Eng J Med* 1981;304:28–33.
7. Albright LA, Meythaler JM, Ivanhoe CB. *Intrathecal baclofen therapy for spasticity of cerebral origin: patient selection guidelines.* Medtronics, Inc., Minneapolis MN, 1997.
8. Katz RT. Mechanisms, measurement, and management of spastic hypertonia after head injury. *Phys Med Clin N Am* 1992;3:319–335.
9. Meythaler JM, Guin-Renfroe S, Johnson A, Brunner RC. Prospective assessment of tizanidine for spasticity due to acquired brain injury. *Arch Phys Med Rehabil* 2001;82:1155–63.
10. Meythaler JM. Physiology of spastic hypertonia. In *Spastic hypertonia*, Meythaler JM, Editor. Saunders, *N Am Clinics of Phys Med Rehabil.* 2001;12:725–32.
11. Davis R. Spasticity following spinal cord injury. *Clin Orthop Relat Res.* 1975;112:66–72.
12. Meythaler JM, Steers WD, Tuel SM, Cross LL, Haworth CS. Continuous intrathecal baclofen in spinal cord spasticity: a prospective study. *Am J Phys Med Rehabil* 1992;71:321–327.
13. Katz RT. Management of spasticity. *Am J Phys Med Rehabil* 1988;67:108–116.
14. Ashby P, Verrier M, Lightfoot E. Segmental reflex pathways in spinal shock and spinal spasticity in man. *J Neurol Neurosurg Psychiatry* 1974;37:1352–1360.
15. Elovic E. Principles of pharmaceutical management of spastic hypertonia. In *Spastic hypertonia*, Meythaler JM, Editor. Saunders, *N Am Clinics of Phys Med Rehabil.* 2001;12:793–816.
16. Glenn MB. Update on pharmacology: antispasticity medications in the patient with TBI. *J Head Trauma Rehabil.* 1986;1:71–72.
17. Meythaler JM, Guin-Renfroe S, Johnson A, Brunner RC. Prospective assessment of tizanidine for spasticity due to acquired brain injury. *Arch Phys Med Rehabil.* 2001;82:1155–63.
18. Meythaler JM. Appendix. In *Spastic hypertonia*, Meythaler JM, Editor. Saunders, *N Am Clinics of Phys Med Rehabil.* 2001;12:953–6.
19. Francisco GE, Kothari S, Huls C. GABA agonists and gabapentin for spastic hypertonia. Meythaler JM, Guest Editor. *Spastic hypertonia.* W.B. Saunders, *N Am Clinics of Phys Med Rehabil.* 2001;12(Issue 4) pp. 875–888.
20. Nance PW. Alpha adrenergic and serotonergic agents in the treatment of spastic hypertonia. In *Spastic hypertonia*, Meythaler JM, Editor. Saunders, *N Am Clinics of Phys Med Rehabil.* 2001;12:889–905.
21. Bloom FE, Inversen LL. Localizing 3H-GABA in nerve terminals of rat cerebral cortex by electron microscopic autoradiography. *Nature* 1971;229:628.
22. Grabb PA, Guin-Renfroe S, Meythaler JM. Midthoracic catheter tip placement for intrathecal baclofen administration

in children with quadriparetic spasticity. *Neurosurgery* 1999;45:833–7.

23. Meythaler JM, Renfroe SG, Grabb PA, Hadley MN. Long-term continuously infused intrathecal baclofen for spastic/dystonic hypertonia in traumatic brain injury: 1-year experience. *Arch Phys Med Rehabil* 1999;80:13–9.

24. Kaplan JP, Raizon BM. New anitconvulsants: shiff bases of gamma-aminobutyric acid and gamma-aminobutyramide. *J Med Chem* 1980;23:702–4.

25. Gracies JM, Nance P, Elovic E, McGuire J, Simpson DM. Traditional pharmacological treatments for spasticity part II: general and regional treatments. *Muscle Nerve* 1997; 21(Suppl.6):S92–120.

26. Hill DR, Bowery NG: [³H]Baclofen and [³H]GABA bind to bicuculline-insensitive GABA_B sites in rat brain. *Nature* 1981;290:149–152.

27. McGeer PL, McGeer EG: Amino acid neurotransmitters. In Siegel GJ, ed. *Basic neurochemistry* (4 ed.), Raven Press, New York, 1989.

28. Hinderer SR, Lehmann JF, Price R, White O, DeLateur BJ, Deitz J: Spasticity in spinal cord injured persons: quantitative effects of baclofen and placebo treatments: *Am J Phys Med Rehabil* 1990;69:311–317.

29. Saichais VA, Lonue JN, Darey MS: Baclofen, a new antispastic drug. *Arch Neurol* 1977;34:422–429.

30. Hattab JR. Review of European clinical trials with baclofen, in Feldman RG, Young RR, Kiella WP (eds.): *Spasticity. Disordered motor control.* Chicago, Year Book Medical Publishers, 1980.

31. MacDonell RAL, Talolla A, Swash M, Grundy D. Intrathecal baclofen and the H-reflex. *J Neurol Neurosurg Psychiatry* 1989;52:1110–1112.

32. Terrence DV, Fromm GH. Complications of baclofen withdrawal. *Arch Neurol* 1981;38:588–589.

33. Wilson PR, Yaksh TL. Baclofen is antinociceptive in the spinal intrathecal space of animals. *Eur J Pharmacol* 1978;51:323–330.

34. Yaksh TL, Ramana Reddy SV. Studies in the primate on the analgetic effects associated with intrathecal actions of opiate, L-adrenergic agonists and baclofen. *Anesthesiology* 1981;54:451–467.

35. Kroin JS, Penn RD, Beissinger RL, Arzbaecher RC. Reduced spinal reflexes following intrathecal baclofen in the rabbit. *Exp Brain Res.*1984;54:191–194.

36. Muller H, Ziersky J, Dralle D, Borner V, Hoffmann O. The effect of intrathecal baclofen on electrical muscle activity in spasticity. *J Neurol* 1987;234:348–352.

37. Knuttson E, Lindblom U, Martensson A. Plasma and cerebrospinal fluid levels of baclofen (Lioresal) at optimal therapeutic responses in spastic paresis. *J Neurol Sci* 1974; 23:473–484.

38. Roy CW, Wakefield IR: Baclofen pseudopsychosis: case report. *Paraplegia* 1986;24:318–321.

39. Sandy KR, Gillman MH. Baclofen-induced memory impairment. *Clin Neuropharmacol* 1985;8:294–295.

40. Lazorthes Y, Sallerin-Caute B, Verdie J, Bastide R, Carillo J. Chronic intrathecal baclofen administration for control of severe spasticity. *J Neurosurg* 1990;72:393–402.

41. Muller H, Zierski J, Dralle D, Krauss D, Mutschler E. Pharmacokinetics of intrathecal baclofen. In : Muller H, Zierski J, Penn RD, eds. *Local-spinal therapy of spasticity.* Berlin: Springer-Verlag, 1988, pp. 223–226.

42. Nance PW, Young RR: Antispasticity medications. In *Rehabilitation pharmacotherapy.* Nance P Ed., N Am Clinics of Phys Med Rehabil 1999;10:337–355.

43. Faigle JW, Keherle H: The chemistry and kinetics of lioresal. *Postgrad Med J* 1972;5:S9–S13.

44. Burke D, Andrews CJ, Knowles L: The action of a GABA derivative in human spasticity. *J Neurol Sci* 1971;14:199–208.

45. Levine IM, Jossmann PB, DeAngelis V: Lioresal, a new muscle relaxant in the treatment of spasticity—a double-blind quantitative evaluation. *Dis Nerv Syst* 1977;1011–1015.

46. Roussan M, Terrence C, Fromm G: Baclofen versus diazepam for the treatment of spasticity and long-term follow-up of baclofen therapy. *Pharmatherapeutica* 1985;4:278–284.

47. Van Hemet JC: A double-blind comparison of baclofen and placebo in patients with spasticity of cerebral origin, *In:* Feldman RG, Young RR, Koella WP (eds): *Spasticity: disordered motor control.* Chicago, Year Book Medical Publishers, 1980, pp. 41–49.

48. Milla PJ, Jackson ADM: A controlled trial of baclofen in children with cerebral palsy. *J Int Med Res* 1977;5:398–404.

49. Pedersen E, Arlien-Soborg P, Grynderup V, Henriksen O: GABA derivative in spasticity. *Acta Neurol Scand* 1979;46:257–266.

50. Duncan GW, Shahani BT, Young RR: An evaluation of baclofen treatment for certain symptoms in patients with spinal cord lesions. *Neurology* 1976;441–446.

51. Feldman RG, Kelly-Hayes M, Donomy JP, Foley JM: Baclofen for spasticity in multiple sclerosis, *Neurology* 1978;25:1094–1099.

52. Eyssette M, Rohmer F, Serratrice G, Warter JM, Doisson D: Multi-centre, double-blind trial of a novel antispastic agent, tizanidine, in spasticity associated with multiple sclerosis. *Curr Med Res Opin* 1988;10:699–707.

53. Bass B, Weinshenker B, Rice GPA, Noseworthy JH, Cameron MGP, Hader W, Bouchard S, Ebers GC: Tizanidine versus baclofen in the treatment of spasticity in patients with multiple sclerosis. *Can J Neurol Sci* 1988;15:15–19.

54. Hudgsdon P, Sedighgmzn D: Baclofen in the treatment of spasticity. *Br Med J* 1971;2:15–27.

55. Cartlidge NEF, Hudgson P, Wrightman D: A comparison of baclofen and diazcpam in the treatment of spasticity. *J Neurol Sci* 1974;23:17–24.

56. From A, Heltberg A: A double blind trial with baclofen (Lioresal) and diazepam in spasticity due to multiple sclerosis. *Acta Neurol Scand* 1975;51:158–166.

57. Rinne UK: Tizanidine treatment of spasticity in multiple sclerosis and chronic myelopathy. *Curr Ther Res* 1980;28:827–836.

58. Sawa GM, Paty DW: The use of baclofen in treatment of spasticity in multiple sclerosis. *Can J Neurol Sci* 1980;6:352–354.

59. Smolenski C, Muff S, Smolenski-Kautz S: A double-blind comparative trial of a new muscle relaxant tizanidine (DS 103-282) and baclofen in the treatment of chronic spasticity in multiple sclerosis. *Curr Med Res Opin* 1981;7:378–383.

60. Newman PM, Nogues M, Newman PK, Weightman D, Hudgson P: Tizanidine in the treatment of spasticity. *Eur J Clin Pharmacol* 1982;23:31–35.

61. Stien R, Nordal HLJ, Ottedal SL, Slettebo M: The treatment of spasticity in multiple sclerosis: a double-blind clinical trial of a new anti-spastic drug tizanidine compared with baclofen. *Acta Neurol Scand* 1987;75:190–194.

62. Hoogstraten RJ, van der Ploeg RJO, Burg W, Vreeling A, van Marte S, Minderhoud JM: Tizanidine versus baclofen in the treatment of spasticity in multiple sclerosis patients. *Acta Neurol Scand* 1988;77:224–230.

63. Orsnes GB, Sorensen PS, Larsen TK, Ravnborg M: Effect of baclofen on gait in spastic MS patients. *Acta Neurol Scand* 2000;101:222–248.

64. Meythaler JM, Guin-Renfro S, Law C, Grabb P, Hadley MN. Continuously infused intrathecal baclofen (ITB) over 12 months for spastic hypertonia in adolescents and adults with cerebral palsy. *Arch Phys Med Rehabil* 2001;82:155–61.

65. Barker I, Grant IS. Convulsions after abrupt withdrawal of baclofen. *Lancet* 1982;2:556–557.

66. Garabedian-Ruffalo SM, Ruffalo RL. Adverse effects secondary to baclofen withdrawal. *Drug Intell Clin Pharm* 1985;19:304–306.

67. Harrison SA, Wood CA. Hallucinations after preoperative baclofen discontinuation in spinal cord injury patients. *Drug Intell Clin Pharm* 1985;19:747–749.

68. Coffey RJ, Edgar TS, Francisco GE, Graziani V. Meythaler JM, Ridgely P, Saddiq SA, Turner M. Abrupt withdrawal from intrathecal baclofen: recognition and management of a potentially life-threatening syndrome. *Arch Phys Med Rehabil* 2002;83:735–41.

69. Meythaler JM, Roper JF, Davis L, Brunner RC. Cyproheptadine in intrathecal baclofen withdrawal: a case series. *Arch Phys Med Rehabil* 2003;84:638–42.

70. Meythaler JM, Yablon S. Antiepileptic drugs. In *Rehabilitation pharmacotherapy*. Nance P (Ed.), *N Am Clinics of Phys Med Rehabil* 1999;10(2):275–300.

71. Henriksen O. An overview of benzodiazepines in seizure management. *Epilepsia* 1998;39(Suppl 1):S2–6.

72. Bezchlibnyk-Butter K Z, Jeffries J J, Martin BA (Eds.). *Clinical handbook of psychotropic drugs* (4th ed.). Seattle, WA: Hogrefe & Huber, 1994.

73. Barbee JG. Memory, benzodiazepines, and anxiety: integration of theoretical and clinical perspectives. *J Clin Psychiatry* 1993;54(Suppl):86–97.

74. Olsen RW: GABA-benzodiazepine-barbiturate receptor interactions. *J Neurochem* 1987;37:1–13.

75. Friedman H, Greenblatt DJ, Peters GR, et al.: Pharmacokinetics and pharmacodynamics oforal diazepam: effect of dose, plasma concentration, and time. *Clin Pharmacol Ther* 1992;52:139–150.

76. Gilman AG, Goodman LS, Rall TW, Gilman AG, Goodman LS, Rall TW, et al. (Eds): *Goodman and Gilman's the pharmacological basis of therapeutics*, 7th. Macmillan Publishing Co, New York, NY, 1985.

77. Locniskar A, Greenblatt DJ, Zinny MA, et al. Absolute bioavailability and effect of food and antacid on diazepam absorption from a slow-release preparation. *J Clin Pharmacol* 1984;24:255–263.

78. Berlin A, Dahlstrom H. Pharmacokinetics of the anticonvulsant drug clonazepam evaluated from single oral and intravenous doses and by repeated oral administration. *Eur J Clin Pharmacol* 1975;9:155.

79. Klonopin(R), Product Information: clonazepam. Hoffman-La Roche Laboratories, 1997.

80. Cardenas DD, Ditunno J, Graziani V, et al. Phase 2 trial of sustained release fampridine in chronic spinal cord injury. *Spinal Cord* 2007;45(2):158–168.

81. Dreifuss FE, Penny JK, Rose SW, et al. Serum clonazepam concentrations in children with absence seizures. *Neurology* 1975;25:255–258.

82. Wilson LA, McKechnie AA: Oral diazepam in the treatment of spasticity in paraplegia a double-blind trial and subsequent impressions. *Scott Med J* 1966;11:46–51.

83. Schmidt RT, Lee RH, Spehlmann R. Comparison of dantrolene sodium and diazepam in the treatment of spasticity. *J Neurol Neurosurg Psychiatry* 1976;39:350–356.

84. Basmajian JV, Shankardass K, Russell D, Yuccel V. Ketazolam treatment of spasticity: double-blind study of a new drug. *Arch Phys Med Rehabil* 1984;65:698–701.

85. Glass A, Hannah A: A comparison of dantrolene sodium and diazepam in the treatment of spasticity. *Paraplegia* 1974;12:170–174.

86. Kendall PH. The use of diazepam in hemiplegia. *Ann Phys Med* 1969;6:225–228.

87. Cocchiarella A, Downey JA, Darling RC: Evaluation of the effect of diazepam on spasticity. *Arch Phys Med Rehabil* 1967;393–396.

88. Rowland T, DePalma L. Current neuropharmacologic interventions for the management of brain injury agitation. *NeuroRehabilitation* 1995;5:219–232.

89. Cendrowski W, Sobczyk W. Clonazepam, baclofen and placebo in the treatment of spasticity. *Eur Neurol* 1977;16:257–62.

90. Dahlin M, Knutsson E, Nergradh A. Treatment of spasticity in children with low dose benzodiazepine. *J Neurol Sci* 1993;11:54–60.

91. Basmajian JV, Shankardass MB, Russell D: Ketazolam once daily for spasticity: double-blind cross-over study. *Arch Phys Med Rehabil* 1986;67:556–557.

92. Ramsey RE. Clinical efficacy and safety of gabapentin. *Neurology* 1994;44(Suppl 5):S23–30.

93. Hendrich J, Van Minh AT, Heblich F, et al. "Pharmacological disruption of calcium channel trafficking by the alpha2delta ligand gabapentin". *Proc Natl Acad Sci U S A* 1008;105(9):3628–33.

94. Pellock JM. Utilization of new antiepileptic drugs in children. *Epilepsia* 1996;37(Suppl 1):S66–73.

95. Shorvon S, Stefan H. Overview of the safety of newer antiepileptic drugs. *Epilepsia* 1997;38(Suppl 1):S45–51.

96. Leppik IE. Antiepileptic drugs in development: prospects for the near future. *Epilepsia* 1994;35(Suppl 4):S29–40.

97. Vollmer KO, Anhur H, Thomann P, et al. Pharmacokinetic model and absolute bioavailability of the new anticonvulsant gabapentijn. *Adv Epileptol* 1987;17:209–211.

98. McLean MJ. Gabapentin. *Epilepsia* 1995;36(Suppl 2):S73–S86.

99. Bruni J: Gabapentin. *Can J Neurol Sci* 1996;23:S10–S12.

100. Satzinger G. Antiepileptics from gamma-aminobutyric acid. *Arzneimitteiforschung* 1994;44:261–6.

101. Mueller ME, Gruenthal M, Olson WL, Olson WH. Gabapentin for relief of upper motor neuron symptoms in multiple sclerosis. *Arch Phys Med Rehabil* 1997;78:521–4.

102. Cutter NC, Scott DD, Johnson JV, Whiteneck G. Gabapentin effect on spasticity in multiple sclerosis: a placebo-controlled, randomized trial. *Arch Phys Med Rehabil* 2000;81:164–169.

103. Gruenthal M, Mueller M, Olson WI, Priebe MM, Sherwood, Olson WH. Gabapentin for the treatment of spasticity in patients with spinal cord injury. *Spinal Cord* 1997;35:686–689.

104. Priebe MM, Sherwood AM, Graves DE, Mueller M, Olson WH: Effectiveness of gabapentin in controlling spasticity: a quantitative study. *Spinal Cord* 1997;35:171–175.

105. Beydoun A. Monotherapy trials of new antiepileptic drugs. *Epilepsia* 1997;38(Suppl 9):S21–S31.

106. Haig GM, Bockbrader HN, Wesche DL, et al: Single-dose gabapentin pharmacokinetics and safety in healthy infants and children. *J Clin Pharmacol* 2001;41:507–514.

107. Chu ML, Sala DA. The use of tiagabine in pediatric spasticity management. *Dev Med Child Neurol* 2006;48:456–9.

108. Fisher R, Blum D. Colbazam, oxcarbazepine, tiagabine, topiramate and other new antiepileptic agents. *Epilepsia* 1995;36(Suppl 2):S105–14.

109. Patsalos PN & Sander WAS: Newer antiepileptic drugs: towards an improved risk-benefit ratio. *Drug Saf* 1994;11:37–67.

110. Brodie MJ. Tiagabine pharmacology in profile. *Epilepsia* 1995;36(Suppl 6):S7–9.

111. So EL, Wolff D, Graves NM, et al. Phamacokinetics of tiagabine as add-on therapy in patients taking enzyme-inducing antiepilepsy drugs. *Epilepsy Res* 1995;22:221–6.

112. Bialer M. Comparative pharmacokinetics of the newer antiepileptic drugs. *Clin Pharmacokinet* 1993;24:441–452.

113. Uldall P, Bulteau C, Pedersen SA, et al. Tiagabine adjunctive therapy in children with refractory epilepsy: a single-blind dose escalating study. *Epilepsy Res* 2000;42:159–168.

114. Holden KR, Titus MO. The effect of tiagabine on spasticity in children with intractable epilepsy: a pilot study. *Pediatr Neurol* 1999;21:728–30.

115. Leppik IE. Tiagabine: the safety landscape. *Epilepsia* 1995;36(Suppl 6):S10–3.

116. Shapel G, Chadwick K. Tiagabine and not-convulsive status epileticus. *Seizure* 1996;5:153–6.

117. Meldrum BS. Identification and preclinical testing of novel antiepileptic compounds. *Epilepsia* 1997;38(Suppl 9):S7–15.

118. Ben-Menachem E. Vigabatrin. *Epilepsia* 1995;36(Suppl 2): S95–104.

119. Rey E, Pons G, Olive G. Vigabatrin: clinical pharmacokinetics. *Clin Pharmacokinet* 1992;23:267–278.

120. Schechter PJ. Clinical pharmacology of vigabatrin. *Br J Clin Pharmacol* 1989;27:19S–22S.

121. Grant SM, Heel RC. Vigabatrin: a review of its phamacodynamic and phamacokinetic properties, and therapeutic potential in epilepsy and disorders of motor control. *Drugs* 1991;41:889–926.

122. Remy C, Beaumont D. Efficacy and safety of vigabatrin in the long-term treatment of refractory epilepsy. *Br J Clin Pharmacol* 1989;27(Suppl):S125–9.

123. Chiron C, Dulac O, Beaumont D, et al. Therapeutic trial of vigabatrin in refractory infantile spasms. *J Child Neurol* 1991;6(Suppl 2):S52–6.

124. Mumford JP. Vigabatrin (Sabril): the strategy for preclinical and clinical evaluation. *Boll Lego It Epil* 1994;86/87:19–23

125. Appleton RE: Guideline may help in prescribing vigabatrin (letter). *BMJ* 1998;317:1322.

126. Koul R, Chacko A, Ganesh A, et al. Vigabatrin associated retinal dysfunction in children with epilepsy. *Arch Dis Child* 2001;85:469–473.

127. Wallace A, Montanez S, Lorio M, et al. Vigabatrin, unlike some anti-convulsants, does not hinder recovery of function. *Epilepsia* 1996;37:27.

128. Perucca E. The new generation of antiepileptic drugs: advantages and disadvantages. *Br J Clin Pharmacol* 1996; 42:531–543.

129. Britton JW, So EL. New antiepileptic drugs: prospects for the future. *J Epilepsy* 1995;8:267–281.

130. Harden CL. New antiepileptic drugs. *Neurology* 1994; 44:787–795.

131. Product Information: Topamax(R), topiramate tablets and sprinkle capsules. Ortho-McNeil Pharmaceutical, Inc, Raritan, NJ, 2008.

132. Doose DR, Walker SA, Gisclon LG, et al. Single-dose pharmacokinetics and effect of food on the bioavailability of topiramate, a novel antiepileptic drug. *J Clin Pharmacol* 1996;36:884–891.

133. Topcu M, Yalnizoglu D, Saatci I, Haliloglu G, Topaloglu H, Senbil N, Onol S, Coskun T. Effect of topiramate on enlargement of head in Canavan disease: a new option for treatment of megalencephaly. *Turk J Pediatr* 2004;46:67–71.

134. Buoni S, Zannolli R, Strambi M, Fois A. Combined treatment with vigabatrin and topiramate in West syndrome. *J Child Neurol* 2004;19:385–6.

135. Gatto EM, Uribe Roca C, Raina G, Gorja M, Folgar S, Micheli FE. Vascular hemichorea/hemiballism and topiramate. *Mov Disord* 2004;19:836–8.

136. Fürst S. Transmitters involved in antinociception in the spinal cord. *Brain Res Bull* 1999;48:129–141.

137. Nance PW, Shears AH, Nance DM: Clonidine in spinal cord injury. *Can Med Assoc J* 1985;133:41–42.

138. Nance PW, Shears AH, Nance DM, et al. Reflex changes induced by clonidine in spinal cord injured patients. *Paraplegia* 1989;27:296–301.

139. Jordan LM, McCrea DA: Analysis of the effects of p-methoxy-phenylethylamine on spinal cord neurones. *Br J Pharmacol* 1976;57:191–199.

140. Powers RK, Rymer WZ: Effects of acute dorsal spinalion on motomeuron discharge in the medial gastrocnemius of the decerebrate cat. *J Neurophysiol* 1988;59:1540–1556.

141. Jankowska E, Gladden MH, Czarkowska-Bauch J: Modulation of responses of feline gamma-motoneurones by noradrenaline, tizanidine and clonidine. *J Physiol* 1998;512:521–531.

142. Skoog B: A comparison of the effects of two antispastic drugs, tizanidine and baclofen, on synaptic transmission from muscle spindle afferents to spinal interneurons in cats. *Acta Physiol Scand* 1996;156:81–90.

143. Kobinger, W, Walland A: Investigations into the mechanisms of the hypotensive effect of 2,(2,6-dichlorophenylamino)2-imidazoline HCl. *Eur J Pharmacol* 1967;2:155–162.

144. Starke K, Borowski E, Endo T: Preferential blockade of presynaptic alpha-adrenoceptors by yohimbine. *Eur J Pharmacol* 1975;34:385–388.

145. Unnerstall JR, Kopajtic TA, et al. Distribution of alpha-2 agonist binding sites in the rat and human central nervous system. *Brain Res Rev* 1984;7:69–101.

146. Donovan WH, Carter RE, Rossi CD, et al. Clonidine effect on spasticity: a clinical trial. *Arch Phys Med Rehabil* 1988;69:193–194.

147. Kooner JS, Edge W, Frankel HL, Peart WS, Mathias CJ. Haemodynamic actions of clonidine in tetraplegia—effects at rest and during urinary bladder stimulation. *Paraplegia* 1988;26(3):200–3.

148. Kooner JS, Birch R, Frankel HL, Peart WS, Mathias CJ. Hemodynamic and neurohormonal effects of clonidine in patients with preganglionic and postganglionic sympathetic lesions. Evidence for a central sympatholytic action. *Circulation* 1991;84:75–83.

149. Davies DS, Dollery CT, Davies DS, et al. Pharmacokinetic and pharmacological studies with clonidine in normal subjects. *Clin Sci Mol Med* 1976;51:639.

150. Dollery CT, Davies DS, Draffan GH, et al. Clinical pharmacology and pharmacokinetics of clonidine. *Clin Pharmacol Ther* 1976;19:11–17.

151. Lopatkin NA, Mazo EB, Guriunov VG, et al. Results of clinical use of atapresan in arterial hypertension. *Ter Arkh* 1974;46:41–44.

152. Krause W, Kramer D, & Grunitz B: Zur Therapie des Hochdrucks mit einem Imidazolinderivat. *Med Klin* 1969; 64:1274–1276.

153. Mroczek WJ, Davidov M, & Finnerty FA Jr: Intravenous clonidine in hypertensive patients. *Clin Pharmacol Ther* 1973;14:847–851.

154. MacGregor TR, Matzek KM, Keirns JJ, et al: Pharmacokinetics of transdermally delivered clonidine. *Clin Pharmacol Ther* 1985;38:278–284.

155. Arndts D & Arndts K: Pharmacokinetics and pharmacodynamics of transdermally administered clonidine. *Eur J Clin Pharmacol* 1984;26:79–85.

156. Boswell G, Bekersky I, Mekki Q, et al. Plasma concentrations and disposition of clonidine following a constant 14-day epidural infusion in cancer patients. *Clin Ther* 1997;19:1024–1030.

157. Ivani G, Bergendahl HT, Lampugnani E, Eksborg S, Jasonni V, Palm C, Mattioli G, Podesta E, Famularo A, Lönnqvist PA. Plasma levels of clonidine following epidural bolus injection in children. *Acta Anaesthesiol Scand* 1998;42:306–11.

158. Catapres package insert (Boehringer Ingelheim—US). Rev Rec 4/92, 9/89.

159. Nishina K, Mikawa K, Shiga M, et al. Clonidine in paediatric anaesthesia. *Paediatr Anaesth* 1999;9:187–202.

160. Maynard FM. Early clinical experience with clonidine in spinal spasticity. *Paraplegia* 1986;24:175–82.

161. Sandford PR, Spengler SE, Sawasky KB. Clonidine in the treatment of brainstem spasticity. Case report. *Am J Phys Med Rehabil* 1992 Oct;71(5):301–3.

162. Yablon SA, Sipski ML. Effect of transdermal clonidine on spinal spasticity. A case series. *Am J Phys Med Rehabil* 1993;72:154–7.

163. Weingarden SI, Belen JG. Clonidine transdermal system for treatment of spasticity in spinal cord injury. *Arch Phys Med Rehabil* 1992;73:876–7.

164. Roche WJ, Nwofia C, Gittler M, Patel R, Yarkony G. Catecholamine-induced hypertension in lumbosacral paraplegia: five case reports. *Arch Phys Med Rehabil* 2000;81: 222–5.

165. Coward DM. Tizanidine: neuropharmacology and mechanism of action. *Neurology* 1994;44 (suppl 9):S6–S11.

166. Wallace JD. Summary of combined clinical analysis of controlled clinical trials with tizanidine. *Neurology* 1994;44 (suppl 9):S60–S69.

167. Meythaler JM, Guin-Renfroe S, Johnson A, Brunner RM. Prospective assessment of tizanidine for spasticity due to acquired brain injury. *Arch Phys Med Rehabil* 2001;82:1155–1163.

168. Nance PW, Bugaresti J, Shellenberger K, Sheremata W, Martinez-Arziala A. Efficacy and safety of tizanidine in the treatment of spasticity in patients with spinal cord injury. *Neurology* 1994;44(suppl 9):S44–S52.

169. Smith C, Birnbaum G, Carter JL, Greenstein J, Lublin FD. Tizanidine treatment of spasticity caused by multiple sclerosis: results of a double-blind, placebo-controlled trial. *Neurology* 1994;44 (suppl 9):S34–S43.

170. Product Information: Zanaflex(R), tizanidine hydrochloride tablets and capsules. Acorda Therapeutics, Inc., Hawthorne, New York, 2005.

171. Wagstaff AJ, Bryson HM: Tizanidine: a review of its pharmacology, clinical efficacy and tolerability in the management of spasticity associated with cerebral and spinal disorders. *Drugs* 1997;53:435–52.

172. Hutchinson DR. Modified release tizanidine: a review. *J Int Med Res* 1989;17:565–573.

173. Gelber DA, Good DC, Dromerick A, Sergay S, Richardson M. Open-label dose-titration safety and efficacy study of tizanidine hydrochloride in the treatment of spasticity associated with chronic stroke. *Stroke* 2001;32:1841–46.

174. Granfors MT, Backman JT, Neuvonen M, et al. Ciprofloxacin greatly increases concentrations and hypotensive effect of tizanidine by inhibiting its cytochrome P450 1A2-mediated presystemic metabolism. *Clin Pharmacol Ther* 2004;76:598–606.

175. Medici M, Pebet M, Ciblis D. A double-blind, long-term study of tizanidine in spasticity due to cerebrovascular lesions. *Curr Med Res Opin* 1989;11:398–407.

176. Johnson TR, Tobias JD. Hypotension following the initiation of tizanidine in a patient treated with an angiotensin converting enzyme inhibitor for chronic hypertension. *J Child Neurol* 2000;15:818–9.

177. Nance PW, Sheremata WA, Lynch SG, Vollmer T, et al. Relationship of the antispasticity effect of tizanidine to plasma concentration in patients with multiple sclerosis. *Arch Neurol* 1997;54:731–736.

178. Mills KC. Serotonin syndrome: a clinical update. *Crit Care Clin* 1997;13:763-83.

179. Carbone JR. The neuroleptic malignant and serotonin syndromes. *Emerg Med Clin North Am* 2000;16:317–25.

180. Barbeau, H, Richards, CL, Bedard, PJ. Action of cyproheptadine in spastic paraparetic patients. *J Neurol Neurosurg Psychiatry* 1982;45:923–926.

181. Wainberg, M, Barbeau, H. Modulatory action of cyproheptadine on the locomotor pattern of spastic paretic patients [Abstract]. *Soc Neurosci* 1986;308.5:1133.

182. Nance P. A comparison of clonidine, cyproheptadine and baclofen in spastic spinal cord injured patients. *J Am Paraplegia Soc* 1994;17:151–157.

183. Product information: cyproheptadine hcl oral tablets, cyproheptadine hcl oral tablets. Cypress Pharmaceuticals,Inc, Madison, MS, 2005.

184. Paton DM, Webster DR. Clinical pharmacokinetics of H1-receptor antagonists (the antihistamines). *Clin Pharmacokinet* 1985;10:477–497.

185. Product information: periactin(R), cyproheptadine hydrochloride. Merck & Co., Inc., West Point, PA, 1999.

186. Baker D, Pryce G, Giovanni G, Thompson AJ. The therapeutic potential of cannabis. *Lancet Neurol* 2003;2:291–8.

187. Product information: MARINOL(R) oral capsules, dronabinol oral capsules. Solvay Pharmaceuticals,Inc, Marietta, GA, 2006.

188. Anderson PO, McGuire GG. Delta-9-tetrahydrocannabinol as an antiemetic. *Am J Hosp Pharm* 1981;38:639-646.

189. Product information: CESAMET(TM) oral capsules, nabilone oral capsules. Valeant Pharmaceuticals,Inc, Costa Mesa, CA, 2006.

190. Rubin A, Lemberger L, Warrick P, et al. Physiologic disposition of nabilone, a cannabinol derivative, in man. *Clin Pharmacol Ther* 1977;22:85–91.

191. Stolp-Smith KA, Wainberg MC. Antidepressant exacerbation of spasticity. *Arch Phys Med Rehabil*. 1999 Mar;80(3):339–42.

192. Consroe P, Musty R, Rein J, et al. The perceived effects of smoked cannabis on patients with multiple sclerosis. *Eur Neurol* 1977;38:44–8.

193. Petro DJ, Ellenberger C Jr. Treatment of human spasticity with delta 9-tetrahydrocannabinol. *J Clin Pharmacol* 1981;21(8-9 Suppl):413S–416S.

194. Malec J, Harvey RF, Cayner JJ. Cannabis effect on spasticity in spinal cord injury. *Arch Phys Med Rehabil* 1982;63:116–8.

195. Consroe P, Sandyk R, Snider SR. Open label evaluation of cannabidiol in dystonic movement disorders. *J Neurosci* 1986;30:277–82.

196. Zajicek J, Fox P, Sanders H, Wright D, Vickery J, Nunn A, Thompson A; UK MS Research Group. Cannabinoids for treatment of spasticity and other symptoms related to multiple sclerosis (CAMS study): multicentre randomised placebo-controlled trial. *Lancet* 2003;362(9395):1517–26.

197. Zajicek JP, Sanders HP, Wright DE, Vickery PJ, Ingram WM, Reilly SM, Nunn AJ, Teare LJ, Fox PJ, Thompson AJ. Cannabinoids in multiple sclerosis (CAMS) study: safety and efficacy data for 12 months follow up. *J Neurol Neurosurg Psychiatry* 2005;76:1664–9.

198. Solowij N, Stephens RS, Roffman RA,Babor T, Kadden R, Miller M, et al. Cognitive functioning of long-term heavy cannabis users seeking treatment. *J Am Med Assoc* 2002; 287:1123–31.

199. Collin C, Davies P, Mutiboko IK, Ratcliffe S; Sativex Spasticity in MS Study Group. Randomized controlled trial of cannabis-based medicine in spasticity caused by multiple sclerosis. *Eur J Neurol* 2007;14:290–6.

200. Brady CM, DasGupta R, Dalton C, Wiseman OJ, Berkley KJ, Fowler CJ. An open-label pilot study of cannabis-based extracts for bladder dysfunction in advanced multiple sclerosis. *Mult Scler* 2004;10:425–33.

201. Van Winkle WB. Calcium release from skeletal muscle sarcoplasmic reticulum: site of action of dantrolene sodium. *Science* 1976;193:1130–1131.

202. Young RR, Emre M, Nance PW, et al. Current issues in spasticity management. *Neurologist* 1997;3:261–275.

203. Katz RT, Campagnolo DI. Pharmocologic management of spasticity. *Phys Med Rehabil State Art Rev* 1994;8:473–480.

204. Alonso RJ, Mancall El. The clinical management of spasticity. *Semin Neurol* 1991;11:215–219.

205. Whyte J, Robinson KM. Pharmacologic management, in Glenn MB, Whyte J (eds): The practical management of spasticity in children and adults. Philadelphia, Lea & Febiger, 1990, 201–226.

206. Davidoff RA. Antispasticity drugs: mechanisms of action. *Ann Neurol* 1981;17:107–116.

207. Merritt JL. Management of spasticity in spinal cord injury. *Mayo Clin Proc* 1981;56:614–622.

208. Monster AW, Herman R, Mees S, et al. Cooperative study for assessing the effect of a pharmacological agent spasticity. *Am J Phys Med* 1973;52:163–188.

209. Herman R, Mayer N, Mecomber SA. Clinical pharmacophysiology of dantrolene sodium. *Am J Phys Med* 1972;51: 296–311.

210. Ward A, Chaffman MO, Sorkin EM. Dantrolene: a review of its pharmacodynamic and pharmacokinetic properties and therapeutic use in malignant hyperthermia, the neuroleptic malignant syndrome and an update of its use in muscle spasticity. *Drugs* 1986;32:130–168.

211. Dykes MHM. Evaluation of a muscle relaxant. Dantrolene sodium (Dantrium). *JAMA* 1975;231:862.

212. Product information: Dantrium®, dantrolene sodium capsules. Proctor and Gamble Pharmaceuticals, Cincinnati, Ohio, USA, 1999.

213. Holllifield RS, Conklin JD. Determination of dantrolene in biological specimens containing drug-related metabolites. *J Pharm Sci* 1973;62:271.

214. Snyder HR, Davis CS, Bickerton RK, et al. 1-(Arylfurfurylodene) amino hydantoins. A new class of muscle relaxants. *J Med Chem* 1967;10:807.

215. Pinder RM, Brogden RN, Speight TM, et al. Dantrolene sodium: a review of its pharmacological properties and therapeutic efficacy in spasticity. *Drugs* 1977;13:3–23.

216. Ketel WB, Kolb ME. Long-term treatment with dantrolene sodium of stroke patients with spasticity limiting the return of function. *Curr Med Res Opin* 1984;9(3):161–169.

217. Zafonte R, Elovic E, Lombard L. Acute care management of post-tbi spasticity. *J Head Trauma Rehabil* 19(2):89–100.

218. Weiser R, Terenty T, Hudgson P, et al. Dantrolene sodium in the treatment of spasticity in chronic spinal cord disease. *Practitioner* 1978;221(1321):123–127.

219. Denhoff E, Feldman S, Smith MG, et al. Treatment of spastic cerebral palsied children with sodium dantrolene. *Dev Med Child Neurol* 1975;17(6):736–742.

220. Gambi d, Rossini PM, Calenda G, et al. Dantrolene sodium in the treatment of spasticity caused by multiple sclerosis or degenerative myelopathies: a double-blind, cross-over study in comparison to placebo. *Curr Ther Res* 1983;33(5):835–840.

221. AMA Department of Drugs. AMA Drug Evaluations, 4th. American Medical Association, Chicago, Il, 1980.

222. Tolman KG. Hepatotoxicity of antirheumatic drugs. *J Rheumatol* 1990;17(Suppl):6–11.

223. Jim LK. Hepatic disorders part I adverse effects of drugs on the liver In:DiPiro JT, Talbert RL, Hayes PE, et al. (Eds): Pharmacotherapy a pathophysiologic approach. Elsevier Science Publishing Co, Inc, New York, NY, 1989.

224. Chan Ch. Dantrolene sodium and hepatic injury. *Neurology* 1990;40:1427–1432.

225. Russo E, Guy GW. A tale of two cannabinoids: the therapeutic rationale for combining tetrahydrocannabinol and cannabidiol. *Med Hypotheses* 2006;66:234–46.

226. Product Information: AMRIX(R) extended-release oral capsules, cyclobenzaprine hcl extended-release oral capsules. FCR Pharmaceuticals, Richmond, VA, 2006.

227. Anon: PDR physicians' desk reference 52nd ed, Medical Economics, Oradell, NJ, 1998, pp 1656–7.

228. Product information: cyclobenzaprine hcl oral tablets, cyclobenzaprine hcl oral tablets. Mutual Pharmaceutical Company,Inc, Philadelphia, PA, 2005.

229. Winchell GA, King JD, Chavez-Eng CM, et al. Cyclobenzaprine pharmacokinetics, including the effects of age, gender, and hepatic insufficiency. *J Clin Pharmacol* 2002;42:61–69.

230. Ashby P, Burke D, Rao S, Jones RF. Assessment of cyclobenzaprine in the treatment of spasticity. *J Neurol Neurosurg Psychiatry*. 1972;35:599–605.

231. Product information: norflex(R), orphenadrine. 3M Pharmaceuticals, Northridge CA, 1998.

232. Labout JJM, Thijssen CT, Keijser GG, et al. Difference between single and multiple dose pharmacokinetics of orphenadrine hydrochloride in man. *Eur J Clin Pharmacol* 1982a; 21:343.

233. Casale R, Glynn C, Buonocore M. Reduction of spastic hypertonia in patients with spinal cord injury: a double blind comparison of intravenous orphenadrine citrate and placebo. *Arch Phys Med Rehabil* 1995;76:660–665.

234. Birket-Smith E. Abnormal involuntary movements induced by anticholinergic therapy. *Acta Neurol Scand* 1974; 50:801–811.

235. Hinderer SR. The supraspinal anxiolytic effect of baclofen for spasicity reduction. *Am J Phys Med Rehabil* 1990; 69(5):254–258.

236. Jones K, Castleden CM. A double-blind comparison of quinine sulfate and placebo in muscle cramps. *Age Ageing* 1983;12(2):155–158.

237. Tarico M, Adone R, Pagliacci C, et al. Pharmacological interventions for spasticity following spinal cord injury. Cochrane Database of Systematic Reviews 2000;(2):CD001131.

238. Corbett M, Frankel HL, Michaelis L. A double blind, cross-over trial of valium in the treatment of spasticity. *Paraplegia* 1972;10:19–22.

239. Hagenbach U, Luz S, et al. The treatment of spasticity with Delta9- tetrahydrocannabinol in persons with spinal cord injury. *Spinal Cord* 2007;45(8):551–562

240. Segal JL, Pathak MS, et al. Safety and efficacy of 4-amino pyridine in humans with spinal cord injury: a long-term , controlled trial. *Pharmacotherapy* 19(6):713–723.

241. Harmon RL, Wooley Sm, Horn LJ. Use of clonidine for spasticity arising from stroke and brain injury: a pilot placebo-controlled trial. *Arch Phys Med Rehabil* 77(9):934.

242. Hulme A, MacLennan WJ, Ritchie RT, et al. Baclofen in the elderly stroke patient its side-effects and pharmacokinetics. *Eur J Clin Pharmacol* 1985;29(4):467–469.

243. Medaer R, Hellebuyk H, Van DBE, et al. Treatment of spasticity due to stroke. A double-blind, cross-over trial comparing baclofne with placebo. *Acta Ther* 1991;17(4):323–331.

244. Maupas E, Marque P, Roques CF, Simonetta-Moreau M. Modulation of the transmission in group II heteronymous pathways by tizanidine in spastic hemiplegic patients. *J Neurol Neurosurg Psychiatry* 2004;75(1):130–135.

245. Groves L, Shellenberger MK, Davis CS. Tizanidine treatment of spasticity: a meta-analysis of controlled, double-blind, comparative studies with baclofen and diazepam. *Adv Ther* 1998;15(4):241–251.

246. Bes A, Eysscttc M, Pierrot-Deseilligny E, Rohmer F, Warter JM. A multi-ccntrc, double trial of tizanidine, a new antispastic agent, in spasticity associated with hemiplegia. *Curr Med Res Opin* 1988;10:709–719

247. Kendall PH. The use of diazepam in hemiplegia. *Ann Phys Med* 1969;6:225–228.

248. Katrak PH, Cole Am, Poulos CJ, et al. Objective assessment of spasticity, strength and function with early exhibition of dantrolene sodium after cerebrovascular accident: a randomized double-blind study. *Arch Phys Med Rehabil* 1992;73(1):4–9.

249. Chyatte SB, Birdsong JH, Bergman BA. The effects of dantrolenc sodium on spasticity and motor performance in hemiplegia. *South Med J* 1971;64(2):180–185.

250. Stamenova P, et al. A randomized, double-blind, placebo-controlled study of the efficacy and safety of tolperisone in spasticity following cerebral stroke. *Eur J Neurol* 2005;12(6):453–61.

251. Scheinberg A, Hall K, Lam LT, O'Flaherty S. Oral baclofen in children with cerebral palsy: a double-blind cross-over pilot study. *J Paediatr Child Health* 2006;42(11):715–720.

252. Lopez SI, Troncoso Sm, De LAABM, Clunes,CA, Hernandez Cm. *Rev Chil Pediatr* 1996;67(5):206–211.

253. Vasquez-Briceno A, et al. The usefulness of tizanidine. A one-year follow-up of the treatment of spasticity in infantile cerebral palsy. *Rev Neurol* 2006;43(3):132–136.

254. Nogen AG. Medical treatment for spasticity in children with cerebral palsy. *Childs Brain* 1976;2(5):304–308.

255. Mathew A, Mathew MC, Thomas M, Antonisamy B. The efficacy of diazepam in enhancing motor function in children with spastic cerebral palsy. *J Trop Pediatr* 2005;51(2):109–113.

256. Chyatte SB, Birdsong JH, Roberson DL. Dantrolene sodium in athetoid cerebral palsy. *Arch Phys Med Rehabil* 1973;54(8):365–368.

257. Haslam RH, Walcher JR, Lietman PS, et al. Dantrolenc sodium in children with spasticity. *Arch Phys Med Rehabil* 1974;55(8):384–388.

258. Joynt RL, Leonard JA Jr. Dantrolene sodium suspension in treatment of spastic cerebral palsy. *Dev Med Child Neurol* 1980;22(6):755–767.

259. Losin S, McKean Cm. Chlorzoxazone (paraflex) in the treatment of severe spasticity. *Dev Med Child Neurol* 1966;8(6):768–769.

260. Bjerre I, Blennow G. Methocarbamol in the treatment of cerebral palsy in children. *Neuropadiatrie* 1971;3(2):140–146.

261. Hurst Dl, Lajara-Nanson W. Use of modafinil in spastic cerebral palsy. *J Child Neurol* 2002;17(3):169–172.

262. Maritz NG, Muller FO, Pompe Van Meerdervoort HF. Piracetam in the management of spasticity in cerebral palsy. *S Afr Med J* 1978;53:889–891.

263. Chu ML, Sala DA. The use of tigabine in pediatric spasticity management. *Dev Med Child Neurol* 2006;48(6):456–459.

264. Brar SP, Smith MB, Nelson LM, et al. Evaluation of treatment protocols on minimal to moderate spasticity in multiple sclerosis. *Arch Phys Med Rehabil* 1991;72(3):186–189.

265. Orsnes G, Crone C, Krarup C, et al. The effect of baclofen on the transmission in spinal pathways in spastic multiple sclerosis patients. *Clin Neurophysiol* 2000;111(8):1372–1379.

266. Basmajian JV. Lioresal (baclofen) treatment of spasticity in multiple sclerosis. *Am J Phys Med* 1975;54(4):175–177.

267. Lapierre Y, Bouchard S, TanseyC, et al. Treatment of spasticity with tizanidine in multiple sclerosis. *Can J Neurol Sci* 1987;14(3 suppl):513–517.

268. Anonymous. A double-blind, placebo-controlled trial of tizanidine in the treatment of spasticity caused by multiple sclerosis. United Kingdom Tizanidine Trial Group. *Neurology* 1994;44(11 Suppl 9):S70–S78.

269. Wilson LA, McKechnie AA. Oral diazepam in the treatment of spasticity in paraplegia: a double-blind trial and subsequent impressions. *Scott Med J* 1966;11:46–51.

270. Gelenberg AJ, Poskanzer DC. The effect of dantrolene sodium on spasticity in multiple sclerosis. *Neurology* 1973;23(12):1313–1315.

271. Tolosa ES, Soll RW, Loewenson RB. Treatment of spasticity in multiple sclerosis with dantrolene. *JAMA* 1975;233(10):1046.

272. Killstein J, Hoogervorst E, et al. Safety, tolerability, and efficacy of orally administered cannabinoids in MS. *American Academy of Neurology* 2002;58(9):1404–1407.

273. Vaney C, et al. Efficacy, safety and tolerability of an orally administered cannabis extract in the treatment of spasticity in patients with multiple sclerosis: a randomized, double-blind, placebo-controlled, crossover study. *Mult Scler* 2004;(4):339–340.

274. Wade DT, Robson P, House H, Makela P, Aram J. A preliminary controlled study to determine whether whole-plant cannabis extracts can improve intractable neurogenic symptoms. *Clin Rehabil* 2003;17(1):21–29.

275. Ungerleider JT, Andyrsiak T, Fairbanks L, Ellison GW, Myers LW. Delta-9-THC in the treatment of spasticity associated with multiple sclerosis. *Adv Alcohol Subst Abuse.* 1987;7(1):39–50.

276. Shakespeare DT, Boggild M, Younc C. Anti-spasticity agents for multiple sclerosis. Cochrane Database of Systemic Reviews 2003, Issue 4. Art. No.:CD001332. DOI: 10.1002/14651858.CD001332.

277. Paisley S, Beard S, Hunn A, Wight J. Clinical effectiveness of oral treatments for spasticity in multiple sclerosis: a systematic review. *Mult Scler* 2002;8(4):319–329.

278. Dunevsky A, Perel AB. Gabapentin for relief of spasticity associated with multiple sclerosis. *Am J Phys Med Rehabil.* 1998;77(5):451–454.

279. Mondrup K, Pedersen E. The clinical effect of the GABA-agonist, progabide on spasticity. *Acta Neurol Scand* 1984;(69)200–206.

280. Rudick RA, Breton D, Krall RL. The GABA-agonist progabide for spasicity in multiple sclerosis. *Arch Neurol* 1987;44:1033–1036.

281. Barbeau H, Richards Cl, Bedard PJ. Action of cyproheptadinein spastic paraparetic patients. *J Neurol Neurosurg Psychiatry* 1982;45:923–926.

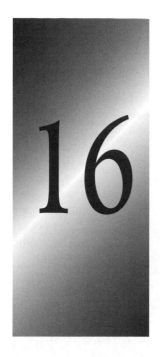

Intrathecal Baclofen for Spasticity

Michael Saulino
Stuart A. Yablon
Elizabeth Moberg-Wolff
John W. Chow
Dobrivoje S. Stokic

Intrathecal baclofen (ITB) therapy is a potent method for the management of spastic hypertonia and related features of the upper motor neuron syndrome. Intrathecal baclofen infusion exerts its therapeutic effect by delivering baclofen directly into the cerebrospinal fluid (CSF) with rapid distribution to target neurons in the spinal cord. Intrathecal administration of baclofen is typically effected through use of an externally programmable, surgically implanted pump, delivering the drug at precise flow rates via a catheter placed in the spinal canal. Studies demonstrate evidence of the effectiveness of the ITB infusion system in reducing hypertonia in patients with cerebral palsy (CP), spinal cord injury, multiple sclerosis, and acquired brain injury due to stroke, trauma, or hypoxia. Although most of the information presented in this chapter is derived from studies of adults treated with ITB for severe spasticity, the discussion also specifically deals with clinical experience in pediatric and ambulatory patient populations. This chapter reviews important aspects of ITB therapy in the treatment of patients with multifocal, dysfunctional spasticity. We specifically address the conceptual framework and indications for ITB therapy, the role of screening trials in patient selection, implantation procedures, post-implantation management, and long-term maintenance, and the evolving experience in ambulatory patients.

HISTORY OF ITB THERAPY

Intrathecal administration facilitates the delivery of neurologically active drugs to target receptors in the central nervous system (CNS) indirectly via diffusion through the CSF. Although this technique has recently attained relatively widespread use, its origins can be traced back more than a century. In 1898, Bier reported the first therapeutic application of intrathecal therapy, performing spinal anesthesia through the use of intrathecal cocaine. In 1901, a Romanian physician, Racoviceanu-Pitesti, described the use of opiates for intrathecal anesthesia. Spinal drug administration subsequently became one of the foundations of modern anesthesiology (1).

Intrathecal drug administration was initially limited to short-term use; however, nearly 8 decades would pass before physicians attempted to implement this therapy for chronic conditions. Onofrio et al. (2) described the beneficial effects of intrathecal morphine administration for the treatment of chronic pain associated with cancer. In 1985, Penn and Kroin (3) described the successful use of continuous ITB (CITB) infusion for reducing spasticity of spinal origin (multiple sclerosis or spinal cord injury). Several clinical trials then preceded the United States Food and Drug Administration (FDA) approval of ITB therapy for spasticity of spinal origin in 1992 (4–7). Subsequent investigations expanded the role of this therapy to spasticity of cerebral origin (stroke, CP, and brain injury) (8–10), with the FDA approval following in 1996.

INTRATHECAL BACLOFEN INFUSION

Neurophysiological Mechanism of Action

As introduced above, the rationale underlying intrathecal infusion therapy is to facilitate the delivery of drugs to their respective sites of action within the CNS. This also reduces certain types of adverse effects because systemic drug exposure is reduced or bypassed entirely. Any drug that exerts a useful pharmacologic effect within the CNS and is capable of being maintained in a stable sterile solution can be considered a potential agent for intrathecal delivery. Although several drugs are commonly used for chronic intrathecal administration, only 3 drugs currently have FDA approval for long-term use: baclofen (for spasticity), morphine (for pain), and ziconotide (for pain).

Intrathecal baclofen's most prominent neurophysiological effect involves the reduction of spinal reflex responses, both monosynaptic (e.g. H reflex) and polysynaptic (e.g. flexion withdrawal reflex) (11), in a dose-dependent manner (12–14). This is consistent with clinical observations of rapid disappearance of tendon taps and decrease in frequency and severity of muscle spasms with ITB. Biomechanical and neurophysiological studies also provide evidence of decreased resistance to imposed passive stretch, accompanied by a decrease in threshold and magnitude of electromyographic response (15). The association of ITB with clinical reduction in muscle hypertonia, while present, is not as straightforward as its effect on reflex activity. Further, convincing data remain elusive regarding the degree to which ITB can improve voluntary motor control. Anecdotal cases of reduced agonist-antagonist electromyographic cocontraction have been reported, documenting improved pattern of voluntary muscle activation during simple motor tasks (14, 16–18), some of which coincided with better functional outcomes (17).

At the neuronal level, baclofen acts as a potent $GABA_B$ receptor agonist. GABA-B receptors are extensively distributed in the spinal cord, making this spinal neuronal network a prime target for this drug's antispastic effects (19–21). Baclofen administered directly to the subarachnoid space has enhanced access to GABA receptors compared to oral administration and thus allows greater reflex inhibition and hypertonia reduction (19, 20). The exact mechanism of

baclofen action, however, remains elusive. Baclofen could interfere with signal transmission along various afferent pathways and with neurotransmitter release (presynaptic) or alter motor neuron physical properties and their excitability (postsynaptic). Although presynaptic mechanisms have been favored, postsynaptic baclofen effects on motor neurons and interneurons have more recently been reported in experimental animals (22–24). These offer a plausible explanation for some neurophysiological studies in humans that favor postsynaptic over presynaptic site of baclofen action. For example, Azouvi et al. (12) reported no discernible effect of baclofen on vibratory inhibition or heteronymous facilitation of the H reflex, thereby challenging assumptions regarding the contribution of presynaptic mechanisms to the inhibition of monosynaptic reflexes. Additional support for the postsynaptic action can be found in decreased F-wave frequency after ITB bolus (25) or CITB administration (26). At clinically achievable ITB doses, the suppressive effect of ITB on monosynaptic and polysynaptic reflex pathways seems to be presynaptic, most probably by interfering with neurotransmitter release, with postsynaptic effects possible at higher doses (27).

Components of ITB Therapy

Intrathecal delivery systems are composed of a few key components. These include an accessible drug

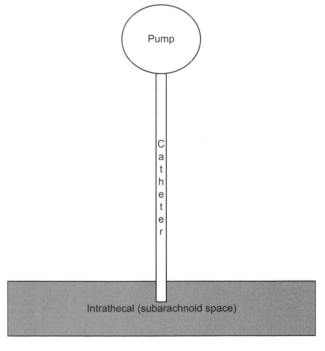

FIGURE 16.1

Schematic diagram of intrathecal delivery system.

reservoir, a method of propelling the drug out of the pump, and a catheter that connects the drug reservoir to the CSF (Figure 16.1). Although constant flow systems are available (28), programmable systems are overwhelmingly preferred due to their adjustability for individual patient need and response (29). Additional components are needed for programmable systems, including an external programming device and a communication method between the programmer and the implanted pump. The propulsion technique for variable controlled pumps is typically electronic, necessitating an energy source to drive the system. In contrast, constant-flow pumps can utilize a pneumatic propulsion technique. Future components may include automated troubleshooting of the system, self-directed patient programming, and integrated sensors to detect patient position and functional activity level.

Intrathecal baclofen infusion systems afford potent relief of spastic hypertonia, although some clinical presentations are better suited for this therapy. Graham et al. (30) used a grid illustration to compare the characteristics of various therapies for spasticity, contrasting reversible versus irreversible options and focal versus global effects (Figure 16.2). In this model, ITB was considered reversible (neural structures are not surgically altered, and the rate of dose administration is adjustable) and global (the CNS effects of ITB distribution are typically observed in all extremities and the trunk). Thus, patients with global or multifocal spasticity who may benefit from an adjustable (versus

permanent) clinical effect are generally considered as better candidates. Further, ITB can be combined with other modalities for synergistic therapeutic effect, including rehabilitative therapies, oral pharmacotherapy, neurolytic procedures, and muscle/tendon lengthening procedures (31). Physical techniques such as stretching, strengthening, bracing, and gait retraining are essential for attaining maximal functional benefit that may follow tone reduction. Patients might continue to utilize oral spasticity agents for a variety of reasons, including ongoing ITB titration, "breakthrough" spasms, an irregular spasticity pattern, disease progression, or residual upper extremity tone. Combining ITB therapy and neurolytic procedures is appropriate for patients manifesting both focal dystonic features and global hypertonicity, or residual upper extremity hypertonia (32). The indications for combining neuro-orthopedic procedures and ITB therapy include correction of fixed deformities in the presence of ongoing spastic hypertonia. Concomitant use of orthopedic surgery and ITB in children with CP may reduce the need for subsequent orthopedic surgery (33).

Patient Selection and the Role of Preimplant Trials

In terms of higher cost, potential benefit, and complication risk, few current spasticity treatments compare with ITB infusion therapy. This form of therapy may be optimal for some patients and yet unsuitable for others with comparable degrees of moderate or severe spasticity. Patient selection and education are important to achieving optimal outcomes. Appropriate candidates need to be counseled regarding that proceeding with this form of therapy represents a long-term commitment.

In general, patients can be considered candidates for ITB therapy when:

- Spasticity is poorly controlled despite maximal therapy with other modalities;
- Spasticity is poorly controlled because of limited patient tolerance of other modalities; and
- Adjustable spasticity reduction afforded by a programmable variable flow pump would be advantageous.

Patients should be clinically stable, understand the risks and benefits of ITB therapy, be able to return to clinic for titration and refills, and have demonstrated a positive response to a test dose of ITB. In severe cases, this therapy can be considered early in the postinjury recovery period (e.g., <12 months [34]). Intrathecal baclofen therapy generally reduces lower limb hypertonia

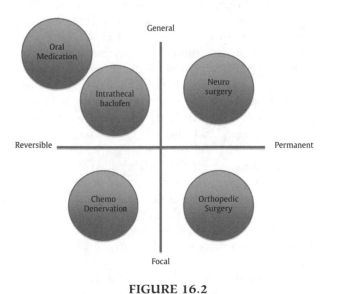

FIGURE 16.2

Characterization of various spasticity treatment modalities. With permission from Graham HK, Aoki KR, Autti-Ramo I, et al., Gait Posture, vol. II, Elsevier, 2000:67–69.

to a greater extent than in the upper extremities. More cephalad catheter tip placement, however, can potentially improve upper limb response (35, 36). The other advantages of ITB therapy include higher potency with potentially less adverse effects compared to oral baclofen, the ability to have a global effect on all the affected limbs, and the possibility of later adjustment with changing patient need or progressive disease. The disadvantages include surgical risks (bleeding, infection, damage of neural structures), the potential for serious adverse effects including overdose and withdrawal, and the requirement for ongoing follow-up with health care professionals for dosing adjustments and pump refills. Ventricular shunting for hydrocephalus is not a contraindication to ITB therapy, but practitioners should be aware of potential interactions between the devices on CSF flow (37). Intrathecal baclofen can also be used in patients with seizures with the understanding that this therapy has been occasionally associated with an increased risk of seizures (38, 39).

For the patient who chooses this form of therapy, the preimplant trial is the first of 4 phases of ITB treatment: (1) trial, (2) surgery, (3) titration, and (4) maintenance. The preimplant trial involves administration of a test dose of ITB to assess the patient's response to this agent. Typically, a lumbar puncture is performed, and a bolus of a baclofen solution is injected into the CSF. Fifty micrograms of baclofen is the most commonly used initial screening dose (40). The onset of clinical effects from a screening bolus occurs within 1 to 3 hours postinjection, and peak effects are typically observed 4 to 6 hours postinjection. The effects of the screening bolus are always temporary, with the effects routinely lasting for 6 to 8 hours (25, 41). Prolonged effects of a single test bolus have been reported (42). Screening boluses can be repeated if the initial injection is unsuccessful. "Positive" responses are reported in 80% to 90% of bolus trials (40). Generally, antibiotic prophylaxis is not needed for a bolus trial (43). For patients on antiplatelet or anticoagulant therapy, recommendations from the American Society of Regional Anesthesia are followed (44). Fluoroscopic guidance can assist needle localization into the intrathecal space (45) because anatomic landmarks for lumbar puncture can be variable.

An alternative method for conducting trials involves the placement of a temporary intrathecal catheter and monitoring the patient response to a short-term continuous infusion of baclofen (46). This technique is more commonly utilized for evaluating chronic pain patients for intrathecal opiate therapy. The specifics of catheter placement are described later in this chapter. The advantages of catheter ITB trials include (1) avoidance of sequential lumbar punctures; (2) presumably improved approximation of chronic postimplant intrathecal infusion response when compared to single bolus injections; (3) ability to control catheter tip placement for the evaluation of upper extremity effects; and (4) ability to adjust the infusion rate while assessing the favorable (and unfavorable) effects of ITB administration. The disadvantages of catheter trials include increased technical difficulty, increased need for observation, and increased risk of meningitis and structural damage. Fluoroscopic guidance is generally considered mandatory for catheter placement. Although antibiotic prophylaxis is usually not needed for bolus trials, it is unclear whether antibiotic prophylaxis is needed for short-duration intrathecal catheter trials. Factors to consider include the duration of the trial, patient immunocompetency, and potential chronic bacterial colonization. Evidence suggests that trial duration is a key risk factor for the development of infectious complications. Thus, the trial should last only as long as required to indicate a potential benefit of chronic ITB therapy (43, 47). There is no consensus regarding the optimal method of anesthesia utilized for catheter placement. Local anesthesia potentially lowers the risk of inadvertent damage to neural structures. However, if excessive patient movement or severe anxiety is anticipated, deep sedation or general anesthesia may be warranted (48). There is little evidence to suggest that catheter trials provide better long-term outcomes compared to bolus trials when utilized as predictors of postimplant response. Prospective data in the pain management literature suggest no difference in outcomes from either intrathecal trial method (49), although the generalizability of these findings to ITB spasticity trials is unclear.

Definitions of "success" for screening trials vary. A more liberal description of a successful trial might be any improvement in spasticity that suggests future benefit from chronic long-term infusion. Subjective patient reports can be used to assess spontaneous spasm frequency and intensity (50). The most commonly cited criterion for a successful ITB trial is a 2-point reduction on the Modified Ashworth Scale (40). Patients may also demonstrate improvement in joint range of motion, both actively and passively. Intrathecal baclofen trials can potentially differentiate range of motion deficits due to severe spasticity, which are potentially reversible without surgery, from fixed contractures.

Although these evaluation techniques are often useful for patients with hypertonia in resting positions, these assessments may be inadequate for the prediction of ITB effect during active functional tasks. In these patients, excessive tone reduction may impede the performance of activities such as transfers and walking. Observation of ambulation, transfers, posture, and wheelchair propulsion during the trial is thus warranted. Adjunctive objective evaluation techniques may be helpful and include neurophysiological assessment (25, 51, 52) and instrumented gait analysis (41, 53). There is an inconsistent correlation between subjective report and objective measures of spasticity (54). During a screening trial, some individuals may experience excessive spasticity reduction during the peak effect of the ITB bolus. This occurrence is not a contraindication for pump implantation because the chronic infusion system has the ability to modulate dose and subsequent desired effect. If excessive or prolonged hypotonia is observed during a screening trial, then a repeat trial at a lower dose or continuous trial may be warranted. Particular care should be paid to patients who demonstrate improvement on "passive" measures of spasticity (thus qualifying for long-term infusion of the basis of trial "success") yet demonstrate functional worsening during the trial. Postimplant rehabilitation in this subset of patients is particularly important.

Adverse effects can occur during the test phase. Spinal headache or postlumbar puncture syndrome is a complication of an injection-related dural leak and is not a direct medication effect. Spinal headaches occur in up to 30% of patients undergoing lumbar puncture and can vary in severity from mild to incapacitating (55). Postlumbar puncture headache typically worsens when the patient sits or stands up, and decreases in the supine position. These headaches typically begin within 2 days but may be delayed for as long as 2 weeks. Spinal headaches can be accompanied by dizziness, neck or arm pain, cranial nerve palsies, tinnitus, nausea, and distorted vision. Spinal headaches are more common in younger women with a low body mass index and in people who have a headache history in general. The risk of spinal headaches increases with the use of larger needles. The headache resolves spontaneously in most patients. Supportive measures include bedrest, caffeine, and abdominal binders. Epidural blood patch is reserved for persistent cases (56). Other procedure-related complications include bacterial and aseptic meningitis. Adverse effects that are more likely related to a pharmacologic effect include nausea/vomiting, urinary retention, hypotension, seizures, drowsiness/sedation, respiratory depression, and coma. Nausea/vomiting and drowsiness/sedation are the most common adverse effects observed during ITB trials, with reported frequency of 2% to 3% (40).

Although the procedural component of the trial should take place in a setting where injection steril-

ity is assured, a number of settings are suitable for monitoring the effects of the trial. Examples include outpatient clinics, ambulatory surgical centers, inpatient hospitals, and inpatient rehabilitation facilities. Further, it is helpful to use practice protocols or pathways to facilitate the consistent assessment of key trial response indicators and reduce the risk of complications. As described above, sequential evaluations of tone, range of motion, and strength are required. For patients who utilize spasticity to assist with functional mobility, similar sequential evaluations of posture, transfers, and gait should be undertaken. Protocols for the management of adverse events should be in place, including spinal headache, bowel and bladder changes, seizures, and respiratory depression. Because the effects of ITB trials are occasionally prolonged, the practice setting should have the capacity for extended observation. Many experienced practitioners of ITB therapy believe that inpatient rehabilitation facilities are an optimal site for trials since these locations offer the best ability to assess functional changes and potentially manage adverse effects.

Some centers proceed directly to pump implantation without a screening trial. For stroke patients, 2 justifications have been proposed: (1) the increased risk of spinal hemorrhage while the patients are in anticoagulation or antiplatelet therapy and (2) the risk of recurrent stroke if these agents are discontinued. This method reduces the ability to differentiate fixed contracture from spasticity before implantation. Although patients may still benefit, it should only be undertaken after a full discussion with the patient and caregivers regarding the risks and benefits of a "no trial" approach.

IMPLANTATION

Once a positive trial response has been observed, a patient may proceed to pump implantation. Patients should be clinically stable before surgery to minimize perioperative complications. Preoperative antibiotics are typically utilized. Patients on chronic anticoagulation will need to discontinue medications in the days preceding the procedure (44). The risks of permanent pump implantation and infusion are similar to those of the screening trial, with the additional risks of drug overdose, drug withdrawal, and device complications.

Various options for pump and catheter placement should be considered before the procedure. The size of the implanted pump should be determined based on the patient's body habitus and anticipated intrathecal dosing. Smaller and thinner individuals might prefer a smaller pump size, either for esthetic reasons or to

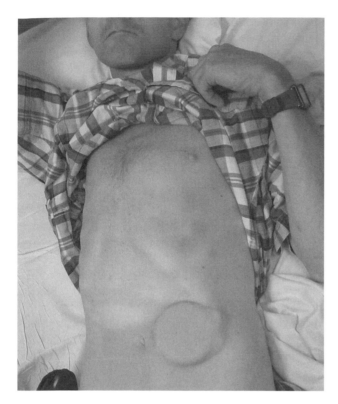

FIGURE 16.3

A picture of a patient after pump implantation.

prevent erosion of the pump through the skin and sub-cutaneous tissue. Similarly, the pump can be placed under abdominal fascia for similar reasons (57) (see Figure 16.3). Patients who are anticipated to require high ITB doses or who reside a great distance from the follow-up clinic will benefit from larger pumps with larger drug reservoirs and longer refill intervals. The tip of the intrathecal catheter is routinely placed in the midlower thoracic region, particularly if reduction of lower extremity spasticity is the primary concern. More rostral tip placement may be attempted to improve upper extremity hypertonicity (35, 36).

Pump implantation and continuous catheter trials are typically performed under general anesthesia. The patient is placed in either prone or lateral decubitus position. Spinal anatomy is confirmed radiographically. The typical site of insertion into the spinal canal is posteriorly at the L2-3 or L3-4 interspace. A spinal needle is inserted through the skin several millimeters lateral to the midline and 1 to 2 spinal levels caudal to the proposed thecal sac penetration. Advancement of the needle should be monitored with fluoroscopic guidance, which ideally permits penetration into the thecal sac on the first attempt. Multiple dural punctures can potentially allow CSF leakage and result in

inadvertent subdural or epidural catheter placement. Once the needle tip in placed in the thecal sac, the inner cannula is removed, and free-flowing CSF should be observed. The intrathecal catheter is then placed through the spinal needle and advanced cephalad (58). The catheter tip is then positioned to the spinal level appropriate for the individual patient, which is usually T10-12 for the paraplegic patient and more rostrally for the tetraplegic or hemiplegic patient (35). The spinal needle is then removed. The catheter should be secured without undue tension to avoid kinking. The pump is generally implanted under the skin or abdominal fascia in the right or left lower quadrant. The catheter is then tunneled subcutaneously and connected to the pump. Liquid, preservative-free baclofen is placed in the pump, and ITB infusion commences intraoperatively. This initial dosage of ITB is often determined by the patient's response due the test dose. A reasonable starting dose is 100% to 200% of the bolus dose divided over a 24-hour period. The patient should continue all oral antispasticity medications until a weaning schedule is prescribed. The duration of acute hospitalization for pump implantation is brief, typically a few days (59).

Titration Phase and Postimplantation Management

Dose adjustments can commence immediately after pump implantation. Further adjustments usually occur no more frequently than every 24 hours. Dose modifications are performed by "interrogating" the pump with a handheld programmer, programming the needed adjustments, and then updating the pump's dosing schedule. The programmer communicates with the pump via radio-telemetry. Various modes of administration include simple continuous (dose delivered continuously throughout the 24-hour cycle), complex continuous (variable dose delivered continuously during the 24-hour cycle), and periodic bolus (regularly scheduled boluses of ITB within the 24-hour cycle). During the titration phase of ITB therapy, the patients are usually weaned from oral antispasticity medications. The amount of each adjustment varies depending on patient tolerability. Nonambulatory patients may tolerate dose adjustments of 20% of the total daily dose, whereas others, especially ambulatory patients, will require lower titration increments (5%–10%). Adverse effects that may be seen during this phase of therapy include excessive hypotonia, changes in bowel (60) and bladder status (61), and increased thromboembolic risk (62, 63). The frequency and size of dosing adjustments should be individualized based on the response to prior changes. Some patients tolerate rapid titration with daily dosing adjustments, whereas others may require longer periods of observation and accommodation before undertaking further adjustments. The titration phase of therapy usually lasts 6 to 9 months after implantation.

If ITB is anticipated to affect the patient's active functional status, then a rehabilitation program after implantation is appropriate. The setting, scope, and complexity of this program will vary depending upon the patient's individual goals. The timing of rehabilitation is also subject to some debate. Some centers defer therapies for a few weeks after the implant due to concerns of catheter fracture or incisional dehiscence, whereas others favor immediate postimplant rehabilitation. Potential disciplines involve in the rehabilitation process include physiatry/neurorehabilitation, physical therapy, occupational therapy, and rehabilitation nursing. Issues that potentially require attention include incisional care, medical management (spinal headache, pain assessment, medication adjustment, dosing changes), mobility, self-care ability, bowel/bladder function, and caregiver training.

Long-Term Maintenance

After the titration phase of ITB therapy, the patient enters the chronic maintenance phase of therapy. Aspects of this treatment period include refilling the pump reservoir with new medication, troubleshooting any infusion system malfunction, and replacing the pump for battery replenishment.

Reservoir refills are a sterile, office-based procedure that occur every few weeks to few months for the duration of treatment. The baclofen solution is stable in the pump reservoir for up to 6 months. The pump has a low residual reservoir volume, which is the lowest volume that supports stable flow through the catheter. The refill interval is the time required for the pump to dispense the volume of solution from a full reservoir to the low reservoir volume. The refill interval will reflect the baclofen concentration and daily dose. Pump refills are scheduled to have sufficient residual reservoir volume before the alarm date to avoid "low reservoir syndrome" and associated symptoms of ITB withdrawal (64, 65). Pump refills are typically accomplished by palpating the pump externally and using a template to guide a needle into the reservoir chamber. Fluoroscopy or ultrasound can be used to assist in guiding the needle through the access port into the reservoir chamber (66). The remaining solution of the previous refill is aspirated and should correspond to the calculated volume by the pump programmer. The new baclofen solution is then instilled through the same needle. The needle tip must be reliably determined to be within the reservoir chamber. Inadvertent injection of an intrathecal solution into the subcutaneous tissue can result in serious adverse events (67).

During titration, some patients require ITB dose increases with a subsequent increase in refill frequency. Under these circumstances, a higher concentration of baclofen solution will extend the refill interval. When changing concentrations, it is imperative to program the pump correctly by incorporating a bridge bolus to compensate for the residual baclofen solution in the pump and catheter (68). Failure to compensate for this residual solution can result in serious underdosing or overdosing.

Two concentrations of ITB (Lioresal Intrathecal) are FDA-approved and commercially available for use in reservoir refills, that is, 500 and 2000 μg/mL. Clinical use of higher concentrations of noncommercially prepared, compounded baclofen has occurred by those seeking lower cost and less frequent pump refills. In a study of 27 samples of compounded baclofen obtained from 7 compounding pharmacies, over 40% were more than 5% above or below their labeled concentration, and 22% deviated more than 10% from its labeled concentration (69). The sterility, duration of stability, and density of the preparations were also not routinely tested or reported as is required for commercial preparations. Thus, compounded baclofen may lead to inaccurate or inconsistent dosing due to concentration variations, causing symptoms of underdose or overdose. There is also anecdotal evidence that baclofen concentrations above 2000 μg/mL can contribute to catheter tip abnormalities (70). Because of the potential for contamination and/or drug precipitation, use of compounded ITB should only be utilized with a full realization of the potential risks associated with this strategy.

Other issues related to long-term intrathecal therapy include precautions for use and battery replacement. The current intrathecal delivery systems are considered magnetic resonance imaging (MRI) compatible and have been formally tested in magnets up to 1.5 T. Intrathecal delivery will automatically stop in the presence of the magnetic field and restart when removed from the magnetic field. An electronic check of the intrathecal delivery can be done with the programmer to insure restart of intrathecal delivery. Normally, the duration of MRI scan is of insufficient duration to result in clinically significant withdrawal (71, 72). Whole-body shock-wave lithotripsy is relatively contraindicated with intrathecal delivery systems due to the potential for electronic damage by the sound waves. Hyperbaric oxygen therapy has been reported to result in a degree of underdosing, and thus, clinicians should proceed with caution with this therapy in patients who have intrathecal pumps (73). Battery replenishment, typically a same day surgical procedure, is undertaken approximately every 5 to 6 years. There may be some benefit in planning a pump replacement before detecting alarm condition in an effort to avoid serious withdrawal symptoms (74).

EXPERIENCE WITH SPECIFIC PATIENT GROUPS

Children

Intrathecal baclofen has been used safely and successfully in pediatric patients with spasticity and dystonia with quadraparetic, hemiparetic, or diplegic distribution patterns (75, 76). The reversibility and adjustability of this therapy in this young age group are seen as an advantage to many families. Pediatric movement disorders may be related to CP, brain injury, and spinal cord injury or less common disorders such as Rett syndrome (77). Early use of ITB in acutely injured patients who manifest "dysautonomia" or "storming" may also produce clinical improvements (78). Intrathecal baclofen may reduce the need for orthopedic surgery and improve comfort, speech, upper extremity use, ease of caregiving, and overall quality of life (79–82). Weight gain, which is often difficult in children with severe spasticity, may be more achievable. Initially used primarily in children with severe spasticity who required wheelchairs for positioning and mobility, recent studies have shown ITB's usefulness in children who are ambulatory, with either diplegia or hemiparesis (83, 84). Reducing the need for assistive devices or improving gait efficiency may lead to improved endurance as well as social integration.

Ambulatory Patients

Over the past 2 decades, a number of studies have reported that CITB administration effectively reduces hypertonia and spasm frequency and improves function, comfort, and ease of caregiving in patients with severe spasticity associated with CNS injury or disease. Most of these studies focus on global measures of tone and function; however, the effects of ITB therapy on specific domains of function, including walking performance, were seldom quantitatively investigated. This is unfortunate, as published reports describe both a potential for improvement in ambulatory function with ITB (85) and a sobering possibility for worsening (86).

From a clinical perspective, 3 related questions are often posed regarding ITB therapy and ambula-

tory function. For patients with CNS injury or disease who are presently unable to walk, will ITB administration permit them to walk or otherwise improve mobility? Similarly, for patients already able to walk with assistance, will ITB help improve their walking ability or permit them to walk independently? Conversely, for those patients who are able to walk, will they experience worsening of their walking ability after ITB? The published scientific literature currently provides few definitive answers to these related questions. Isolated case reports describe nonambulatory individuals with spasticity who regained an ability to walk after implantation of the ITB pump (87, 88). It appears, however, that such occurrences are relatively infrequent and that prognosis for improving ambulatory function appears to favor those who have better baseline ambulatory function over those with slower baseline gait velocity (41). Most of the larger studies (84, 89–91) report mixed results, with some patients significantly improving in walking outcomes, a smaller percentage significantly worsening, with the largest subgroup demonstrating nonsignificant changes overall (84, 90, 91).

In summary, most studies addressing ambulatory function after bolus or continuous administration of ITB report either positive effects or no overall significant changes in ambulatory status or gait function. At present, these studies provide only tentative support and limited guidance for recommendations that clinicians have offered previously based on anecdotal experience. For patients whose locomotor function is impaired by spasticity, a reduction in spasticity through ITB therapy may improve the ambulation status or gait performance with concurrent intensive therapy. On the other hand, diminished spasticity may be counterproductive to patients who rely on spastic cocontraction for support during walking and standing, particularly at larger doses among patients with multiple sclerosis and incomplete spinal cord injury. For domains of passive function, ITB effectively reduces spasticity and thus provides relief in positioning, pain, and discomfort and facilitates caregiving. Improvement in walking function, however, currently cannot be reliably assured to a prospective patient before ITB pump implantation.

APPARENT LOSS OF DRUG EFFECT, WITHDRAWAL, SYSTEM MALFUNCTIONS, AND TROUBLESHOOTING

For patients with chronic, nonprogressive neurologic conditions, ITB dosing should be relatively stable during the maintenance phase of therapy. Individuals with progressive diseases, such as amyotrophic lateral sclerosis or multiple sclerosis, may require more frequent evaluation and dose adjustments. Patients with previously well-controlled hypertonia on a stable dosing regimen who present with increased spasticity should be examined carefully (92). Comorbidities of neurological disease can serve as noxious stimuli that act as "triggers" for increased spasticity (e.g. urinary tract infection, bladder distention, urolithiasis [61]). If no cause for increased spasticity is discovered, then an investigation for system malfunction should be promptly undertaken. An approach to this exploration will be discussed below.

Abrupt reduction or cessation of ITB delivery can result in withdrawal, a serious and potentially fatal complication. Perhaps the most common symptomatic presentation for withdrawal includes return of the patient's "baseline" degree of hypertonia. Other symptoms of ITB withdrawal include pruritus, seizures, hallucinations, and autonomic dysreflexia. Some patients will demonstrate a life-threatening syndrome characterized by exaggerated/rebound spasticity (ie, greater than baseline degree of hypertonia), fever, hemodynamic instability, and altered mental status. If not treated aggressively, this syndrome can progress over 24 to 72 hours to include rhabdomyolysis (with associated elevation of creatine kinase or creatine phosphokinase), elevated transaminase levels, hepatic and renal failure, disseminated intravascular coagulation, multiorgan system failure, and rarely death (93). Typically, the withdrawal symptoms will abate in several days, although there are reports of prolonged ITB withdrawal syndrome (94). After recognition of ITB withdrawal, initial treatment includes supportive care, careful observation and replacement of baclofen either via enteral, or preferably through restoration of intrathecal delivery. Adjunctive pharmacotherapy includes administration of benzodiazepines (enteral or intravenous [95]), dantrolene (96), or cyproheptadine (97, 98).

Potential causes for loss of effectiveness of ITB therapy include programming errors and mechanical problems involving the pump or catheter (eg, kinks, holes, occlusions) (99, 100) (Table 16.1). Some of these problems are readily detectable, whereas the others are more challenging to identify. Programming and refilling errors tend to be easily identified and corrected. Malfunctions involving the pump mechanism are rare, but when present, these malfunctions are also rather simply confirmed. Catheter problems are relatively frequent, however, and may vary in their presentations and ease of diagnostic identification. Figure 16.4 illustrates potential sites of catheter disruption. Approaches to pump and catheter malfunction will be

TABLE 16.1
*Possible Causes of Intrathecal
Drug Deliver Failure*

Pump
- Mechanical failure: rotor stall, computer error
- No/low drug in reservoir
- Battery failure

Catheter
- Migration: subcutaneous, subdural, epidural space
- Fracture: micro versus macro leak
- Kink/Occlusion: connection points, suture points, pump flip, catheter tip loculations
- Disconnection of catheter from pump

Human Error
- Programming error for bolus dose, maintenance dose, reservoir volume, catheter length
- Refill error: subcutaneous refill, incorrect drug or concentration

presented next. It is important to note that no consensus exists regarding an optimal diagnostic algorithm. Physicians should make decisions based upon their individual resources and familiarity with each diagnostic technique. Prompt identification of the underlying problem is important, if possible, so timely restoration of drug delivery can ensue.

Pharmacodynamic tolerance refers to the adaptive changes that have taken place within systems affected by the drug so that clinical response to the drug is reduced (101). Tolerance has been implicated as a cause of acquired loss of response to ITB despite escalating ITB doses, often in the context of failure to demonstrate radiological evidence of an ITB system malfunction. Controversy exists, however, regarding

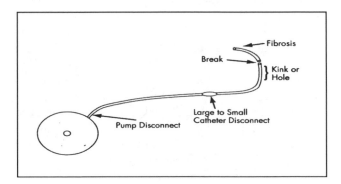

FIGURE 16.4

Potential catheter disruptions.

whether ITB response failure in such scenarios represents undiagnosed problems with drug administration through the pump and catheter system rather than actual pharmacodynamic tolerance (102) in GABA-ergic target neurons of the spinal cord. Accordingly, a thorough analysis of any potential system malfunction should be undertaken before attributing dose escalation to tolerance. Neurophysiological assessment may be helpful in this scenario (52, 103). Assuming that these steps have been unsuccessfully attempted, interventions for tolerance include decreasing the concentration of baclofen solution with a concomitant increase in flow rate (104), utilization of periodic bolus delivery (105), and substitution with intrathecal morphine (106).

Two initial techniques for the investigation of pump malfunction include pump "interrogation" and checking the pump residual reservoir volume. Detection of an audible alarm during pump interrogation, or discovery of an unexpected "extra" residual volume in the reservoir, suggests a pump-related malfunction. The most common culprit is the pump rotor. Rotor failure will result in loss of drug delivery with a residual volume on reservoir aspiration that exceeds the predicted reservoir volume. Rotor failure is diagnosed with a "rotor test." This involves imaging of the pump rotors, then programming a specific bolus that rotates the rotor axis 90°, and then repeating the x-ray. Failure to rotate the expected amount is an indication of possible rotor failure. Rotor stall can also be seen with a severely kinked catheter. A temporary rotor stall will occur when a patient enters an MRI scanner, but the pump will self-restart as soon as the patient leaves the magnetic field. A low battery alarm will sound when the battery has reached significant discharge. The presence of a permanent rotor stall or a low-battery condition should prompt urgent replacement of the pump.

Imaging evaluation of the catheter typically begins with plain radiography. A KUB, anteroposterior and lateral lumbar and thoracic spine series should be obtained to visualize all tubing, connectors, and entrance of the catheter into the spinal canal. If the films are normal, then a catheter access port (CAP) aspiration can be undertaken. This procedure involves accessing a port that is in direct continuity with the catheter (the CAP). Because the distal end of the catheter lies with the subarachnoid space, the CSF should be readily withdrawn through the catheter. Aspiration of at least 2 to 3 mL is necessary for the determination of a "normal" aspiration since the volume of the catheter is typically less than 0.25 mL. Failure to aspirate fluid strongly suggests catheter disruption or occlusion. Once the catheter has been cleared of the

drug solution and the CSF is obtained, a contrast medium can be injected and visualized fluoroscopically or with computed tomography. Extravasation of dye out of catheter can diagnose catheter breaks, catheter tip loculations, and migration of the catheter into the subdural or epidural spaces. Contrast should not be injected if 2 to 3 mL of CSF cannot be easily aspirated since this can potential expose the patient to ITB overdose from infusion of drug remaining in the catheter (107).

Other imaging techniques for the diagnosis of catheter malfunction include radionuclide scintigraphy and MRI. Indium I-111 DTPA can be injected into the pump reservoir and used as a tracer to determine the patency of the infusion system. After injection, serial sequential scanning occurs every 24 hours for 2 to 3 days. Normal studies should demonstrate an intact catheter and a full ventriculogram. This technique can detect evidence of catheter occlusion, pump malfunctions, and large leaks. The disadvantages of this procedure include cost, the need for 2 to 3 days to confirm the abnormality, and limited anatomic resolution (108). The MRI imaging of the thoracic spine can demonstrate spinal hemorrhage, abscess, and other soft tissue abnormalities near the catheter tip. Rarely, granulomas can develop at the catheter tip, but these have only been pathologically confirmed with intrathecal opiate therapy for chronic pain. Although rare, granulomas have the potential to cause serious neurologic injury from spinal cord compression. The MRI imaging of the catheter tip with gadolinium contrast is the diagnostic test of choice for granuloma detection (109).

The enhanced sensitivity of the H/M ratio to the presence of baclofen in the CSF contributes to the potential application of this technique as an objective adjunctive troubleshooting technique (51, 52). It is reliably sensitive to both time-dependent and dose-dependent changes after bolus or CITB administration (13, 25). The absence of response to bolus doses of ITB, whether administered via lumbar puncture or programmed through the pump and catheter, constitutes an objective evidence of dose delivery failure to target receptors in the spinal cord (52) that is more sensitive than clinical assessment with the Ashworth scale (25). For patients receiving CITB administration, the greatest diagnostic yield of H/M ratio measurement, particularly in troubleshooting scenarios, is achieved with serial assessment (52). The assessment ideally includes bilateral recordings of baseline H reflexes before ITB bolus administration, on 2 to 3 occasions after ITB bolus injection, immediately after pump implantation, followed by repeated recordings during dose titration until its disappearance.

This occurs in many patients within a dose range of 150 to 200 µg/d or less (13). Conversely, the reemergence of an elevated H/M ratio that has previously been suppressed suggests that spinal reflex hyperexcitability has been reestablished by loss or reduction of ITB exposure. Although some limitations warrant consideration (51, 52), particularly in children (110), the sensitivity and reliability of this neurophysiological technique suggest that catheter problems can be detected early, often before clinically or radiographically verifiable changes occur.

In contrast to withdrawal, which can occur despite vigilant attention, ITB overdose is generally due to human miscalculation during dosing adjustments or concentration changes. Mechanical difficulties with the pump are exceedingly rare. There are rare reports of inadvertent injection of a refill solution into the CAP that results in massive overdose (111). Overdose more commonly occurs during catheter patency studies without emptying the catheter. Clinical evidence of baclofen overdose includes profound hypotonia or flaccidity, hyporeflexia, respiratory depression, apnea, seizures, coma, autonomic instability, hallucinations, hypothermia, and cardiac rhythm abnormalities (112). The plasma and CSF levels of baclofen can be obtained, but the results may be misleading because there is no direct correlation between the programmed intrathecal dosing and the CSF baclofen levels (113). Initial management of ITB overdose is supportive and includes maintenance of airway, respiration, and circulation. Intubation and ventilatory support may be necessary. Secondary measures include interruption of ITB delivery. Optional measures for ITB overdose include CSF drainage via CAP aspiration or lumbar puncture and administration of an "antidote." Although not true antidotes, both physostigmine and flumazenil have been reported to reduce central side effects, such as somnolence and respiratory depression. Physostigmine is the more commonly utilized agent but may produce adverse affects such as bradycardia, seizures, and increased respiratory secretions. Patients who are treated for baclofen overdose must be watched closely for rebound ITB withdrawal once the pump is stopped and the drug load is decreased (112).

SUMMARY

Intrathecal baclofen therapy has evolved from an investigational therapeutic modality to a mainstay for spasticity management. Yet after almost 2 decades of widespread clinical use, there remain aspects of this therapy that challenge even experienced clinicians. Many of the interventions described in this chapter are based upon expert consensus and large clinical series. Further investigations, especially well-designed randomized trials, are warranted to refine the role of ITB therapy within spasticity management. Because neurotransmitters other than GABA can influence the spastic condition, other molecules may be worthy of study for chronic intrathecal delivery. Lastly, as with many aspects of rehabilitative care, a dedicated team approach can maximize the achievable outcomes with ITB therapy.

References

1. Brill S, Gurman GM, Fisher A. A history of neuraxial administration of local analgesics and opioids. *Eur J Anaesthesiol* 2003;20:682–9.
2. Onofrio BM, Yaksh TL, Arnold PG. Continuous low-dose intrathecal morphine administration in the treatment of chronic pain of malignant origin. *Mayo Clin Proc* 1981;56:516–20.
3. Penn RD, Kroin JS. Continuous intrathecal baclofen for severe spasticity. *Lancet* 1985 Jul 20; 2(8447):125–7.
4. Penn RD, Savoy SM, Corcos D, Latash M, Gottlieb G, Parke B, Kroin JS. Intrathecal baclofen for severe spinal spasticity. *N Engl J Med* 1989;320:1517–21.
5. Ochs G, Struppler A, Meyerson BA, Linderoth B, Gybels J, Gardner BP, Teddy P, Jamous A, Weinmann P. Intrathecal baclofen for long-term treatment of spasticity: a multi-centre study. *J Neurol Neurosurg Psychiatry* 1989;52:933–9.
6. Lazorthes Y, Sallerin-Caute B, Verdie JC, Bastide R, Carillo JP. Chronic intrathecal baclofen administration for control of severe spasticity. *J Neurosurg* 1990;72:393–402.
7. Loubser PG, Narayan RK, Sandin KJ, Donovan WH, Russell KD. Continuous infusion of intrathecal baclofen: long-term effects on spasticity in spinal cord injury. *Paraplegia* 1991;29:48–64.
8. Saltuari L, Schmutzhard E, Kofler M, Baumgartner H, Aichner F, Gerstenbrand F. Intrathecal baclofen for intractable spasticity due to severe brain injury. *Lancet* 1989 Aug 26; 2(8661):503–4.
9. Albright AL, Cervi A, Singletary J. Intrathecal baclofen for spasticity in cerebral palsy. *JAMA* 1991;265:1418–22.
10. Albright AL, Barron WB, Fasick MP, Polinko P, Janosky J. Continuous intrathecal baclofen infusion for spasticity of cerebral origin. *JAMA* 1993;270:2475–7.
11. Latash ML, Penn RD, Corcos DM, Gottlieb GL. Short-term effects of intrathecal baclofen in spasticity. *Exp Neurol* 1989;103:165–72.
12. Azouvi P, Roby-Brami A, Biraben A, Thiebaut JB, Thurel C, Bussel B. Effect of intrathecal baclofen on the monosynaptic reflex in humans: evidence for a postsynaptic action. *J Neurol Neurosurg Psychiatry* 1993;56:515–9.
13. Stokic DS, Yablon SA, Hayes A, Vesovic-Potic V, Olivier J. Dose-response relationship between the H-reflex and continuous intrathecal baclofen administration for management of spasticity. *Clin Neurophysiol* 2006;117:1283–9.
14. Bowden M, Stokic DS. Clinical and neurophysiologic assessment of strength and spasticity during intrathecal baclofen titration in incomplete spinal cord injury: single-subject design. *J Spinal Cord Med* 2009;32:183–90.
15. Schmit BD, Gaebler-Spira D. Mechanical measurements of the effects of intrathecal baclofen dosage adjustments in cerebral palsy: a pilot study. *Am J Phys Med Rehabil* 2004;83: 33–41.
16. Latash ML, Penn RD, Corcos DM, Gottlieb GL. Effects of intrathecal baclofen on voluntary motor control in spastic paresis. *J Neurosurg* 1990;72:388–92.

17. Almeida GL, Campbell SK, Girolami GL, Penn RD, Corcos DM. Multidimensional assessment of motor function in a child with cerebral palsy following intrathecal administration of baclofen. *Phys Ther* 1997;77:751–64.

18. Sgouros S, Seri S. The effect of intrathecal baclofen on muscle co-contraction in children with spasticity of cerebral origin. *Pediatr Neurosurg* 2002;37:225–30.

19. Abbruzzese G. The medical management of spasticity. *Eur J Neurol* 2002;9 (Suppl 1):30–34.

20. Orsnes G, Crone C, Krarup C, Petersen N, Nielsen J. The effect of baclofen on the transmission in spinal pathways in spastic multiple sclerosis patients. *Clin Neurophysiol* 2000; 111:1372–9.

21. Yang K, Wang D, Li Y. Distribution and depression of the GABAb receptor in the spinal dorsal horn of adult rat. *Brain Res Bull* 2001;55:479–85.

22. Russo RE, Nagy F, Hounsgaard J. Inhibitory control of plateau properties in dorsal horn neurons in the turtle spinal cord in vitro. *J Physiol* 1998;506:795–808.

23. Svirskis G, Hounsgaard J. Transmitter regulation of plateau properties in turtle motoneurons. *J Neurophysiol* 1998;79: 45–50.

24. Voisin DL, Nagy F. Sustained L-type calcium currents in dissociated deep dorsal horn neurons of the rat: characteristics and modulation. *Neuroscience* 2001;102:461–72.

25. Stokic DS, Yablon SA, Hayes A. Comparison of clinical and neurophysiologic responses to intrathecal baclofen bolus administration in moderate-to-severe spasticity after acquired brain injury. *Arch Phys Med Rehabil* 2005;86: 1801–6.

26. Dressnandt J, Auer C, Conrad B. Influence of baclofen upon the alpha-motoneuron in spasticity by means of F-wave analysis. *Muscle Nerve* 1995;18:103–7.

27. Li Y, Li X, Harvey PJ, Bennett DJ. Effects of baclofen on spinal reflexes and persistent inward currents in motoneurons of chronic spinal rats with spasticity. *J Neurophysiol* 2004;92: 2694–703.

28. Ethans KD, Schryvers OI, Nance PW, Casey AR. Intrathecal drug therapy using the codman model 3000 constant flow implantable infusion pumps: experience with 17 cases. *Spinal Cord* 2005;43:214–8.

29. Krach LE, Kriel RL, Nugent AC. Complex dosing schedules for continuous intrathecal baclofen infusion. *Pediatr Neurol* 2007;37:354–9.

30. Graham HK, Aoki KR, Autti-Ramo I, Boyd RN, Delgado MR, Gaebler-Spira DJ, et al. Recommendations for the use of botulinum toxin type A in the management of cerebral palsy. *Gait Posture* 2000;11:67–79.

31. Kunz KD, Ames SL, Saulino MF. Multimodality approach to spasticity management—how patients treated with intrathecal baclofen also utilize other spasticity interventions. *Am J Phys Med Rehabil* 2009;88:S57. (abstract)

32. Gill CE, Andrade EO, Blair CR, Taylor HM, Charles D. Combined treatment with BTX-A and ITB for spasticity: *case report. Tenn Med* 2007;100:41–2, 44.

33. Gerszten PC, Albright AL, Johnstone GF. Intrathecal baclofen infusion and subsequent orthopedic surgery in patients with spastic cerebral palsy. *J Neurosurg* 1998;88:1009–13.

34. Francisco GE, Hu MM, Boake C, Ivanhoe CB. Efficacy of early use of intrathecal baclofen therapy for treating spastic hypertonia due to acquired brain injury. *Brain Inj* 2005;19: 359–64.

35. Burns AS, Meythaler JM. Intrathecal baclofen in tetraplegia of spinal origin: efficacy for upper extremity hypertonia. *Spinal Cord* 2001;39:413–9.

36. Motta F, Stignani C, Antonello CE. Upper limb function after intrathecal baclofen treatment in children with cerebral palsy. *J Pediatr Orthop* 2008;28:91–6.

37. Fulkerson DH, Boaz JC, Luerssen TG. Interaction of ventriculoperitoneal shunt and baclofen pump. *Childs Nerv Syst* 2007;23:733–8.

38. Buonaguro V, Scelsa B, Curci D, Monforte S, Iuorno T, Motta F. Epilepsy and intrathecal baclofen therapy in children with cerebral palsy. *Pediatr Neurol* 2005;33:110–3.

39. Schuele SU, Kellinghaus C, Shook SJ, Boulis N, Bethoux FA, Loddenkemper T. Incidence of seizures in patients with multiple sclerosis treated with intrathecal baclofen. *Neurology* 2005;64:1086–7.

40. Stempien L, Tsai T. Intrathecal baclofen pump use for spasticity: a clinical survey. *Am J Phys Med Rehabil* 2000;79: 536–41.

41. Horn TS, Yablon SA, Stokic DS. Effect of intrathecal baclofen bolus injection on temporospatial gait characteristics in patients with acquired brain injury. *Arch Phys Med Rehabil* 2005;86:1127–33.

42. Baguley IJ, Bailey KM, Slewa-Younan S. Prolonged antispasticity effects of bolus intrathecal baclofen. *Brain Inj* 2005; 19:545–8.

43. Rathmell JP, Lake T, Ramundo MB. Infectious risks of chronic pain treatments: injection therapy, surgical implants, and intradiscal techniques. *Reg Anesth Pain Med* 2006;31: 346–352.

44. Horlocker TT, Wedel DJ, Benzon H, Brown DL, Enneking FK, Heit JA, Mulroy MF, Rowenquist RW, Rowlingson J, Tryba M, Yuan CS. Regional anesthesia in the anticoagulated patient: defining the risks (The Second ASRA Consensus Conference on Neuraxial Anesthesia and Anticoagulation). *Reg Anesth Pain Med* 2003;28:172–97.

45. Eskey CJ, Ogilvy CS. Fluoroscopy-guided lumbar puncture: decreased frequency of traumatic tap and implications for the assessment of CT-negative acute subarachnoid hemorrhage. *AJNR Am J Neuroradiol* 2001;22:571–76.

46. Bleyenheuft C, Filipetti P, Caldas C, Lejeune T. Experience with external pump trial prior to implantation for intrathecal baclofen in ambulatory patients with spastic cerebral palsy. *Neurophysiol Clin* 2007;37:23–28.

47. Burgher AH, Barnett CF, Obray JB, Mauck WD. Introduction of infection control measures to reduce infection associated with implantable pain therapy devices. *Pain Pract* 2007; 7:279–284.

48. Staats PS. Complications of intrathecal therapy. *Pain Med* 2008;9 (suppl):S102–S107.

49. Deer T, Chapple I, Classen A, Javery K, Stoker V, Tonder L, Burchiel K. Intrathecal drug delivery for treatment of chronic low back pain: report from the National Outcomes Registry for low back pain. *Pain Med* 2004;5:6–13.

50. Hsieh JC, Penn RD. Intrathecal baclofen in the treatment of adult spasticity. *Neurosurg Focus* 2006;21:e5.

51. Yablon SA, Stokic DS. Neurophysiologic evaluation of spastic hypertonia; implications for management of the patient with the intrathecal baclofen pump. *Am J Phys Med Rehabil* 2004;83 (10 Suppl):S10–S18.

52. Stokic DS, Yablon SA. Neurophysiological basis and clinical applications of the H-reflex as an adjunct for evaluating response to intrathecal baclofen for spasticity. *Acta Neurochir Suppl* 2007;97:231–241.

53. Horn TS, Yablon SA, Chow JW, Lee JE, Stokic DS. Effect of intrathecal baclofen bolus injection on lower extremity joint range of motion during gait in patients with acquired brain injury. *Arch Phys Med Rehabil* 2009 Nov 12. [Epub ahead of print]

54. Lechner HE, Frotzler A, Eser P. Relationship between self- and clinically rated spasticity in spinal cord injury. *Arch Phys Med Rehabil* 2006;87:15–19.

55. Evans RW, Armon C, Frohman EM, Goodin DS. Assessment: prevention of post-lumbar puncture headaches: report of the Therapeutics and Technology Assessment Subcommittee of the American Academy of Neurology. *Neurology* 2000;55: 909–14.

56. Ahmed SV, Jayawarna C, Jude E. Post lumbar puncture headache: diagnosis and management. *Postgrad Med J* 2006;82:713–16.

57. Kopell BH, Sala D, Doyle WK, Feldman DS, Wisoff JH, Weiner HL. Subfascial implantation of intrathecal baclofen pumps in children: technical note. *Neurosurgery* 2001;49:753–56.

58. Albright AL, Turner M, Pattisapu JV. Best-practice surgical techniques for intrathecal baclofen therapy. *J Neurosurg* 2006;104 (4 Suppl):233–39.

59. Penn RD. Intrathecal medication delivery. *Neurosurg Clin N Am* 2003;14:381–87.

60. Kofler M, Matzak H, Saltuari L. The impact of intrathecal baclofen on gastrointestinal function. *Brain Inj* 2002;16:825–36.

61. Vaidyanathan S, Soni BM, Oo T, Hughes PL, Singh G, Watt JW, Sett P. Bladder stones - red herring for resurgence of spasticity in a spinal cord injury patient with implantation of medtronic synchromed pump for intrathecal delivery of baclofen—a case report. *BMC Urol* 2003;3:3.

62. Murphy NA. Deep venous thrombosis as a result of hypotonia secondary to intrathecal baclofen therapy: a case report. *Arch Phys Med Rehabil* 2002;83:1311–12.

63. Carda S, Cazzaniga M, Taiana C, Pozzi R. Intrathecal baclofen bolus complicated by deep vein thrombosis and pulmonary embolism. A case report. *Eur J Phys Rehabil Med* 2008;44:87–88.

64. Rigoli G, Terrini G, Cordioli Z. Intrathecal baclofen withdrawal syndrome caused by low residual volume in the pump reservoir: a report of 2 cases. *Arch Phys Med Rehabil* 2004;85:2064–66.

65. Taha J, Favre J, Janszen M, Galarza M, Taha A. Correlation between withdrawal symptoms and medication pump residual volume in patients with implantable SynchroMed pumps. *Neurosurgery* 2004;55:390–94.

66. Hurdle MF, Locketz AJ, Smith J. A technique for ultrasound-guided intrathecal drug-delivery system refills. *Am J Phys Med Rehabil* 2007;86:250–51.

67. Coyne PJ, Hansen LA, Laird J, Buster P, Smith TJ. Massive hydromorphone dose delivered subcutaneously instead of intrathecally: guidelines for prevention and management of opioid, local anesthetic and clonidine overdose. *J Pain Symptom Manage* 2004;28:273–6.

68. Elovic E, Kirschblum SC. Managing spasticity in spinal cord injury: safe administration of bridge boluses during intrathecal baclofen pump refills. *J Spinal Cord Med* 2003;26:2–4.

69. Moberg-Wolff E. Potential clinical impact of compounded versus noncompounded intrathecal baclofen. *Arch Phys Med Rehabil* 2009;90:1815–20.

70. Deer TR, Raso LJ, Coffey RJ, Allen JW. Intrathecal baclofen and catheter tip inflammatory mass lesions (granulomas): a reevaluation of case reports and imaging findings in light of experimental, clinicopathological, and radiological evidence. *Pain Med* 2008;9:391–95.

71. Sawyer-Glover AM, Shellock FG. Pre-MRI procedure screening: recommendations and safety considerations for biomedical implants and devices. *J Magn Reson Imaging* 2000;12:92–106.

72. von Roemeling R, Lanning RM, Eames FA. MR imaging of patients with implanted infusion pumps. *J Magn Reson Imaging* 1991;1:77–81.

73. Akman MN, Loubser PG, Fife CE, Donovan WH. Hyperbaric oxygen therapy: implications for spinal cord injury patients with intrathecal baclofen infusion pumps. *Case report. Paraplegia* 1994;32:281–84.

74. Leong M, Carpenter W. Pump battery assessment: cold, old, or dead! *Neuromodulation* 2001;4:117–19.

75. Meythaler JM, Guin-Renfroe S, Law C, Grabb P, Hadley MN. Continuously infused intrathecal baclofen over 12 months for spastic hypertonia in adolescents and adults with cerebral palsy. *Arch Phys Med Rehabil* 2001;82:155–61.

76. Campbell WM, Ferrel A, McLaughlin JF, Grant GA, Loeser JD, Graubert C, Bjornson K. Long-term safety and efficacy of continuous intrathecal baclofen. *Dev Med Child Neurol* 2002;44:660–65.

77. Kadyan V, Clairmont AC, George FJ, Johnson EW. Intrathecal baclofen for spasticity management in Rett syndrome. *Am J Phys Med Rehab* 2003;82:560–2.

78. Turner MS. Early use of intrathecal baclofen in brain injury in pediatric patients *Acta Neurochir Suppl* 2003;87:81–3.

79. Murphy NA, Irwin MC, Hoff C. Intrathecal baclofen therapy in children with cerebral palsy: efficacy and complications. *Arch Phys Med Rehabil* 2002;83:1721–5.

80. Gooch JL, Oberg WA, Grams B, Ward LA, Walker ML. Care provider assessment of intrathecal baclofen in children. *Dev Med Child Neurol* 2004;46:548–52.

81. Krach LE, Kriel RL, Gilmartin RC, et al. Hip status in cerebral palsy after one year of continuous intrathecal baclofen infusion. *Pediatr Neurol* 2004;30:163–68.

82. Bjornson KF, McLaughlin JF, Loeser JD, Nowak-Cooperman KM, Russel M, Bader KA, Desmond SA. Oral motor, communication and nutritional status of children during intrathecal baclofen therapy: a descriptive pilot study. *Arch Phys Med Rehabil* 2003;84:500–506.

83. Brochard S, Remy Neris O, Filipetti P, Bussel B. Intrathecal baclofen in ambulant children with cerebral palsy. *Pediatr Neurol* 2009;40:265–270.

84. Gerszten PC, Albright AL, Barry MJ. Effect on ambulation of continuous intrathecal baclofen infusion. *Pediatr Neurosurg* 1997;27:40–44.

85. Francisco GE, Boake C. Improvement in walking speed in poststroke spastic hemiplegia after intrathecal baclofen therapy: a preliminary study. *Arch Phys Med Rehabil* 2003;84:1194–99.

86. Kofler M, Quirbach E, Schauer R, Singer M, Saltuari L. Limitations of intrathecal baclofen for spastic hemiparesis following stroke. *Neurorehabil Neural Repair* 2009;23:26–31.

87. Meythaler JM, Guin-Renfroe S, Hadley MN. Continuously infused intrathecal baclofen for spastic/dystonic hemiplegia. *Am J Phys Med Rehabil* 1999;78:247–54.

88. Dario A, Di Stefano MG, Grossi A, Casagrande F, Bono G. Long-term intrathecal baclofen infusion in supraspinal spasticity of adulthood. *Acta Neurol Scand* 2002;105:83–87.

89. Zahavi A, Geertzen JH, Middel B, Staal M, Rietman JS. Long term effect (more than 5 years) of intrathecal baclofen on impairment, disability, and quality of life in patients with severe spasticity of spinal origin. *J Neurol Neurosurg Psychiatry* 2004;75:1553–57.

90. Chow J, Yablon S, Horn T, Hemleben M, Stokic D. Effects of intrathecal baclofen administration on gait kinematics in patients with acquired brain injury. *Proceedings of the 13th Annual Meeting of the Gait & Clinical Movement Analysis Society* 2008; pp. 244–245.

91. Plassat R, Perrouin Verbe B, Menei P, Menegalli D, Mathé JF, Richard I. Treatment of spasticity with intrathecal baclofen administration: long-term follow-up, review of 40 patients. *Spinal Cord* 2004;42:686–93.

92. Francisco GE, Saulino MF, Yablon SA, Turner M. Intrathecal baclofen therapy; an update. *PM R* 2009;1:852–858.

93. Coffey RJ, Edgar TS, Francisco GE, Graziani V, Meythaler JM, Ridgely PM, Sadiq SA, Turner MS. Abrupt withdrawal from intrathecal baclofen; recognition and management of a potentially life-threatening syndrome. *Arch Phys Med Rehabil* 2002;83:735–41.

94. Hansen CR, Gooch JL, Such-Neibar T. Prolonged, severe intrathecal baclofen withdrawal syndrome: a case report. *Arch Phys Med Rehabil* 2007;88:1468–71.

95. Cruikshank M, Eunson P. Intravenous diazepam infusion in the management of planned intrathecal baclofen withdrawal. *Dev Med Child Neurol* 2007;49:626–628.

96. Khorasani A, Peruzzi WT. Dantrolene treatment for abrupt intrathecal baclofen withdrawal. *Anesth Analg* 1995;80:1054–1056.

97. Meythaler JM, Roper JF, Brunner RC. Cyproheptadine for intrathecal baclofen withdrawal. *Arch Phys Med Rehabil* 2003;84:638–42.

98. Savelka JA, Shelton JE. Cyproheptadine for pediatric intrathecal baclofen withdrawal. A case report. *Am J Phys Med Rehabil* 2007;86:994–997.

99. Albright AL, Gilmartin R, Swift D, Krach LE, Ivanhoe CB, McLaughlin JF. Long-term intrathecal baclofen therapy for severe spasticity of cerebral origin. *J Neurosurg* 2003;98:291–5.

100. Follett KA, Naumann CP. A prospective study of catheter-related complications of intrathecal drug delivery systems. *J Pain Symptom Manage* 2000;19:209–215.

101. O'Brien CP. Drug addiction and drug abuse. In: Hardman JG, Limbird LE, Molinoff PB, Buddon RW, Gilman AG, eds. The pharmacological basis of therapeutics. 9th ed. New York: McGraw-Hill; 1996:557–580.

102. Francisco GE, Yablon SA, Schiess MC, Wiggs L, Cavalier S, Grissom S. Consensus panel guidelines for the use of intrathecal baclofen therapy in poststroke spastic hypertonia. *Top Stroke Rehabil* 2006;13:74–85.

103. Yablon SA, Hayes A, Stokic DS. The utility of the h-reflex for monitoring the delivery of continuous intrathecal baclofen (CITB) in patients with dysfunctional spasticity. Dose adjustment and troubleshooting. *Neurorehabil Neural Repair* 2001;15:328. (abstract)

104. Heetla HW, Staal MJ, Kliphuis C, van Laar T. The incidence and management of tolerance in intrathecal baclofen therapy. *Spinal Cord* 2009;47:751–6.

105. Heetla HW, Staal MJ, van Laar T. Tolerance to continuous intrathecal baclofen infusion can be reversed by pulsatile bolus infusion. *Spinal Cord* 2009 Nov 17. [Epub ahead of print]

106. Soni BM, Mani RM, Oo T, Vaidyanathan S. Treatment of spasticity in a spinal cord-injured patient with intrathecal morphine due to intrathecal baclofen tolerance—a case report and review of literature. *Spinal Cord* 2003;41:586–9.

107. Lew SM, Psaty EL, Abbott R. An unusual cause of overdose after baclofen pump implantation: case report. *Neurosurgery* 2005;56:E624.

108. Stinchon JF, Shah NP, Ordia J, Oates E. Scintigraphic evaluation of intrathecal infusion systems: selection of patients for surgical or medical management. *Clin Nucl Med* 2006;31:1–4.

109. Coffey RJ, Burchiel K. Inflammatory mass lesions associated with intrathecal drug infusion catheters: report and observations on 41 patients. *Neurosurgery* 2002;50:78–86.

110. Hoving MA, van Raak EP, Spincemaille GH, Palmans LJ, Sleypen FA, Vles JS; Dutch Study Group on Child Spasticity. *Dev Med Child Neurol* 2007;49:654–9. Intrathecal baclofen in children with spastic cerebral palsy: a double-blind, randomized, placebo-controlled, dose-finding study.

111. Sauter K, Kaufman HH, Bloomfield SM, Cline S, Banks D. Treatment of high-dose intrathecal morphine overdose. Case report. *J Neurosurg* 1994;81:143–6.

112. Shirley KW, Kothare S, Piatt JH Jr, Adirim TA. Intrathecal baclofen overdose and withdrawal. *Pediatr Emerg Care* 2006;22:258–61.

113. Albright AL, Thompson K, Carlos S, Minnigh MB. Cerebrospinal fluid baclofen concentrations in patients undergoing continuous intrathecal baclofen therapy. *Dev Med Child Neurol* 2007;49:423–5.

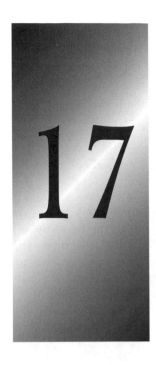

Surgery in the Management of Spasticity

David A. Fuller

PHILOSOPHY OF SURGERY FOR SPASTICITY

Spasticity occurs as a result of injury to the central nervous system (CNS). Existing surgical techniques do not repair the injury to the CNS but rather aim to improve or modulate the output of the CNS to improve a person's function. Surgical intervention may be targeted at the brain, spinal cord, peripheral nerves, or musculoskeletal system (Table 17.1). The goal of this chapter is for the reader to gain understanding of surgical options for spasticity and understand the challenges in the evolving field.

History of Surgical Interventions in Spasticity

The success rate of surgical intervention for spasticity has typically utilized as a secondary option failing more conservation treatments covered elsewhere in this text. Although peripheral musculoskeletal surgery will be the focus of this chapter, a brief review of other past uses of surgery for spasticity is useful for the reader.

Of the 3 techniques used in the past, that is, brain surgery, rhizotomy, neurectomy, each has a unique role to play in a very specialized patient population. Brain surgery utilizing temperature control electrocoagulation and cerebellar stimulation has been attempted with poor results (1–3). The most popular form of spinal cord surgery for spasticity is selective posterior rhizotomy. Typically, posterior rhizotomy is done for patients with cerebral palsy who have pure spasticity, good strength and motor control, minimal fixed contractures, and good intelligence. Posterior rhizotomy is currently utilized with variable success in very limited patients (4, 5). Neurectomy has been used with some success for very specific problems. However, neurectomy, particularly of mixed motor and sensory nerves, can have the unfortunate consequence of permanent painful dysesthetic pain (6). These techniques will be discussed more completely elsewhere in this text. The greatest success and the majority of surgical interventions for the management of spasticity are performed on the peripheral muscles and tendons (7) and will be the focus of this discussion as techniques and examples of musculoskeletal surgery will be discussed in detail.

Spasticity is a motor disorder characterized by a velocity-dependent increase in tonic stretch reflexes (muscle tone) with exaggerated tendon jerks, resulting from hyperexcitability of the stretch reflex (8–13). The result manifested in the musculoskeletal system is altered limb function. When this affects the upper extremity, one's ability to interact with the environment and perform many of his or her activities of daily living is impaired. Although deficits are noted in the lower extremities, the greatest impact is noted in ambulation and position. Surgery for spasticity is

TABLE 17.1
Surgery for Spasticity

TARGET ORGAN	PROCEDURE
Brain	Stereotactic neurosurgery
	Cerebellar stimulation
Spinal cord	Posterior rhizotomy
Peripheral nerve	Neurectomy
Muscle or tendon	Lengthening
	Release
	Transfer

directed at correcting these deficits. Sometimes, it can be highly effective, providing permanent correction. Other times, the procedure is not successful, perhaps even worsening a difficult situation. To be an appropriate option, a procedure needs to be as effective, predictable, permanent, and painless as possible. The more that is known about the CNS injury and the pathology and residual function of the muscles that are being treated, the better is the potential outcome.

Surgery can alter the force that a muscle exerts, either by decreasing, redirecting, or eliminating the muscle force (14, 15). It can also increase a muscle's effect by eliminating or decreasing the force from an antagonist muscle (16). Mobilization of stiff joints resulting from spasticity by removing passive restraints to movement such as heterotopic ossification, adhesions, or contracted ligaments can also be treated in the operating room. Although surgery cannot increase the force that a muscle generates, nor impart volitional control to a muscle with no underlying motor control, it can sometimes unmask motor control in a muscle that may not have been evident initially (Figure 17.1).

Surgery should be thought of as an important component of the paradigm for the management of the upper motor neuron syndrome. As a result, it has an important place in a comprehensive spasticity management program. Even after surgical intervention, there may be a need for other treatment interventions, including physical therapy, oral medications, chemodenervation, chemoneurolysis, and intrathecal medications. The challenge for clinicians is to pick the best modality or combination of them to treat the problems related to a person's spasticity. Each available treatment for spasticity has unique benefits, costs, and risks. Surgery has historically been viewed as a last resort, but this view is now antiquated and can be costly to patients. For some patients, especially those

with a focal presentation, surgical intervention should be considered earlier perhaps as the first treatment.

For some patients, an operative procedure has many advantages over many of the other treatment modalities available for spasticity, and for some patients, it may be considered ahead of other modalities. In the right patient, when properly planned and performed by a skilled clinician, the results are predictable as well as permanent, which is in contrast to many other interventions that are commonly used. In this chapter, the reader will have examples of proven surgical techniques provided to familiarize them with conditions amenable to surgical treatment. The primary focus will be on principles of surgical management, which will be discussed first, followed by specific surgical procedures later. Spasticity is encountered in many disorders including traumatic brain injury (TBI), stroke (cerebrovascular accident [CVA]), cerebral palsy, and multiple sclerosis (12, 17) The principles discussed in this chapter are applicable to all of these disorders in all age ranges.

Goals of Surgery for Spasticity

The goals of surgery for spasticity are no different than those of nonsurgical treatment. Some goals focus on improving function and active movement. These goals are classified as active goals. Examples of these include better forward flexion of the shoulder for grooming, better opening and closing of the hand for grasping and releasing objects, or an improved overall gait. In other cases, where patients have more advanced spasticity and demonstrate no or very limited active movement, the goals consist of passive functional improvement, and treatment addresses improving passive function and movement. Examples of these include increased

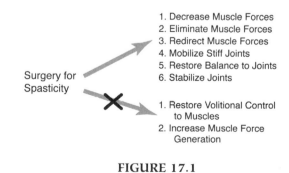

FIGURE 17.1

Although surgery cannot increase the force that a muscle generates nor impart volitional control to a muscle with no underlying motor control, it can sometimes unmask motor control in a muscle that may not have been evident initially.

TABLE 17.2
Surgical Goals

1. Improved function
   – Active function
   – Passive function
2. Pain relief
3. Decreased reliance on systemic medications
4. Permanent solution rather than temporizing treatment
5. Improved cosmesis

ease for the patient or caregiver to position the patient or limb more easily, easier hip abduction for perineal care, improved elbow extension for ease of dressing, or easier finger extension for improved hygiene of palm (18).

Other goals of surgery for spasticity include pain relief, improved cosmesis, decreased reliance on systemic medication, or chemodenervation. In regards to pain, spastic muscles can be a source of pain, which can be addressed by eliminating the spasticity (19). Cosmesis can be an important issue to a person's self-esteem and quality of life; surgical management of spasticity can address many of the balance and aesthetics to the limb and person. Sedation is a side effect of many of the oral medications prescribed for the treatment of spasticity. Sedating medications can exacerbate the already impaired sensorium of a person with TBI or CVA, and they can also hinder recovery. Many of the interventions for the management

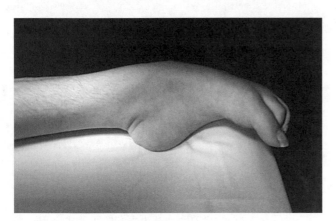

FIGURE 17.2

A severe, long-standing equinus contracture due to spasticity such as this is unlikely to respond to nonsurgical treatment.

of muscle overactivity have a limited duration of effect. Physical therapy and serial casting may be very effective at stretching out a mildly contracted joint, but once the treatment is stopped, the deformity often returns. Chemodenervation with the botulinum toxins can provide treatment for muscle overactivity, but the results last months and not a lifetime (Table 17.2). Muscle overactivity can also exacerbate other conditions. Examples of this include exacerbation of posttraumatic elbow osteroarthrosis by increased elbow tone or exacerbation of median nerve compression and carpal tunnel syndrome as a result of flexor spasticity at the wrist and or finger flexors (20).

Factors Important the Decision-Making Process

Surgery is indicated when nonoperative options have failed. It may also be indicated when nonsurgical options can be expected to fail, such as a rigid, long-standing equinus contracture at the ankle (Figure 17.2). Attempts at managing this condition by physical therapy or chemodenervation would not be successful and would be inadvisable for a number of reasons. They would consume valuable resources, require time, potentially promote prolongation and exacerbation of the deformity, and with a potentially high risk/benefit ratio potentially, hurt the patient without a realistic expectation of clinical improvement. An operation to address equinus deformity is safe, effective, and cost-effective and should be the treatment of choice in cases such as this (21).

Medical stability is important for a person to safely undergo a procedure and is an important factor in the decision to take a person to the operating room. Some patients with spasticity are healthier than others. Often, people with TBI-related spasticity are younger and healthier than those with spasticity from CVA. Preoperative evaluation should ensure that the patient has adequate vascularity to heal lower extremity surgical wounds. In addition, a cardiovascular evaluation is usually necessary before operating on a patient with a prior CVA. A person's medication regimen must be carefully reviewed when planning surgery; management of diabetic treatment and anticoagulants need to be considered and managed appropriately perioperatively.

The sensory component of a person's deficits is often overlooked in the assessment of spasticity and the development of a treatment program. Profound sensory loss can significantly limit functional improvement even after the motor control issues are addressed successfully. This is true for both the upper and lower extremities. In the upper extremity, severe sensory loss may prevent a patient from using the limb even if they are capable. Similarly, in the lower extremity, sensory deficit may put the patient at risk for skin ulceration with increased weight-bearing and no change in gait function. Profound sensory loss can be a contraindication to either upper or lower extremity surgery.

Appropriate Timing for Intervention

Selecting the appropriate time for a surgical intervention for spasticity is critical because operating too early or too late can lead to inferior outcomes. Some variables influencing the timing of surgery are specific to a patient, such as age, overall health, motivation, and cognition. Other considerations are procedure-specific. An operation to rebalance soft tissue structure is a good demonstration of this concept. It will only be successful if the underlying joints are supple, which may only exist for a short period after the onset of spasticity. Surgical arthrodesis, on the other hand, can be expected to yield good results even when performed a long period after onset. Figure 17.3 demonstrates a person with a significant equinovarus deformity involving the right foot. Addressing this condition early on will ensure greater success and enable the person to begin ambulating more comfortably earlier.

For many patients with spasticity, an injury occurs to the CNS at a discreet point in time, regardless of etiology. After the initial event, a period of neurologic recovery occurs, which can potentially continue for years. At some point in the recovery, a plateau is reached. However, in some patients, even before reaching this plateau, the manifestations of spasticity and its effect on their function are known. A pattern of movement, impairment, and disability becomes evident as demonstrated in Figure 17.4; surgery should only be contemplated after it is apparent what pattern will result after neurologic recovery is near complete.

Performing surgery, when there is a reasonable likelihood that the spasticity and disability will resolve with time, is not indicated. Complicating this issue is that the natural history of recovery is not always known early after the injury, and therefore, a period of observation is appropriate. During this period of early recovery when surgery is relatively contraindicated, observation and temporizing treatments are essential to maintain supple joints and surgery. For many patients, this dynamic period will last about 6 months or perhaps a little more. During this period, extensive rehabilitation and recovery can take place, and multimodal nonsurgical treatments are indicated.

In many patients, approximately 6 months after the initial event, the examination and pattern of spastic muscles will begin to stabilize (Figure 17.2) Surgery can be contemplated at this point depending

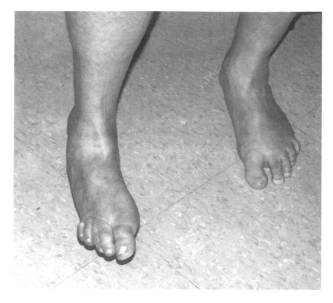

FIGURE 17.3

A spastic equinovarus deformity with associated cavus and claw toes prevents comfortable weight-bearing and gait. Patients often desire return to function as quickly as possible. Delay of treatment will prolong disability. A single surgery can predictably and permanently correct this deformity.

on other patient-specific issues. Some of these issues include nutrition, pain tolerance, cognition, ability to cooperate with rehabilitation, and comorbidities such as cardiovascular disease. Some operations require more patient cooperation and rehabilitation

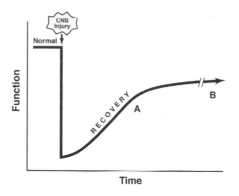

FIGURE 17.4

An example of functional recovery is shown graphically after an injury to the CNS. If functional recovery is incomplete, a plateau is reached at some point in time. At the time point A that a plateau of recovery is beginning, surgery can be done to recover additional function. Surgery can also be done later in time B, but surgery should not be delayed too long. Typically, surgery should be done between 6 and 18 months after the injury to the CNS.

afterwards than others. If the patient is not capable of participating in postoperative rehabilitation, then surgery may need to be delayed. Malnutrition, poor skin integrity, and poor pain control may be the other relative contraindications to surgery. Significant vascular disease may also preclude surgery, particularly on the lower extremities where wound healing may be compromised.

Conversely, delaying an operation for too long may also problematic and limit the best outcome. The result of waiting for surgery may in some cases do nothing more than increase and/or prolong disability and suffering. It is also possible that by letting too much time pass, the performance of the procedure may make it more difficult if not impossible to perform. Many of the interventions for spasticity involve rebalancing the muscle forces around a joint. If the activity has been out of balance for a prolonged period, then it is possible that rigid contractures will have developed in the joint precluding attempts at rebalancing. Spasticity at the foot/ankle serves as an excellent example of this issue. Waiting too long for the treatment of equinovarus deformity may result in a contracture that would have responded well to tendon rebalancing earlier in recovery but may only be amenable to an ankle arthrodesis later in recovery. Advanced, rigid deformities also put neurovascular structures at higher risk when a surgical procedure stretches a contracted joint. Waiting too long to release or lengthen the hamstrings can allow the popliteal artery to contract, and attempts to straighten the knee late in recovery will stretch the artery beyond its limits, possibly leading to ischemia in the leg. A patient with advanced knee flexion contracture is shown in Figure 17.5, where the window of opportunity for effective soft tissue releases has been missed.

Typically, the ideal timing for surgery for spasticity is usually between 6 and 18 months after the injury to the CNS; however, it is occasionally done earlier in some extreme cases that are not responding to nonsurgical treatment. A procedure can also be performed later than 18 months after injury with good results, but the 6- to 18-month time frame is a good general guideline. The decision to take a patient to the operating room should be made after input from all of the clinicians and other stakeholders. This includes the patient, family, physiatrist, neurologist, therapists, nurses, and surgeon. Table 17.3 highlights advantages and disadvantages of early and late surgery.

Planning Surgery for Spasticity

Planning is especially critical for this type of surgery. The author will discuss the process in depth for the

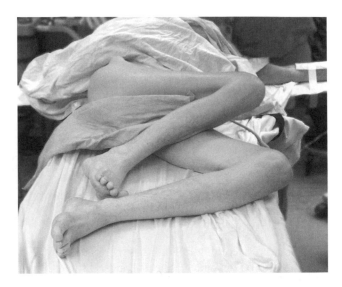

FIGURE 17.5

A patient with advanced flexion contractures of the hips and knees. Passive function is severely compromised. Sitting posture, clothing, and hygiene are impossible in this patient. Too much time has passed for effective soft tissue releases to treat the spasticity in this patient.

management of spastic elbow flexion contracture in 3 different patients (see Table 17.4). For each of these patients, the goal is the same: improved elbow extension. However, the goal is achieved in a very different manner for each of these patients. Lessons from these 3 patient examples are applicable for any joint with spastic muscles producing disability. Reproducible surgical techniques are necessary, and reasonable goals are always requisite for a successful outcome.

Information is necessary to plan a successful surgery. Knowledge regarding both the underlying structure (bones and joints) and the motors (muscles) is necessary to proceed. Once the skeleton has been evaluated, then the muscles need to be considered because a muscle-specific approach is necessary at the time of surgery. Physical examination alone is not adequate to understand individual muscle activity. The 3 main flexors of the elbow are the biceps brachii, brachialis, and brachioradialis, and these may demonstrate varying degrees of spasticity and volitional control. Instrumented, dynamic electromyography (EMG) serves this role, providing critical muscle-specific information regarding activation, volitional control, and spasticity of each muscle (22–26).

Although dynamic EMG does provide some critical information, it does not currently provide force generation data for each muscle. Force generation may be estimated based on the size of the muscle and its moment arm related to the joint under consideration.

TABLE 17.3
Timing of Surgery

Early Surgery (Time Point A, Figure 17.4)	Later Surgery (Time Point B, Figure 17.4)
Advantages: – Supply joints – Shorter duration of disability	Advantages: – Natural history of recovery more clearly known – Greater healing of initial injury
Disadvantages: – Neurologic condition may stir be dynamic and unpredictable – Medical morbidities and initial injury are relatively recent	Disadvantages: – Stiffer joints – Longer disability

Once each muscle that can contribute to the deformity, both agonists and antagonists, is understood, then treatment can be planned. Each muscle can be left alone, lengthened, shortened, released, or transferred based on it function and contribution to the deformity.

In addition to understanding the function of the agonist muscles with muscle activity, it is also critical to have a good understanding of the function of antagonist muscles, the elbow extensors. If there is no volitional control or force generation of the elbow extensors, then it is unlikely the patient will ever be able to actively extend the elbow even if the elbow flexors are lengthened and weakened. A surgery that lengthens the elbow flexors reduces their force genera-

tion, but if there is no antagonist extension force, the flexion deformity will recur with certainty. Balance at the joint can never be achieved if the extension force is zero until the flexion force equals zero also and then the elbow has no motors and this is not desirable either.

In our first patient example (see Figure 17.6), the joint does not have a passive block to motion, and the dynamic EMG for the 3 elbow flexors is illustrated in Figure 17.7. Interpretation of this figure reveals all 3 muscles to have spasticity but also underlying volitional control with phasic activation with elbow flexion and extension.

The dynamic EMG for the triceps is also shown in Figure 17.8 for patient 1. There is demonstrated appropriate activation of the elbow extensors with no spasticity. The patient is able to voluntarily activate and relax the triceps muscle. Based on this analysis, a plan for surgical lengthening of all 3 flexor muscles should be made. Figure 17.9 summarizes these considerations when planning a surgery to improve elbow extension with a spastic elbow flexion contracture. The goal of this planned surgery, as described, is to improve active elbow extension.

In a patient with a spastic elbow flexion contracture, the presentation is somewhat diffcrent, but the goal remains the same. For patient 2, the physical examination reveals lack of full passive extension with a rigid end point. The clinical picture of patient 2 at full active extension may look similar to patient 1. Radiographs, however, for patient 2 are necessary due to the passive limitations to movement and may reveal a structural problem with the joint such as heterotopic ossification as shown in Figure 17.10. Computed tomography scans are occasionally necessary to define subtle or complex structural deformities. If a struc-

TABLE 17.4
Three Examples of Patients With Spastic Elbow Flexion Contracture

Patient 1	Patient 2	Patient 3
– Age 58 – CVA – Supple elbow – Full passive extension – Active control	– Age 23 – TBI – Limited passive movement – Active control	– Age 17 – Anoxic brain injury – Rigid elbow – Active infection antecebral fossa

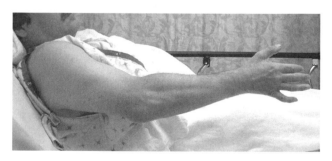

FIGURE 17.6

A patient with a spastic elbow flexion contracture lacks full active extension of the elbow. Physical examination alone does not allow identification of the offending muscles, and dynamic EMG is necessary as shown in Figures 17.7 and 17.8.

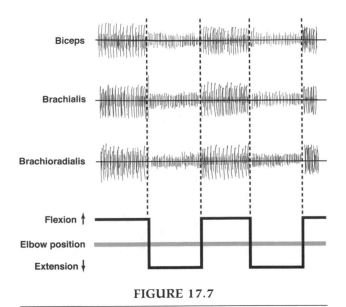

FIGURE 17.7

A dynamic EMG is shown for patient 1 with a spastic elbow flexion contracture. Phasic activation of all three elbow flexors is seen. When elbow flexion occurs, all three flexors are active. Spasticity is also seen in all three elbow flexors. When the elbow is extended, muscle activity is recorded in all three elbow flexors, which should be silent.

tural problem is identified, then it must be addressed at the time of surgery. All passive restraints to motion need to be eliminated before achieving improved motion. Surgical incisions need to be made to allow access to the structural block.

Sometimes elbow motion can be so limited that through physical examination it is difficult to ascertain whether volitional muscle control is present or not. In these cases, dynamic EMG can be helpful to ensure that the patient is able to activate the appro-

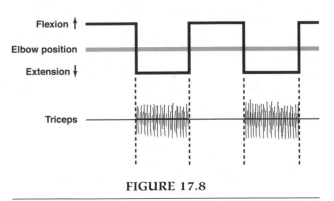

FIGURE 17.8

A dynamic EMG for patient 1 is shown for the elbow extensors. Phasic activation is seen for the triceps. When the elbow is extended, the triceps are activated. No spasticity is noted during elbow flexion.

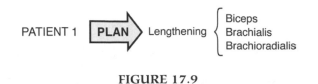

FIGURE 17.9

Surgical plan for patient 1.

priate muscles at the appropriate times. The dynamic EMG for patient 2 is shown in Figure 17.11, and it has a different appearance than the one seen in Figure 17.4 for patient 1. No volitional control is evident in the brachioradialis of Figure 17.11, rather just baseline spasticity. The goal of improved elbow extension can still be achieved, but a different procedure will be required. Rather than lengthening all 3 elbow flexors as was done for patient 1, the brachioradialis should be released for patient 2 and the other 2 elbow flexors lengthened. Different incisions are necessary for patient 2 to accomplish the goal of increased elbow extension, particularly for the resection of the heterotopic bone. The surgical plan for patient 2 is shown in Figure 17.12.

In the third patient (Figures 17.13 and 17.14) with a spastic elbow flexion deformity, the clinical problem appears differently. In this patient with no volitional control of the elbow, skin breakdown has occurred in the antecubital fossa, and an abscess has developed. The deformity is more severe and longer standing, and the patient has had poor access to the antecubital fossa for hygiene. Radiographs shown in Figure 17.13 demonstrate prior trauma, heterotopic ossification, and ankylosis of the joint. The goal remains the same: improved elbow extension. Two surgical options exist for this patient: complete release of all 3 flexors and resection of the heterotopic bone or amputation. This represents an extreme case, but one that if left untreated will result in advanced spasticity at the elbow. Figure 17.14 represents the surgical plan for this patient.

In planning surgery, these 3 examples have all examined the clinical problem of elbow flexor spasticity. Three different surgeries have been planned and hopefully executed successfully with predictable, lasting, excellent outcomes. The principles and thought that went into planning these surgeries at the elbow are applicable to deformity at any joint in the upper or lower extremity. At the different joints, the anatomy and the surgical approaches will vary but the principles remain the same. Spastic muscles with volitional control should be lengthened. Spastic muscles without volitional control should be released or potentially transferred to redirect the force.

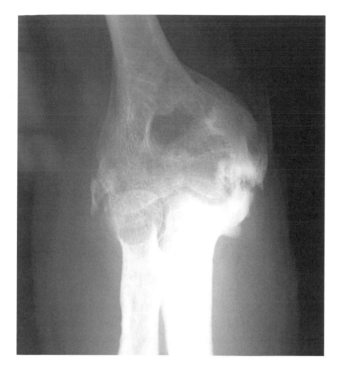

FIGURE 17.10

For patient 2, passive elbow motion is limited, and radiographs demonstrate heterotropic ossification. To improve motion, a resection of this passive block to motion is required at the time of surgery.

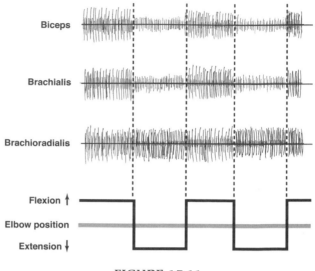

FIGURE 17.11

A dynamic EMG is shown for patient 2 with a spastic elbow flexion contracture. Phasic activation is observed for only the biceps and brachialis. When the elbow is extended, muscle activity is also noted in both biceps and brachialis. Spasticity is present in these 2 muscles. Brachioradialis shows no alteration in activity during either flexion or extension and therefore does not contribute to effective functional movement. Spasticity is present in brachioradialis. Brachioradialis does not and will not contribute to functional elbow movement. Brachioradialis should be released.

Specific Surgical Techniques for Treatment of Spasticity

Spasticity is in part due to the stretch reflex of the muscle. A principle of surgery for spasticity is to lengthen the spastic muscle, therefore decreasing the tension in the muscle and hence decreasing the spastic stretch response. By lengthening a muscle or tendon, the tension in the intrafusal muscle spindle is decreased and the stretch reflex is diminished (7, 12). Different techniques have evolved to effectively lengthen muscles (Table 17.5).

The most valuable and versatile lengthening technique in spasticity surgery is called a fractional lengthening. Most muscles have a region wherein there exists overlap between the muscle and the tendon. At this level where there is overlap between the muscle and the tendon, the fractional lengthening is performed. The tendon is simply transected within the substance of the muscle. The muscle at the myotendinous junction is then able to stretch in the region where the tendon was cut, allowing overall lengthening of the structure. Clinical pictures of a fractional lengthening

of a superficial finger flexor in the forearm are shown in Figure 17.15.

The amount of lengthening that occurs with a fractional lengthening will be proportional to the amount of tension in the muscle or the amount of passive stretch that is applied. This is depicted in Figure 17.16 using a spring mechanism analogy. In a muscle with greater spasticity, more lengthening will occur, whereas one with less will have a smaller amount of lengthening. This allows the intrinsic spasticity of the specific muscle to determine the amount of lengthening that will occur. If greater passive stretch is applied either intraoperatively or postoperatively with reha-

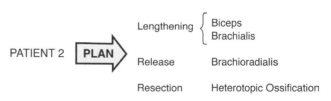

FIGURE 17.12

Surgical plan for patient 2.

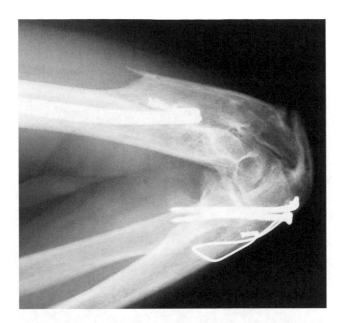

FIGURE 17.13

For patient 3, a profound rigid flexion contracture prevents movement. This contracture also makes hygiene in the antecubital fossa impossible. Fractures were associated with the original trauma. Uncontrolled spasticity was present after the initial injury. Heterotopic ossification formed with the elbow in a severely flexed position. Early effective treatment of the spasticity and heterotopic ossification may have prevented this outcome.

bilitation, then greater lengthening will also occur. If there is no adequate muscle surrounding the tendon, then it is possible for the myotendinous junction to overlengthen and rupture.

After some period (approximately 3 months) after a fractional lengthening has been performed, a new tendon will heal, filling in gap that was created with the surgery. Before the tendon gap is filled with a new tendon, the lengthening can be increased with passive stretch of the muscle or due to the spasticity. During this period of rehabilitation, it is important not to overstretch the muscle and excessively weaken or rupture the muscle.

Another surgical technique to decreases spasticity is a muscle slide or advancement. In this procedure, the entire origin of the muscle is advanced and is done occasionally with the thenar muscles in the hand for a thumb contracture. By advancing the muscle origin, the distance across which a muscle works is shortened, in effect lengthening the muscle relative to its task. Lengthening techniques are directed at the tendon portion of the muscle and require a long healthy tendon. Three such techniques that lengthen the tendon include a V-to-Y lengthening, a Z lengthening, or a lengthening with multiple hemitenotomies. These additional 4 lengthening techniques differ from a fractional lengthening and are shown Figure 17.17. Choosing one technique over another usually is based on specific anatomical constraints.

A difficulty of the Z lengthening or the V-to-Y lengthening is that the surgeon is required to pick a new length for the tendon at the time of surgery. This is not an ideal situation because there is no way to make a precise decision intraoperatively, and the surgeon is forced to guess the appropriate length. When a person with muscle overactivity undergoes surgery, they are under anesthesia, which reduces to making it near impossible to judge. Once a new length is set with the Z lengthening or the V-to-Y lengthening, it is established and cannot be changed. It takes about 3 months for the tendon to heal at its new established length during which time it must be protected or risk rupture. The lengthening with multiple hemitenotomies has similar disadvantages and is primarily used for the Achilles tendon. Achieving substantial lengthening with the V-to-Y lengthening, Z lengthening, or hemitenotomy lengthening technique is very difficult with small or weak tendons.

Tendon transfer is another important potential technique to treat spasticity. Tendon transfer is a technique that has shown great value in the treatment of peripheral nerve injuries but has limited utility in the management of spasticity. Because of the unpredictable nature of spasticity, the tendon transfer may lead to overcorrection or undercorrection of a deformity

---

TABLE 17.5
Surgical Lengthening Techniques

1. Fractional lengthening
2. Muscle slide or advancement
3. V-to-Y lengthening
4. Z lengthening
5. Hemitenotomy lengthening

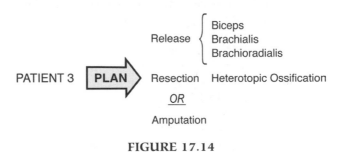

FIGURE 17.14

Surgical plan for patient 3.

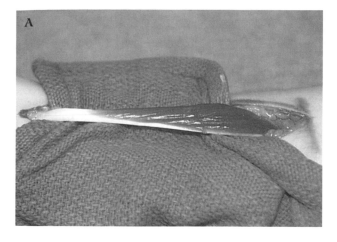

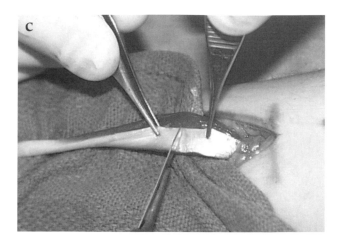

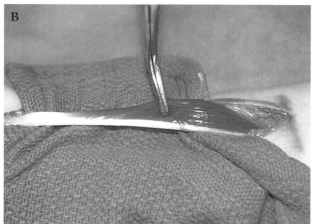

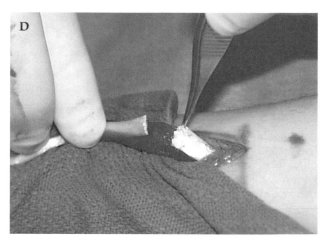

FIGURE 17.15

A fractional lengthening of a superficial finger flexor is shown. (A) A flexor digitorum superficialis is pictured at the time of surgery. The muscle belly is to the right and the tendon to the left of the figure. The myotendinous junction is the overlap region of muscle and tendon. (B) A surgical instrument is gently probing the muscle. (C) The tendon is being cut. There is extensive overlapping of the muscle in the region where the tendon is being cut. After cutting the tendon, the muscle will elongate, effectively lengthening the overall length of the muscle tendon unit.

and thus failure of the surgery. In this procedure, the surgeon detaches a tendon from one location and re-attaches it to another. The intention of transfer is to redirect the force of the muscle. A deforming or desta-bilizing force can potentially be redirected into a use-ful, functional force. An example of a tendon transfer for spasticity is the split anterior tibialis tendon trans-fer for the equinovarus foot and ankle. In this transfer, the anterior tibialis tendon is split and the lateral half of the tendon is detached from the medial foot and is newly attached to the lateral foot (Figure 17.18). When performed properly, the anterior tibialis tendon becomes a neutral dorsiflexor of the ankle. This pro-cedure can be successfully performed even with un-derlying spasticity being present.

In addition to the techniques of lengthening and transfers, other surgical techniques that can be potentially useful include neurectomy and joint arthrodesis. Neu-rectomy is the cutting of a nerve. This is irreversible, and once a nerve is cut, no recovery can be expected. This can be valuable with a pure motor nerve, such as the obturator nerve in the thigh or the ulnar motor nerve in the palm. When performing neurectomies, it is important to avoid interrupting significant sensory nerves. Sensory denervation increases the risk for skin breakdown in patients that may already have other risk factors for skin ulceration.

Joint fusion procedures are performed occasion-ally when it is not possible or unnecessary to rebal-ance the joint. This is most commonly done at the

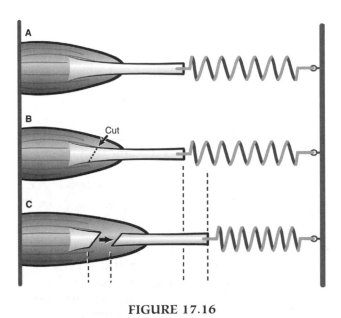

FIGURE 17.16

(A) The intrinsic spasticity of a muscle will determine the amount of lengthening that occurs with a fractional lengthening. (B) Once the tendon is cut, the amount of lengthening that occurs will be proportion to the tension in the muscle. (C) A muscle with little spasticity will exert only a small pull on the spring, and only a little lengthening will occur. For a muscle with a high degree of spasticity, once the tendon is cut, a stronger pull is exerted and a greater lengthening will occur.

wrist, ankle, or foot. For severe wrist or foot/ankle deformity, a fusion or arthrodesis can be done to permanently place the joint in one position for function. In the ankle for example, a severe equinovarus deformity due to spasticity can be corrected with an ankle fusion placing the ankle in a permanent plantigrade (foot flat on the ground) position for sitting comfort, standing, or gait.

Surgery Management of Specific Conditions

Some clinical deformities are seen frequency in patients with spasticity. This section will review many of these common clinical presentations and discuss their most appropriate surgical treatment. Patients have their own unique pattern of movement and spasticity, and as a result of this, each requires a program tailored to them. It is critical to have a thorough knowledge of anatomy, kinesiology, and surgical approaches to the involved muscles. However, the decision of which technique to choose, which muscles and joints to treat, and which to leave alone will depend on each individual patient. At the time of surgery, the surgeon

Other Muscle Tendon Lengthening Techniques

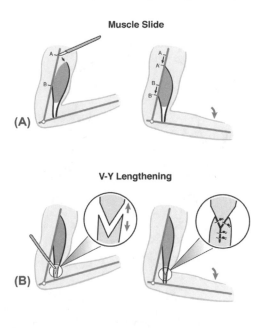

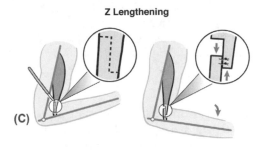

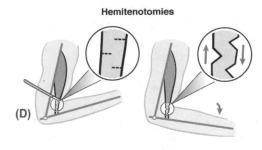

FIGURE 17.17

Four other lengthening techniques are depicted, including (A) muscle slide, (B) V-to-Y lengthening, (C) Z lengthening or (D) hemitenotomy lengthening. Choosing between a fractional lengthening and one of these other techniques is often dictated by anatomical constraints for each specific muscle.

must ensure that there is no passive restraint to motion at every joint treated. Multiple surgeries can be done in combination, and multiple joints can be operated on at the same time.

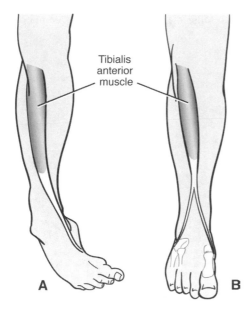

Tibialis
anterior
muscle

A   B

FIGURE 17.18

A split anterior tibialis tendon transfer is shown. The tendon transfer redirects the deforming force. In this example, (A) the anterior tibialis tendon is causing a varus deformity of the foot before transfer. (B) By transferring the lateral half of the tendon into the lateral foot, balance is restored to the foot.

Typically, if more that one joint or deformity is to be treated in a limb at one surgery, the incisions are made from proximal to distal on the limb. For example, if both an elbow and a shoulder require surgery, the surgery is done at the shoulder before the elbow. Usually, correcting the more proximal deformity first allows easier access and positioning for the more distal deformity, whereas the reverse is not true. Sometimes, it is even necessary to perform the more proximal surgery first before the more distal surgery can even be done. Bilateral surgery is occasionally necessary as well. In addition to the specific surgeries discussed below, a brief discussion of rehabilitation priorities is included with each example as necessary.

Upper Extremity

Shoulder Adduction, Internal Rotation Spasticity

The spasticity observed in the shoulder commonly produces an adducted, internally rotated position for the shoulder. This position can limit a patient's ability to move the arm in the environment and position their hand for function. For patients with a more advanced deformity, this shoulder position can make hygiene of the axilla difficult and puts the humerus at risk for fracture with aggressive manipulation of the arm.

The surgical approach for this deformity is typically made through an incision in the anterior shoulder, usually along the anterior axillary line. Through this incision, the spastic muscles contributing to the shoulder deformity can be accessed. The pectoralis major, latissimus dorsi, teres major, and subscapularis can all be accessed. Each of these muscles has the requisite myotendinous junction necessary for a fractional lengthening. Selective lengthenings or releases can be performed to increase external rotation and abduction of the shoulder. Once the muscles have been lengthened, the anterior capsule is easily accessible if anterior capsular release can also be performed.

If fractional lengthenings have been performed, some care must be taken with postoperative passive stretching to reduce the risk of rupture particularly of the pectoralis major muscle. The pectoralis major muscle does not have a large myotendinous overlap and may rupture if stretched too aggressively after a fractional lengthening, and generally active motion with only gentle assistance is allowed after the fractional lengthening. If muscle releases are performed for a more advanced deformity where simply access to the axilla with improvement in passive movement is the goal, then typically passive stretching is allowed postoperatively (27–32).

Elbow Flexion Spasticity

Lack of elbow extension limits a patient's ability to extend the arm for activities. The surgery is typically directed at the spasticity in the 3 primary elbow flexors: the biceps brachii, the brachialis, and the brachioradialis. Whether a release or lengthening of each muscle is necessary has been discussed previously under planning of surgery. This decision is often dependent on dynamic EMG data for the elbow flexor muscles. For the biceps brachii, if a lengthening is to be done, a proximal fractional lengthening at the myotendinous junction is recommended. The biceps brachii has a large myotendinous junction proximally and an incision over the anterior shoulder will allow access to it. The muscle of the biceps brachii has only a very short myotendinous junction distally, and if surgery is done at the distal end, then only the Z lengthening of the muscle can be performed. If a distal Z lengthening is done, then early postoperative motion cannot be allowed as the tendon requires time for healing. The brachialis muscle, on the other hand, has a broad myotendinous junction distally that can be approached through a transverse incision over the antecubital fossa. The brachioradialis should be lengthened in the midforearm with a longitudinal incision over the radial border of the brachioradialis. The tendon of the brachioradialis is on the undersurface of the muscle. Figure 17.19 shows a fractional lengthening of the brachioradialis in the forearm. After a fractional lengthening of each of the 3 elbow flexors, early active movement is encouraged. Gentle passive stretching can be done as well because the muscles are unlikely to rupture or overlengthen due to their broad and long myotendinous junctions.

Figure 17.20 shows an advanced flexion contracture of the elbow with no volitional control of the muscles at the elbow. If a release of the elbow muscles is necessary for advanced flexion contracture of the elbow, such as this due to spasticity, then a lateral incision over the elbow is recommended. Surgery is usually being done in situations such as this to improve access to the antecubital fossa for improved hygiene. The lateral skin incision is preferred over an anterior incision. An anterior incision is often difficult to perform with the elbow flexed, and the anterior incision does not tolerate aggressive postoperative stretching well. Through a lateral incision at the elbow, the 3 major elbow flexors can be released. First, the bicep brachii tendon is identified anteriorly and released. Next, the brachioradialis is released by cutting through the muscle belly with electrocautery while protecting the radial nerve. The brachialis is then released by cutting its muscle belly across the anterior humerus. The anterior capsule can be easily released from this approach as well. Once these muscles are released, the elbow can be passively stretched intraoperatively. After the 3 elbow flexor muscles have been released, the skin,

brachial artery, and median nerve will then limit extension. Attention should be paid to not injure these structures acutely with overzealous stretching. Typically at the time of surgery, about a 50% improvement can be realized with releases without compromising the skin or neurovascular structures. Stretching postoperatively can slowly realize more significant gains.

On rare occasions, other muscles can contribute to the spastic elbow flexion deformity, such as the origin of the flexor-pronator muscles, which are attached to the medial epicondyle. These muscles, or others, occasionally require releases also at the elbow for very advanced deformity due to spasticity. For most of cases, simply releasing the 3 primary elbow flexors is adequate (27–31).

Forearm Pronation Spasticity

Spasticity involving the pronator muscles makes it difficult for a patient to supinate the arm and may complicate one's ability to use the hand. A flexed and pronated forearm can be treated in selected patients by simply releasing the flexor pronator origin (33). Alternatively, a more functional, muscle-specific approach requires selective lengthening of the 2 pronator muscles: the pronator quadratus and the pronator teres. The pronator quadratus is a short broad muscle in the distal forearm. Its ulnar attachment is usually approached for the lengthening. Either a fractional lengthening or muscle slide can be done at its origin on the ulna. For a more severe deformity, a release of its entire attachment into the ulna can be done, which allows the muscle attachment to slide radially.

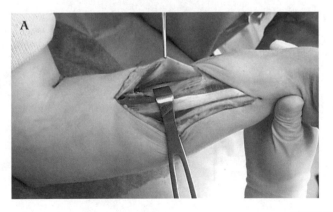
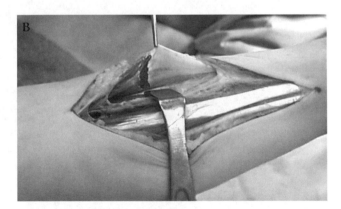

FIGURE 17.19

Preoperative (A) and postoperative (B) images of a fractional lengthening of the brachioradialis are shown. The broad tendon is on the undersurface of the brachioradialis muscle in the mid forearm. The ultimate amount of lengthening that occurs to this muscle will be determined by the amount of spasticity in the muscle and the passive stretch that may be applied after fractional lengthening.

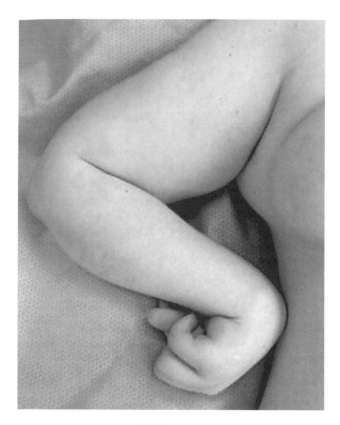

FIGURE 17.20

Advanced spasticity has led to deformity in this arm. Elbow flexion, forearm pronation, wrist flexion, and finger flexion lead to the typical posture. Normally, more adduction and internal rotation of the shoulder are seen, but this patient has had a chronically anteriorly dislocated shoulder since the time of her trauma. Difficulty with control of her spasticity after the initial injury lead to inability to maintain the shoulder in a reduced position, and ultimately, it required an arthrodesis to control pain.

The ulnar origin of the pronator quadratus is shown in Figure 17.21(A). The pronator teres is approached through an incision over the volar and radial aspect of the midforearm. A fractional lengthening can be done at the myotendinous junction, or if desired, it can simply be released from the radius. A fractional lengthening of the pronator teres is shown in Figure 17.21(B). Postoperatively, for either a fractional lengthening or a release, gentle stretching is appropriate. When a contracture has been long standing, other structures may contribute to the deformity. Other potential contributing structures include the interosseous ligament or the capsule of the distal radioulnar joint. Addressing these other restraints to rotation can be difficult for some patients.

Wrist Flexion Spasticity

Wrist flexion spasticity is often encountered in combination with finger flexion spasticity and exacerbates difficulties with the use of one's hand. It may also contribute to symptoms of carpal tunnel syndrome. For mild wrist flexion deformity, in which active wrist extension is present, myotendinous lengthening of the wrist flexors is possible through a volar incision over the forearm. The flexor carpi radialis, flexor carpi ulnaris, and palmaris longus can all be treated with fractional lengthening. Dynamic EMG can be particularly helpful in determining which muscles are firing appropriately and which are contributing to the deformity and can also establish the presence of wrist extensor activation when it is a very weak wrist. For patients with no active wrist extension or very weak extension, the wrist flexion deformity will recur after lengthening of the wrist flexors, and a wrist arthrodesis should be considered as the primary treatment.

For severe wrist flexion contractures, a wrist arthrodesis is recommended. Arthrodesis will provide a permanent neutral position of the wrist that is desirable for patients with severe deformity. This will place the hand in a better position for both active function and passive care needs. Preoperative and postoperative images of a wrist arthrodesis are shown in Figure 17.22. At the time of arthrodesis, typically a skeletal shortening is also done to relax tension on the volar skin and neurovascular structures. The skeletal shortening can be accomplished by resection of the distal radius and ulna or resection of the proximal carpal row at the time of surgery. A dorsal incision is made over the wrist, and a wrist fusion plate is used bridging and compressive from the third metacarpal to the distal radius. Typically, iliac crest bone graft is not necessary. The wrist arthrodesis also prevents development of a hyperextension deformity of the wrist, which can occur if wrist flexors are simply released and spasticity exists in the wrist extensors. This is a greater concern for a patient with a longer life expectancy, for example, a young person with a TBI, rather than someone with a shorter life expectancy, such as a stroke patient.

Finger Flexion Spasticity (Extrinsic Hand Spasticity)

Extrinsic finger flexion spasticity severely impairs hand function. Patients have difficulty with grasp and release activity as well as difficulties performing their activities of daily living both active and passive. Selective fractional lengthening is a very powerful tool for

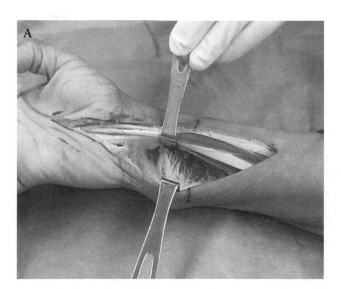 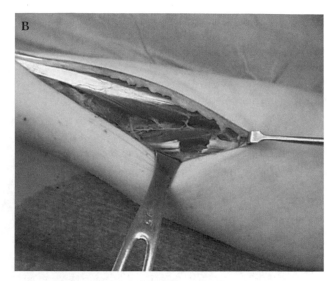

FIGURE 17.21

The origin of the pronator quadratus (A) is amenable to either fractional lengthening, muscle slide, or release in the distal forearm. The pronator teres (B) has undergone a fractional lengthening in this picture to improve active forearm supination.

lengthening the extrinsic finger flexors, improving finger flexor spasticity. All the superficialis and profundus finger flexors have generous myotendinous junctions in the midforearm that can be reached through a longitudinal incision over the midforearm for lengthening. Images of a selective fractional lengthening of an individual extrinsic finger flexor have been shown previously in Figure 17.15. Alternatively, for an advanced contracture, where the goal is simply passive opening of the hand, a superficialis to profundus tendon transfer is an extremely effective surgical tool. The choice of active or passive finger opening is entirely dependent on the underlying motor control of both the extrinsic finger flexors and extensors.

Dynamic EMG is valuable in planning surgical interventions to treat this deformity. Evaluating with EMG enables the identification of which muscles are firing appropriately or demonstrating spasticity, co-contraction, or other components of the upper motor neuron syndrome. It increases the surgeon's knowledge of the underlying motor control and assist him or her in muscle and procedure selection (34). If one muscle group of finger flexors exhibits spasticity with volitional control and the other muscle group is normal, then a selective fractional lengthening of only the one spastic group is all that is necessary (35). Operating unnecessarily on the normal, nonspastic muscle group will produce iatrogenic, undesirable weakness in the muscles that were otherwise normal. Alternatively, if some of the muscles studied showed no voli-

tional control, then selective releases may be indicated to treat the deformity. After fractional lengthenings of the extrinsic finger flexors, immediate postoperative active finger movement is allowed and encouraged. Passive extension stretching of the fingers is discouraged after a fractional lengthening of the extrinsic finger flexors for the first 6 weeks postoperatively because it can cause overlengthening or rupture of the muscles.

For an advanced finger flexion deformity, a superficialis to profundus tendon transfer is recommended (36–39). This requires an extended volar incision including a carpal tunnel release. All of the superficialis tendons are transected in the palm at the level of the carpal tunnel. All of the profundus tendons are transected proximally in the forearm just distal to their myotendinous junctions. The fingers are then maximally extended intraoperatively. Figure 17.23 shows an intraoperative image of a superficialis to profundus transfer. A wrist arthrodesis (see Figure 17.22) was performed at the same time.

The superficialis to profundus tendon transfer does not necessarily provide active control to the fingers, but it does provide a small amount of antagonist force in case extensor tendon spasticity exists. In rare cases, some active finger flexion may be observed if there exists underlying motor control of the superficialis muscles. If the thumb has a spastic flexion contracture, its tendon should be released and transferred also to the superficialis tendons proximally and also when a superficialis to profundus transfer is performed. Generally, extension splinting is done for about 6 weeks after the procedure. Often, this superficialis to profundus transfer is performed in combination with a wrist arthrodesis and an ulnar motor neurectomy used to treat intrinsic hand spasticity.

Hand Spasticity (Intrinsic Spasticity)

Finger Flexion Spasticity

If the intrinsic muscles of the hand are contracted, either a lengthening or denervation can be done. A hand with mild intrinsic spasticity is shown in Figure 17.24. Lengthening can be done of the palmar intrinsic muscles at the myotendinous junction through selective palmar incisions. The dorsal intrinsics can be approached through dorsal longitudinal incisions over the metacarpals. Dorsally, the muscle origins are released and advanced distally to lengthening the dorsal intrinsics. Early active finger motion is encouraged after the lengthening procedures (40).

For a more severe hand intrinsic contracture due to spasticity with no volitional control, an ulnar motor nerve neurectomy can be done at Guyon canal. The ulnar motor branch runs deep around the hook of the hamate where it can be isolated and transected. Resection of a 1-cm segment of the nerve is recommended to reduce the risk of regeneration of the nerve. Passive splinting with the fingers in extension is done postoperatively after the neurectomy.

Thumb Spasticity (Intrinsic Spasticity)

Patients with thumb spasticity have difficulty extending the thumb for opposition. This is seen in Figure 17.24 and is called a thumb-in-palm deformity. When there is underlying volitional control of the thenar muscles, the Matev slide is the recommended lengthening technique. The thenar muscle slide is performed using a longitudinal palmar incision, through which the origin of the thenar muscles is identified as they arise off of the palmar fascia. Using a surgical blade, the thenar muscles are then elevated and advanced radially. Protection of the recurrent motor branch is essential so that the muscles are not denervated. Early active movement is allowed during rehabilitation after the muscle slide has been performed. If the patient also has extrinsic spasticity of the flexor pollicis longus, a fractional lengthening should be done simultaneously in the forearm for extrinsic thumb flexor (41–43).

For a severe intrinsic contracture of the thumb with uncontrolled spasticity, it is also possible to simply cut the recurrent motor nerve in the palm at the same time that the muscles are advanced. The influence of any ulnar innervated muscle must also be considered. If an ulnar motor neurectomy is performed concomitantly, then the active contribution from the ulnar innervated muscles is also eliminated. Release of the adductor pollicis tendon may be necessary if an advanced, rigid contracture is present. Occasionally, a fusion of the thumb interphalangeal joint is necessary if the flexion deformity is advanced due to extrinsic flexor spasticity. Selective temporary nerve blocks at the wrist with lidocaine can help determine the rela-

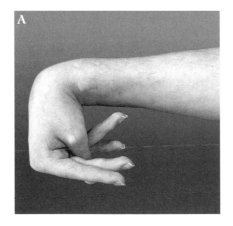
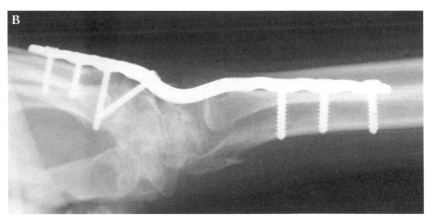

FIGURE 17.22

A severe wrist flexion contracture is shown (A). Despite the spasticity in the wrist and intrinsic muscles, the extrinsic finger flexors have not contracted the interphalangeal joints in this position. Once the wrist is straightened however, the tension in the extrinsic finger flexors will become apparent also. Mild wrist flexion contractures may be amenable to selective lengthening, but severe contractures such as this one are treated surgically with fusion (B).

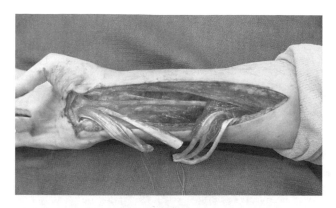

FIGURE 17.23

An intraoperative photograph of a superficialis to profundus tendon transfer for extrinsic finger flexor spasticity. The profundus tendons have been released from their muscles proximally and remain attached to the fingers distally. The superficialis tendons have been released from the fingers distally and remain attached to their muscles proximally. Full passive extension of the fingers is now possible.

tive contribution of the median and ulnar innervate muscles (41–43).

Lower Extremity (30, 44–50)

Hip Flexion and Adduction Spasticity

Deformities secondary to muscle overactivity in the hip muscles are encountered in patients with both higher and lower levels of function. In the ambulatory patient, it results in the impairment of gait. Hip flexor spasticity can contribute to a crouched gait deformity, with a resultant much energy-consuming gait

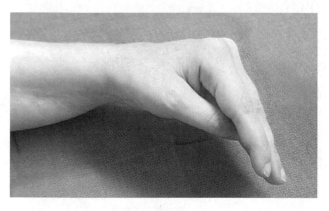

FIGURE 17.24

A hand with intrinsic spasticity is shown. In addition to the intrinsic-plus position of the fingers, a thumb-in-palm deformity is also seen.

than one with normal extension of the hip and knee. Adductor spasticity leads to a scissoring gait deformity. In this gait deformity, the width of stance is compromised and one leg can strike the other as limb advancement is attempted, which results in greater instability and greater risk of falls. For the lower-level patient, these deformities can greatly complicate positioning, personal hygiene sitting posture, transfers, and hygiene.

The muscles that contribute to this deformity can be approached surgically through a longitudinal incision over the proximal, medial thigh. Through this incision the adductor muscles are easily approached and can be either lengthened or released. The adductor muscles that can be addressed through this incision include the gracillis, adductor longus, adductor brevis, and adductor magnus. Also accessible through this incision is the obturator nerve. Rather than releasing the muscles, an obturator nerve neurectomy can be performed through this same incision. The neurectomy at this level will not completely denervate the adductors but only partially due to its many proximal branches to these muscles.

Once the adductors have been corrected, deeper dissection through this same incision will expose several of the critical hip flexors at the level of the proximal femur. Once the femur can be palpated, retractors should be placed above and below the femur at the level of the lesser trochanter to expose the pectineus and the iliopsoas. Both of these muscles can be released under direct vision at this point. The iliospoas is released off of the lesser trochanter. Because of the soft tissue attachments of the iliospoas to the anterior hip capsule and to the presence of other hip flexor muscles, this surgery will not eliminate all active hip flexion. A patient with severe adductor spasticity with scissoring of the legs is shown in Figure 17.25(A). In this example, a hip flexion contracture is demonstrated. Figure 17.25(B) shows a postoperative image after the release of the spastic hip adductors and flexor muscles.

Physical therapy begins immediately after surgery. Early active motion and weight-bearing are encouraged after the procedure. Often, an abduction pillow is used between the legs for about 6 weeks postoperatively while the patient is in bed. This surgical incision is at an increased risk of wound infection due to its proximity to the perineum. A drain should be left in this proximal thigh wound postoperatively, and close attention to wound hygiene is necessary.

Hip Extension Spasticity

Occasionally, spasticity in the hip extensors can lead to functional problems for patients. For active, ambulatory patients, hip extensor spasticity can limit forward progression of the limb and limit stride length. For the nonambulatory patient, limited forward flexion of the hip can impair sitting posture. If the patient cannot flex adequately at the hip, attempts to flex the hip and seat the patient will transmit forces and motion to the lumbar spine. To treat this problem surgically, a lengthening of the hip extensors can be performed.

With the patient in the prone position, a longitudinal incision is made over the proximal hamstring tendon. While protecting the sciatic nerve, the proximal hamstring tendons are released off of the ischium. This allows the origin of the muscle to retract distally, thus decreasing the hip extensor pull of the hamstrings. In addition, the gluteal muscles can be

lengthened or selectively released if necessary. A risk of this operation is that it places a surgical wound in a weight-bearing area during seating and is at risk for breakdown during healing.

Knee Flexion Spasticity

Flexor spasticity at the knee makes it difficult for a patient to straighten the knee. For the ambulatory patient, this leads to the high-energy gait crouched gait pattern. When a person's knees are bent at 30°, his quadriceps are required to perform twice the work they have to do normally. This can have deleterious effects on a person's ambulation, ability to stand, and transfer. Often, hip and knee spasticity occur in

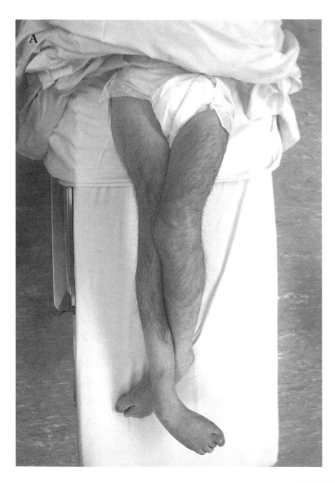
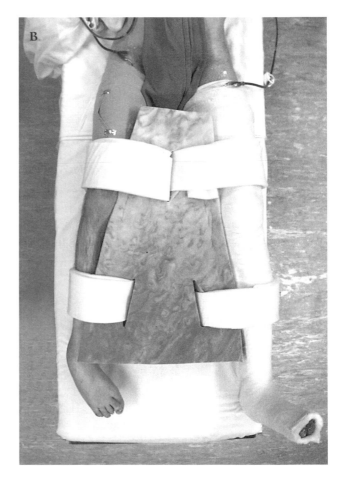

FIGURE 17.25

A patient with spastic hip adduction contracture is shown both preoperatively (A) and postoperatively (B). The hip adductors and flexors have been released through incisions in the proximal medial thigh, and surgical drains have been left in the wounds. In the left leg, the knee flexion deformity was treated with hamstring release as well, and the foot was corrected with soft tissue rebalancing. A hip adduction pillow is used, postoperatively and a long leg cast was chosen for the left knee and ankle.

combination, and surgery is necessary at both joints to improve posture. For the less-active patient, advanced deformity at the knee can lead to hygiene problems in the popliteal fossa. Sitting posture can be compromised because rigid knee flexion deformities can exceed 90° for some patients with spasticity. An advanced knee flexion contracture is shown in Figure 17.26.

Surgical treatment of knee flexor spasticity needs to consider all of the muscle forces posterior to the knee flexion axis that can contribute to this deformity. These muscles are approached surgically through medial and lateral incisions over the distal hamstring tendons. Through the medial incision, the sartorius, gracillis, semitendinosus, and semimembranosis can be isolated and either lengthened or released. Through the lateral incision, the biceps femoris can be isolated and treated. Importantly, through the lateral incision, the posterior portion of the iliotibial band, which can contribute to the knee flexion deformity, should be incised (51, 52).

Typically, dynamic EMG data are not available on the individual knee flexors. Therefore, decisions regarding treatment of the knee flexors, whether to release or lengthen, require a degree of intraoperative decision making coupled with knowledge of preoperative analysis. A lengthening or release of each muscle can be done. Once the muscles have been treated, if there is also a posterior knee capsular contracture, then a posterior knee capsulotomy can be done to increase knee extension. Through the lateral incision, an elevator is advanced across the posterior aspect of the knee joint, releasing the posterior capsule off of the distal femur. This needs to be done carefully to protect the neurovascular structure behind the knee. Occasionally, for severe contractures at the knee, an amputation should be considered (53). Figure 17.5 shows severe knee flexion contractures for which amputation may be the appropriate surgical treatment to prevent ulceration of the popliteal fossa.

Postoperative physical therapy can begin immediately whether lengthenings or releases of the hamstrings have been done. Daily stretching, gait retraining, and ambulation are allowed for patients with mild deformity. Occasionally, a knee immobilizer is used for about 6 weeks. For patients with advanced deformity, a period of extension casting or use of an external fixator that is adjusted weekly can slowly stretch a firm contracture. Figure 17.25(B) shows a postoperative cast for the left leg after release of the knee flexors. Neurovascular structures posterior to the knee are at risk of injury not only during performance of the procedure but also during the postoperative period from stretching.

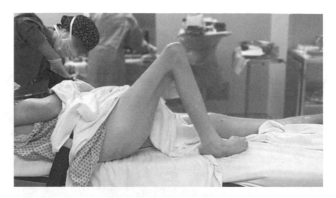

FIGURE 17.26

A severe knee flexion contracture due to spasticity is shown. The ipsilateral leg also has a hip flexion contracture and an equinovarus deformity at the foot and ankle.

Knee Extension Spasticity

Muscle overactivity can be a problem for both ambulatory and nonambulatory patients. Although ambulatory patients may have active goals, the latter may have more passive goals. Knee extensor spasticity leads to a slow and energy-costly pattern that makes it challenging for a person to maneuver on stairs and other obstacles. For the nonambulatory, a spastic knee can make comfortable sitting difficult. A well-designed operative procedure can address issues in both of these groups.

For mild knee extension spasticity, a selective fractional lengthening of the quadriceps muscle can be performed. This is typically done through an anterior midline incision just proximal to the patella. The different sections of the quadriceps can be isolated and fractional lengthenings performed. In about one quarter of patients, the spasticity is due to the central portion of the quadriceps, the rectus femoris, which is shown in Figure 17.27(A). For these patients, the rectus femoris can be selectively lengthened (Figure 17.27(B)), released, or even transferred (Figure 17.27(C)) to the medial hamstrings to act as a knee flexor during swing phase of gait (54–56). A fractional lengthening of the vastus lateralis and medialis can also be performed if necessary.

The transfer of the rectus femoris should be done if the rectus femoris demonstrates phasic EMG activity synchronous with appropriate hamstring activation. A second incision is necessary over the distal, medial hamstrings to accomplish this procedure. Typically, enough length of tendon can be harvested with the rectus femoris anteriorly to weave it through the gracillis muscle in the medial thigh. The defect left in the quadriceps tendon anteriorly can be closed in a side-to-side

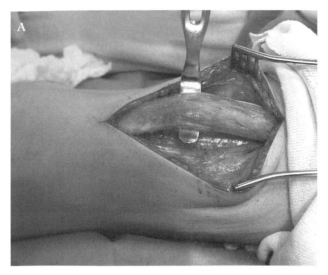

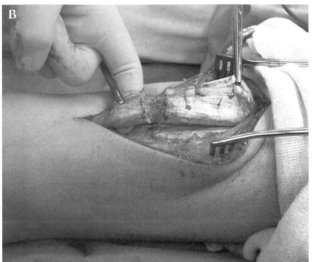
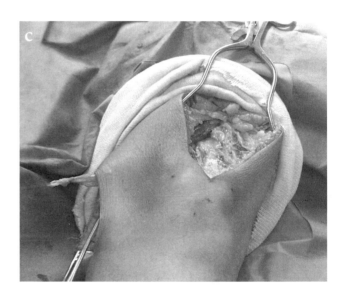

FIGURE 17.27

Spastic knee extension contracture can often be due to isolated spasticity in the rectus femoris. In (A), the rectus femoris has been isolated. In (B), a myotendinous lengthening of the rectus femoris has been performed to help a patient with a mild stiff knee gait. (C) demonstrates another patient where the rectus femoris is being transferred into the medial thigh and attached to the gracillis.

fashion. Immediate weight-bearing and knee flexion are typically allowed after such a procedure.

For nonambulatory patients where the goal is simply better knee flexion for improved sitting posture, a V-to-Y lengthening of the distal quadriceps tendon is recommended. Significant gains in flexion can be realized with this tendon lengthening. Preoperative and postoperative images of a knee treated with a V-to-Y lengthening of the quadriceps are shown in Figure 17.28. A reverse deformity, that is, a flexion deformity of the knee, can be created with excessive lengthening

of the quadriceps tendon in a V-to-Y fashion, particularly if underlying hamstring spasticity exists.

Foot and Ankle Spasticity

Surgery is an incredibly powerful tool in the lower extremity especially around the foot and ankle. For effective ambulation, a plantigrade foot is necessary. Surgery is very effective at accomplishing this goal. A supple, well-balanced, well-aligned active foot is the highest goal. However, this goal may not always be

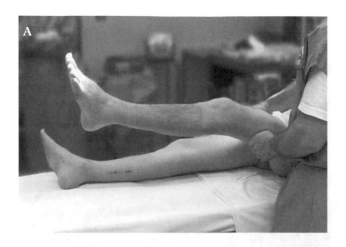
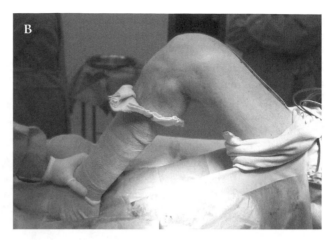

FIGURE 17.28

A more severe knee extension contracture is seen (A), and a V-to-Y lengthening of the quadriceps tendon was performed to improve passive knee flexion (B) for better sitting posture.

attainable, in which case an arthrodesis provides an excellent alternative goal to provide a stable, painless foot for weight-bearing. The flexibility of the patient's foot and ankle, as well as the underlying motor control of the muscles, often determines whether a soft tissue reconstruction or an arthrodesis is the surgical goal. Achieving either goal can provide significant improvement in patient function.

Equinus Ankle Spasticity

Equinus spasticity leads to significant alterations in gait. An equinus posture contracture of the ankle will prevent forward progression of the tibia during stance phase. Acutely, this will limit stride length and gait, and over time, compensatory deterioration of the midfoot and knee can be observed in response to the deformity. The majority of equinus deformity is a result of overactivity of the soleus and gastrocnemius muscles; however, other muscles that cross the ankle can also contribute to this deformity and need to be considered during corrective surgery (57, 58).

There are several different procedures that have demonstrated efficacy in the management of equinus ankle spasticity. Two of them utilize a lengthening technique and include a fractional lengthening at the myotendinous junction and percutaneous hemitenotomies through the tendon. To perform fractional lengthening of the soleus and gastrocnemius, a longitudinal incision is made over either the medial or the lateral calf. The interval between the gastrocnemius and soleus muscles is identified and developed. Through this interval, the myotendinous junctions of

both muscles are identifiable and can be lengthened. The interval between the 2 muscles is shown at mid-calf level in Figure 17.29 (57, 58).

Alternatively, the Achilles tendon can be lengthened percutaneously distally using 3 hemitenotomies. Once the hemitenotomies are performed, the ankle is

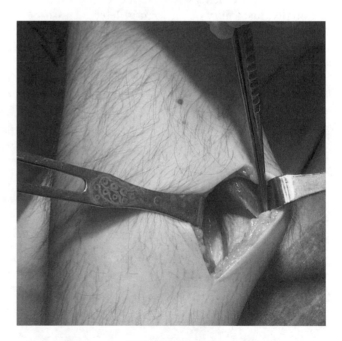

FIGURE 17.29

A longitudinal incision is shown in the midportion of the calf. The broad tendons of the gastrocnemius and soleus are evident through this incision and can be selectively lengthened.

passively dorsiflexed, effectively tearing the weakened tendon. The hemitenotomies allow the tendon to tear longitudinally, thus leaving some residual tendon fibers in continuity for healing if performed correctly. This percutaneous, distal technique does not allow selective lengthening of the soleus and gastrocnemius (57, 58).

Immediate weight-bearing is allowed after either lengthening techniques. The ankle must be protected for 8 to 12 weeks after surgery with either a cast or orthotic to prevent overlengthening or rupture of the calf muscles. If there is no active dorsiflexion, the equinus contracture will likely recur unless bracing and stretching are continued into the future (57, 58).

Varus Foot Spasticity

Mild deformity can be treated with orthotics, but unfortunately for many patients, the varus foot deformity progresses. The foot may develop such advanced deformity that weight-bearing is impossible on the plantar surface. Over time, a very rigid contracture can develop and will only be treatable with arthrodesis. A patient with bilateral equinovarus deformities is shown in Figure 17.30. Before advanced rigid deformity development, it may be possible to rebalance the spastic muscles and produce a supple, plantigrade foot. Radiographs are essential to ensure no structural problems with the underlying joint. Occasionally, instability of the joint is detected as shown in Figure 17.31. Before attempts at soft tissue rebalances, these structural problems need to be recognized (58–60).

The varus foot is seen most commonly in conjunction with an equinus deformity. Spasticity in any

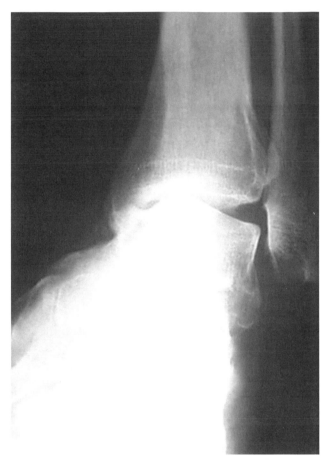

FIGURE 17.31

A weight-bearing radiograph of a patient with a clinical equinovarus deformity is shown. In addition to surgical correction of the spasticity, it is necessary to reconstruct the lateral collateral ligament of the ankle to improve the posture of the foot and ankle.

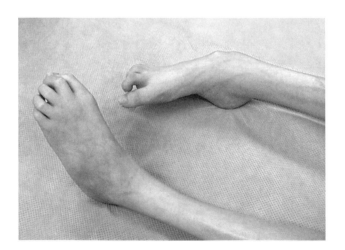

FIGURE 17.30

A patient with bilateral equinovarus deformity is shown. The deformity on the right limb is more advanced.

muscle on the medial aspect of the foot can contribute to the varus deformity including the anterior tibialis, posterior tibialis, extensor hallucis longus, or flexor digitorum longus. As the heel shifts into increasing varus, the spasticity in the ankle plantar flexors will also exacerbate the varus deformity (58–60).

Fractional lengthenings can be performed to any of the muscles that contribute to a varus foot. Fractional lengthening is the recommended treatment when the deformity is mild. When performing this procedure, the myotendinous junctions of many of these muscles should be approached through longitudinal incisions over the mid to distal tibia. The posterior tibialis muscle is accessed via an incision just posterior to the medial tibia. The anterior tibialis and extensor hallucis longus can be lengthened in the anterior compartment. If the muscles have moderate to severe spasticity, the addition of a tendon transfer is also recommended to treat the deformity. Dynamic EMG assists in the muscle selection process for the performance of any procedure (22, 61).

Tendon transfers are routinely performed through very small incisions over the distal insertions of the appropriate tendons. The detached tendons are then tunneled and transferred into bone and secured with bone anchors (62, 63). For the varus foot, if the anterior tibialis is involved, then a split anterior tibialis tendon transfer is recommended (Figure 17.18). In this transfer, the lateral half of the anterior tibialis tendon is detached from the medial foot, tunneled subcutaneously across the foot, and reattached into the cuboid. Figure 17.32 demonstrates the attachment of the lateral limb of the tendon into the cuboid using a bone anchor. If the 2 limbs of the tendon are tensioned equally, then the muscle should produce neutral dorsiflexion without a varus or valgus torque (58–60).

If the posterior tibialis tendon is also contributing to the varus deformity, then a fractional lengthening of this muscle is recommended at the same time that the split anterior tibialis transfer is done. If the extensor hallucis and flexor digitorum longus are also contributing to the varus deformity, then they may be lengthened, released, or transferred. The flexor digitorum longus has been used as a transfer into the medial calcaneus to increase calf strength. The extensor hallucis longus has been transferred into the midfoot to supplement ankle dorsiflexion during swing phase.

When soft tissue rebalancing has been done, whether with lengthenings or tendon transfers, immediate weight-bearing is allowed in a short leg cast. The position of the foot and ankle must be held in a neutral position for 12 weeks after surgery. The cast can be converted to a molded orthotic or a well-fitting cast boot during early recovery if the patient is compliant with removable devices. Using a removable device allows daily monitoring of the soft tissues, whereas a cast for the 12-week tendon-healing period ensures compliance (58–60).

If soft tissue rebalancing is not possible, then it is usually possible to restore proper position to the foot and ankle with bone surgery. An ankle arthrodesis can restore a plantigrade ankle, and a triple arthrodesis can restore a neutrally aligned heel. Occasionally, a plantar arthrodesis is necessary with fusion of the tibia, talus, calcaneus, cuboid, and navicular. Such an arthrodesis is shown in Figure 17.33 using an intramedullary fibula strut graft. If arthrodesis is done, basic soft tissue rebalancing should also be performed to help maintain the position of the foot and ankle during healing and subsequent ambulation. Immediate weight-bearing is often allowed after arthrodesis also in a well-molded short leg walking cast (58–60).

Valgus Foot Spasticity

Spasticity with a resultant valgus foot (outward angulation of the foot at the ankle) is much less common than equinovarus deformity. The main deforming force in this presentation is a result of spasticity involving the peroneal muscles (Figure 17.34). Muscle overactivity from the plantar flexors also contributes to the deformity, as the heel moves into an increasingly valgus position. Depending in the severity of the deformity, the spastic muscles can be treated with either fractional lengthening or transfer. The peroneal muscles are accessible through a longitudinal incision over lateral compartment of the calf. For more advanced spasticity, the peroneus longus, if it is the main contributing muscle to the valgus, should be transferred to the medial aspect of the midfoot. Rigid valgus deformities can be salvaged with arthrodesis (64).

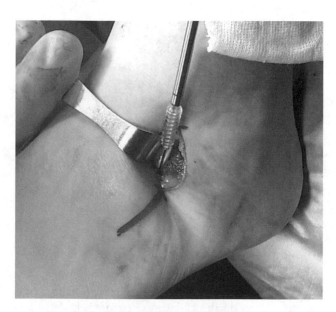

FIGURE 17.32

Tendon transfers can be done through very small incisions using bioabsorbable bone anchors (interference screws) to secure the tendons into the bone. Shown here is a bone anchor being inserted into the cuboid to secure the lateral half of the anterior tibialis tendon that has been transferred. The tendon has been pulled through the cuboid and is secured with the screw.

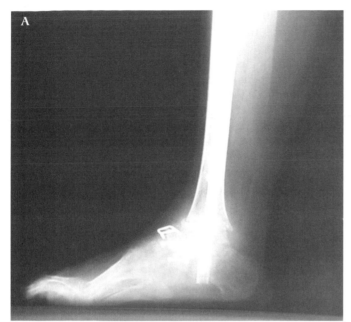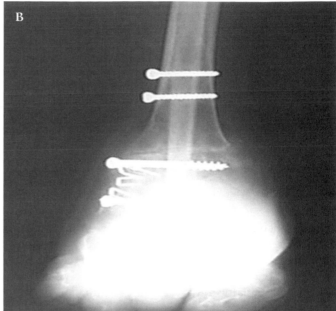

FIGURE 17.33

When soft tissue rebalancing is not possible, ankle arthrodesis can restore a plantigrade foot. Lateral (A) and anteroposterior (B) radiographs of an ankle arthrodesis using an intramedullary fibula are shown.

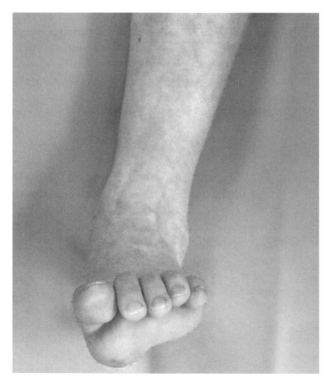

FIGURE 17.34

A mild spastic valgus foot as shown may be corrected with either tendon lengthening or transfer.

Cavus Spasticity

A cavus foot (a high-arched foot that does not flatten with weight-bearing) can be very painful to a patient and may not be amenable to support with orthotics. A supple cavus deformity due to spasticity can be treated with soft tissue releases. Through a medial incision over the foot, the spastic abductor tendon can be lengthened or released. Dissection across the plantar aspect of the foot will allow a release of the plantar fascia. For a more rigid deformity as shown in Figure 17.35, a dorsal closing wedge osteotomy of the foot is necessary in addition to the soft tissue releases to correct the cavus deformity.

Toe Spasticity

Toe flexor spasticity can be a source of significant pain and functional disability because painful clawed toes make walking difficult. As shown in Figure 17.30, spasticity involving the toe flexors forces the toes into a claw pattern and the tips of the toes drive into the sole of the shoe. Toe flexion deformity can be due to either intrinsic (flexor digitorum brevis) or extrinsic spasticity (flexor digitorum longus). Typically, treatment of this condition is performed through release of the spastic muscles causing the deformity. The ex-

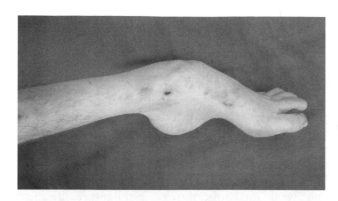

FIGURE 17.35

A severe cavus foot as shown is not likely to respond to soft tissue release alone.

trinsic flexors are released through an incision over the medial foot at the knot of Henry. The intrinsic toe flexors are released through a longitudinal incision under the plantar aspect of each toe. If the spasticity has been long-standing and rigid contractures have developed, then resection of the bone may be necessary. Usually, the bone is shortened at the proximal phalanx by resection of the distal condyles and shortening the shaft as much as is necessary to allow full extension of the toe.

Hyperextension deformity of the great toe can be extremely painful because the toe extends into the top of the shoe. With hyperextension, paronychia and skin breakdown can result due to chronic irritation of the nail. This can be addressed surgically with lengthening, release, or transfer of the extensor hallucis longus. A lengthening of the extensor hallucis longus can be done in the anterior compartment of the calf in a fractional manner or a Z lengthening can be done in the foot. If the tendon is released or transferred, the distal stump of the tendon can be sutured into the dorsal capsule of the metatarsophalangeal joint of the great toe to reduce the risk of a reverse hyperflexion deformity (65).

The Role of Rehabilitation After Surgery for Spasticity

Pain Management

Effective perioperative pain management is essential for obtaining optimal results from surgical intervention. The entire surgical process can be considered noxious stimuli. In addition to operative site-specific pain, there is also an overall increase in generalized spasticity throughout the body for at least the first few days after the procedure. Recent advances in pain management have been developed to ease a person's recovery. Adequate pain relief facilitates early therapy and functional retraining process.

Oral medications have been used with regularity and continue to have a valuable role in postoperative treatment. Oral analgesics, muscle relaxants, and antispasticity medications can provide relief to patients. Newer modalities of perioperative pain management include continuous intravenous or transdermal analgesics, indwelling postoperative pain pumps, and perioperative use of botulinum toxin injections. All of these treatments have been shown to be useful and can be used on an individual basis. Patients with limited cognition may require a pain management program independent of patient input. Transdermal and continuous intravenous delivery have the advantage of maintaining a constant level of analgesia independent of patient input. A risk of a continuous, systemic delivery, however, is overdose and toxicity. This can be avoided by using indwelling pain catheters. These pain catheters are left in the surgical wound and deliver a continuous infusion of analgesics to the surgical site. This technique has been shown to be safe and effective. Recently, botulinum toxin injections have been used as an adjunct to surgery for pain relief and rehabilitation. Perioperative use of botulinum toxin injections may decrease spasticity and pain from the muscles. Bone procedures (arthrodesis, arthroplasty) typically are more painful than soft tissue procedures, and longer duration of treatment should be anticipated.

Mobilization

Patients with spasticity and movement disorders often suffer from disuse osteopenia. A prolonged period of immobilization or limited weight-bearing should be avoided, if at all possible, after surgery. Many of the patients with spasticity have very limited ability to follow partial weight-bearing protocols. Therefore, full weight-bearing should be anticipated postoperatively once weight-bearing is allowed.

Some surgical procedures for spasticity do require protection postoperatively. In these situations, a lightweight cast or orthotic should be used while maximizing mobilization of other joints. Early weight-bearing has been employed regularly in the rehabilitation population even for surgeries that are typically treated with prolonged non–weight-bearing, such as ankle arthrodesis. Prolonged non–weight-bearing situations and bed rest are to be discouraged.

Physical and occupational therapy typically begin immediately after surgery. Communication between surgeon, therapist, and patient is essential. The therapist must know what muscles have been lengthened and which muscles may be at risk for passive stretch rupture. Active movement is encouraged at any joint where fractional lengthenings have been performed. Passive stretch is done at the joint where releases have been done. It must be done cautiously and sometimes avoided where fractional lengthenings have been performed because of the risk of tendon or muscle injury. In some muscles that have undergone a fractional lengthening, passive stretch should not be performed for a period of 8 to 12 weeks after the procedure due to a risk of overlengthening. This is particularly true of the finger flexors, which are at particular risk for overlengthening and overweakening. Other muscle groups such as the elbow flexors and knee flexors can tolerate gentle passive stretching after a fractional lengthening early after the procedure.

Skin Integrity

Patients with spasticity and movement disorders are predisposed to skin breakdown. Before surgery, the skin requires full inspection to understand areas at risk or preexisting ulceration. A history of skin difficulties needs to be obtained, particularly if a patient has had prior flaps done for breakdown. During and after surgery, skin integrity needs to be monitored closely. Pressure-relieving padding should be placed at the bony prominences. Patients that are bedridden require frequent turning after surgery.

Nutrition

Although sometimes overlooked, it is important that a patient's nutritional status be optimized before they undergo an operation. Malnutrition can lead to poor wound healing and infection, and unfortunately, a well-executed surgery may fail if the patient does not have the ability to heal after surgery. Optimizing the nutritional status is also critical postoperatively. Patients should be well hydrated and have caloric needs met as they recover. Caloric demands increase as a result of the surgery and the postoperative mobilization. Many patients that were once nonambulatory will experience nutritional demands well beyond preoperative levels as a result of intervention.

Future Considerations in Surgery for Spasticity

Most of the current strategies that were reviewed in this chapter are directed at the peripheral structures: nerves, muscles, tendons, and joints. There are limitations in the current procedures, and hopefully, some of these inadequacies will be addressed. Ideally, in the future, interventions will directly address the injury more centrally at the CNS level, and perhaps, it will be possible to repair the CNS lesion itself.

Hopefully, techniques will be developed to mitigate the problems and expand the scope of limb deformities amendable to surgical correction. One of the current limitations is that the procedures used for lengthening spastic muscles routinely weaken muscles. It may be possible in the future to strengthen or reanimate weak antagonist muscles. In the future, this may possibly be addressed through stem cell transplants, reconstruction of the neurologic system with implantable neurologic systems, or nerve transfers. Perhaps, improvements in the available techniques for tendon transfers will be developed that will enable the rebuilding of weak antagonist muscles. Better understanding of the forces generated by the existing spastic muscles may facilitate these developments.

In the meantime, in an appropriately selected patient, surgery for spasticity remains a safe, effective, and predictable technique for providing permanent correction of many deformities with an acceptable risk-benefit ratio. Well-established surgical techniques are available that restore function for many patients. It is important that all patients suffering from the sequela of spasticity who would benefit from surgical intervention should have access to it. The opportunity for improved lifelong function and improved quality of life continues to motivate patients and physicians alike.

References

1. Broggi F, Angelini L, Bono R, et al. Long-term results of steroetactic thalamotomy for cerebral palsy. *Neurosurgery* 1973; 12:195–202.
2. Broggi F, Angelini L, Giorgi C. Neurological and psychological side effects after stereotactic thalamotomy in patients with cerebral palsy. *Neurosurgery* 1980;7:127–134.
3. Gahm NJ, Russman BS, Cerciello RL, et al. Chronic cerebellar stimulation for cerebral palsy; a double blind study. *Neurology* 1981;31:87–90.
4. Peacock WJ, Arens LJ, Berman B. Cerebral palsy spasticity: selective posterior rhizotomy. *Pediatr Neurosci* 1987;13: 61–66.
5. Peacock WJ, Staudt. Functional outcomes following selective posterior rhizotomy in children with cerebral palsy. *J Neurosurg* 1991;74:380–385.
6. Stoffel A. The treatment of spastic contractures. *Am J Orthop Surg* 1913;10:611–644.
7. Chambers HG. The surgical treatment of spasticity. *Muscle Nerve* 1997; suppl 6:S121–S125.
8. Lieber RL, Friden J. Spasticity causes a fundamental rearrangement of muscle-joint interaction. *Muscle Nerve* 2002; 25:265–270.
9. Lieber RL, Runesson E, Einarsson F, et al. Inferior mechanical properties of spastic muscle bundles due to hypertrophic

but compromised extracellular matrix material. *Muscle Nerve* 2003b;28:464–471.

10. Lieber RL, Steinman S, Barash IA, et al. Structural and functional changes in spastic skeletal muscle. *Muscle Nerve* 2004; 29:615–627.

11. Smeulders MJ, Kreulen M, Hage JJ, et al. Spastic muscle properties are affected by length changes of adjacent structures. *Muscle Nerve* 2005;32:208–215.

12. Mayer NH. Clinicophysiologic concepts of spasticity and motor dysfunction in adults with an upper motorneuron lesion. *Muscle Nerve* 1997;Supp 6:S1–S13.

13. Carey JR. Manual stretch: effect on finger movement control and force control in stroke subjects with spastic extrinsic finger flexor muscles. *Arch Phys Med Rehabil* 1990;71:888.

14. Smeulders MJ, Kreulen. Myofascial force transmission and tendon transfer for patients suffering from spastic paresis: a review and some new observations. *J Electromyogr Kinesiol* 2007;17:644–656.

15. Smeulders MJ, Kreulen M. Adaptation of the properties of spastic muscles with wrist extension deformity. *Muscle Nerve* 2006;34:65–368.

16. Reimers J. Functional changes in the antagonists after lengthening the agonists in cerebral palsy. I. Triceps surae lengthening, *Clin Orthop Relat Res*, 1990; Apr(253):30–34.

17. O'Dwyer NJ, Ada L, Neilson PD. Spasticity and muscle contracture following stroke. *Brain* 1996;119:1737.

18. Atiyeh BS, Hayek SN. Pressure sores with associated spasticity: a clinical challenge. *Int Wound J*, 2005;2(1):77–80.

19. Gellman H, Keenan MA, Stone L, et al. Reflex sympathetic dystrophy in brain-injured patients. *Pain* 1992;51(3):307–311.

20. Orcutt SA, Kramer WG, Howard MW, et al. Carpal tunnel syndrome secondary to wrist and finger flexor spasticity. *J Hand Surg Am* 1990;15(6):940–944.

21. Reddy S, Kusuma S, Hosalkar H, et al. Surgery can reduce the nonoperative care associated with an equinovarus foot deformity. *Clin Orthop Relat Res*, 2008;466(7):1683–1687.

22. Fuller DA, Keenan MA, Esquenazi A, et al. The impact of instrumented gait analysis on surgical planning: treatment of spastic equinovarus deformity of the foot and ankle. *Foot Ankle Int* 2002;23(8):738–743.

23. Keenan MA, Fuller DA, Whyte J, et al. The influence of dynamic poly-EMG in formulating a surgical plan in treatment of spastic elbow flexion deformity. *Arch Phys Med Rehabil* 2003;84:291–296.

24. Kozin SH, Keenan MA. Using dynamic electromyography to guide surgical treatment of the spastic upper extremity in the brain-injured patient. *Clin Orthop Relat Res*, 1993;Mar (288):109–117.

25. Keenan MA, Haider TT, Stone LR. Dynamic electromyography to assess elbow spasticity. *J Hand Surg Am* 1990; 15(4): 607–614.

26. Mayer NH. Choosing upper limb muscles for focal intervention after traumatic brain injury. *J Head Trauma Rehabil* 2004;19(2):119–142.

27. Kolessar DJ, Keenan MA. Surgical management of upper extremity deformities following traumatic brain injury. *Phys Med Rehabil* 1993;7(3):623–635.

28. Keenan MA. Management of the spastic upper extremity in the neurologically impaired adult. *Clin Orthop Relat Res*, 1988; Aug (233):116–125.

29. Waters RL. Upper extremity surgery in stroke patients. *Clin Orthop* 1978;133:30.

30. Keenan MA, Kozin SH, Berlet AC. Manual of surgery for spasticity. New York; Raven Press, 1993.

31. Tafti MA, Cramer SC, Gupta R. Orthopaedic management of the upper extremity of stroke patients. *J Am Acad Orthop Surg* 2008;16:462–470.

32. Keenan MA, Mehta S. Neuro-orthopaedic management of shoulder deformity and dysfunction in brain injured patients: a novel approach. *J Head Trauma Rehabil* 2004;19(2): 143–154.

33. Braun RM, Mooney V, Nickel. Flexor-origin release for pronation-flexion deformity of the forearm. *J Bone Joint Surg Am* 1970;52:907.

34. Keenan MA, Romanelli RR, Lunsford BR. The use of dynamic electromyography to evaluate motor control in the hands of adults who have spasticity caused by brain injury. *J Bone Joint Surg Am* 1989;71(1):120–126.

35. Keenan MA, Abrams RA, Garland DE, et al. Results of fractional lengthening of the finger flexors in adults with upper extremity spasticity. *J Hand Surg Am* 1987;12(4):575–581.

36. Palma D, Fuller DA, Keenan MA. Superficialis to profundus tendon transfer. *Atlas of Hand Clinics* 2002;7(1):153–162.

37. Pomerance JF, Keenan MA. Correction of severe spastic flexion contractures in the nonfunctional hand. *J Hand Surg Am* 1996;21(5):823–833.

38. Keenan MA, Korchek JI, Botte MJ, et al. Results of transfer of the flexor digitorum superficialis tendons to the flexor digitorum profundus tendons in adults with acquired spasticity of the hand. *J Bone Joint Surg Am* 1987;69(8): 1127–1132.

39. Braun RM, Vise GT. Sublimus-to-profundus tendon transfers in the hemiplegic upper extremity. *J Bone Joint Surg Am* 1973;55:873.

40. Keenan MA, Todderud EP, Henderson R, et al. Management of intrinsic spasticity in the hand with phenol injection of neurectomy of the motor branch in the ulnar nerve. *J Hand Surg Am* 1987;12(5):734–739.

41. Botte MJ, Keenan MA, Gellman H, et al. Surgical management of spastic thumb-in-palm deformity in adults with brain injury. *J Hand Surg Am* 1989;14(2):174–182.

42. Matev I. Surgical treatment of spastic "thumb-in-palm" deformity, *J Bone Joint Surg Br* 1963;45:703.

43. Matev I. Surgery of the spastic thumb-in-palm deformity. *J Hand Surg Br* 1991;16:127.

44. Anmuth CJ, Esquenazi A, Keenan MA. Lower extremity surgery for the spastic patient. *Phys Med Rehabil* 1994;8(3): 547–564.

45. Patrick JH, Keenan MA. Gait analysis to assist walking after stroke. *Lancet* 2007;369(9558):256–257.

46. Keenan MA, Esquenazi A, Mayer NH. Surgical treatment of common patterns of lower limb deformities resulting from upper motoneuron syndrome. *Adv Neurol* 2001;87:333–346.

47. Keenan MA, Perry J, Jordan C. Factors affecting balance and ambulation following stroke. *Clin Orthop Relat Res* 1984; Jan-Feb(182):165–171.

48. Esquenazi A. Evaluation and management of spastic gait in patients with traumatic brain injury. *J Head Trauma Rehabil* 2004;19(2):109–118.

49. Perry J. Determinants of muscle function in the spastic lower extremity. *Clin Orthop* 1993;131:10.

50. Pinzur MS. Surgical correction of lower extremity problems in patients with brain injury. *J Head Trauma Rehabil* 1996;44:69.

51. Keenan MA, Ure K, Smith CW, et al. Hamstring release for knee flexion contracture in spastic adults. *Clin Orthop Relat Res*, 1988;Nov(236):221–226.

52. Grujic H, Asparisi R. Distal hamstring release in knee flexion deformity. *Int Orthop* 1982;6:103.

53. Cipriano C, Keenan MA. Knee disarticulation and hip release for severe lower extremity contractures. *Clin Orthop Relat Res* 2007;462:150–155.

54. Punpuu MS, Muik E, David III RB, et al. Rectus femoris surgery in children with cerebral palsy. Part II: a comparison between the effect of transfer and release of the distal rectus femoris on knee motion. *J Pediatr Orthop* 1993;13:331.

55. Murray HH. The stiff knee gait in hemiplegia. *Orthopaedic Seminars* 1972;5:329–333.

56. Waters RL, Garland DE, Perry J, et al. Stifflegged gait in hemiplegia: surgical correction. *J Bone Joint Surg Am* 1979;61: 929–933.

57. Pinzur MS, Sherman R, DiMonte-Levine P, et al. Adult-onset hemiplegia: changes in gait after muscle-balancing

procedures to correct the equinus deformity. *J Bone Joint Surg Am* 1986;68:1249–1257.

58. Roper BA, Williams A, King JB. The surgical treatment of equinovarus deformity in adults with spasticity. *J Bone Joint Surg Br* 1978;60:533–535.

59. Waters RL, Frazier J, Garland DE, et al. Electromyographic gait analysis before and after operative treatment for hemiplegic equinus and equinovarus deformity. *J Bone Joint Surg Am* 1982;64:284–288.

60. Perry J, Waters RI, Perrin T. Electromyographic analysis of equinovarus following stroke. *Clin Orthop* 1978; 131, 47.

61. Perry J. *Gain analysis. Normal and pathologic function.* Thororfare; Slack Inc., 1992.

62. Fuller DA, McCarthy JJ, Keenan MA. The use of bioabsorbable interference screw for a split anterior tibialis tendon (SPLATT) transfer procedure. *Orthopedics* 2004;27:372–374.

63. Hosalkar H, Goebel J, Reddy S, et al. Fixation techniques for split anterior tibialis transfer in spastic equinovarus feet. *Clin Orthop Relat Res*, 2008;466(10):2500–2506.

64. Young S, Keenan MA, Stone LR. The treatment of spastic planovalgus foot deformity in the neurologically impaired adult. *Foot Ankle* 1990;10(6):317–324.

65. Keenan MA, Gorai AP, Smith CW, et al. Intrinsic toe flexion deformity following correction of spastic equinovarus deformity in adults. *Foot Ankle* 1987;7(6):333–337.

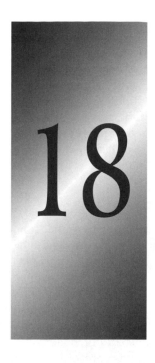

Diagnostic Evaluation of Adult Patients With Spasticity

18

Geoffrey Sheean

This chapter will discuss the diagnostic approach to the patient with spasticity and associated forms of motor overactivity. It will begin with a discussion of the upper motor neuron (UMN) syndrome and the types of motor overactivity that can arise from it, of which spasticity is only one. Next, there is a discussion of other neurologic and nonneurologic disorders that could mimic these UMN motor overactivities, a kind of phenomenological differential diagnosis. Following that is a discussion of the approach to making an etiological diagnosis using history, examination, and investigations.

UPPER MOTOR NEURON SYNDROME

The UMNs are descending motor pathways that originate in the cortex or brainstem that influence excitability of the lower motor neurons (cranial motor neurons or anterior horn cells). Damage to the UMNs results in the UMN syndrome, which has clinical features that are classified as either negative (loss of function or motor underactivity, eg, weakness) or positive (gain of function or motor overactivity). The forms of motor overactivity include spasticity, as classically defined, and can be further grouped into hyperkinetic (involuntary movements) and hypokinetic (impairment of movement) (Table 18.1).

Thus, a variety of motor overactivities can be seen in the UMN syndrome, and so the differential diagnosis will depend upon which are present (Table 18.2). For example, the differential diagnosis of spastic hypertonia (spasticity or spastic dystonia) will include all other causes of hypertonia, neurologic and musculoskeletal, and will differ considerably from the differential diagnosis of, say, extensor spasms. Differentiating spastic hypertonia from other causes of hypertonia will be based on velocity and length dependence and a pattern favoring extensors over flexors or vice versa, and a tendency to be greater in adductors and pronators than in abductors and supinators. Other clues that motor overactivity is due to the UMN syndrome might come from associated positive features such as deep tendon hyperreflexia, an extensor plantar response, and from associated negative features, such as weakness in a UMN distribution, associated sensory loss, loss of superficial abdominal reflexes, aphasia, and so on.

CAUSES OF SPASTICITY

Very often, the cause of spasticity in an adult is already apparent because it follows a known event, such as a stroke, head injury, spinal cord injury, or episode of anoxia, or it occurs in the course of a known disease,

TABLE 18.1
Positive Features of the UMN Syndrome

HYPERKINETIC (INVOLUNTARY MOVEMENTS)	HYPOKINETIC (IMPAIRED MOVEMENT[a])
Spasms—flexor, extensor	Spasticity
Action-induced spastic dystonia (dynamic)	Spastic dystonia (static)
Positive support reaction	Spastic cocontraction
Associated movements	
Extensor toe response	

[a]Active or passive.

such as multiple sclerosis (MS). If not, the cause is frequently found with neuroimaging of the brain or spinal cord with magnetic resonance imaging (MRI), which reveals spinal cord compression, a brain or spinal cord tumor, hydrocephalus, myelomalacia, plaques of MS, diffuse demyelination of a leukodystrophy, and so on. This chapter will deal with causes of spasticity that are not so readily apparent, as well as uncommon causes that have nonspecific features on neuroimaging (Table 18.3).

Spasticity usually does not develop rapidly but rather gradually. The sudden onset of something that appears to be spasticity is probably some other type or motor overactivity, for example, tetanus, strychnine poisoning, or decerebrate rigidity. Furthermore, most of the occult causes of spasticity are slowly progressive disorders.

EVALUATION OF THE PATIENT WITH SPASTICITY

History

History taking might reveal a family history of a spastic disorder (eg, hereditary spastic paraparesis [HSP]) or another genetic neurologic disorder that can cause spasticity. Previous transient neurologic symptoms might suggest MS. A history of electrocution or irradiation might be relevant. Excessive alcohol consumption, a strict vegan diet (vitamin B12), and a history of tick bite and a rash (Lyme disease) could point to the cause. A history of cirrhosis, especially with a portosystemic shunt (spontaneous or surgical), might suggest a diagnosis of hepatic myelopathy. Alcoholism can result in spasticity in several ways. Adults with phenylketonuria who abandon their diet can present with spasticity. A history of spinal injury in the past

could raise concern for a delayed posttraumatic complication. A history of repair of myelomeningocele or other congenital abnormality in childhood would make one consider a tethered cord. Some unusual causes of spasticity have symptoms of autonomic dysfunction or dementia. A history of urinary or fecal incontinence would also narrow the field of possibilities.

Examination

The examination should include testing of muscle tone at different velocities of muscle stretch to determine whether the hypertonia is velocity-dependent or not. Observation of whether hypertonia affects some muscle groups more than their antagonists (eg, wrist flexors more than extensors) should be made to help distinguish spasticity from rigidity. The clasp-knife phenomenon might be present in the elbow flexors or quadriceps, for example, rapid flexion of the knee proceeds until it soon meets sudden strong resistance (a "catch") slowing movement, but under a continuing stretching force, the resistance gradually "melts away." Brisk deep tendon reflexes and clonus at the knees or ankles are sup-

TABLE 18.2
Differential Diagnosis of Spastic Motor Overactivity

TYPE OF SPASTIC MOTOR OVERACTIVITY	DIFFERENTIAL DIAGNOSIS
Spasticity/spastic dystonia (static)	Rigidity (extrapyramidal)
	Myotonia
	Neuromyotonia
	Stiff person syndrome
	Encephalomyelitis with rigidity
	Soft tissue stiffness or contracture
	Joint calcification
	Decerebrate or decorticate posturing
Spasms	Stiff person syndrome
	Decerebrate or decorticate posturing
	Tetany
	Paroxysmal tonic spasms in MS
Dynamic spastic dystonia	Extrapyramidal dystonia
Extensor toe response	"Striatal" toe
Spastic cocontraction	Dystonic cocontraction
Clonus	Tremor
	Seizure

TABLE 18.3
Nonobvious Causes of Spasticity

Genetic
Friedreich ataxia (1)
Spinocerebellar ataxia (especially SCA3 types II and IV (2), SCA7 (3)
Adrenomyeloneuropathy/Adrenoleukodystrophy (4) (including females (5))
Adult Alexander disease (6)
HSP
Inborn errors of metabolism (7)
  Dopa-responsive dystonia (8)
  Sjogren-Larsson Syndrome, etc (9)
Huntington disease (10, 11)
Adult GM2-gangliosidosis (12)
Adult polyglucosan body disease (13)
Mitochondrial (e.g., Leigh disease (14), Leber (15))
Hallervorden-spatz (16)
Fragile X syndrome (17)
Phenylketonuria (18, 19)
Hereditary motor-sensory neuropathy type 5 (20)
Charlevoix-Saguenay syndrome (spastic ataxia) (21)

Infectious
HIV
HTLV 1, 2
Neurosyphilis
Neuroborreliosis (22)
Spinal tuberculosis
Neurocysticercosis (23)
Neurobrucellosis (24)
Prion diseases (e.g., Creutzfeld-Jacob disease (25), Gerstmann-Sträussler-Scheinker (GSS) (26)
Whipple disease (27)
Subacute sclerosing panencephalitis (28)

Neurodegenerative
Amyotrophic lateral sclerosis/ Primary lateral sclerosis (ALS/PLS)
Alzheimer disease (29)
Multiple system atrophy
Corticobasal degeneration
Progressive supranuclear palsy

Physical
Electrocution (30)
Irradiation (31)
Congenital or acquired tethered cord (32–34)
Posttraumatic progressive myelomalacia (35) or syringomyelia (36)
Basilar impression and impacted cisterna magna (38)
Spinal epidural venous engorgement during pregnancy (39)

Toxic/Metabolic
Lathyrism
Cassava ingestion (Konzo) (40)
Nitrous oxide
Hepatic (portosystemic) myelopathy/hepatocerebral degeneration (41, 42)
Alcoholic myelopathy (43)
Solvents (e.g., n-hexane (44), 1-bromopropane (45))
Organophosphates (e.g., triorthocresyl phosphate: Jamaican ginger paralysis (46), trichloronate (47))
Opiates (48, 49)
Cyclosporine (50)
Methanol (51)

Nutritional
B12 deficiency (52)
Copper deficiency (53)
Vitamin E deficiency (54)

Demyelinating
Transverse myelitis (55)
Central nervous system myelinolysis

Other
Spinal Sarcoidosis (56)
Sjogren syndrome (57)
Spinal dural ateriovenous malformation (AVM) (58)
Hashimotos encephalopathy (59)
Paraneoplastic disorder (eg, anti-Yo (60), breast cancer (61)
Superficial siderosis (62)

portive of a UMN syndrome but can be physiological or due to other disorders such as hyperthyroidism. Similarly, radiation of reflexes, crossed adductor reflexes, and Hoffman sign only indicate hyperreflexia, which is not necessarily pathological. Clonus at the wrists can be difficult to distinguish from the cog-wheeling of parkinsonism, but the latter would be associated with rigidity rather than spasticity. The absence of superficial abdominal reflexes supports a UMN syndrome but can be absent in multiparous women, obese people, and those with extensive abdominal surgery. Extensor toe responses, whether obtained by plantar stimula-

tion (Babinski sign) or otherwise, indicate pathology of the corticospinal tract: an astute observer might notice that pulling off the patient's socks elicits an extensor great toe response. There may or may not be evidence of the negative features of the UMN syndrome, such as a UMN pattern of weakness. Fine finger movements might be impaired, and there may be a pronator drift in the outstretched upper limbs.

Active movement may elicit spastic cocontraction, for example, cocontraction of the finger or elbow flexors when attempting extension. Standing and walking might reveal the abnormal posturing of spastic dystonia (eg, the "hemiplegic posture or gait" or the 'spastic diplegic gait"). Some patients do not have spasticity (at rest) and only develop motor over-activity during active movement.

Clues might also be obtained from the topography of the spasticity. Affliction of the lower limbs only suggests a spinal cord lesion below T1 or a parasagittal frontal lesion. A hemibody pattern suggests a lesion above C5, whereas facial or bulbar involvement places the lesion above the brainstem, as does a brisk jaw jerk.

Involvement of other neurologic systems and other bodily systems can also yield clues to the etiology (Table 18.4).

Investigations

In some cases, tests might be performed simply to distinguish spasticity from other types of motor overactivity. For example, electromyography (EMG) would distinguish myotonia or neuromyotonia from spasticity, or soft tissue stiffness from muscle contraction. Prolongation of central motor conduction time measured by transcranial magnetic stimulation would favor spasticity over rigidity. Diffusion tensor imaging (DTI) might show abnormalities of the UMN tracts that strongly suggest amyotrophic lateral sclerosis. However, transcranial magnetic stimulation and DTI are not readily available.

If after MRI scanning of the relevant areas of the brain and spinal cord the cause of the spasticity remains unknown, other tests could be performed, which follow directly from the etiological differential diagnosis (Table 18.5).

Depending on the presentation, a trial of levodopa for Dopa-responsive dystonia might be warranted, although this is unlikely to present as spasticity in an adult.

Cerebrospinal fluid (CSF) examination might reveal evidence suggestive of MS when the MRI scan does not. Cerebrospinal fluid abnormalities might lead to a discovery of spinal tuberculosis, Lyme disease, neurosyphilis, or sarcoidosis.

Genetic testing for HSP is commercially available (eg, Athena Daignostics), but unfortunately, not all types are covered. Other diagnoses that might be revealed by readily available DNA analysis include Friedreich ataxia and SCA3, among others.

Other tests might be performed to look for involvement of other systems, such as EMG for lower motor neuron disease, nerve conduction testing for polyneuropathy (demyelinating or axonal), and evoked potentials for involvement of special sensory and somatosensory fibers. Liver function tests could supply a clue to cirrhosis, alcoholism, Wilson disease, or mito-

chondrial disease. A chest x-ray might lead to a diagnosis of sarcoidosis. Elevated creatine phosphokinase could be due to a myopathy, such as might be seen in a mitochondrial disorder.

Basic tests include (MRI) scans of the neuraxis, serum B12 levels, and possibly routine CSF examination, including electropheresis for oligoclonal bands. Table 18.5 is a list of suggestions for advanced tests that could be run to investigate for the cause of spasticity. As always, investigation must include looking

---

TABLE 18.4
Signs to Look for During an Examination as Clues to Etiology

REGION OR SYSTEM	SIGNS
Cognitive function	Dementia Psychiatric disorder
Motor system	Chorea, dystonia, myoclonus, parkinsonism, tremor Muscle atrophy, fasciculations Oculomasticatory or oculofacialskeletal myorhythmia
Sensory system	Polyneuropathy Dorsal column dysfunction Dissociated sensory loss over shoulders
Cerebellar	Cerebellar signs
Ocular	Retinitis pigmentosa other retinal degenerations Optic atrophy Cataracts Kayser-Fleischer (KF) rings Jaundice Ocular motility disorders (gaze palsies)
Skin	Icthyosis Hyperpigmentation Spider naevi, palmar erythema, leuconychia Radiation changes Cutaneous signs of spina bifida occulta
Musculoskeletal	Scoliosis Pes cavus Tendon xanthomas
Oral	Dental abnormalities Glossitis Xerostomia Palatal myoclonus
Autonomic	Orthostatic hypotension
Other	Lymphadenopathy

for potentially treatable causes, no matter how rare or unlikely, assuming the cost (medical or otherwise) is not too great.

After all this, the cause may still be unknown. The development of additional symptoms or signs over time may ultimately reveal the cause.

Worsening Spasticity

Another aspect of dealing with patients with spasticity is the workup of patients in whom spasticity is worsening unexpectedly, that is, in patients with usually nonprogressive disorders. This usually occurs because the underlying spasticity is aggravated by other factors or because of an additional cause of spasticity.

Table 18.6 is a list of common factors that can aggravate existing spasticity, often through noxious stimulation, which should be considered in the evaluation. Additional causes of spasticity could be spondylotic cervical myelopathy in patients with cervical dystonia and spasticity, which might arise in cerebral palsy, Huntington disease, and Wilson disease. Another might be a patient with a Chiari malformation and syringomyelia, an unrecognized congenital tethered cord that becomes symptomatic later, or an acquired tethered cord that developed after meningomyelocoele repair. Patients with spinal cord injury can develop posttraumatic progressive myelomalacia (or cystic myelopathy) or a tethered cord from adhesions, or syringomyelia, which can aggravate underlying spasticity.

TABLE 18.5
Advanced Investigations[a]

INVESTIGATION	CONDITION
Serology—blood or CSF	Lyme, syphilis, HIV, HTLV 1,2, brucellosis, measles
Vitamin E levels	Vitamin E deficiency
Serum copper and ceruloplasmin, 24 hour urinary copper	Wilson disease, copper deficiency
Serum ammonia	Hepatic myelopathy
Magnetic resonance angiography (MRA) or spinal angiography	Spinal dural AVM
Lactate, pyruvate	Mitochondrial disorders
Hexosaminidase A levels	Adult GM2 gangliosidosis
Serum angioconverting enzyme levels	Sarcoidosis
Sural nerve biopsy	Polyglucosan body disease, leucodystrophies
Thyroid peroxidase antibodies	Hashimoto disease
Serum phytanic acid level	Refsum disease
Computed tomography myelogram of spine	Arachnoid cyst (may not be seen on MRI)
Muscle biopsy	Mitochondrial disorders
Small bowel biopsy	Whipple disease
CSF polymerase chain reaction	Whipple disease
Electroencephalogram	Prion diseases, SSPE
CSF 14-3-3	Prion diseases
DTI	ALS
Nerve conduction testing	Polyglucosan body disease, B12 deficiency, vitamin E deficiency, leucodystrophies, spinocerebellar ataxias, some types of HSP, copper deficiency, hereditary motor-sensory neuropathy type 5, Charlevoix-Saguenay syndrome
EMG	ALS, GM2-gangliosidosis, mitochondrial myopathy, sarcoid myopathy, myopathy associated with polyglucosan body disease
Somatosensory-evoked potentials	Dorsal column dysfunction
Chest x-ray	Sarcoidosis
Creatine phosphokinase	Myopathy
Paraneoplastic antibodies (e.g., anti-Yo)	Paraneoplastic syndrome
Mammography	Primary lateral sclerosis associated with breast cancer
Specific metabolic testing	Inborn errors of metabolism

[a]Does not include numerous genetic tests possible.

TABLE 18.6
Factors Aggravating Spasticity

Medications (eg, SSRIs) (63)
Urinary tract infections
Constipation
Ingrown toenail
Inflamed skin creases
In-dwelling catheter
Tight clothing
Poor positioning
Tight orthoses
Pressure sores
Joint subluxation

CONCLUSION

The clinician should first satisfy themselves that they are dealing with spasticity or some form of spastic motor overactivity, whether hyperkinetic or hypokinetic. In most cases, the cause will already be obvious or readily found with neuroimaging. In the remaining cases, a thoughtful approach to the history and examination is needed together with a judicious application of diagnostic testing. In some situations, time alone will deliver the answer.

CASE STUDIES

Case 1: Woman With Primary Lateral Sclerosis

A 39-year-old Hispanic woman presented with a year-long history of progressive dysarthria and dysphagia. In recent months, she had developed difficulty moving her left upper and lower limbs. On examination, she was unable to speak and had drooling. She was unable to protrude her tongue or to make voluntary facial movements. However, emotional facial expressions were intact and apparently exaggerated. The jaw jerk was increased. Tone was increased in the left upper and lower limbs with normal strength, but movements, especially fine finger movements, were slow. The deep tendon reflexes were brisk throughout but symmetrical. Plantar responses were extensor. There was no tremor or atrophy and no fasciculations. Sensory examination was intact. Cognitive function was difficult to examine, but her family maintained that it was intact.

Magnetic resonance imaging scans of the brain and cervical cord were normal. Electromyography and nerve conduction testing found no abnormalities. Blood testing was negative or normal for B12, syphilis, Lyme disease, HIV, HTLV-1 and HTLV-2, ANA,

angiotensin-converting enzyme, and antiphospholipids. Cerebrospinal fluid examination was normal.

A trial of levodopa, 750 mg per day, made no difference.

Her condition gradually deteriorated, with worsening hypertonia and reduced and slow voluntary movements now affecting all limbs but still worse on the left. Strength appeared to remain intact.

A provisional diagnosis of primary lateral sclerosis beginning as pseudobulbar palsy was made.

Case 2: Myotonia Congenita Woman

A 35-year-old woman was referred for evaluation of difficulty in walking, which was thought to be due to spasticity or dystonia. Since her teenaged years, she had experienced difficulty in walking due to stiffness of her legs, particularly after resting for a while and especially if she started to move quickly. She described herself as walking "like a robot." With continued walking, her legs would loosen up somewhat. The symptoms were worse in cold weather.

Examination revealed normal strength and tone in her upper limbs and in her lower limbs, which were quite muscular. Deep tendon reflexes were normal, and plantar responses were flexor. Her gait was stiff and awkward and did resemble spastic diplegia mildly. There was a delayed release of her handgrip, slow relaxation after strong eye closure, and percussion myotonia in her thenar eminence.

Needle EMG examination revealed profuse myotonia in her upper and lower limbs. A diagnosis was made of myotonia congenita, and her symptoms improved on mexiletine.

Case 3: Possible MS

A previously healthy 31-year-old man was referred for EMG to evaluate muscle stiffness and weakness in his arms, which was thought to be due to myotonia congenita. The symptoms began in the right upper limb 6 months beforehand, first with loss of sensation, paresthesias, and pain 6 in proximal to his elbow. These symptoms lasted about 1 week. He next developed "stiffness" in his right upper limb described as his tendon being shorter on the right. These symptoms progressed to involve the left upper limb in the succeeding month. The proximal arm and shoulder girdle muscles were most affected, but he had some loss of grip strength. Symptoms were worse in morning and after rest. The symptoms improve partially with use and are not worse in cold weather. His legs were unaffected.

Examination revealed a very muscular young man with normal strength in the upper and lower limbs. Muscle tone was mildly increased in the arms, with a "catch" in the elbow flexors. He had great difficulty flexing and extending his elbows. Deep tendon reflexes were brisk throughout the upper and lower limbs, but the plantar responses were flexor. Muscle tone and strength were normal in the lower limbs. Sensory examination was normal.

Nerve conduction studies were normal. Needle EMG examination revealed no myotonia in the arms, but there was evidence of a tonic stretch reflex and cocontraction of the biceps and triceps muscles during flexion and extension of the elbows. An UMN lesion was considered most likely.

Blood tests were normal or negative for ESR, ANA, B12, homocysteine, angiotensin-converting enzyme, syphilis and Lyme serology, HIV, HTLV-1, and HTLV-2.

An MRI of the cervical cord was normal. The MRI of the brain with contrast revealed multifocal abnormal, somewhat subtle, nonenhancing supratentorial white matter lesions that demonstrate T2 prolongation and are predominantly "smudgy" in appearance on a background of slightly "dirty" white matter (Figure 18.1). There was no abnormal restricted diffusion in the brain. Cerebrospinal fluid had a mildly elevated protein of 54 (<45 g/dL) and a mild lymphocytic pleocytosis (WCC = 27). Oligoclonal bands were present, and IgG synthesis was elevated. Myelin basic protein was normal.

He had mildly prolonged prothrombin time and partial thromboplastin time, with an abnormal diluted Russell viper venom test indicating the presence of a lupus anticoagulant. Anticardiolipin antibodies were absent.

A provisional diagnosis of MS was made, with an associated antiphospholipid syndrome.

This case demonstrates that severe spastic cocontraction can occur with only mild resting hypertonia (spasticity).

References

1. Castelnovo G, Biolsi B, Barbaud A, Labauge P, Schmitt M. Isolated spastic paraparesis leading to diagnosis of Friedreich. *J Neurol Neurosurg Psychiatry.* 2000;69(5):693.
2. Junck L, Fink JK. Machado-Joseph disease and SCA3: the genotype meets the phenotypes. *Neurology.* 1996;46:4–8.
3. Linhares Sda C, Horta WG, Cunha FM, Castro JD, Santos AC, et al. Spastic paraparesis as the onset manifestation of spinocerebellar ataxia type 7. *Arq Neuropsiquiat.* 2008; 66(2A):246–8.
4. Crum BA, Carter JL. 26-Year-old man with hyperpigmentation of skin and lower extremity spasticity. *Mayo Clin Proc.* 1997;72(5):479–82.
5. H. H. Jung, I. Wimplinger, S. Jung, K. Landau, A. Gal, F. L. Heppner. Phenotypes of female adrenoleukodystrophy. *Neurology.* 2007;68:960–961.
6. Balbi P, Seri M, Ceccherini I, Uggetti C, Casale R, et al. Adult-onset Alexander disease: report on a family. *J Neurol.* 2008;255(1):24–30.
7. Sedel F, Fontaine B, Saudubray JM, Lyon-Caen O. Hereditary spastic paraparesis in adults associated with inborn errors of metabolism: a diagnostic approach. *J Inherit Metab Dis.* 2007;30(6):855–64.
8. Bandmann O, Marsden CD, Wood NW. Atypical presentations of Dopa-responsive dystonia. *Adv Neurol.* 1998;78:283–90
9. Alió AB, Bird LM, McClellan SD, Cunningham BB. Sjögren-Larson syndrome: a case report and literature review. *Cutis.* 2006;78(1):61–5.
10. Frucht S, Fahn S, Shannon KM, Waters CH. A 32-year-old man with progressive spasticity and parkinsonism. *Mov Dis.* 1999;14(2):350–7.
11. Katafuchi Y, Fujimoto T, Ono E, Kuda N. A childhood form of Huntington's disease associated with marked pyramidal signs. *Eur Neurol.* 1984;23:296–299.
12. Johnson WG. The clinical spectrum of hexosaminidase deficiency diseases. *Neurology.* 1981;31(11):1453–6.
13. Cafferty MS, Lovelace RE, Hays AP, Servidei S, DiMauro S, Rowland LP. Polyglucosan body disease. *Muscle Nerve.* 1991; 14:102–107.
14. Clarençon F, Touzé E, Leroy-Willig A, Turmel H, Naggara O, et al. Spastic paraparesis as a manifestation of Leber. *J Neurol.* 2006;253(4):525–6.
15. Beltran RS, Coker SB. Familial spastic paraparesis: a case of a mitochondrial disorder. *Pediatr Neurosurg.* 16(1):40–2.
16. Hayflick SJ, Westaway SK, Levinson B, Zhou B, Johnson MA, et al. Genetic, clinical, and radiographic delineation of Hallervorden-Spatz syndrome. *N Engl J Med.* 2003;348(1): 33–40.
17. Cellini E, Forleo P, Ginestroni A, Nacmias B, Tedde A, et al. Fragile X premutation with atypical symptoms at onset. *Arch Neurol.* 2006;63(8):1135–8.
18. Kasim S, Moo LR, Zschocke J, Jinnah HA. Phenylketonuria presenting in adulthood as progressive spastic paraparesis with dementia. *J Neurol Neurosurg Psychiatry.* 2001;71(6): 795–7.
19. McCombe PA, McLaughlin DB, Chalk JB, Brown NN, McGill JJ, et al. Spasticity and white matter abnormalities in adult phenylketonuria. *J Neurol Neurosurg Psychiatry.* 1992;55(5): 359–61.
20. L. Schols, R. Schule, B. Mauko, M. Auer-Grumbach, L. Schols, Hereditary motor and sensory neuropathy type V or complicated form of spastic paraplegia? *Clin Neurophysiol.* Volume 118, Issue 4, April 2007, Pages e90–e91.
21. Bouchard JP, Richter A, Mathieu J, Brunet D, Hudson TJ, et al. Autosomal recessive spastic ataxia of Charlevoix-Saguenay. *Neuromuscul Disord.* 1998;8(7):474–9.
22. Logigian EL, Kaplan RF, Steere AC. Chronic neurologic manifestations of Lyme disease. *N Engl J Med.* 1990;323(21): 1438–44.
23. Hamed SA, El-Metaal HE. Unusual presentations of neurocysticercosis. *Acta Neurol.* Scand 2007;115(3):192–8.
24. Karaca S, Demiroglu YZ, Karataş M, Tan M. Acquired progressive spastic paraparesis due to neurobrucellosis: a case report. *Acta Neurol Belg.* 2007;107(4):118–21.
25. Yamada M, Satoh S, Sodeyama N, Fujigasaki H, Kaneko K, et al. Spastic paraparesis and mutations in the prion protein gene. *J Neurol Sci.* 1995;134(1–2):215–6.
26. De Michele G, Pocchiari M, Petraroli R, Manfredi M, Caneve G, et al. Variable phenotype in a P102L Gerstmann-Sträussler-Scheinker Italian family. *Can J Neurol Sci.* 2003;30(3):233–6.
27. Fenollar F, Puechal X, Raoult D. Whipple's disease. *N Engl J. Med* 2007;356:55–66.
28. Singer C, Lang AE, Suchowersky O. Adult-onset subacute sclerosing panencephalitis: case reports and review of the literature. *Mov Dis.* 1997;12(3):342–53.
29. Verkkoniemi A, Somer M, Rinne JO, Myllykangas L, Crook R, et al. Variant Alzheimer's disease with spastic paraparesis. *Neurology.* 2000;54(5):1103–9.

30. Kalita J, Jose M, Misra UK. Myelopathy and amnesia following accidental electrical injury. *Spinal Cord.* 2002;40(5):253–5.

31. New P. Radiation injury to the nervous system. *Curr Opin Neurol.* 2001;14(6):725–34.

32. George TM, Fagan LH. Adult tethered cord syndrome in patients with postrepair myelomeningocele: an evidence-based outcome study. *J Neurosurg.* 2005;102(2 Suppl):150–6.

33. Lapsiwala SB, Iskandar BJ. The tethered cord syndrome in adults with spina bifida occulta. *Neurol Res.* 2004;26(7):735–40.

34. Lee TT, Arias JM, Andrus HL, Quencer RM, Falcone SF, et al. Progressive posttraumatic myelomalacic myelopathy: treatment with untethering and expansive duraplasty. *J Neurosurg.* 1997;86(4):624–8.

35. Lee TT, Alameda GJ, Gromelski EB, Green BA. Outcome after surgical treatment of progressive posttraumatic cystic myelopathy. *J Neurosurg.* 2000;92(2 Suppl):149–54.

36. Lee TT, Alameda GJ, Camilo E, Green BA. Surgical treatment of post-traumatic myelopathy associated with syringomyelia. *Spine.* 2001;26(24 Suppl):S119–27.

37. Merwick A, O SS. A role for myelography in assessing paraparesis. *Ir Med J.* 2008;101(1):21–2. (arachnoid cyst)

38. Gonçalves da Silva JA, de Almeida Holanda MM, do Desterro Leiros M, Melo LR, de Araújo AF, et al. Basilar impression associated with impacted cisterna magna, spastic paraparesis and distress of balance: case report. *Arq Neuropsiquiat.* 2006;64(3A):668–71.

39. Franco MJ, Vendrame M, Haneef Z, Azizi SA. Teaching neuroimage: acute spastic monoplegia secondary to spinal epidural venous engorgement in pregnancy. *Neurology.* 2008;71(1):e1.

40. Carod-Artal FJ, Vargas AP, del Negro C. [Spastic paraparesis due to long term consumption of wild cassava (*Manihot esculenta*): a neurotoxic model of motor neuron disease]. *Rev Neurol.* 1999;29(7):610–3.

41. Mendoza G, Marti-Fabregas J, Kulisevsky J, Escartin A. Hepatic myelopathy: a rare complication of portocaval shunt. *Eur Neurol.* 1994;34:209–212.

42. Utku U, Asil T, Balci K, Uzunca I, Celik Y. Hepatic myelopathy with spastic paraparesis. *Clin Neurol Neurosurg.* 2005;107(6):514–6.

43. Sage JI, Van Uitert RL, Lepore FE. Alcoholic myelopathy without substantial liver disease. A syndrome of progressive dorsal and lateral column dysfunction. *Arch Neurol.* 1984;41(9):999–1001.

44. Passero S, Battistini N, Cioni R, Giannini F, Paradiso C, et al. Toxic polyneuropathy of shoe workers in Italy. A clinical, neurophysiological and follow-up study. *Ital J Neurol Sci.* 1983;4(4):463–72.

45. Majersik JJ, Caravati EM, Steffens JD. Severe neurotoxicity associated with exposure to the solvent 1-bromopropane (*n*-propyl bromide). *Clin Toxicol.* 2007;45(3):270–6.

46. Morgan JP, & Penovich P. Jamaica ginger paralysis. Forty-seven-year follow-up. *Arch Neurol.* 1978;35(8):530–2.

47. Jedrzejowska H, Rowińska-Marcińska K, Hoppe B. Neuropathy due to phytosol (agritox). Report of a case. *Acta Neuropathol.* 1980;49(2):163–8.

48. Kloke M, Bingel U, Seeber S: Complications of spinal opioid therapy: myoclonus, spastic muscle tone and spinal jerking. *Support Care Cancer.* 1994;2:249–252

49. Manfredi PL, Gonzales GR, Payne R. Reversible spastic paraparesis induced by high-dose intravenous methadone. *J Pain.* 2001;2(1):77–9.

50. Rai M, Srinivasan A, Sundar S, Singh VP. Cyclosporine-induced reversible pure motor spastic paraparesis in a patient with aplastic anaemia. *J Assoc Physicians India.* 2002;50:1337.

51. Hageman G, van der Hoek JA, Faber CG. Spastic paraparesis without optic atrophy after occupational methanol exposure. *J Neurol.* 2003;250(7):876–7.

52. Cheng SH, Chang MH, Soong BW, Chen CW, Lee YC. Spastic paraparesis as a manifestation of metabolic vitamin B12 deficiency: a case report. *J Neurol.* 2005;252(9):1125–6.

53. Kumar N, Gross JB, Ahlskog JE. Copper deficiency myelopathy produces a clinical picture like subacute combined degeneration. *Neurology* 2004;63(1):33–9.

54. Verma V, Dhar A, Chinnery PF. Occult gastro-intestinal cause of spastic paresis of the legs. *Gut.* 2008;57(8):1064. Vitamin E

55. Brinar VV, Habek M, Zadro I, Barun B, Ozretić D, et al. Current concepts in the diagnosis of transverse myelopathies. *Clin Neurol Neurosurg.* 2008;110(9):919–27.

56. Perdigão S, Arantes M, Pinheiro L, Costa M. [Atypical presentation of intramedullary sarcoidosis: report of two cases]. *Rev Neurol.* 2007;45(7):406–8.

57. Delalande S, de Seze J, Fauchais AL, Hachulla E, Stojkovic T, et al. Neurologic manifestations in primary Sjögren syndrome: a study of 82 patients. *Medicine.* 2004;83(5):280–91.

58. Lev N, Maimon S, Rappaport ZH, Melamed E. Spinal dural arteriovenous fistulae—a diagnostic challenge. *Isr Med Assoc J.* 2001;3(7):492–6.

59. George A, Abdurahman P, James J. Spastic paraparesis, abnormal muscle biopsy and positive antithyroid antibodies. *J Assoc Physicians India.* 2007;55:585–6.

60. Finsterer J, Bodenteich A, Drlicek M. Atypical paraneoplastic syndrome associated with anti-Yo antibodies. *Clin Neuropathol* 2003;22(3):137–40.

61. Forsyth PA, Dalmau J, Graus F, Cwik V, Rosenblum MK, et al. Motor neuron syndromes in cancer patients. *Ann Neurol.* 1997;41(6):722–30.

62. Carod-Artal FJ, Viana-Brandi I, de Melo CM. [Superficial siderosis of the central nervous system: an uncommon cause of spastic paraparesia]. *Rev Neurol.* 2001;33(6):548–52.

63. Stolp-Smith KA, Wainberg MC. Antidepressant exacerbation of spasticity. *Arch Phys Med Rehabil.* 1999;80(3):339–42.

IV

EVALUATION AND MANAGEMENT OF DISEASES INVOLVING SPASTICITY

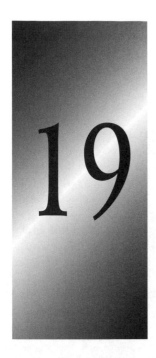

Overview of Genetic Causes of Spasticity in Adults and Children

19

Donald McCorquodale, III
Stephan Züchner

Spasticity is a common symptom in neurology and has a direct genetic cause in the clinically simple and complex forms of hereditary spastic paraplegias (HSPs). Hereditary spastic paraplegia comprises a group of clinically and genetically heterogeneous diseases that affect the upper motor neurons and their axonal projections. To date, 39 chromosomal loci have been identified for autosomal dominant, recessive, and X-linked HSP. The underlying genes for 17 of these loci have been described. The molecular dissection of the cellular functions of the related gene products has already greatly advanced our understanding of the most critical pathways involved in HSP. This chapter will give a detailed overview of the current state of genetic and molecular research and its applications for genetic testing. It is hoped that in the foreseeable future, this knowledge will begin to translate into novel pharmacologic approaches for this devastating disease.

INTRODUCTION

Spasticity as a neurologic symptom has many faces. Instead of being a disease entity in itself, spasticity more often accompanies complex conditions that involve the upper motor neuron. Diseases as heterogeneous as multiple sclerosis, stroke, trauma, inflammation, tumors, and amyotrophic lateral sclerosis (ALS) are able to cause spasticity. In most cases, spasticity is a more

or less voluntary symptom in neurologic disorders that are clinically defined by other lead symptoms. Probably the only disease where spasticity is viewed as the defining symptom is HSP, also known as familial spastic paraplegia. Utilizing spasticity to define and categorize HSP has been extremely successful for the identification of phenotypically similar families and the identification of underlying genes (1, 2). From this clinical and genetic work, it became evident that HSP is indeed a very heterogeneous group of diseases (1, 3). Hereditary spastic paraplegia can be accompanied by a number of additional neurologic and nonneurologic symptoms. This brings some complex HSP forms in close relationship to motor neuron diseases, ataxias, and axonopathies. This clinical, pathological, and genetic overlap of diseases, such as ALS, distal hereditary motor neuropathy (dHMN), and hereditary motor and sensory neuropathy type 2, will ultimately be advantageous for the understanding of the biology of HSP and the development of new therapies (4). Ultimately, the underlying gene defects will provide the basis of classifying such conditions. This book chapter will focus on the HSPs and describe the spectrum of genes identified thus far. The molecular genetic findings of each gene are summarized, and the major cell biological pathways involved in HSP are being discussed. Finally, a perspective is provided on new developments in this field, and potential approaches to therapeutic intervention are laid out.

HEREDITARY SPASTIC PARAPLEGIAS

Hereditary spastic paraplegia affects approximately 1.2 to 9.6 in every 100,000 individuals (5, 6). This makes it a rare neurodegenerative disease. Traditionally, HSPs are divided into "pure" and "complicated" forms. The latter are characterized by additional neurologic and nonneurologic symptoms. In complicated HSP, clinical examination frequently reveals mental retardation, epilepsy, cerebellar ataxia, or optic atrophy (1). Some of these complex phenotypes are clinically quite characteristic, and the genetic diagnosis can be greatly facilitated by careful clinical assessment (e.g. Silver syndrome in SPG17). This distinction is usually not possible in uncomplicated HSP forms, although frequent nonspasticity symptoms may include scoliosis, sphincter disturbances, and mild sensory loss at the distal lower limbs. The few exceptions include SPG3A (atlastin), where families often have an earlier onset than in the most prevalent form SPG4 (spastin) (7). A bimodal age of onset distribution has been suggested for SPG31 (REEP1), but this has not yet been confirmed by additional studies (8). As seen in other monogenic neurodegenerative diseases, age of onset, clinical course, and degree of disability often vary between the different subtypes and even within families. This is probably due to additional genetic risk factors or environmental influences.

Generally, the diagnosis of HSP is made by the presence of gait disturbance, spasticity of the lower extremities, hyperreflexia, weakness, and often urinary urgency. The presence of a family history of similar conditions can confirm the familial nature of the condition and provide information of the Mendelian trait (e.g. X-linked, autosomal recessive, or autosomal dominant disorder) (9).

GENETIC HETEROGENEITY IN HSP

Genetic studies have revealed as many as 39 different chromosomal HSP loci (9). Of the 17 identified genes, 9 cause autosomal dominant disease, 4 recessive, and 2 X-linked forms. The autosomal dominant HSP represents the most prominent forms. Mutations in the genes spastin (SPG4) and atlastin (SPG3A) account for 40% and 10% of all HSP cases, respectively (10). Mutations in REEP1 (SPG31) account for 4% to 8.2% of autosomal dominant HSP (8, 11). All other dominant genes (KIF5A, HSP60, NIPA1, KIAA1096, BSCL2, ZFYVE27) seem to cause HSP in less than 1%, respectively (12, 13).

Recessive HSPs are rare causes for disease in the outbred white population but are more frequent in regions such as Northern Africa and the Near East (14). Mutations in recessive genes are often associated with complicated forms of HSP. Some forms are more reminiscent of a genetic syndrome. For example, SPG21, also known as mast syndrome, was defined in an Amish family, and the underlying (founder-) mutation was later identified in the gene maspardin (ACP33) (15). The affected patients have dementia, developmental delay, pseudobulbar, cerebellar, and extrapyramidal abnormalities (16).

Two genes are known to cause X-linked HSP: L1CAM and PLP1 (Table 19.1). Both genes cause complicated forms of HSP. Other examples of rare, and not yet clarified loci, are SPG23 and SPG29 (17, 18). SPG23 is a recessive HSP form with skin pigmentary abnormalities, and SPG29 is complicated by hearing impairment and persistent vomiting due to hiatal hernia (18).

Most genetic defects in HSP are point mutations or small insertions and deletions. However, Beetz et al. (19) showed recently that small copy number variations in spastin at the subgene level are a relatively frequent cause for SPG4. It remains to be seen whether this mutation mechanism does apply to other HSP genes. Another novel molecular mechanism causing HSP has been proposed that involves variations in highly conserved binding sites for micro-RNAs (20). These binding or target sites are generally present only in the 3 untranslated regions of genes. Micro-RNAs confer another means of gene expression by controlling translation and mRNA stability (21). Several SPG31 (REEP1) families have been reported that carried mutations in the target site of micro-RNA140 (miR140) in REEP1 (8, 11, 22).

EMERGING PATHWAYS IN HSP

The remarkable heterogeneity of HSP, although posing a considerable obstacle to clinical genetic diagnoses, has provided invaluable genetic data, which appear to converge on several important cellular pathways (23, 24). Unlike other neurodegenerative diseases such as Alzheimer and Parkinson, in which genetic data have yielded an important but less coherent understanding of the underlying pathogenic pathways as of yet, the growing identified HSP genes continue to highlight the same or similar molecular pathways. The growing body of molecular work on the 17 genes identified from the 39 SPG loci has provided the first cogent models of how mutations in a wide variety of genes might explain the neuronal specificity and complex clinical manifestation of HSP.

Moreover, when the molecular genetics of HSP is incorporated into a broader understanding of other hereditary axonopathies, a more general concept regarding cell-specific vulnerabilities becomes apparent. Although genetic neurodegenerative diseases such as Charcot-Marie-Tooth disease type 2, dHMN, spinal muscle atrophy, and familial ALS are clinically differentiated based on neurologic diagnostic schemes, they all share important elements. Chiefly, both the upper and lower motor neurons, particularly in the case of neurons innervating the most distal sites, have axon projections that extend over distances 1,000 times the diameter of a neuronal cell body. Such a morphological arrangement makes distal molecular processes exceedingly dependent on efficient transport. The genetics of HSP and other hereditary axonopathies point more to the importance the cellular logistics and less to genes associated with the sophisticated molecular strategies underlying neurotransmission and synaptic function. The exceptionally long axons affected in HSP and other genetic forms of axonal degeneration serve in a sense as a model system in which the extreme axonal length pushes cellular processes to limits not reached in other cells types. Small inefficiencies in transport and trafficking result in the manifestation of disease. Because these axonal transport processes are shared by shorter neurons in the central and peripheral nervous system, a greater understanding of the molecular processes underlying HSP will likely shed light on other axonal degenerative diseases and neurodegeneration in general. Most importantly, a unified understanding of the cellular pathways deranged in HSP will allow for the development of new therapeutic approaches (see Figure 19.1).

AUTOSOMAL DOMINANT HSP

SPG3, Atlastin-1 (ATL1). SPG3 is caused by mutations in the gene atlastin-1 (ATL1) (25). SPG3 is an uncomplicated HSP form with symptoms usually beginning in early childhood (26). Durr et al. (7) studied 12 SPG3 families and found that scoliosis was present in 22% of patients, mild pes cavus in 15%, and brisk upper limb reflexes in 10%, although sensation was not impaired and only 13% of patients reported decreased vibration sense in the ankles. In another study, 17% of 36 affected individuals exhibited an axonal, predominantly motor polyneuropathy (27). SPG3 mutations account for up to 10% of all autosomal cases, and the characteristic early age at onset should guide the genetic testing efforts.

Before its association with SPG3, ATL1 was called guanylate-binding protein 3 or GBP3 (28). GBP3 was found to interact with the hydrophobic leucine-rich CHN domain of mitogen-activated

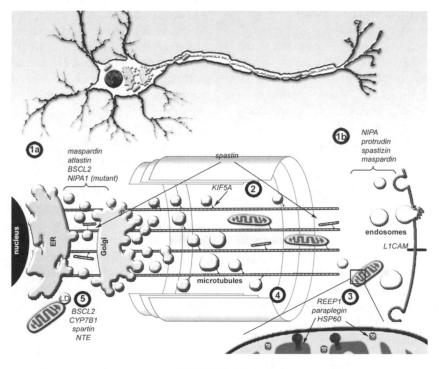

FIGURE 19.1

Model of HSP. See color insert.

protein kinase 4, a known activator of the SAPK/ JNK cascade (28). Subsequent to the identification of mutations in ATL1 in SPG3, molecular studies revealed that ATL1 is an oligomeric integral membrane GTPase with 2 putative transmembrane domains projecting the N- and C-terminals into the cytoplasm (29). Two additional members of the atlastin family were identified, alastin-2 and atlastin-3, that have a similar membrane orientation and high sequence homology. The atlastin family shares membrane topology and has high sequence homology with other dynamin-like GTPase, such as *mitofusin,* which causes axonal degeneration in peripheral nerves (29, 30). Examination atlastin in rat brain showed that it is enriched in the lamina V pyramidal neurons of the cerebral cortex, which is selectively affected in HSP (31, 32). Two independent groups reported yeast 2-hybrid screens using SPG4 (spastin) as bait, with subsequent identification of atlastin as a binding partner of spastin (31, 32). These experiments thus linked the 2 most common HSP genes. SPG3 has also been shown to regulate vesicular traffic at the ER/Golgi interface, making it likely that its dynamin-like GTPase domain regulates vesicular budding or severing from the ER and/or subsequent fusion with the Golgi (33). Highly relevant to HSP, mutations in the GTPase domain halted vesicle budding from the ER and resulted in the formation of aggregates, positive for ER markers, which most likely represent "aborted vesiculation" (33). SPG3 was also shown to interact with p24, a protein thought to act as a scaffold in the trafficking of cargo vesicles and controlling the integrity of cholesterol-poor membranes in the Golgi (33–35). These finding add experimental weight to a regulatory function of SPG3 in the vesicular trafficking at the ER/Golgi interface, where mutations in SPG3 may alter ER to Golgi vesicular trafficking along microtubules.

SPG4, Spastin (SPAST). SPG4 is caused by mutations in the gene spastin (36). This HSP form is uncomplicated, and symptoms start from age 2 to 75 (37). The clinical expression of the disorder within a family may include asymptomatic patients who are unaware of their condition, mildly affected individuals who have a spastic gait but are able to walk independently, and severely affected patients who are wheelchair-bound (37). Urinary urgency or other symptoms compatible with a neurogenic bladder, leg weakness, and decreased vibration sense can be present in some but not all SPG4 patients (38). Few reports have implicated a possible link to dementia in SPG4 (39, 40). Orlacchio et al. reported a large family from Italy with additional symptoms that included pes cavus and weak intrinsic hand muscles with severe amyotrophy of the thenar eminence (41). Most importantly, SPG4

accounts for up to 45% of all autosomal dominant HSP (42, 43). Testing of SPG4 is therefore the first step in a molecular-genetic evaluation.

The identification of mutations in SPAST was accompanied with the immediate recognition of spastin as a member of the AAA protein family (like SPG7, paraplegin). Other conserved protein domains in spastin suggested interaction with nuclear protein complexes (25, 36). Although the molecular function of spastin was at the time unknown, unique splice site mutations were reported to be partially penetrant or "leaky," as expressions of both mutant and wild-type splice variants were observed (44). Such a phenomena suggested that the function of spastin was highly dependent on expression levels (44). In experiments with controlled spastin expression, it was confirmed that different levels of spastin have pleiotropic effects on neuronal morphology (45). Two alternative transcription start sites within spastin result in 2 spastin isoforms of 68 and 60 kDa, whereas alternative splicing of both isoforms can include or skip exon 4, yielding a 64- and 55-kDa protein (46). It is still debated which isoform is the more abundant or predominant player in HSP (46, 47).

Cell models and molecular analysis revealed that spastin functions in a very similar way to the microtubule-severing protein, katanin (47–49). Overexpression of exogenous spastin in cultured cells resulted in the localizing of spastin to microtubule asters (48, 49). Disease-associated mutations in the ATPase domain abrogate ATPase activity and are sufficient to ablate the microtubule-severing activity of spastin in mammalian cell models and *Drosophila* (47, 50, 51). As a consequence, microtubule-dependent transport is disrupted as indicated by perinuclear clustering of mitochondria and peroxisomes (49). Spastin and spartin (SPG2) contain a conserved microtubule-interacting and trafficking domain (MIT), within which disease-causing mutations are found (52).

Silencing of *spg4* in zebra fish caused widespread defects in neuronal connectivity and extensive neuronal apoptosis, with specific defects in motor neuron outgrowth and disorganized axonal microtubule arrays (53). *Drosophila* models of spastin revealed irregularities in microtubules of neurons, severe reduction of the synaptic terminal area at the neuromuscular junction, and subsequent neurotransmission defects (54–56). The so-called cut-and-run hypothesis describes a system of mobile short microtubule segments, severed by spastin from intact microtubule lattices, that are transported, anchored, and immobilized again as they elongate microtubules in a treadmill-like process (57, 58). In this model, the mobility of severed microtubules is inversely proportional to its length providing a potential explanation for the length-dependent defects in HSP (57, 58). Interestingly, in spastin null flies, administration of the vinca alkaloid vinblastin, which inhibits microtubule assemble, diminishes phenotypes associated with loss of spastin in *Drosophila* (55). Although this observation suggests a potential therapeutic mechanism for HSP, it directly conflicts with important published reports of vincristine administration exacerbating axonal neuropathies in peripheral nerves (59–64).

Mice deficient in spastin are viable and show no motor deficiencies until 2 years of age (65). However, examination of corticospinal neurons demonstrated an age-dependent progressive increase in focal axonal swellings, accumulations of organelles, and intermediate filaments within the regions where stable and dynamic microtubule lattices meet (65). Conversely, spastin overexpression resulted in more microtubule branching and shorter severed microtubule segments (66). It has also been suggested that the role of spastin at microtubules is linked to protein tau (66). This is interesting because brain lesions from spastin patients stain positively for tau (67, 68).

SPG6, Nonimprinted in Prader-Willi/Angelman 1 (NIPA1). NIPA1 was named for "nonimprinted in Prader-Willi/Angelman," as a 1 of 4 genes falling within the centromeric end of a 4mb deletion within 15q11-q13 associated with Prader-Willi/Angelman syndrome (69). Its association with SPG6 was identified by Rainier et al. (70). SPG6 represents an uncomplicated HSP form, often with late onset but severe progression (9, 70, 71). Some patients may have pes cavus and tonic-clonic seizures (72). Genetic screens have suggested that NIPA is a relatively rare cause for HSP (73, 74).

The NIPA protein contains conserved domains that suggest a role as a membrane-based receptor or transporter (75). A screen for up-regulated genes in epithelial cells in conditions of low magnesium (Mg+) identified NIPA2, and subsequently NIPA1, as a magnesium response gene. Expression of NIPA1 in Xenopus oocytes and electrophysiological recording of Mg+ indicator dyes demonstrated that NIPA1 selectively conducts Mg+ (75). The mouse equivalent of 2 clinically observed mutations, T45R (mouse T39R) and G106R (mouse G100R), were tested in different mouse models (75). The T39R mutation reduced Mg+ current by 30% when expressed in the same experimental model, whereas the G106 mutant resulted in a complete loss of Mg+ conduction. When the cellular distribution of the 2 mutated NIPA1 isoforms were examined, it appeared that the T39R mutation reduced the transport of NIPA1 to the plasma membrane, whereas the G100R mutation caused complete

retention of NIPA1 in the ER. These results suggest that mutations in NIPA1 alter the folding and subsequent insertion of NIPA1 proteins into membranes. Wild-type NIPA1 was found to colocalize with the trafficking proteins EEA1 and Rab5, and functional studies suggested that NIPA1 is actively recycled from the plasma membrane and the early endosomal compartment in response to Mg+ levels (75). In vivo overexpression of the wild-type *Caenorhabditis elegans* homologue of NIPA1 was well tolerated in *C elegans*, but the T45R and G106R mutations caused progressive motor paralysis (76). The motor paralysis phenotype was rescued in mutants deficient of the unfolded protein response (UPR) machinery (76). The authors suggested that NIPA1 mutations created a toxic gain of function, caused ER stress, and elicited the UPR to initiate cell death pathways (76). The *Drosophila* homologue of NIPA1 is also localized to early endosomes. Flies expressing mutated NIPA1 have longer and overgrown neuromuscular junctions with increased numbers of synaptic boutons (77). Thus, although *Drosophila* models suggest a role in presynaptic growth (via BMP signaling), mammalian and *C elegans* models suggest that mutations in NIPA1 cause toxic gain of functions, caused by misfolding and subsequent ER stress.

SPG8, Strumpellin (KIAA0196). Mutations in KIAA0196 cause SPG8 (78). This HSP form is relatively new, and clinical data are scarce. SPG8 is considered a clinically uncomplicated HSP form with adult onset (79). Mutations in KIAA0196 are likely to be a rare cause of HSP.

There are no detailed functional analyses reported on strumpellin. KIAA0196 is composed of 28 exons, encoding a 1159 amino acid protein. The European Bioinformatics Institute InterProScan predicts a spectrin-repeat–containing domain in amino acids 434–518, within which a mutation at position 471 may interfere (78). The secondary structure is predicted to be 74% alpha-helical, with 2 mutations within the amino acids 606–644 making up an alpha helix (78). Injection of wild-type, but not mutant strumpellin, into zebrafish is sufficient to rescue the phenotype associated with strumpellin knockdown (enlarged heart cavity and curly tail) (78). In addition, increased expression of KIAA0196 was found in prostate tumors (80).

SPG10, Kinesin 5A (KIF5A). SPG10 is caused by mutations in the gene KIF5A (12). Only few families with KIF5A mutations have been reported to date (81, 82). Recently, Goizet et al. (83) reported several new KIF5A families with additional clinical features including peripheral neuropathy, severe upper limb amyotrophy (Silver syndrome–like), mental impairment, parkinsonism, deafness, and retinitis pigmentosa. They concluded that KIF5A accounts for 10%

of complicated HSP forms in their sample making KIF5A the most important from of complicated autosomal dominant HSP (83). If confirmed, this would be important for future decisions on medical genetic testing. The age of onset in uncomplicated SPG10 ranges from 8 to 40 years (82).

Kinesin motor proteins are microtubule-dependent trafficking machines. Axonal transport genes are very good candidates for spastic paraplegia, as some of the longest axons in the human body are involved in the disease. Studies found that KIF5A-/- mice were neonatal lethal (84). In a conditional knockout model, the postnatal loss of KIF5A caused sensory neuron degeneration and seizures, with no morphological abnormalities in the spinal cord (84). Fast axonal transport appeared to be normal in the absence of KIF5A (84). However, slow axonal transport and, more specifically, the transport of neurofilaments were profoundly disrupted in KIF5A-/- mice (84). Neurofilaments are thought to play an important role in the increase in caliber of large axons during development, as heavy neurofilament (NF-H) -/- mice exhibit a severe axonal hypotrophy (85). Mutations in neurofilaments are also associated with forms of axonal degeneration in the peripheral nerve, suggesting that these disease pathways converge (86).

Two models of how mutations in KIF5A cause HSP have been suggested. The first model proposes that mutant KIF5A are slower motor proteins, with slower transport rates having retarding effects on axonal transport (87). Alternatively, mutations may abrogate microtubule binding, allowing free mutant KIF5A to compete with microtubule-bound wild-type KIF5A for cargo (87). Using in vitro homodimeric motor gliding assays, it was determined that both these models may be true depending on the exact mutation. The K253N and R280S mutations diminished the fraction of transported cargo, suggesting they competed with wild-type KIF5A for cargo, statistically sequestering it from transport (87). The N256S mutant still binds to microtubules but slowed down the transport of cargo (87).

SPG13, Heat Shock Protein 60 (HSP60). Mutations in HSP60 cause SPG13 (88). Only few SPG13 families have been identified since the description of the underlying gene (88, 89). SPG13 is a rare, late-onset, and uncomplicated HSP form.

Hereditary spastic paraplegia 60 represents a mitochondrial heat shock protein that prevents other proteins from misfolding; this protein family is also known as chaperones. The correct folding of proteins is crucial to their function. Cellular environments that are rich with free radicals, such as mitochondria, are prone to induce misfolding of proteins. To investigate the function of HSP60, in vitro chaperone assays were applied to measure the ability of wild-type and mutant forms to refold denatured malate dehydrogenase (90). The V98I mutation causes severe reduction in refolding capacity, whereas the G67S mutation was similar to wild-type HSP60 (90). ATPase assays revealed that the V98I mutation decreases rates of ATP hydrolysis, as compared to wild-type HSP60. Using primary patient fibroblasts from a patient with HSP with the V98I mutation, no differences were found in mitochondrial functions, including mitochondrial membrane potential, cell viability, and sensitivity toward oxidative stress (89). However, the authors observed a downregulation of mitochondrial proteases (89). Interestingly, SPG7 (paraplegin) is a mitochondrial protease, which suggests that mitochondrial protein turnover may represent a pathogenic mechanism in HSP (89).

SPG17, Seipin (BSCL2). SPG17 or Silver syndrome is caused by mutations in BSCL2 (91). Silver et al. (92) reported 2 families with spastic paraplegia and amyotrophy of the hands inherited in an autosomal dominant pattern. However, mutations in the BSCL2 gene are associated with a broader array of diseases, including the recessive Berardinelli-Seip congenital lipodystrophy type 2 (BSCL2 or CGL2), dHMN type V, and variants of axonal Charcot-Marie-Tooth disease (93–95). Additional symptoms of SPG17 include distal motor neuropathy and pes cavus (96–99). The age of onset varies from childhood to the fourth decade of live (92). Few families have been reported so far with SPG17 and BSCL2 mutations.

The involvement of upper motor neurons, lower motor neurons, and peripheral nerves has led Ito and Suzuki (100) to propose the term *seipinopathies* to describe this collection of related diseases. Seipin has no closely related homologue genes. The highly conserved amino acids 1 to 280 encode a leucine zipper domain motif. The predicted secondary structure of the zipper domain is similar to sterol regulatory element binding proteins, which regulate cholesterol and lipid metabolism (100). Seipin also contains 2 transmembrane domains and has been shown in multiple studies to be an ER membrane protein (91, 100, 101). Two seipin transcripts (1.8 and 2.4 kb) are ubiquitously expressed, whereas the 2.0-kb transcript is expressed at high levels in the central nervous system (CNS) and testis (91). Molecular studies have demonstrated that seipinopathies associated with mutations in BSCL2 are diseases resulting from problems with dysfunctional protein folding within the endoplasmic reticulum (102). Eventually, misfolded mutant proteins undergo a conformational change that leads to aggregation, a phenomena common to other neurodegenerative diseases of the CNS (102, 103). The N88S and S90L BSCL2 mutations, which are associated with "seipinopathic" motor neuron diseases, alter the N-glycosylation site of seipin and cause accumulation of unfolded protein in the ER (102). It was demonstrated that expression of mutant seipin in cultured cells activates UPR stress and induces ER stress–mediated apoptosis (103).

Recent reports suggest a function for seipin in the interface between the ER and lipid droplets, or adiposomes. Deletion of yeast seipin results in irregular adiposome formation (104). Fibroblasts from patients with congenital lipodystrophy type 2 also form irregular lipid droplets (104). Other reports have revealed a role of seipin in the adipogenesis, with obvious relevance to the lack of adipose tissue observed in Berardinelli-Seip congenital lipodystrophy type 2 (105).

SPG31, Receptor Expression Enhancing Protein 1 (REEP1). SPG31 is caused by mutations in REEP1 (11). An increasing number of families have recently been reported with SPG31, and it is suggested that this HSP form accounts for up to 8.2% of all autosomal dominant cases (8, 22, 106, 107). Most cases are clinically uncomplicated, but additional symptoms may include scoliosis, peripheral neuropathy, spastic tetraparesis, and bulbar dysfunction (8, 22). The age of onset appears to be bimodal, with a subgroup of patients showing early onset in childhood and a second peak in the third and fourth decade of life (8).

REEP1 was first reported as a protein, which associated with odorant receptor proteins and enhanced the receptor response to odorant ligands (108). Along with its identification as the gene mapping to SPG31, REEP1 was shown to be ubiquitously expressed and localized to mitochondria in a number of cell types (11). Interestingly, mutation analysis has revealed mutations in highly conserved predicted micro-RNA binding sites (8). REEP1 also contains a TB2/DP1/HVA22 domain common to heat-shock proteins. Recent work in our laboratory suggests that REEP1 may have alternative splice isoforms, which are expressed and have contrasting subcellular localization patterns (unpublished data). Along with HSP60 (SPG13) and paraplegin (SPG7), mutations in REEP1 point to the importance of mitochondria in the pathogenesis of HSP.

SPG33, Protrudin (ZFYVE27). This form of spastic paraplegia may be caused by mutation in the ZFYVE27 gene (109). The only family reported to date had a pure form of HSP with a late onset of symptoms. More genetic screening studies are necessary to verify the phenotypic spectrum and evaluate the frequency of this HSP form. A recent report suggested that the G191C change in protrudin is a polymorphism (rs35077384) with higher than expected allele frequencies in multiple populations (110).

Protrudin was identified in a yeast 2-hybrid screen as a binding partner of spastin (109). There are, however, conflicting reports regarding how mutations, specifically the single G191V change, affect interactions with spastin (SPG4) (110, 111). Protrudin contains a FYVE-finger domain, which is thought to mediate interactions with phosphoinositide during regulation of vesicular trafficking. Protrudin also has a Rab11 binding domain (RBD11), a guanosine diphosphate dissociation inhibitor consensus sequence, 2 hydrophobic domains, a FFAT endoplasmic reticulum–targeting signal, and a coiled-coil domain (111). Protrudin also plays a critical role in adhesion molecule expression, membrane trafficking, and neurite formation (111). Recently, protrudin was also shown to interact with vesicle-associated membrane protein–associated protein A (VAP-A) (112). Interestingly, mutations in VAP-B, a protein very similar to VAP-A, are associated with ALS (113).

AUTOSOMAL RECESSIVE HSP

SPG5, Cytochrome P450, Family 7, Subfamily B, Polypeptide 1 (CYP7B1). SPG5 is caused by mutations in CYP7B1 (114–121). All patients reported had a pure form of motor neuron degeneration with progressive spastic paraplegia and variable bladder and sensory impairment (121). The findings indicated a pivotal role of altered cholesterol metabolism in the pathogenesis of motor neuron degenerative disease. Recent genetic screens identified additional mutations in CYP7B1, with some families expressing symptoms of the complicated HSP spectrum, including optic atrophy, cerebellar abnormalities, and white matter lesions (122, 123). However, other reports suggested that screening for mutations in CYP7B1 in sporadic and familial cases is of low diagnostic yield (123).

The majority of work on CYP7B1 relate to its function as the first catabolic enzyme in the degradation of cholesterol to bile acids in extrahepatic tissue. CYP7B1 is also thought to function in the pathogenic cholesterol pathways involved in atherosclerosis and act as a metabolic enzyme of neurosteroids and sex hormones. How cholesterol metabolism is related to the pathogenesis of HSP remains an intriguing and unanswered question.

SPG7, Paraplegin. SPG7 is caused by mutations in paraplegin (124). SPG7 presents an autosomal recessive complicated HSP characterized by progressive weakness and spasticity of the lower limbs, diminished vibratory sense, and urinary incontinence. Additional symptoms include peripheral neuropathy, optic atrophy, supranuclear palsy, and cerebelar and cortical atrophy (124–126). SPG7 accounts for about 4% of the autosomal recessive HSP forms. Recently, Brugman et al. (127) screened apparently sporadic HSP cases and found that 8.2% of uncomplicated patients had compound heterozygous paraplegin mutations. However, caution should be taken in interpreting paraplegin sequencing results, as the gene contains a number of common coding changes, some of them were questioned whether they have a direct, causative role in SPG7 (125, 128). These variants may nevertheless amount to modulating or risk alleles for HSP (2).

Paraplegin encodes a mitochondrial inner-membrane ATP-dependent protease. Paraplegin also shows high sequence homology to a family of well-studied yeast ATP-dependent zinc metalloproteases, which suggested a role as a mitochondrial chaperone and proteolytic enzyme (129). In muscle biopsies and cultured primary fibroblasts from SGP7 patients, paraplegin causes defects in oxidative phosphorylation (124, 130, 131). Furthermore, it has been shown that paraplegin interacts with AFG3L2 in the mitochondrial inner membrane to form a high molecular mass complex known as the matrix AAA ATP-dependent protease (m-AAA protease) (130). In cultured SPG7 patient fibroblasts, the paraplegin-AFG3L2 complex fails to function and results in reduced complex I activity and increased sensitivity to oxidative stress (130). Paraplegin knockout mice develop normally up to the age of 1 year, when they begin to show loss of body weight (131). By 17 months, paraplegin null mice display a profound scoliosis along with an uncoordinated movement of the hindlimbs leading to an abnormal gait (131). Histological analysis of spinal cord sections showed axonal degeneration and axon swelling (131). Electron microscopy revealed that mitochondrial abnormalities preceded axonal degeneration and correlated with the appearance of motor impairments (131). Mitochondrial abnormalities and neurofilament aggregates were also seen in optic and sciatic nerve, and retrograde axonal transport was impaired (131). Interestingly, and of potential future therapeutic value, intramuscular injection of adeno-associated virus encoding wild-type paraplegin into paraplegin null mice significantly delayed the onset of motor (132). Regarding the occurrence of optic atrophy in SPG7, it is of interest that the mitochondrial gene OPA1, which causes the most common pure form of optic atrophy, is processed by the m-AAA protease paraplegin.

SPG11, Spatacsin (KIAA1840). Mutations in spatacsin are associated with complicated forms of HSP with mental impairment, thinning of the corpus callosum, among other neurologic findings (133–136). One case of juvenile parkinsonism was associated with

mutations in spatacsin (137). Mutations in KIAA1840 account for up to 21% of all autosomal recessive HSP, which makes SPG11 the most important recessive HSP (133). Recently, it has been shown that large genomic rearrangements can disrupt KIAA1840 (138).

In his original report, Stevanin et al. (133) provided the first description of spatacsin as a 40-exon gene with a ubiquitously expressed full-length 8-kb transcript, encoding a predicted protein of 2,443 amino acids. Spatacsin is highly conserved, but the transcript or protein sequence does not show any significant sequence similarity to known cDNA or protein sequences (133). It is predicted to have 4 putative transmembrane domains. Cell-based experiments also suggested that spatacsin is associated with membranes (133). However, the diffuse staining demonstrated partial overlap with multiple organelles, including mitochondria, ER, but not with Golgi structures, transport vesicles, or alpha-tubulin (133).

SPG15, Spastizin (ZFYVE26). Complicated HSP with pigmentary maculopathy, also known as Kjellin syndrome, is associated with mutations in spastizin (139). Clinical features can also include saccadic pursuit, cognitive impairment, cerebellar signs, dysarthria, peripheral neuropathy, and thin corpus callosum (140, 141). As most recessive HSP forms, the disorder starts in early childhood. HSP15 is a rare recessive HSP form.

Spastizin is a member of the FYVE-finger family, which includes the early endosome antigen 1 and protrudin (SPG33), is thought to mediate interactions with phosphoinositides in endocytic membrane trafficking. The gene is widely expressed in many adult tissues but appears to be more highly expressed in embryonic cells (139). In cell-based experiments, spastizin was found to colocalize with markers of early endosomes and the ER (139). More detailed functional analyses of spastizin will shed light on how endosomal pathways are related to the pathogenesis of HSP.

SPG20, Spartin (KIAA0610). Frameshift mutations in spartin cause this complicated form of HSP, known as Troyer syndrome (142, 143). The disorder has its onset in early childhood with dysarthria, distal muscle wasting, and difficulty in learning to walk. Lower limb spasticity and contractures usually make walking impossible by the third or fourth decade. The syndrome also includes weakness and atrophy of thenar, hypothenar, and dorsal interosseous muscles (143–145).

Both spastin and spartin share an 80 amino acid sequence, which has been termed MIT (contained within microtubule-interacting and trafficking molecules), which is thought to mediate interactions with microtubules in both proteins (52). Initial functional studies showed spartin is a cytosolic protein with some association with membranes (146). In a yeast 2-hybrid screen spartin interacted with the endocytotic protein Eps15, which suggests that it has a role in endosomal trafficking (146). Two spartin isoforms are expressed and show different subcellular localizations (147). In humans, the major cytosolic or membranous spartin isoform is 85 kDa with a larger 100-kDa isoform present in the nucleus (147). Spartin is also present in distal neuronal processes, which appear to partially colocalize with synaptotagmin-positive vesicles (147). Studies of EGF receptor trafficking in HeLa cells also suggest that spartin functions in intracellular trafficking (148). Contrastingly, other reports using mouse and human neuroblastoma cell lines demonstrated mitochondrial localization for spartin (149). Spartin was also identified in a screen for proteins interacting with "homologous to the E6AP C terminus" (HECT) ubiquitin ligase WWP1. Ubiquitination of spartin will target it for degradation and appeared to limit its association to lipid droplets or adiposomes in a number of cell lines (150). This latter report, along with data from seipin mutations, suggests that lipid droplet formation and regulation may have special significance in the pathogenesis of HSP.

SPG21, Maspardin (ACP33). Much like SPG20 and Troyer syndrome, SPG21 and mast syndrome were first described in an Amish family as a slowly progressing form of complicated HSP, including presenile dementia, thin corpus callosum, white matter abnormalities, and cerebellar and extrapyramidal signs (15). Genetic mutations in masparadin were described by Simpson et al. (16). SPG21 presents a rare, clinically complex HSP form (2).

Maspardin has been shown to localize to the endosomal and trans-Golgi network, where it negatively regulates the expression of CD4 in T cells, most likely via endocytosis (151). Subsequent reports confirmed its localization to endosomal and Golgi structures, and mass spectrometry of immunoprecipitated complex identified interactions with aldehyde dehydrogenase ALDH16A1 (152). At this time, no data have been reported that might suggest how mutations in maspardin cause HSP.

SPG39, Neuropathy Target Esterase (NTE). Triaryl phosphates have been use in many commercial and industrial applications, and growing evidence suggest that they may potentially cause organophosphate-induced delayed neuropathy (114). Although acute organophosphate toxicity is associated with a cholinergic crisis, the neurologic syndromes resulting from organophosphate toxicity are highly variable but may lead to progressive spastic paraplegia (115–117). NTE is thought to be the target of neurotoxic organophosphates, which inhibit its catalytic actions or forms a neurotoxic complex. NTE is a lipase that acts to cleave acyl chains from phospholipids in neurons and has been shown to have important roles in cell proliferation and differentiation (118–120). Exogenously expressed NTE is localized to the endoplasmic reticulum and Golgi in mammalian cell lines and is thought to be an important regulator of organelle membrane composition (118). Mutations in the catalytic domains of NTE were found in the genetic analysis of 2 families with HSP resembling organophosphate-induced delayed neuropathy and Troyer syndrome (SPG20) (117). This exciting finding suggests that NTE may contribute to other forms of upper and lower motor neuron disease. A more detailed functional understanding of NTE will be important in our understanding of how membrane and lipid metabolism support axonal processes. The identification of NTE along with BSCL2 and CYP7B1 highlight the potential importance of lipid metabolism in HSP.

X-LINKED HSP

SPG1, L1 Cellular Adhesion Molecule (L1CAM). SPG1 is allelic with the MASA syndrome (mental retardation, aphasia, shuffling gait, and adducted thumbs) and caused by mutations in L1CAM (153). Spastic paraplegia is found in 90% of patients, however (154). Another allelic disorder is X-linked aqueductal stenosis (HSAS). Another acronym that has been suggested is CRASH syndrome (corpus callosum hypoplasia, retardation, adducted thumbs, spastic paraplegia, and hydrocephalus) (155). X-linked spastic paraplegia is a rare disease. HSAS, SPG1, and MASA syndrome occur very early in infancy and neuropathological examination of HSAS patient spinal cord reveals the absence of the corticospinal tract (153). It is thought that mutations associated with SPG1 cause a slightly less severe loss of function, which allows for the development, but not for the proper function, of the corticospinal tract (153). With such a severe and early presentation, the identification of L1CAM as the cause of SPG1 highlights its importance in the development of the corticospinal tract but reveals little about the more slowly progressing HSP forms occurring later in life. L1CAM is an important cell adhesion molecule in the central neurons and was shown to stimulate axon growth (156).

SPG2, Proteolipid Protein 1 (PLP). Pelizaeus-Merzbacher disease (PMD) and SPG2 share the common features of cerebellar ataxia, mental retardation, congenital nystagmus, and seizures (157). Histological analysis of PMD patient CNS tissues revealed diffuse loss of myelin across the brain (157). The clinical and neuropathogial similarities between PMD and SPG21 led investigators to analyze the PLP gene in SPG2 families (157). Indeed, unique mutations were identified in SPG2 patients, suggesting that different mutations in PLP alter the pathogenesis and explain the differences in clinical presentation between PMD and SPG2 (157–159). A mouse line with a spontaneous mutation in PLP coined "rumpshaker" indicates increased rates of myelin degradation (160). Interestingly, it was also found that the UPR, which appears to be activated in response to mutations in PLP in specific strains of mice but not others, modifies the severity of the resulting phenotype (161). It is suggested that genetic background may have a strong influence in the phenotypes resulting from PLP mutations (161).

PERSPECTIVE

With the rapid expansion of known genes in HSP, the key proteins in the pathology of the disease come into focus of molecular research. There is cautious optimism that we will further dissect the major pathways for HSP in the coming decade. Examples of these emerging pathways in HSP are given in the paragraphs above. The main two pathways discussed at the current stage of knowledge are axonal transport/trafficking and mitochondrial function. Yet, these two basic cellular functions involve hundreds if not thousands of proteins and cascades of regulatory and signaling factors. The next aim should therefore be to further specify which functions are inhibited in axonal transport in long axons. This will hopefully shed light on the old question why ubiquitously expressed genes cause such specific phenotypes. Moreover, deciphering the molecular biology of HSP will likely help research on other form of spasticity that are not necessarily genetic in origin. This includes spasticity due to stroke, trauma, or inflammation, as well as spasticity as a symptom within a broader phenotype. Genetic research on a rare condition could therefore well produce the most significant initial pieces of this puzzle. With its unbiased methods, it often leads the investigator to unexpected targets that offer new opportunities of studying this condition.

As for most monogenic neurodegenerative diseases, one should be careful about predicting the appearance of an effective pharmacotherapy. The complicated architecture of the CNS, which does not show significant capacity for regeneration, makes it hard to imagine reparative pharmacologic strategies. The current treatment of HSP consists of symptomatic medical management and physical therapy. No therapies that slow the progression of HSP or even prevent or reverse the symptoms are known. A reduction of muscle spasticity can be achieved with a skeletal muscle relaxant such as the GABA receptor agonist baclofen. Another skeletal muscle relaxant that may improve spasticity is dantrolene. The dose has to be adjusted individually to each patient because variations in drug response exist. In addition, not all patients with HSP exhibit the same degree of spasticity. Other medications include zanaflex, which has been approved to treat muscle spasms, diazepam, and clonazepam. Oxybutynin, a smooth muscle relaxant, is given to reduce the urinary urgency that some patients with HSP complain about. Some patients may be candidates for "chemodenervation," This approach may help to reduce muscle overactivity and can be achieved by intramuscular injections of botulinum toxin. In some patients, neuro-orthopedic surgery to lengthen the ankle plantar flexors or hip adductors may be appropriate. Although physical therapy does not prevent or reduce degenerative changes, it is important to maintain and improve the range of motion and muscle strength.

Hereditary spastic paraplegia probably starts long before recognition of the first clinical symptoms; thus, the availability of comprehensive genetic testing will be important to begin therapy as early as possible for at-risk individuals. This goes in hand with the need to further improve the existing genotype/phenotype data to better predict the actual risk and course of a certain mutation. The variability of the clinical course, even within families, is not well understood. Besides environmental factors, additional genetic susceptibility genes are likely to play a role. The identification and pharmacologic targeting of HSP susceptibility genes might allow for modulation of the clinical course toward milder phenotypes.

For the initial evaluation of new compounds, it will be necessary to focus on one HSP form or on a circumscript pathway. Otherwise, the genetic heterogeneity could be a serious confound for clinical trials. Thus, future clinical trials will require the cooperation of many specialized centers because of the low prevalence of even the most frequent forms of HSP. Specific HSP subtypes might turn out to be better accessible for future compounds, yet another reason for genetic testing. However, the existence of key pathways, such as axonal trafficking, could allow for therapeutic strategies that will improve not just one but several different types of HSP. A potential problem is that many HSP genes are expressed in different tissues but cause specific neurologic disease. Drugs that directly interact with these molecules might have unexpected side effects in other tissues. Animal models will guide the way to successful drug development. Substances such as Vinca alkaloids have already proven potential in *Drosophila* models. However, *Drosophila* is not a full substitute for mammalian models and can only be a first step.

As mentioned above, the potential involvement of micro-RNA binding sites in some cases of HSP could lead the way to new experimental therapeutic strategies. Micro-RNAs are small RNA genes that have only very recently been discovered. Those RNAs target specific conserved regions in the 3'-UTR of many, but not all mRNAs. The disruption of such sites interferes with the binding of micro-RNA's and causes abnormal translation or altered stability of the particular mRNA. Beyond this being the likely mechanism of action for a very limited number of cases in SPG31, it might be possible to develop artificial micro-RNAs that interfere with natural occurring binding sites and thereby change the availability of specific mRNAs that encode for HSP genes. This mechanism would preferentially target loss-of-function HSP genes.

Taken together, the scientific progress in HSP has never been faster than in the last 15 years. This was largely possibly through the advances of human genetics and the availability of ever more detailed maps of the human genome. We are still in the phase of exploring the full spectrum of contributing genes and molecules. The genes identified to date explain about 50% to 60% of all HSP cases, and we might end up with up to 100 HSP genes. Consequently, genetic diagnosis of HSP will become much more complicated as it is today. The molecular deciphering of HSP has already narrowed the focus to a few major pathways, and with the increasing availability of cell and animal models, the evaluation of pharmacologic compounds should progress faster in the near future.

References

1. Harding AE. Classification of the hereditary ataxias and paraplegias. *Lancet* 1983;833:1151–1155.
2. Stevanin G, Ruberg M, Brice A. Recent advances in the genetics of spastic paraplegias. *Curr Neurol Neurosci Rep* 2008;3:198–210.
3. Fink JK. Advances in hereditary spastic paraplegia. *Curr Opin Neurol* 1997;4:313–318.
4. Zuchner S, Vance JM. Emerging pathways for hereditary axonopathies. *J Mol Med* 2005;1:935–943.
5. Filla A, De Michele G, Marconi R, Bucci L, Carillo C, Castellano AE, Iorio L, Kniahynicki C, Rossi F, Campanella G. Prevalence of hereditary ataxias and spastic paraplegias in Molise, a region of Italy. *J Neurol* 1992;239(6):351–353.
6. Polo JM, Calleja J, Combarros O, Berciano J. Hereditary ataxias and paraplegias in Cantabria, Spain. An epidemiological and clinical study. *Brain* 1991;114(2):855–866.
7. Durr A, Camuzat A, Colin E, Tallaksen C, Hannequin D, Coutinho P, Fontaine B, Rossi A, Gil R, Rousselle C, et al. Atlastin1 mutations are frequent in young-onset autosomal

dominant spastic paraplegia 1. *Arch Neurol* 2004;1:1867–1872.
8. Beetz C, Schule R, Deconinck T, Tran-Viet KN, Zhu H, Kremer BP, Frints SG, van Zelst-Stams WA, Byrne P, Otto S. et al. REEP1 mutation spectrum and genotype/phenotype correlation in hereditary spastic paraplegia type 31. *Brain* 2008;131(Pt 4):1078-1086.
9. Fink JK. Advances in the hereditary spastic paraplegias. *Exp Neurol* 2003;184:S106–S110.
10. Soderblom C, Blackstone C. Traffic accidents: molecular genetic insights into the pathogenesis of the hereditary spastic paraplegias. *Pharmacol Ther* 2006;1:42–56.
11. Zuchner S, Wang G, Tran-Viet KN, Nance MA, Gaskell PC, Vance JM, Ashley-Koch AE, Pericak-Vance MA. Mutations in the novel mitochondrial protein REEP1 cause hereditary spastic paraplegia type 31. *Am J Hum Genet* 2006; 79(2):365–369.
12. Reid E, Kloos M, Ashley-Koch A, Hughes L, Bevan S, Svenson IK, Graham FL, Gaskell PC, Dearlove A, Pericak-Vance MA et al. A kinesin heavy chain (KIF5A) mutation in hereditary spastic paraplegia (SPG10). *Am J Hum Genet* 2002;71(5):1189–1194.
13. Hansen JJ, Durr A, Cournu-Rebeix I, Georgopoulos C, Ang D, Nielsen MN, Davoine CS, Brice A, Fontaine B, Gregersen N. et al. Hereditary spastic paraplegia SPG13 is associated with a mutation in the gene encoding the mitochondrial chaperonin Hsp60. *Am J Hum Genet* 2002;70(5):1328–1332.
14. Boukhris A, Stevanin G, Feki I, Denis E, Elleuch N, Miladi MI, Truchetto J, Denora P, Belal S, Mhiri C, et al. Hereditary spastic paraplegia with mental impairment and thin corpus callosum in Tunisia: SPG11, SPG15, and further genetic heterogeneity. *Arch Neurol* 2002;3:393–402.
15. Cross HE, McKusick VA. The mast syndrome. A recessively inherited form of presenile dementia with motor disturbances. *Arch Neurol* 1967;1:1–13.
16. Simpson MA, Cross H, Proukakis C, Pryde A, Hershberger R, Chatonnet A, Patton MA, and Crosby AH. Maspardin is mutated in mast syndrome, a complicated form of hereditary spastic paraplegia associated with dementia. *Am J Hum Genet* 2003;73(5):1147–1156.
17. Blumen SC, Bevan S, Abu-Mouch S, Negus D, Kahana M, Inzelberg R, Mazarib A, Mahamid A, Carasso RL, Slor H, et al. A locus for complicated hereditary spastic paraplegia maps to chromosome 1q24-q32. *Ann Neurol* 2003; 54(6):796–803.
18. Orlacchio A, Kawarai T, Gaudiello F, George-Hyslop PH, Floris R, Bernardi G. New locus for hereditary spastic paraplegia maps to chromosome 1p31.1-1p21.1. *Ann Neurol* 2005;58(3):423–429.
19. Beetz C, Nygren AO, Schickel J, Auer-Grumbach M, Burk K, Heide G, Kassubek J, Klimpe S, Klopstock T, Kreuz F. et al. High frequency of partial SPAST deletions in autosomal dominant hereditary spastic paraplegia. *Neurology* 2006;1:1926–1930.
20. Zuchner S, Wang G, Tran-Viet KN, Nance MA, Gaskell PC, Vance JM, Ashley-Koch AE, and Pericak-Vance MA. Mutations in the novel mitochondrial protein REEP1 cause hereditary spastic paraplegia type 31. *Am J Hum Genet* 2006;2:365–369.
21. Bartel DP. MicroRNAs: genomics, biogenesis, mechanism, and function. *Cell* 2004;116(2):281–297.
22. Hewamadduma C, McDermott C, Kirby J, Grierson A, Panayi M, Dalton A, Rajabally Y, Shaw, P. New pedigrees and novel mutation expand the phenotype of REEP1-associated hereditary spastic paraplegia (HSP). *Neurogenetics* 2009;2:105–110.
23. Reid E. Science in motion: common molecular pathological themes emerge in the hereditary spastic paraplegias. *J Med Genet* 2003;40(2):81–86.
24. Zuchner S. The genetics of hereditary spastic paraplegia and implications for drug therapy. *Expert Opin Pharmacother* 2007;10:1433–1439.

25. Zhao X, Alvarado D, Rainier S, Lemons R, Hedera P, Weber CH, Tukel T, Apak M, Heiman-Patterson T, Ming L. et al. Mutations in a newly identified GTPase gene cause autosomal dominant hereditary spastic paraplegia. *Nat Genet* 2001;29(3):326–331.

26. Abel A, Fonknechten N, Hofer A, Durr A, Cruaud C, Voit T, Weissenbach J, Brice A, Klimpe S, Auburger G, et al. Early onset autosomal dominant spastic paraplegia caused by novel mutations in SPG3A 1. *Neurogenetics* 2004;5(4):239–243.

27. Ivanova N, Claeys KG, Deconinck T, Litvinenko I, Jordanova A, Auer-Grumbach M, Haberlova J, Lofgren A, Smeyers G, Nelis E, et al. Hereditary spastic paraplegia 3A associated with axonal neuropathy. *Arch Neurol* 2007; 5:706–713.

28. Luan Z, Zhang Y, Liu A, Man Y, Cheng L, Hu G. A novel GTP-binding protein hGBP3 interacts with NIK/HGK. *FEBS Lett* 2002;1-3:233–238.

29. Zhu PP, Patterson A, Lavoie B, Stadler J, Shoeb M, Patel R, Blackstone, C. Cellular localization, oligomerization, and membrane association of the hereditary spastic paraplegia 3A (SPG3A) protein atlastin. *J Biol Chem* 2003;4:49063–49071.

30. Zuchner S, Mersiyanova IV, Muglia M, Bissar-Tadmouri N, Rochelle J, Dadali EL, Zappia M, Nelis E, Patitucci A, Senderek J, et al. Mutations in the mitochondrial GTPase mitofusin 2 cause Charcot-Marie-Tooth neuropathy type 2A. *Nat Genet* 2004;36(5):449–451.

31. Sanderson CM, Connell JW, Edwards TL, Bright NA, Duley S, Thompson A, Luzio JP, and Reid E. Spastin and atlastin, two proteins mutated in autosomal-dominant hereditary spastic paraplegia, are binding partners. *Hum Mol Genet* 2006;15(2):307–318.

32. Evans K, Keller C, Pavur K, Glasgow K, Conn B, Lauring B. Interaction of two hereditary spastic paraplegia gene products, spastin and atlastin, suggests a common pathway for axonal maintenance. *Proc Natl Acad Sci U S A* 2006; 2:10666–10671.

33. Namekawa M, Muriel MP, Janer A, Latouche M, Dauphin, A, Debeir T, Martin E, Duyckaerts C, Prigent A, Depienne C, et al. Mutations in the SPG3A gene encoding the GTPase atlastin interfere with vesicle trafficking in the ER/Golgi interface and Golgi morphogenesis. *Mol Cell Neurosci* 2007; 1:1–13.

34. Rojo M, Emery G, Marjomaki V, McDowall AW, Parton RG, Gruenberg J. The transmembrane protein p23 contributes to the organization of the Golgi apparatus. *J Cell Sci* 2000;pt 6:1043–1057.

35. Emery G, Parton RG, Rojo M, Gruenberg J. The transmembrane protein p25 forms highly specialized domains that regulate membrane composition and dynamics. *J Cell Sci* 2003;Pt 23:4821–4832.

36. Hazan J, Fonknechten N, Mavel D, Paternotte C, Samson D, Artiguenave F, Davoine CS, Cruaud C, Durr A, Wincker P, et al. Spastin, a new AAA protein, is altered in the most frequent form of autosomal dominant spastic paraplegia. *Nat Genet* 1999;23(3):296–303.

37. Durr A, Davoine CS, Paternotte C, von Fellenberg J, Cogilinicean S, Coutinho P, Lamy C, Bourgeois S, Prud'homme JF, Penet C, et al. Phenotype of autosomal dominant spastic paraplegia linked to chromosome 2. *Brain* 1996;Pt 5:1487–1496.

38. Nance MA, Raabe WA, Midani H, Kolodny EH, David WS, Megna L, Pericak-Vance MA, Haines JL. Clinical heterogeneity of familial spastic paraplegia linked to chromosome 2p21. *Hum Hered* 1998;3:169–178.

39. Reid E, Grayson C, Rubinsztein DC, Rogers MT, Rubinsztein JS. Subclinical cognitive impairment in autosomal dominant "pure" hereditary spastic paraplegia. *J Med Genet* 1999; 10:797–798.

40. McMonagle P, Byrne PC, Fitzgerald B, Webb S, Parfrey NA, Hutchinson M. Phenotype of AD-HSP due to mutations in the SPAST gene: comparison with AD-HSP without mutations. *Neurology* 2000;12:1794–1800.

41. Orlacchio A, Patrono C, Gaudiello F, Rocchi C, Moschella V, Floris R, Bernardi G, Kawarai T. Silver syndrome variant of hereditary spastic paraplegia: a locus to 4p and allelism with SPG4. *Neurology* 2008;21:1959–1966.

42. Svenson IK, Ashley-Koch AE, Gaskell PC, Riney TJ, Cumming WJ, Kingston, HM, Hogan EL, Boustany RM, Vance JM, Nance MA, et al. Identification and expression analysis of spastin gene mutations in hereditary spastic paraplegia. *Am J Hum Genet* 2001;68(5):1077–1085.

43. Crippa F, Panzeri C, Martinuzzi A, Arnoldi A, Redaelli F, Tonelli A, Baschirotto C, Vazza G, Mostacciuolo ML, Daga A, et al. Eight novel mutations in SPG4 in a large sample of patients with hereditary spastic paraplegia. *Arch Neurol* 2006;5:750–755.

44. Svenson IK, Ashley-Koch AE, Pericak-Vance MA, Marchuk, DA. A second leaky splice-site mutation in the spastin gene. *Am J Hum Genet* 2001;69(6):1407–1409.

45. Riano E, Martignoni M, Mancuso G, Cartelli D, Crippa F, Toldo I, Siciliano G, Di Bella D, Taroni F, Bassi MT, et al. Pleiotropic effects of spastin on neurite growth depending on expression levels. *J Neurochem* 2009;5:1277–1288.

46. Claudiani P, Riano E, Errico A, Andolfi G, and Rugarli EI. Spastin subcellular localization is regulated through usage of different translation start sites and active export from the nucleus. *Exp Cell Res* 2005;2:358–369.

47. Salinas S, Carazo-Salas RE, Proukakis C, Cooper JM, Weston AE, Schiavo G, Warner, TT. Human spastin has multiple microtubule-related functions. *J Neurochem* 2005;5:1411–1420.

48. Errico A, Ballabio A, Rugarli EI. Spastin, the protein mutated in autosomal dominant hereditary spastic paraplegia, is involved in microtubule dynamics. *Hum Mol Genet* 2002;11(2):153–163.

49. McDermott CJ, Grierson AJ, Wood JD, Bingley M, Wharton SB, Bushby, KM, and Shaw, P.J. Hereditary spastic paraparesis: disrupted intracellular transport associated with spastin mutation. *Ann Neurol* 2003;54(6):748–759.

50. Evans KJ, Gomes ER, Reisenweber SM, Gundersen GG, Lauring, BP. Linking axonal degeneration to microtubule remodeling by spastin-mediated microtubule severing. *J Cell Biol* 2005;168(4):599–606.

51. Roll-Mecak A, Vale, RD. The *Drosophila* homologue of the hereditary spastic paraplegia protein, spastin, severs and disassembles microtubules. *Curr Biol* 2005;7:650–655.

52. Ciccarelli FD, Proukakis C, Patel H, Cross H, Azam S, Patton MA, Bork P, Crosby, AH. The identification of a conserved domain in both spartin and spastin, mutated in hereditary spastic paraplegia. *Genomics* 2003;81(4):437–441.

53. Wood JD, Landers JA, Bingley M, McDermott CJ, Thomas-McArthur V, Gleadall LJ, Shaw PJ, Cunliffe VT. The microtubule-severing protein spastin is essential for axon outgrowth in the zebrafish embryo. *Hum Mol Genet* 2006;1:2763–2771.

54. Trotta N, Orso G, Rossetto MG, Daga A, Broadie K. The hereditary spastic paraplegia gene, spastin, regulates microtubule stability to modulate synaptic structure and function. *Curr Biol* 2004;1:1135–1147.

55. Orso G, Martinuzzi A, Rossetto MG, Sartori E, Feany M, Daga A. Disease-related phenotypes in a *Drosophila* model of hereditary spastic paraplegia are ameliorated by treatment with vinblastine. *J Clin Invest* 2005;1:3026–3034.

56. Sherwood NT, Sun Q, Xue M, Zhang B, Zinn K. *Drosophila* spastin regulates synaptic microtubule networks and is required for normal motor function. *PLoS Biol* 2004;12, e429.

57. Baas PW, Karabay A, Qiang, L. Microtubules cut and run. *Trends Cell Biol* 2005;1:518–524.

58. Roll-Mecak A, Vale RD. Making more microtubules by severing: a common theme of noncentrosomal microtubule arrays? *J Cell Biol* 2006;6:849–851.

59. Nishikawa T, Kawakami K, Kumamoto T, Tonooka S, Abe A, Hayasaka K, Okamoto Y, Kawano, Y. Severe neurotoxicities in a case of Charcot-Marie-Tooth disease type 2 caused by vincristine for acute lymphoblastic leukemia. *J Pediatr Hematol Oncol* 2008;7:519–521.

60. Weimer LH, Podwall D. Medication-induced exacerbation of neuropathy in Charcot Marie Tooth disease. *J Neurol Sci* 2006;1-2:47–54.

61. Orejana-Garcia AM, Pascual-Huerta J, Perez-Melero A. Charcot-Marie-Tooth disease and vincristine. *J Am Podiatr Med Assoc* 2003;3:229–233.

62. Hogan-Dann CM, Fellmeth WG, McGuire SA, Kiley VA. Polyneuropathy following vincristine therapy in two patients with Charcot-Marie-Tooth syndrome. *JAMA* 1984;20:2862–2863.

63. Chauncey TR, Showel JL, Fox JH. Vincristine neurotoxicity. *JAMA* 1985;4:507.

64. Griffiths JD, Stark RJ, Ding JC, Cooper IA. Vincristine neurotoxicity in Charcot-Marie-Tooth syndrome. *Med J Aust* 1985;7:305–306.

65. Tarrade A, Fassier C, Courageot S, Charvin D, Vitte J, Peris L, Thorel A, Mouisel E, Fonknechten N, Roblot N, et al. A mutation of spastin is responsible for swellings and impairment of transport in a region of axon characterized by changes in microtubule composition. *Hum Mol Genet* 2006;24:3544–3558.

66. Yu W, Qiang L, Solowska JM, Karabay A, Korulu S, Baas PW. The microtubule-severing proteins spastin and katanin participate differently in the formation of axonal branches. *Mol Biol Cell* 2008;4:1485–1498.

67. White KD, Ince PG, Lusher M, Lindsey J, Cookson M, Bashir R, Shaw PJ, Bushby KM. Clinical and pathologic findings in hereditary spastic paraparesis with spastin mutation. *Neurology* 2000;1:89–94.

68. Wharton SB, McDermott CJ, Grierson AJ, Wood JD, Gelsthorpe C, Ince PG, Shaw PJ. The cellular and molecular pathology of the motor system in hereditary spastic paraparesis due to mutation of the spastin gene. *J Neuropathol Exp Neurol* 2003;11:1166–1177.

69. Chai JH, Locke DP, Greally JM, Knoll JH, Ohta T, Dunai J, Yavor A, Eichler EE, Nicholls RD. Identification of four highly conserved genes between breakpoint hotspots BP1 and BP2 of the Prader-Willi/Angelman syndromes deletion region that have undergone evolutionary transposition mediated by flanking duplicons. *Am J Hum Genet* 2003;4:898–925.

70. Rainier S, Chai JH, Tokarz D, Nicholls RD, and Fink JK. NIPA1 gene mutations cause autosomal dominant hereditary spastic paraplegia (SPG6). *Am J Hum Genet* 2003;73(4):967–971.

71. Kaneko S, Kawarai T, Yip E, Salehi-Rad S, Sato C, Orlacchio A, Bernardi G, Liang Y, Hasegawa H, Rogaeva E, et al. Novel SPG6 mutation p.A100T in a Japanese family with autosomal dominant form of hereditary spastic paraplegia. *Mov Disord* 2006;9:1531–1533.

72. Reed JA, Wilkinson PA, Patel H, Simpson MA, Chatonnet A, Robay D, Patton MA, Crosby AH, Warner TT. A novel NIPA1 mutation associated with a pure form of autosomal dominant hereditary spastic paraplegia. *Neurogenetics* 2005;2:79–84.

73. Klebe S, Lacour A, Durr A, Stojkovic T, Depienne C, Forlani S, Poea-Guyon S, Vuillaume I, Sablonniere B, Vermersch P, et al. NIPA1 (SPG6) mutations are a rare cause of autosomal dominant spastic paraplegia in Europe. *Neurogenetics* 2007;2:155–157.

74. Beetz C, Schule R, Klebe S, Klimpe S, Klopstock T, Lacour A, Otto S, Sperfeld AD, van de Warrenburg B, Schols L, et al. Screening of hereditary spastic paraplegia patients for alterations at NIPA1 mutational hotspots. *J Neurol Sci* 2008; 1-2:131–135.

75. Goytain A, Hines RM, El-Husseini A, Quamme GA. NIPA1(SPG6), the basis for autosomal dominant form of hereditary spastic paraplegia, encodes a functional Mg2+ transporter. *J Biol Chem* 2007;11:8060–8068.

76. Zhao J, Matthies DS, Botzolakis EJ, Macdonald RL, Blakely RD, Hedera P. Hereditary spastic paraplegia-associated mutations in the NIPA1 gene and its *Caenorhabditis elegans* homolog trigger neural degeneration in vitro and in vivo through a gain-of-function mechanism. *J Neurosci* 2008;51:13938–13951.

77. Wang X, Shaw WR, Tsang HT, Reid E, O'Kane CJ. *Drosophila* spichthyin inhibits BMP signaling and regulates synaptic growth and axonal microtubules. *Nat Neurosci* 2007;2:177–185.

78. Valdmanis PN, Meijer IA, Reynolds A, Lei A, Macleod P, Schlesinger D, Zatz M, Reid E, Dion PA, Drapeau P, et al. Mutations in the KIAA0196 gene at the SPG8 locus cause hereditary spastic paraplegia. *Am J Hum Genet* 2007;80:152–161.

79. Rocco P, Vainzof M, Froehner SC, Peters MF, Marie SK, Passos-Bueno MR, Zatz M. Brazilian family with pure autosomal dominant spastic paraplegia maps to 8q: analysis of muscle beta 1 syntrophin. *Am J Med Genet* 2000;2:122–127.

80. Porkka KP, Tammela TL, Vessella RL, Visakorpi T. RAD21 and KIAA0196 at 8q24 are amplified and overexpressed in prostate cancer. *Genes Chromosomes Cancer* 2004;1:1–10.

81. Tessa A, Silvestri G, de Leva MF, Modoni A, Denora PS, Masciullo M, Dotti MT, Casali C, Melone MA, Federico A. et al. A novel KIF5A/SPG10 mutation in spastic paraplegia associated with axonal neuropathy. *J Neurol* 2008;7:1090–1092.

82. Reid E, Dearlove AM, Rhodes M, Rubinsztein DC. A new locus for autosomal dominant "pure" hereditary spastic paraplegia mapping to chromosome 12q13, and evidence for further genetic heterogeneity. *Am J Hum Genet* 1999;3:757–763.

83. Goizet C, Boukhris A, Mundwiller E, Tallaksen C, Forlani S, Toutain A, Carriere N, Paquis V, Depienne C, Durr A, et al. Complicated forms of autosomal dominant hereditary spastic paraplegia are frequent in SPG10. *Hum Mutat* 2009;2:E376–85.

84. Xia CH, Roberts EA, Her LS, Liu X, Williams DS, Cleveland DW, Goldstein LS. Abnormal neurofilament transport caused by targeted disruption of neuronal kinesin heavy chain KIF5A. *J Cell Biol* 2003;161(1):55–66.

85. Zhu Q, Couillard-Despres S, Julien JP. Delayed maturation of regenerating myelinated axons in mice lacking neurofilaments. *Exp Neurol* 1997;1:299–316.

86. Mersiyanova IV, Perepelov AV, Polyakov AV, Sitnikov VF, Dadali EL, Oparin RB, Petrin AN, Evgrafov OV. A new variant of Charcot-Marie-Tooth disease type 2 is probably the result of a mutation in the neurofilament-light gene. *Am J Hum Genet* 2000;67(1):37–46.

87. Ebbing B, Mann K, Starosta A, Jaud J, Schols L, Schule R, Woehlke G. Effect of spastic paraplegia mutations in KIF5A kinesin on transport activity. *Hum Mol Genet* 2008;9:1245–1252.

88. Hansen JJ, Bross P, Westergaard M, Nielsen MN, Eiberg H, Borglum AD, Mogensen J, Kristiansen K, Bolund L, Gregersen N. Genomic structure of the human mitochondrial chaperonin genes: HSP60 and HSP10 are localised head to head on chromosome 2 separated by a bidirectional promoter. *Hum Genet* 2003;1:71–77.

89. Hansen J, Corydon TJ, Palmfeldt J, Durr A, Fontaine B, Nielsen MN, Christensen JH, Gregersen N, Bross, P. Decreased expression of the mitochondrial matrix proteases Lon and ClpP in cells from a patient with hereditary spastic paraplegia (SPG13). *Neuroscience* 2008;2: 474–482.

90. Bross P, Naundrup S, Hansen J, Nielsen MN, Christensen JH, Kruhoffer M, Palmfeldt J, Corydon TJ, Gregersen N, Ang D, et al. The Hsp60-(p.V98I) mutation associated

with hereditary spastic paraplegia SPG13 compromises chaperonin function both in vitro and in vivo. *J Biol Chem* 2008;23:15694–15700.

91. Windpassinger C, Auer-Grumbach M, Irobi J, Patel H, Petek E, Horl G, Malli R, Reed JA, Dierick I, Verpoorten N, et al. Heterozygous missense mutations in BSCL2 are associated with distal hereditary motor neuropathy and Silver syndrome. *Nat Genet* 2004;36(3):271–276.

92. Silver JR. Familial spastic paraplegia with amyotrophy of the hands. *Ann Hum Genet* 1966;1:69–75.

93. Bienfait HM, Baas F, Koelman JH, de Haan RJ, van Engelen BG, Gabreels-Festen AA, Ongerboer de Visser BW, Meggouh F, Weterman MA, De Jonghe P, et al. Phenotype of Charcot-Marie-Tooth disease Type 2. *Neurology* 2007;20:1658–1667.

94. Rohkamm B, Reilly MM, Lochmuller H, Schlotter-Weigel B, Barisic N, Schols L, Nicholson G, Pareyson D, Laura M, Janecke AR, et al. Further evidence for genetic heterogeneity of distal HMN type V, CMT2 with predominant hand involvement and Silver syndrome. *J Neurol Sci* 2007;1-2:100–106.

95. Irobi J, Van den Bergh P, Merlini L, Verellen C, Van Maldergem L, Dierick I, Verpoorten N, Jordanova A, Windpassinger C, De Vriendt E, et al. The phenotype of motor neuropathies associated with BSCL2 mutations is broader than Silver syndrome and distal HMN type V. *Brain* 2004;Pt 9:2124–2130.

96. van de Warrenburg BP, Scheffer H, van Eijk JJ, Versteeg MH, Kremer H, Zwarts MJ, Schelhaas HJ, van Engelen BG. BSCL2 mutations in two Dutch families with overlapping Silver syndrome-distal hereditary motor neuropathy. *Neuromuscul Disord* 2006;2:122–125.

97. Bruyn RP, Scheltens P, Lycklama a Nijeholt J, de Jong, JM. Autosomal recessive paraparesis with amyotrophy of the hands and feet. *Acta Neurol Scand* 1993;6:443–445.

98. Cafforio G, Calabrese R, Morelli N, Mancuso M, Piazza S, Martinuzzi A, Bassi MT, Crippa F, Siciliano G. The first Italian family with evidence of pyramidal impairment as phenotypic manifestation of Silver syndrome BSCL2 gene mutation. *Neurol Sci* 2008;3:189–191.

99. Cho HJ, Sung DH, Ki CS. Identification of de novo BSCL2 Ser90Leu mutation in a Korean family with Silver syndrome and distal hereditary motor neuropathy. *Muscle Nerve* 2007;3:384–386.

100. Ito D, Suzuki N. Seipinopathy: a novel endoplasmic reticulum stress-associated disease. *Brain* 2009;Pt 1:8–15.

101. Ito D, Fujisawa T, Iida H, Suzuki N. Characterization of seipin/BSCL2, a protein associated with spastic paraplegia 17. *Neurobiol Dis* 2008;2:266–277.

102. Ito D, Suzuki N. Molecular pathogenesis of seipin/BSCL2-related motor neuron diseases. *Ann Neurol* 2007;3:237–250.

103. Ito D, Suzuki N. Seipin/BSCL2-related motor neuron disease: seipinopathy is a novel conformational disease associated with endoplasmic reticulum stress. *Rinsho Shinkeigaku* 2007;6:329–335.

104. Szymanski KM, Binns D, Bartz R, Grishin NV, Li WP, Agarwal AK, Garg A, Anderson RG, Goodman JM. The lipodystrophy protein seipin is found at endoplasmic reticulum lipid droplet junctions and is important ;for droplet morphology. *Proc Natl Acad Sci U S A* 2007;52 20890–20895.

105. Payne VA, Grimsey N, Tuthill A, Virtue S, Gray SL, Dalla Nora E, Semple RK, O'Rahilly S, Rochford JJ. The human lipodystrophy gene BSCL2/seipin may be essential for normal adipocyte differentiation. *Diabetes* 2008;8:2055–2060.

106. Liu SG, Che FY, Heng XY, Li FF, Huang SZ, Lu de G, Hou SJ, Liu SE, Wang Q, Wang HP, et al. Clinical and genetic study of a novel mutation in the REEP1 gene. *Synapse* 2009;3:201–205.

107. Schlang KJ, Arning L, Epplen JT, Stemmler S. Autosomal dominant hereditary spastic paraplegia: novel mutations in the REEP1 gene (SPG31). *BMC Med Genet* 2008;9:71.

108. Saito H, Kubota M, Roberts RW, Chi Q, Matsunami H. RTP family members induce functional expression of mammalian odorant receptors. *Cell* 2004;119(5):679–691.

109. Mannan AU, Krawen P, Sauter SM, Boehm J, Chronowska A, Paulus W, Neesen J, Engel W. ZFYVE27 (SPG33), a novel spastin-binding protein, is mutated in hereditary spastic paraplegia. *Am J Hum Genet* 2006;79(2):351–357.

110. Martignoni M, Riano E, Rugarli, EI. The role of ZFYVE27/protrudin in hereditary spastic paraplegia. *Am J Hum Genet* 2008;1, 127-8;author reply:128–30.

111. Shirane M, Nakayama KI. Protrudin induces neurite formation by directional membrane trafficking. *Science* 2006; 5800:818–821.

112. Saita S, Shirane M, Natume T, Iemura SI, Nakayama KI. Promotion of neurite extension by protrudin requires its interaction with VAMP-associated protein (VAP). *J Biol Chem* 2009;284:13766–13777.

113. Mitne-Neto M, Ramos CR, Pimenta DC, Luz JS, Nishimura AL, Gonzales FA, Oliveira CC, Zatz M. A mutation in human VAP-B–MSP domain, present in ALS patients, affects the interaction with other cellular proteins. *Protein Expr Purif* 2007;1:139–146.

114. Weiner ML, Jortner BS. Organophosphate-induced delayed neurotoxicity of triarylphosphates. *Neurotoxicology* 1999; 4:653–673.

115. Morgan JP. The Jamaica ginger paralysis. *JAMA* 1982;15: 1864–1867.

116. Inoue N, Fujishiro K, Mori K, Matsuoka M. Triorthocresyl phosphate poisoning—a review of human cases. *J UOEH* 1988;4:433–442.

117. Rainier S, Bui M, Mark E, Thomas D, Tokarz D, Ming L, Delaney C, Richardson RJ, Albers JW, Matsunami N. et al. Neuropathy target esterase gene mutations cause motor neuron disease. *Am J Hum Genet* 2008;3:780–785.

118. van Tienhoven M, Atkins J, Li Y, Glynn P. Human neuropathy target esterase catalyzes hydrolysis of membrane lipids. *J Biol Chem* 2002;23:20942–20948.

119. Chang PA, Liu C, Chen R, Wu YJ. Effect of over-expression of neuropathy target esterase on mammalian cell proliferation. *Cell Prolif* 2006;5:429–440.

120. Chang PA, Wu YJ, Chen R, Li M, Li W, Qin QL. Inhibition of neuropathy target esterase expressing by antisense RNA does not affect neural differentiation in human neuroblastoma (SK-N SH) cell line. *Mol Cell Biochem* 2005;1-2: 47–54.

121. Tsaousidou MK, Ouahchi K, Warner TT, Yang Y, Simpson MA, Laing NG, Wilkinson PA, Madrid RE, Patel H, Hentati F, et al. Sequence alterations within CYP7B1 implicate defective cholesterol homeostasis in motor-neuron degeneration. *Am J Hum Genet* 2008;2:510–515.

122. Schule R, Brandt E, Karle KN, Tsaousidou M, Klebe S, Klimpe S, Auer-Grumbach M, Crosby AH, Hubner CA, Schols L. et al. Analysis of CYP7B1 in non-consanguineous cases of hereditary spastic paraplegia. *Neurogenetics* 2009;2:97–104.

123. Biancheri R, Ciccolella M, Rossi A, Tessa A, Cassandrini D, Minetti C, Santorelli FM. White matter lesions in spastic paraplegia with mutations in SPG5/CYP7B1. *Neuromuscul Disord* 2009;1:62–65.

124. Casari G, De Fusco M, Ciarmatori S, Zeviani M, Mora M, Fernandez P, De Michele G, Filla A, Cocozza S, Marconi R, et al. Spastic paraplegia and OXPHOS impairment caused by mutations in paraplegin, a nuclear-encoded mitochondrial metalloprotease. *Cell* 1998;6:973–983.

125. Elleuch N, Depienne C, Benomar A, Hernandez, AM, Ferrer X, Fontaine B, Grid D, Tallaksen CM, Zemmouri R, Stevanin G, et al. Mutation analysis of the paraplegin gene (SPG7) in patients with hereditary spastic paraplegia. *Neurology* 2006;5:654–659.

126. Warnecke T, Duning T, Schwan A, Lohmann H, Epplen JT, Young P. A novel form of autosomal recessive hereditary spastic paraplegia caused by a new SPG7 mutation. *Neurology* 2007;4:368–375.

127. Brugman F, Scheffer H, Wokke JH, Nillesen WM, de Visser M, Aronica E, Veldink JH, van den Berg LH. Paraplegin mutations in sporadic adult-onset upper motor neuron syndromes. *Neurology* 19:1500–1505.
128. Arnoldi A, Tonelli A, Crippa F, Villani G, Pacelli C, Sironi M, Pozzoli U, D'Angelo MG, Meola G, Martinuzzi A, et al. A clinical, genetic, and biochemical characterization of SPG7 mutations in a large cohort of patients with hereditary spastic paraplegia. *Hum Mutat* 2008;4:522–531.
129. Pearce DA. Hereditary spastic paraplegia: mitochondrial metalloproteases of yeast. *Hum Genet* 1999;6:443–448.
130. Atorino L, Silvestri L, Koppen M, Cassina L, Ballabio A, Marconi R, Langer T, Casari G. Loss of m-AAA protease in mitochondria causes complex I deficiency and increased sensitivity to oxidative stress in hereditary spastic paraplegia. *J Cell Biol* 2003;163(4):777–787.
131. Ferreirinha F, Quattrini A, Pirozzi M, Valsecchi V, Dina G, Broccoli V, Auricchio A, Piemonte F, Tozzi G, Gaeta L, et al. Axonal degeneration in paraplegin-deficient mice is associated with abnormal mitochondria and impairment of axonal transport. *J Clin Invest* 2004;113:231–242.
132. Pirozzi M, Quattrini A, Andolfi G, Dina G, Malaguti MC, Auricchio A, Rugarli EI. Intramuscular viral delivery of paraplegin rescues peripheral axonopathy in a model of hereditary spastic paraplegia. *J Clin Invest* 2006;1:202–208.
133. Stevanin G, Santorelli FM, Azzedine H, Coutinho P, Chomilier J, Denora PS, Martin E, Ouvrard-Hernandez AM, Tessa A, Bouslam N, et al. Mutations in SPG11, encoding spatacsin, are a major cause of spastic paraplegia with thin corpus callosum. *Nat Genet* 2007;39(3):366–372.
134. Del Bo R, Di Fonzo A, Ghezzi S, Locatelli F, Stevanin G, Costa A, Corti S, Bresolin N, Comi GP. SPG11: a consistent clinical phenotype in a family with homozygous spatacsin truncating mutation. *Neurogenetics* 2007;4:301–305.
135. Hehr U, Bauer P, Winner B, Schule R, Olmez A, Koehler W, Uyanik G, Engel A, Lenz D, Seibel A, et al. Long-term course and mutational spectrum of spatacsin-linked spastic paraplegia. *Ann Neurol* 2007;6:656–665.
136. Crimella C, Arnoldi A, Crippa F, Mostacciuolo ML, Boaretto F, Sironi M, D'Angelo MG, Manzoni S, Piccinini L, Turconi AC, et al. Point mutations and a large intragenic deletion in SPG11 in complicated spastic paraplegia without thin corpus callosum. *J Med Genet* 2009;46(5):345–351.
137. Anheim M, Lagier-Tourenne C, Stevanin G, Fleury M, Durr A, Namer IJ, Denora P, Brice A, Mandel JL, Koenig M, et al. SPG11 spastic paraplegia. A new cause of juvenile parkinsonism. *J Neurol* 2009;1:104–108.
138. Denora PS, Schlesinger D, Casali C, Kok F, Tessa A, Boukhris A, Azzedine H, Dotti MT, Bruno C, Truchetto J, et al. Screening of ARHSP-TCC patients expands the spectrum of SPG11 mutations and includes a large scale gene deletion. *Hum Mutat* 2009;3:E500–19.
139. Hanein S, Martin E, Boukhris A, Byrne P, Goizet C, Hamri A, Benomar A, Lossos A, Denora P, Fernandez J, et al. Identification of the SPG15 gene, encoding spastizin, as a frequent cause of complicated autosomal-recessive spastic paraplegia, including Kjellin syndrome. *Am J Hum Genet* 2008;4:992–1002.
140. Elleuch N, Bouslam N, Hanein S, Lossos A, Hamri A, Klebe S, Meiner V, Birouk N, Lerer I, Grid D, et al. Refinement of the SPG15 candidate interval and phenotypic heterogeneity in three large Arab families. *Neurogenetics* 2007;4:307–315.
141. Boukhris A, Feki I, Denis E, Miladi MI, Brice A, Mhiri C, Stevanin G. Spastic paraplegia 15: linkage and clinical description of three Tunisian families. *Mov Disord* 2008;3:429–433.
142. Patel H, Cross H, Proukakis C, Hershberger R, Bork P, Ciccarelli FD, Patton MA, McKusick VA, Crosby AH. SPG20 is mutated in Troyer syndrome, an hereditary spastic paraplegia. *Nat Genet* 2002;31(4):347–348.
143. Cross HE, McKusick VA. The Troyer syndrome. A recessive form of spastic paraplegia with distal muscle wasting. *Arch Neurol* 1967;5:473–485.
144. Bakowska JC, Wang H, Xin B, Sumner CJ, Blackstone C. Lack of spartin protein in Troyer syndrome: a loss-of-function disease mechanism? *Arch Neurol* 2008;4:520–524.
145. Proukakis C, Cross H, Patel H, Patton MA, Valentine A, Crosby AH. Troyer syndrome revisited. A clinical and radiological study of a complicated hereditary spastic paraplegia. *J Neurol* 2004;9:1105–1110.
146. Bakowska JC, Jenkins R, Pendleton J, Blackstone C. The Troyer syndrome (SPG20) protein spartin interacts with Eps15. *Biochem Biophys Res Commun* 2005;4:1042–1048.
147. Robay D, Patel H, Simpson MA, Brown NA, Crosby, AH. Endogenous spartin, mutated in hereditary spastic paraplegia, has a complex subcellular localization suggesting diverse roles in neurons. *Exp Cell Res* 2006;15:2764–2777.
148. Bakowska JC, Jupille H, Fatheddin P, Puertollano R, Blackstone C. Troyer syndrome protein spartin is mono-ubiquitinated and functions in EGF receptor trafficking. *Mol Biol Cell* 2007;5:1683–1692.
149. Lu J, Rashid F, Byrne PC. The hereditary spastic paraplegia protein spartin localises to mitochondria. *J Neurochem* 2006;98(6):1908–1919.
150. Eastman SW, Yassaee M, Bieniasz PD. A role for ubiquitin ligases and Spartin/SPG20 in lipid droplet turnover. *J Cell Biol* 2009;6:881–894.
151. Zeitlmann L, Sirim P, Kremmer E, Kolanus W. Cloning of ACP33 as a novel intracellular ligand of CD4. *J Biol Chem* 2001;12:9123–9132.
152. Hanna MC, Blackstone, C. Interaction of the SPG21 protein ACP33/maspardin with the aldehyde dehydrogenase ALDH16A1. *Neurogenetics* 2009;10(3):217–228.
153. Jouet M, Rosenthal A, Armstrong G, MacFarlane J, Stevenson R, Paterson J, Metzenberg A, Ionasescu V, Temple K, Kenwrick S. X-linked spastic paraplegia (SPG1), MASA syndrome and X-linked hydrocephalus result from mutations in the L1 gene. *Nat Genet* 1994;3:402–407.
154. Schrander-Stumpel C, Howeler C, Jones M, Sommer A, Stevens C, Tinschert S, Israel J, Fryns JP. Spectrum of X-linked hydrocephalus (HSAS), MASA syndrome, and complicated spastic paraplegia (SPG1): clinical review with six additional families. *Am J Med Genet* 1995;1:107–116.
155. Fransen E, Lemmon V, Van Camp G, Vits L, Coucke P, Willems PJ. CRASH syndrome: clinical spectrum of corpus callosum hypoplasia, retardation, adducted thumbs, spastic paraparesis and hydrocephalus due to mutations in one single gene, L1. *Eur J Hum Genet* 1995;3(5):273–284.
156. Lagenaur C, Lemmon V. An L1-like molecule, the 8D9 antigen, is a potent substrate for neurite extension. *Proc Natl Acad Sci U S A* 1987;21:7753–7757.
157. Saugier-Veber P, Munnich A, Bonneau D, Rozet JM, Le Merrer M, Gil R, Boespflug-Tanguy O. X-linked spastic paraplegia and Pelizaeus-Merzbacher disease are allelic disorders at the proteolipid protein locus. *Nat Genet* 1994;3:257–262.
158. Hodes ME, Zimmerman AW, Aydanian A, Naidu S, Miller NR, Garcia Oller JL, Barker B, Aleck KA, Hurley TD, Dlouhy SR. Different mutations in the same codon of the proteolipid protein gene, PLP, may help in correlating genotype with phenotype in Pelizaeus-Merzbacher disease/X-linked spastic paraplegia (PMD/SPG2). *Am J Med Genet* 1999;2:132–139.
159. Cailloux F, Gauthier-Barichard F, Mimault C, Isabelle V, Courtois V, Giraud G, Dastugue B, Boespflug-Tanguy O. Genotype-Phenotype correlation in inherited brain myelination defects due to proteolipid protein gene mutations. Clinical European Network on Brain Dysmyelinating Disease. *Eur J Hum Genet* 2000;11:837–845.
160. McLaughlin M, Barrie JA, Karim S, Montague P, Edgar JM, Kirkham D, Thomson CE, Griffiths IR. Processing of PLP in a model of Pelizaeus-Merzbacher disease/SPG2 due to the rumpshaker mutation. *Glia* 2006;53(7):715–722.
161. McLaughlin M, Karim SA, Montague P, Barrie JA, Kirkham D, Griffiths IR, Edgar JM. Genetic background influences UPR but not PLP processing in the rumpshaker model of PMD/SPG2. *Neurochem Res* 2007;2:167–176.

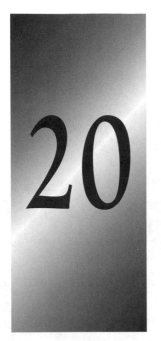

20 Spasticity Affecting Those With Neuromuscular Diseases: Pathology, Epidemiology, and Treatment

Rachel M. Dolhun
Peter D. Donofrio

Neuromuscular disorders are defined as those whose pathology affects any process in the motor unit, including the anterior horn cells, motor roots, peripheral nerve, neuromuscular junction, and muscle. The common presentation of neuromuscular disorders is weakness. Atrophy is frequently observed in neuromuscular disorders but may not be present in the initial phase of the illness. The weakness and atrophy are often asymmetric in anterior horn cell disorders and radiculopathy and typically symmetric in diseases of the peripheral nerve, neuromuscular junction, and muscle. Fasciculations are random discharges of motor units and are most commonly associated with amyotrophic lateral sclerosis (ALS) but can be seen in radiculopathy and peripheral neuropathy. Sensory symptoms and sensory loss are observed in peripheral neuropathies and radiculopathy but are not seen in diseases of the anterior horn cell, neuromuscular junction, or muscle unless a superimposed neuropathy, radiculopathy, myelopathy, or other central nervous system disorder is present.

Spasticity is not detected in most patients presenting with neuromuscular disorders. This chapter discusses 6 conditions where spasticity may play a role in the disability of the patient. Spasticity is very common in ALS and is the predominate feature in patients with primary lateral sclerosis (PLS) and hereditary spastic paraparesis (HSP) or paraplegia. It is not uncommonly detected in patients with Friedreich

ataxia (FA), B12 deficiency, and copper deficiency but may not be present in many patients, and often, it is not a distinctive feature of the neurologic presentation or examination.

AMYOTROPHIC LATERAL SCLEROSIS

Overview

Amyotrophic lateral sclerosis is a progressive neurodegenerative disease that targets both upper and lower motor neurons in the motor cortex, brainstem, and spinal cord. Amyotrophic lateral sclerosis is sometimes referred to as Lou Gehrig disease, after the famous baseball player who died of the disease and who raised awareness of the illness. Clinical symptoms involve limb and bulbar weakness, the latter manifesting as dysarthria and dysphagia, along with fasciculations and spasticity. Signs include atrophy, hyperreflexia, clonus, and extensor plantar responses; the demonstration of hyperreflexia in a weak and wasted extremity is highly suggestive of ALS. Figure 20.1 demonstrates severe atrophy of the hands in a young woman who has ALS. Figure 20.2 shows atrophy of the tongue in the same person. The illness is relentlessly progressive and debilitating. The combination of weakness and spasticity eventually interferes with ambulation, impairs performance of activities of daily living, and causes significant pain.

The diagnosis of ALS is made on clinical grounds after mimicking illnesses have been excluded. The revised El Escorial Criteria (1) provide a framework for diagnosis, dividing the clinical presentation into categories ranging from definite to possible ALS based on the presence of upper and lower motor neuron degeneration, progressive spread of symptoms or signs within or to additional anatomically defined regions (craniobulbar, cervical, thoracic, and lumbosacral), and absence of electrophysiologic, pathological, and neuroimaging evidence of alternate etiologies to explain symptoms and signs. The differential diagnosis of ALS is broad. A limited list is as follows: for bulbar symptoms—myasthenia gravis, brainstem lesions, progressive bulbar palsy, and oculopharyngeal dystrophy; for upper motor neuron dysfunction—cervical spondolytic myeloradiculopathy, multiple sclerosis, PLS, hereditary spastic paraplegia, infectious myelopathy (HIV or HTLV-1), and subacute combined degeneration of the spinal cord; and for lower motor neuron disease—spinal or progressive muscular atrophy, multifocal motor neuropathy, chronic inflammatory demyelinating neuropathy, and spinobulbar muscular atrophy (2).

No single diagnostic test is confirmatory for ALS. Electrophysiologic testing documents lower motor neuron dysfunction in the setting of normal sensory studies. Magnetic resonance imaging of the brain and spine excludes structural causes for symptoms; T2 hyperintensity in the corticospinal tracts, most likely secondary to Wallerian degeneration, has been demonstrated in some patients. Additional laboratory studies to rule out infectious, inflammatory, metabolic, or nutritional etiologies may be necessary in

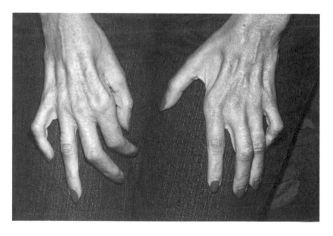

FIGURE 20.1

Photo of the hands of a young woman with ALS showing pronounced atrophy of intrinsic hand muscles and finger contractures.

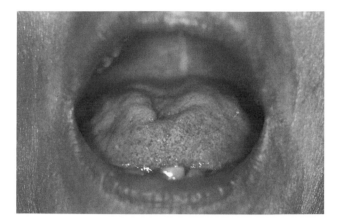

FIGURE 20.2

Photo of the tongue of the same young woman with ALS in Figure 20.1. Tongue atrophy and fissuring are observed.

patients whose clinical presentation is not compelling for ALS.

Amyotrophic lateral sclerosis is inevitably fatal, usually due to failure of respiratory function. Population studies have reported the cumulative probability of survival after diagnosis as 78% at 12 months, 56% at 24 months, and 32% at 36 months. Only 25% live beyond 5 years (3, 4). Median survival is approximately 3 to 5 years from symptom onset. Negative prognostic factors for survival are older age, rapid progression of symptoms, site of disease onset, and low compound muscle action potential amplitudes on motor conduction studies. Bulbar onset disease comprises 25% of cases and portends a poorer prognosis than spinal onset (4).

Amyotrophic lateral sclerosis is currently without an adequate disease-modifying therapy to halt or reverse the progression of disease. As such, treatment efforts are concentrated on symptom management to optimize the quality of life.

Epidemiology

Amyotrophic lateral sclerosis is a relatively rare disease. In population studies from Europe and North America, the reported incidence is 1.5 to 2.5 per 100,000 individuals per year (3), whereas the prevalence is 4 to 6 per 100,000 (4). The incidence is 50 to 150 times higher in the Western Pacific where ALS is associated with the parkinsonism-dementia complex, and environmental, rather than genetic, factors are thought to play a role.

The incidence of ALS increases after the age of 40 years, peaks in the 7th and 8th decades, and then rapidly declines. Approximately 15% of patients are diagnosed at an age younger than 40. In this setting, a positive family history is often present. Familial cases associated with superoxide dismutase 1 (SOD1) mutations present, on average, 10 years earlier than sporadic cases with an average age of onset of 46 versus 56 years (5). Gender studies indicate nearly equal incidence with a male-to-female ratio of 1.3-1.6:1 (4). The incidence of ALS appears to be lower among African, Asian, and Hispanic ethnicities than among whites (6). The current hypothesis is that ALS is a complex genetic condition with significant variability in presentation ranging from sporadic cases without any family history to families displaying a typical autosomal dominant inheritance pattern (4). Sporadic cases account for 90% of all ALS diagnoses; any prior family history denotes familial ALS in the remaining 10%. Thus far, the SOD1 gene has been the most thoroughly investigated in familial ALS. Mutations of this gene, localized to chromosome 21, lead to a toxic gain-of-function pathology, which accounts for 10% to 20% of the autosomal dominant familial ALS cases (5).

Pathogenesis of ALS

Familial ALS

As stated above, SOD1 mutations have been implicated in familial autosomal dominant ALS. Despite the identification of genetic defects in juvenile-onset disease and in families displaying autosomal dominant inheritance patterns, the SOD1 mutations are the only ones that lead specifically and exclusively to classic ALS (4, 5). Superoxide dismutase 1 works as an antioxidant to transform superoxide anions into hydrogen peroxide. Oxidation and subsequent misfolding of SOD1 are believed to lead to an extracellular protein secreted by neurons and glial cells, which is selectively toxic to cortical and spinal motor neurons, cortical and certain spinal interneurons, and dopaminergic neurons (5).

Sporadic ALS

Several mechanisms, which are not mutually exclusive, have been hypothesized in the initiation and propagation of the neurodegeneration in ALS. The major theories include excitotoxicity, oxidative stress, mitochondrial dysfunction, immune or inflammatory mechanisms, neurofilament abnormalities, and microglial-mediated neurotoxicity (7, 8).

The excitotoxicity model is based on glutamate. Excitotoxicity leads to neuronal cell death by repetitive firing or elevation of intracellular calcium by calcium-permeable glutamate receptors.

Glutamate is released by presynaptic terminals and then diffuses across synaptic clefts to induce receptors on postsynaptic dendrites. Glutamate transporters facilitate the reuptake of glutamate to prevent repetitive motor firing. Excitatory amino acid transporter type 2 is the main glial glutamate transporter; loss of this protein and subsequently reduced transport and elevated cerebrospinal fluid (CSF) glutamate have been implicated in the pathogenesis of ALS (7, 8).

The hypothesis of oxidative stress involves the failure of antioxidant defenses in motor neurons to limit the attack of subcellular components by oxygen free radicals, which causes lipid peroxidation, cytoskeletal disruption, and mitochondrial damage (8, 9–17).

Mitochondrial dysfunction is proposed as an additional cause of neurodegeneration. Morphologic studies have demonstrated mitochondrial abnormalities in patients with sporadic ALS and in familial ALS mice (with SOD1 mutation) in which mitochondrial swelling and vacuolization were seen early in the course of the disease (8, 18–20).

Environmental factors, including cycad seeds and mineral imbalances in the ALS-parkinsonism-dementia complex of the Western Pacific and pesticides and heavy metals, have been proposed to play a role in the development of ALS (5). In most patients, however, the contribution of environmental factors to the pathogenesis of ALS is unclear.

Pathogenesis of Spasticity

Amyotrophic lateral sclerosis encompasses a combination of upper and lower motor neuron symptoms and signs. The upper motor neuron features are the negative signs of weakness and loss of dexterity and positive signs of hyperreflexia, clonus, flexor spasms, and spasticity. Spasticity is thought to arise from hyperexcitability of lower motor neurons and abnormal processing of proprioceptive input in the spinal cord. The increased excitability of lower motor neurons is a result of damage in the descending modulatory tracts, which include the corticospinal, reticulospinal, vestibulospinal, and tectospinal tracts. Corticospinal tract axons provide both excitatory and inhibitory influences through the alpha motor neurons, gamma motor neurons, and Ia inhibitory interneurons. A pure pyramidal lesion, however, is thought to have a minimal contribution to spasticity as demonstrated extensively in animal studies. Rather, it is the dorsal reticulospinal tract that appears to be the main inhibitory pathway, providing tonic inhibition of flexor reflex afferents and spinal stretch reflexes. Excitatory pathways are conducted through the medial reticulospinal and vestibulospinal tracts; lesions of these axons seem to have some contribution to spasticity.

Normal tone thus consists of a balance between inhibitory effects on stretch reflexes mediated by the dorsal reticulospinal tract and excitatory effects on extensor tone modulated by the medial reticulospinal and vestibulospinal tracts. Lesions of these upper motor neurons therefore disturb this delicate balance, which produces a state of net disinhibition of the spinal reflexes (9–11).

Pathology

On gross examination, there is atrophy of the precentral gyrus of the motor cortex and ventral spinal roots. Microscopically, there is a loss of anterior horn neurons, anterior root myelinated fibers, and brainstem motor nuclei with specific involvement of the hypoglossal, ambiguus, and motor trigeminal cranial nerves. Destruction of these and other upper motor neurons leads to Wallerian degeneration in the corticospinal tracts. Characteristic Bunina bodies, Periodic Acid Schiff-positive cytoplasmic inclusions, and ubiquinated inclusions are present in remaining neurons. The sensory system is typically spared.

Neurofibrillary tangles composed of hyperphosphorylated tau protein are often seen in patients with the ALS-parkinsonism-dementia complex of Guam (11, 12).

Treatment

Disease Modifying

Riluzole is currently the only disease-modifying agent approved for the treatment of ALS. This medication works on 3 separate mechanisms to inhibit glutamate release, block postsynaptic N-methyl-D-aspartic acid receptor-mediated responses, and inactivate voltage-sensitive sodium channels (8).

The use of riluzole is based on the results of 2 large randomized, double-blind, placebo-controlled clinical trials. Bensimon et al. (13) analyzed the primary outcome measures of survival and rate of change in functional outcomes and the secondary outcome of change in muscle strength as assessed manually using the Medical Research Council Scale in 155 patients with ALS taking either riluzole 100 mg per day or placebo for 12 months. After a median follow-up of 18 months, the drug appeared to slow the progression of the disease, showing a more prominent therapeutic benefit in patients with bulbar versus those with limb onset. For patients with bulbar-onset disease, the 1-year survival rate was 73% (compared to 35%

in placebo), and for those with limb-onset disease, 1-year survival was 74% (vs 64% in placebo). A beneficial effect on rate of muscle strength deterioration was also noted to be significant in the riluzole group (13).

A second dose-ranging trial of riluzole was performed by Lacomblez et al. (14) to evaluate a primary outcome of survival without tracheostomy and secondary outcomes of rates of change of functional measures including muscle strength (as manually measured by the Medical Research Council Scale), functional status, respiratory function, and the participant's subjective assessments of fasciculations, cramps, stiffness, and tiredness. Patients with ALS (959 patients) were followed up for a median period of 18 months after being randomized to receive placebo, or 50, 100, or 200 mg per day for 12 months. The results demonstrated a small but significant survival prolongation in patients receiving riluzole compared to placebo with an inverse dose response in the risk of death (50.4% of placebo patients alive at 18 months compared to 55.3%, 56.8%, and 57.8% in those taking 50, 100, and 200 mg riluzole per day, respectively). Notably, functional scales did not differentiate between treatment groups, and the trial was unable to confirm a difference in therapeutic response based on site of disease onset, a result different from the original trial by Bensimon et al. (14).

Bensimon et al undertook another study of riluzole 100 mg per day versus placebo in 168 more advanced patients with ALS (age >75, disease duration >5 years, forced vital capacity <60%). This study failed to demonstrate a significant survival advantage in the riluzole-treated patients based on survival analysis at 12 months (15).

Pooling data from these pivotal trials, the authors of the Cochrane Collaboration concluded that riluzole offers a modest prolongation of median survival of 2 to 3 months. The drug is well tolerated; the most common adverse effects are gastrointestinal upset, asthenia, and transaminase elevation (16).

Based on the previously described theories for the pathogenesis of ALS and successful results in the mouse model of the SOD1 mutation, a variety of drugs have been investigated in large placebo-controlled trials. Unfortunately, none has been able to show additional disease-modifying benefits. One example is gabapentin. Gabapentin has been hypothesized to reduce the pool of releasable glutamate, and any benefit could be explained by the glutamate excitotoxicity theory of ALS. Several studies have been completed with this drug. Miller et al. (17) administered gabapentin 800 mg 3 times per day versus placebo for 6 months to 152 patients with ALS in a randomized, double-blind trial. The primary outcome measure was the slope of the arm megascore, the average maximum voluntary isometric contraction strength from 8 arm muscles standardized against a reference ALS population. The secondary outcome measure was forced vital capacity. The results did not show a statistically significant trend toward a slower rate of decline of arm strength in the gabapentin-versus-placebo group; in addition, there was no observed treatment effect on forced vital capacity (17). The authors thereafter initiated a randomized, double-blind, placebo-controlled trial of 128 patients with ALS who took gabapentin 3600 mg per day for 9 months; the same outcome measures were utilized. Once again, there was no difference in the rate of decline of arm scores between the groups (18). A combined analysis of the phase II and phase III studies showed a more rapid rate of decline of the forced vital capacity in patients treated with gabapentin (8).

Topiramate, which also possesses anti-excitatory properties, was proposed as a potential ALS therapy. This drug reduces glutamate release from neurons and antagonizes kainate activation of the α-amino-3-hydroxy-5-methyl-isoxazole-4-propionic acid glutamatergic excitatory amino acid receptor. Cudkowicz et al. (19) randomized 296 patients with ALS to either placebo or topiramate (maximum 800 mg per day) for 12 months of treatment in a double-blind trial. The primary end point was rate of change in the upper extremity motor function measured by the maximum voluntary isometric contraction strength; surprisingly, subjects in the topiramate group showed a faster decrease in arm and grip strength compared to placebo. There was no significant effect on secondary outcomes of rates of decline in forced vital capacity, ALS Functional Rating Scale (ALSFRS), and survival. In addition, a large number of adverse effects were reported with the medication (19).

Cyclooxygenase-2 is thought to play a key role in both glutamate-mediated excitotoxicty and inflammation. The enzyme catalyzes the synthesis of prostaglandins, which trigger neuronal and astrocytic glutamate release. As for inflammation, the enzyme is involved in the production of reactive oxygen species, free radicals, and pro-inflammatory cytokines (8). Cudkowicz et al. conducted a double-blind, placebo-controlled trial of 300 patients with ALS, administering celecoxib, a selective cyclooxygenase-2 inhibitor, in a dose of 800 mg per day versus placebo for 12 months. The primary outcome was rate of change of upper extremity motor function measured by the maximum voluntary isometric contraction strength; secondary outcomes were safety, survival, change in CSF prostaglandin E_2 levels, and changes in the rate of decline of leg and grip strength, forced vital capacity, ALSFRS-Revised,

and motor unit number estimates. Although celecoxib was well tolerated, it did not significantly affect survival nor did it slow decline in muscle strength, forced vital capacity, motor unit estimates, or scores on the Functional Rating Scale (20).

Minocycline, a tetracycline antibiotic with anti-inflammatory and antiapoptotic properties, was evaluated in several randomized, double-blind, placebo-controlled trials by Gordon et al. (21). The initial trial demonstrated that minocycline could be taken safely in combination with riluzole (21). A subsequent randomized, placebo-controlled study was conducted in 412 patients who received either placebo or escalating doses of minocycline to 400 mg per day for 9 months. The study organizers selected the rate of change of the ALSFRS as the primary outcome and analyzed forced vital capacity, manual muscle testing, quality of life, survival, and safety as secondary outcomes. The final result was a 25% faster rate of deterioration of the ALSFRS score and a nonsignificant tendency toward faster decline in functional vital capacity, manual muscle testing, and increased mortality in the group receiving minocycline (21, 22).

To evaluate the role of oxidative stress in the pathogenesis of ALS, vitamin E has been tested in conjunction with riluzole. Desnuelle et al. (23) studied 289 patients with ALS taking riluzole 50 mg per day in a randomized, double-blind trial of placebo versus vitamin E 500 mg, BID. There was no significant difference in the primary outcome measure of the Norris Limb Scale at 12 months (23). A subsequent randomized, double-blind trial of 160 patients with ALS on riluzole, done by Graf et al. (24), compared placebo to vitamin E 5000 mg per day. At 18 months, a significant difference could not be shown in the survival rate (the primary outcome) or in the secondary outcomes of rate of deterioration of function, manual muscle testing, or spasticity scale (24).

Creatine plays a significant role in mitochondrial ATP production; thus, its use in ALS might attenuate mitochondrial dysfunction and neurodegeneration. The supplement also has direct antioxidant effects, may contribute to prevention of excitotoxicity and apoptosis, and has been shown to improve muscle strength in healthy individuals. However, 2 randomized, double-blind, placebo-controlled trials failed to identify a beneficial effect on survival or disease progression in ALS. Groeneveld et al. (25) performed a double-blind placebo controlled trial in 175 patients with ALS randomized to either creatine monohydrate 5 g, BID, or placebo. The authors failed to identify a difference in survival, the primary outcome, at 12 months; secondary outcome measures, including rate of decline of isometric arm muscle strength, forced vital capacity, functional status, and quality of life, similarly did not demonstrate a difference in treatment groups (25). Shefner et al. (26) conducted a randomized, placebo-controlled, double-blind trial of 104 patients with ALS to evaluate the efficacy of creatine 5 g per day. The authors also were unable to observe a significant effect of creatine on maximum voluntary isometric contraction of upper extremity muscles, grip strength, ALSFRS-Revised scores, and motor unit number estimates when analysis was completed at 6 months (26).

Motor neuron degeneration is the cornerstone of ALS. A lack of trophic factors, molecules that support cell survival and promote cell differentiation, has been hypothesized as a causative factor. One example is the ciliary neurotrophic factor (CNTF), an endogenous protein of Schwann cells in the peripheral nervous system that is released in response to injury purportedly to limit neuronal damage (27, 28). In ALS wobbler mouse models, CNTF slowed disease progression and improved muscle strength (29). Miller et al. (27) conducted a placebo-controlled trial of escalating doses of recombinant human CNTF (rhCNTF) in 570 patients with ALS. Participants received either placebo or rhCNTF 0.5, 2, or 5 μg/kg per day for 6 months. Primary outcomes were based on changes in maximum voluntary isometric contraction in the upper and lower extremities and pulmonary function; secondary outcomes included survival among other measures. The authors found no beneficial effects of the medication. In fact, more deaths and adverse events were observed in the group receiving the highest dose of rhCNTF (27). The ALS Study Group completed a trial of rhCNTF 15 or 30 μg/kg or placebo injected 3 times weekly for 9 months in 730 patients with ALS. The authors found no statistically significant difference between the treatment and placebo groups (28). Side effects were noted to limit dosing of rhCNTF.

Another neutrophic factor, insulin-like growth factor-1 (IGF-1), is a naturally occurring peptide that exerts its influence on motor neurons, neuromuscular junctions, and muscles and has been shown to promote motor neuron survival in vitro and to improve strength in the wobbler mouse model of ALS. The combined results of 2 important trials provide a small statistically significant benefit after taking IGF-1 based on a change in the score of the Appel Amyotrophic Lateral Sclerosis Rating Scale; the clinical relevance of this remains unclear (30). In the first study of 266 patients, subjects were randomized to placebo, recombinant human IGF-1 (rhIGF-1) 0.5 mg/kg per day, or rhIGF-1 0.10 mg/kg per day for 9 months. The treated groups displayed a slowed progression of functional impairment and health-related quality of life (31). A second trial, done by Borasio et al. (32), compared 183 patients who either received placebo or rhIGF-1 0.10 mg/kg per day for 9 months. The outcome was a nonsignificant difference in the treatment group (32).

Other drugs and therapies have been proposed as disease-modifying agents but have failed to show a beneficial effect. Using the concept that a serum factor might be playing a role in ALS, plasmapheresis has been proposed as a disease-modifying therapy. In at least 2 small case studies, the treatment did not alter the course of the disease (33, 34).

Symptomatic (Spasticity)

Spasticity is a major component of ALS and leads to functional impairment and pain. Usually, a multimodal symptomatic treatment plan is needed, combining medications and physical therapy to improve the quality of life in patients with ALS. Oral medications form the mainstay of therapy despite the absence of large studies specifically showing that the drugs are useful in patients with ALS (35). The most commonly utilized medications include baclofen, diazepam, tizanidine, and dantrolene. Additional therapies include intrathecal baclofen (ITB) and botulinum toxin A injections.

Baclofen stimulates the $GABA_B$ receptor to suppress excitatory neurotransmitter release and to enhance presynaptic inhibition. Its use is limited by side effects of central nervous system depression, such as sedation, confusion, and dizziness, as well as weakness. In those patients with severe spasticity who experience dose-limiting side effects or are otherwise refractory to medical management, ITB may be an option. This therapy involves the long-term delivery of baclofen, at a dose 1% of the typical oral dose, directly into the intrathecal space through an implanted programmable pump. Potential complications of this procedure include infection, pump dysfunction, and baclofen withdrawal symptoms such as seizures (36–38). The literature in ALS is limited to small cohorts, but 2 specific studies suggest that a decrease in spasticity and pain, improved quality of life, and improved function can result from ITB, even in the terminal stages of ALS (39–41).

Benzodiazepines, primarily diazepam, are often used as an adjunct to baclofen. These medications work centrally to increase presynaptic inhibition by binding to $GABA_A$ receptors. Side effects are similar to those listed for baclofen; dependence and tolerance can develop in high doses (36, 37).

Tizanidine, a centrally acting alpha-2 agonist, inhibits the release of excitatory amino acids in spinal interneurons (36, 37). Tizanidine in certain trials reduces spasticity without significantly altering muscle strength and has a similar efficacy and better tolerability as compared to baclofen and diazepam (42, 43). Side effects include sedation, dizziness, and dry mouth.

Dantrolene is the only antispasticity agent that works peripherally to inhibit calcium release from the sarcoplasmic reticulum in skeletal muscle and thereby interferes with the excitation-coupling reaction to decrease the force of muscle contraction. Adverse reactions are gastrointestinal symptoms, hepatotoxicity, generalized weakness, and sedation (36, 37, 44–46).

Botulinum toxin A (botox), derived from the anaerobic bacteria *Clostridium botulinum*, acts presynaptically in the neuromuscular junction to prevent the release of acetylcholine. Injections of botox are widely used to treat spasticity secondary to stroke and multiple sclerosis. They are less commonly utilized in ALS but have been shown to be effective for trismus and stridor in case reports (46, 47). The injections exert a local effect; there remains a risk of generalized weakness if injected intravenously.

Medications should be coupled with exercise and physical therapy. A randomized, controlled trial found that moderate-intensity, endurance-type exercises for the trunk and limbs may reduce spasticity and impact positively disability in ALS (48).

PRIMARY LATERAL SCLEROSIS

Overview

Primary lateral sclerosis is a rare, nonhereditary, neurodegenerative disorder targeting only upper motor neurons. The main clinical manifestation is spasticity, which is accompanied by symptoms and signs of upper motor neuron dysfunction, including hyperreflexia, clonus, and extensor plantar responses. The disease has an insidious onset, typically beginning with spasticity of one or both lower limbs. Patients complain of loss of dexterity, slowness, and stiffness along with gait abnormalities; weakness may be present but is not as prominent as in ALS (49). Often, patients with PLS complain of weakness, yet the neurologic examination demonstrates little if any true weakness, and the predominant sign is profoundly increased tone. Primary lateral sclerosis has the tendency to gradually ascend and evolve into a tetrapyramidal syndrome including pseudobulbar involvement characterized by unprovoked and inappropriate emotional displays. In some instances, the disease presents initially in the upper extremities or the bulbar region (50). The course is very slowly progressive, often with periods of stabilization, but eventually leading to debilitating spasticity. Median survival rate is not well defined; it is generally accepted to be much longer than survival in ALS. Survival ranges from 1 to 15 years from disease onset and has been described as approximately 8 years in a number of studies (51). Sensory symptoms are usually absent. Urinary incontinence, most likely due to detrusor hyperreflexia and internal sphincter spasticity, is fairly common in later stages of the illness (49, 51, 52).

The diagnosis is made on clinical grounds, when other disorders causing spasticity are excluded. Criteria for PLS were originally proposed by Pringle et al. (53, 54), but modifications have been suggested based on additional research. The initial guidelines permitted occasional fibrillation potentials and increased insertional activity on electrophysiologic testing to be included in the diagnosis of PLS, but subsequent guidelines have categorized patients with those electrographic abnormalities to clinical or suspected, rather than classic, PLS (54). Pringle et al. in his criterion required only 3 years of monitoring for the development of lower motor neuron symptoms before establishing the formal diagnosis of PLS, whereas Gordon et al. (55) extended this observation period to 4 years.

Corticospinal spasticity with or without corticobulbar symptoms can be observed in many illnesses including structural disorders (Arnold-Chiari malformation, cervical spondylotic myelopathy, spinal arteriovenous malformation, or hydrocephalus), degenerative diseases (multiple sclerosis and spinocerebellar ataxia), leukodystrophy, toxic/metabolic illnesses (subacute combined degeneration, vitamin E deficiency), and infectious etiologies (syphilitic hypertrophic pachymeningitis, tropical spastic paraparesis, AIDS) (56). However, when patients present with an isolated syndrome of progressive spinobulbar spasticity, the list is substantially narrowed to PLS, hereditary spastic paraplegia, and upper motor neuron-onset ALS (49).

Nearly all patients with suspected PLS undergo electrophysiologic testing to determine the presence of subclinical lower motor neuron disease. Further evaluation for alternate explanations of generalized upper motor neuron disease is individually tailored to the specifics of the clinical presentation.

Hematologic and CSF testing is performed to exclude infectious etiologies of myelopathy (syphilis, Lyme disease, HTLV-1, HIV), nutritional (vitamin B12, folic acid, copper deficiencies), and genetic disorders (specific mutations for HSP, spinocerebellar ataxia, and hexosaminidase A deficiency and very long chain fatty acids for adrenomyeloneuropathy) (1). In rare cases, PLS symptoms have been associated with HIV infection, paraneoplastic syndromes, sprue, and Sjogren syndrome (57).

Imaging of the brain and spine are performed to eliminate structural anomalies (Chiari malformation, spondylosis, and intrinsic spinal cord lesions), compressive etiologies, and T2 hyperintensities of multiple sclerosis (1). Cortical atrophy, either diffuse or focal in the primary motor region, has been observed in PLS but is not a consistent feature (58–60).

Debate continues as to whether PLS is a distinct pathological entity or represents one point on a spectrum of motor neuron disease between ALS with its upper and lower motor neuron involvement and a pure upper motor neuron syndrome, which has not yet been clearly defined. Features that differentiate this disease from ALS are the prolonged course and lack of impressive weakness and lower motor neuron signs. Occasionally, patients with suspected PLS demonstrate electrophysiologic evidence of lower motor neuron dysfunction or clinical evidence of cramps, fasciculations, or amyotrophy either at the time of diagnosis or at follow-up (52, 53, 58, 59). Several authors have attributed these signs, particularly atrophy, to disuse, whereas others judge them to be a signal that the disease has evolved into classic ALS. Still, others believe that the lower motor neuron dysfunction is either transient or a product of the chronicity of PLS as it progresses (61).

Similarities between ALS and PLS are the age of onset, presence of spinal and bulbar forms of the disease, and lack of sensory disturbances. Additional clues to a continuous relationship between the 2 motor neuron diseases and to other neurodegenerative disorders are the presence of frontal lobe dementia or neuropsychological impairment and ocular movement abnormalities (49, 54, 58).

Epidemiology

Primary lateral sclerosis is rare, comprising only 2% of 5% of all patients with motor neuron disease. Symptoms begin in the fifth to sixth decade; the mean age of onset is 45.4 to 53.7 years. There may be a slight male predominance, but this is based on small population studies (49, 52).

Pathophysiology of Spasticity

As in ALS, the increased tone of PLS is thought to be a manifestation of the disturbed balance between inhibitory input of the dorsal reticulospinal tract and facilitatory input of the medial reticulospinal and vestibulospinal tracts on lower motor neurons (62–64).

Pathology

Only a few patients with PLS have gone to autopsy. In PLS, there is degeneration of the frontal and prefrontal motor cortex with selective loss of Betz cells and giant pyramidal neurons located in layer 5. Laminar gliosis is seen in layers 3 and 5. Atrophy of the precentral gyrus can be visualized on gross examination (58, 65). Loss of these upper motor neurons results in secondary demyelination and degeneration of the descending corticospinal and corticobulbar pathways (59). Anterior horn motor neurons are typically preserved in classic PLS, but loss of these neurons, to a lesser extent than that in ALS, has been documented (60, 65). Bunina bodies and ubiquinated inclusions, previously thought to be the hallmark of ALS, have also been noted in patients with PLS (49, 53).

Treatment

Primary Lateral Sclerosis

No disease-modifying therapy for PLS has been found based on the lack of clinical trials showing any therapy to be useful for the illness. Patients may be offered high doses of the antioxidants, vitamins C and E, and beta carotene (49).

Spasticity

Therapy is directed at symptomatic management. As in ALS, oral baclofen, a $GABA_B$ agonist, and tizanidine, a central alpha-2 agonist, are first-line medications; benzodiazepines and dantrolene are utilized less frequently. Intrathecal baclofen is an option in refractory cases. In case reports, ITB has been shown to partially relieve spasticity and improve quality of life without causing excessive weakness out of proportion to that expected by disease progression itself (49, 66, 67).

HEREDITARY SPASTIC PARAPARESIS

Overview

The term *hereditary spastic paraparesis* encompasses a heterogeneous group of inherited disorders characterized by progressive gait dysfunction secondary to symmetric lower extremity spasticity (68). The disease is classified by clinical presentation into pure and complicated forms.

Pure HSP is a syndrome of insidiously progressive and symmetric lower extremity spasticity that leads to gait disturbances (69). The age of onset spans from infancy into the eighth decade (68), although most develop symptoms between the second and fourth decades (70). Patients initially present with difficulty walking, stumbling, and tripping along with stiffness and cramping (69). Childhood onset may present as a delay in walking (68). Frequently associated symptoms are urinary urgency, hesitancy, and frequency (in up to 50%) and mildly impaired distal vibratory sense (10%–65%), especially in long-standing disease (68, 69). Pes cavus deformities, absence of ankle reflexes, upper extremity ataxia, and mild distal amyotrophy, particularly of the shins, have also been noted (68). The latter muscle wasting is usually attributed to disuse atrophy, as it is primarily present in patients with a prolonged disease course. In general, strength and dexterity of the upper extremities, speech, and swallowing remain unaffected in pure HSP (71).

Complicated HSP is diagnosed when HSP is associated with neurologic symptoms and signs not commonly observed in a myelopathy such as epilepsy, cataracts, amyotrophy, extrapyramidal disease, cutaneous abnormalities, mental retardation, peripheral neuropathy, and dementia (68, 69). Of note, cognitive impairment has been described in some families with HSP (69).

Although gait disturbance is a universal symptom, the severity ranges from one of no functional consequence to spastic diplegia requiring a cane, walker, or wheelchair (69, 71). Severity and prognosis cannot be reliably predicted given the extent of variation in disease progression between and within families with the same genetic mutation. It has been observed that a younger age of disease onset (<35 years) tends to be associated with slow progression and preservation of ambulation (68). Regardless of the age of presentation, patients with HSP have a normal life expectancy (68).

Autosomal dominant, autosomal recessive, and X-linked forms of the disease have been delineated, and at least 20 genetic loci have been identified (72). An autosomal dominant pattern is the most common, and among these, the spastin mutation of the spastic paraplegia loci (SPG) 4 gene on chromosome 2p accounts for approximately 40% of the autosomal dominant forms (68). In the majority, the spastin mutation confers a phenotypic pattern of pure HSP (73).

Neurologic examination reveals bilateral lower extremity spasticity, particularly in the hamstrings, quadriceps, and ankles, hyperreflexia, and extensor plantar responses (68). Weakness is present, often in the tibialis anterior, hamstrings, and iliopsoas muscles, but is often mild in comparison to the degree of spasticity (69). The upper extremities may display hyperreflexia but are otherwise unaffected, as is function of cranial nerves. Sensory testing may reveal decreased vibratory sense in the distal lower extremities. Gait testing demonstrates short stride length due to limited thigh flexion and foot dorsiflexion, leg circumduction, and often toe walking or a tendency to keep the legs partially flexed (68).

Hereditary spastic paraparesis is a diagnosis of exclusion and is based on the distinctive symptoms of gait disturbance, positive family history, and typical features on examination (70). Mimicking disorders include subacute combined degeneration, vitamin E deficiency, copper deficiency, Dopa-responsive dystonia, structural disorders (cervical spondylosis, Chiari malformation, tethered cord, spinal cord ateriovenous malformation) and compressive spinal cord disorders, progressive multiple sclerosis, motor neuron disorders (PLS and upper motor neuron-onset ALS), spinocerebellar ataxia type 3, Friedrich ataxia, inherited leukodystrophies, HIV or HTLV-1 myelopathy, and neurosyphilis (68, 69).

The necessity of laboratory and imaging investigation varies depending on the clinical presentation and physical findings. Electrophysiologic testing is not routinely performed but is typically normal in pure HSP. Magnetic resonance imaging of the brain is negative; spinal imaging may reveal minor atrophy, particularly in the thoracolumbar segments of the cord (68, 69). Genetic testing for the common forms of dominantly inherited HSP is commercially available (71).

Epidemiology

The prevalence of the disease ranges from 2.0 to 9.6 per 100,000 people. An accurate estimate is made difficult by the indolent nature of the disease (68, 70).

Pathophysiology

Hereditary spastic paraparesis is transmitted through autosomal dominant, autosomal recessive, and X-linked inheritance modes.

The spastin mutation, responsible for an autosomal dominant form of HSP, has been the most widely characterized. Spastin belongs to a group of proteins known as the ATPases, which are involved in diverse cellular activities (AAA). These proteins participate in cell cycle regulation, protein degradation, organelle biogenesis, and vesicle-mediated protein function (68). All spastin mutations elucidated thus far confer a loss of function of the protein and have been shown to disrupt microtubule regulation and intracellular transport (73). The SPG3A mutations cause a dominant form of HSP; this and the SPG4 mutation account for 50% of dominantly inherited HSP (71).

Paraplegin, like spastin, is a member of an AAA subgroup but encodes a mitochondrial metalloprotease.

Mutations at SPG7 have been linked to autosomal recessive forms of HSP (71, 74).

Axonal degeneration is a common pathological finding. The molecular mechanisms underlying this pathologic process are still poorly understood, but in different genetic subtypes may involve intrinsic central nervous system myelin protein composition, embryonic development of the corticospinal tracts, deficits of oxidative phosphorylation, axonal transport, and cytoskeletal disturbance (71).

Pathology

The major neuropathological feature in HSP is axonal degeneration, which is maximal in the terminal portions of the corticospinal and dorsal column pathways. In most patients, this is apparent in the thoracolumbar regions of corticospinal tracts and the fasciculus gracilis of the dorsal columns at the cervicomedullary region. Secondary demyelination and gliosis are observed. Spinocerebellar tracts are involved in about half of autopsy cases of HSP. Anterior horn cell and Betz cell loss has been reported but is rare (68, 69, 73, 74).

Treatment

Presently, only symptomatic therapies are available. Physical therapy and oral medications, such as baclofen, dantrolene, and tizanadine, are utilized. Intrathecal baclofen has also been tried in small cohorts of patients with HSP with good functional improvement and maintenance of ambulation (75), decreased muscle tone (76), and improved joint coordination (77). Botulinum toxin A injections can be administered to lessen lower extremity spasticity in patients who have suboptimal responses to oral medications. In a small open-label study, botulinum injections were shown to significantly reduce spasticity in specific lower extremity muscle groups, improve range of motion at the ankle, and increase gait velocity without worsening of weakness (78). Another study showed improvement in gait pattern in a small number of patients with HSP (79). Physical therapy is advocated to improve muscle flexibility, strength, and range of motion and to maintain walking reflexes (69, 71).

FRIEDREICH ATAXIA

Overview

Friedreich ataxia is an autosomal recessive hereditary ataxia. The age of onset ranges from 5 to 25 years, but the disease most often manifests around the time of puberty. Essential criteria for the clinical diagnosis are autosomal recessive inheritance, age of onset prior to 25 years, cerebellar ataxia, lower extremity areflexia, extensor plantar responses, and electrophysiologic evidence of a sensory axonal neuropathy (80). The classical phenotype is characterized by progressive gait and limb cerebellar and sensory ataxia associated with dysarthria, mild lower extremity weakness, and oculomotor abnormalities (81). Loss of ambulation occurs on average about 10 to 15 years after disease onset; life expectancy is somewhat shortened (81, 82).

The disease is associated with scoliosis and hypertrophic cardiomyopathy, the latter being the most common cause of death (82). Other less commonly associated features are nystagmus, optic atrophy, sensorineural hearing loss, distal amyotrophy, pes cavus, and diabetes mellitus (83).

Because of the availability of testing for the genetic mutation of FA, the clinical phenotype has been broadened to include patients with atypical features, a characteristic of approximately 25% of patients (84). These atypical features include late-onset disease (25–39 years) or very-late-onset (40 years) disease, slow progression, lack of classical features, and retained reflexes or spasticity (83–85). In a study comparing patients with typical FA to those with late-onset disease, the latter group was found to have fewer skeletal anomalies and a longer period from disease onset to wheelchair confinement. Those patients were also more likely to display lower limb spasticity and retained reflexes (86). Several cases of patients with FA presenting with adult-onset spastic paraparesis or tetraparesis are reported in the literature (84, 85, 87).

In the most common clinical presentation, neurologic examination demonstrates absence of lower extremity reflexes, extensor plantar responses, and impaired distal vibration and proprioception (83).

Electrophysiologic studies reveal absent or reduced sensory nerve action potentials and normal motor nerve conduction studies. Imaging of the brain is usually normal in the early course of the disease, although mild cerebellar atrophy has been noted in late-onset FA and in advanced disease (81, 86). Spinal imaging shows significant atrophy, particularly in the cervical region of the spinal cord (82).

Differential diagnosis of progressive ataxia includes posterior fossa tumors and malformations, multiple sclerosis, and autoimmune and paraneoplastic disorders (81). The differential of the FA phenotype includes ataxia with vitamin E deficiency, abetalipoproteinemia, and Refsum disease (88). Diseases that have a similar phenotype but prominent cerebellar atrophy are late-onset Tay-Sachs disease, cerebrotendinous xanthomatosis, mitochondrial recessive ataxia syndrome, spinocerebellar ataxia with axonal neuropathy and infantile-onset spinocerebellar ataxia, ataxia telangiectasia, autosomal recessive spastic ataxia of Charlevoix-Saguenay, posterior column ataxia with retinal pigmentary changes, and early-onset cerebellar atrophy with retained reflexes (83, 88).

Epidemiology

Friedreich ataxia is the most common hereditary ataxia. The prevalence of the disease varies from 1 person in 30,000 to 1 in 50,000 in most populations (88).

Pathophysiology

The illness results from a deficiency of the protein frataxin, which is involved in mitochondrial iron homeostasis and is essential for normal mitochondrial function. Loss of frataxin disturbs mitochondrial iron homeostasis resulting in iron accumulation and respiratory chain dysfunction, which leads to oxidative stress and cellular damage (88–90).

The genetic abnormality in FA is located in chromosome 9, and mutations most often involve GAA expansions. Ninety-five percent of patients are homozygous for this trinucleotide repeat expansion; the remaining are heterozygotes with GAA expansion and point mutations (85, 90). Larger expansions are linked to atypical features such as spasticity, earlier age of onset, and more rapid disease progression (83, 85).

Pathology

There is loss of dorsal root ganglion neurons and degeneration of the dorsal columns. Corticospinal and spinocerebellar tracts are affected, as is Clarke's column (83). The dentate nucleus and other deep cerebellar nuclei are severely affected; there is mild loss of purkinje cells, yet cerebellar atrophy itself is not prominent (83, 86). Loss of large pyramidal cells in the primary motor areas is a late finding (86). Macroscopically, the spinal cord is small, primarily affecting the posterior and lateral columns (82).

Treatment

Given the current theory of FA pathogenesis, treatment attempts have focused on antioxidants. Studies of the coenzyme Q analogue, idebenone, have shown a decrease in cardiac hypertrophy but no improvement in neurologic symptoms (91–94). A small uncontrolled, open-label study of a combination of coenzyme Q and vitamin E also demonstrated improvement in cardiac function. Although certain neurologic symptoms stabilized in this study, gait, posture, and hand dexterity continued to decline (95). No disease-modifying therapy has been found; treatment remains largely supportive focusing on management of cardiomyopathy, arrhythmias, scoliosis, and diabetes.

VITAMIN B12 DEFICIENCY

Overview

Vitamin B12 deficiency can present as a myelopathy with or without a peripheral neuropathy, cognitive impairment, optic neuropathy, and paresthesias (96, 97). The myelopathy, termed *subacute combined degeneration*, involves the dorsal columns, which interferes with proprioception and vibration sense, and the lateral columns, which manifests as a spastic paraparesis and extensor plantar responses. Onset is subacute; symptoms typically begin symmetrically in the distal lower extremities (96, 97). If the disease is severe, patients may have weakness, spasticity, clonus, paraplegia, and rarely, bowel and fecal incontinence (96). Lhermitte phenomenon, a feature commonly associated with multiple sclerosis, can be seen in cobalamin deficiency. Patients may have subtle neuropsychiatric symptoms such as impaired memory, irritability, and changes in personality and behavior (96, 97). Often taught as the classical presentation of cobalamin deficiency is an elderly white woman of northern European decent who has light-colored skin, blue eyes, blonde hair, a shiny tongue, a wide-based gait, and paresthesias in the legs.

Laboratory investigation usually shows low vitamin B12 levels. In the case of borderline values, methylmalonic acid and homocysteine can be measured. Both are elevated in B12 deficiency, although homocysteine elevation is not specific for the disorder. Hematologic anomalies, including megaloblastic anemia and neutrophil hypersegmentation, are also present but not necessarily in conjunction with neurologic symptoms (96, 97). Other hematologic abnormalities sometime observed in cobalamin deficiency include a low reticulocyte count, high serum iron, mild hemolysis, low haptoglobin level, high lactic acid dehydrogenase, and elevated bilirubin. In the severest patients, thrombocytopenia and neutropenia will be observed.

Magnetic resonance imaging of the spine typically shows T2 hyperintensity in the posterior and lateral columns. Contrast enhancement of both columns, T1 hypointensity in the dorsal columns, spinal cord atrophy, and anterior column involvement have all been reported in B12 deficiency. Treatment may reverse imaging abnormalities, but the radiologic changes do not always correlate with clinical improvement. Nerve conduction studies may reveal a peripheral axonal sensorimotor polyneuropathy (96).

Epidemiology

Neurologic dysfunction secondary to vitamin B12 deficiency is common and occurs more often in elderly persons. In one study, the incidence of pernicious anemia was 4.1% in white and black women and 2.1% in white and black men (96). It occurs in both sexes primarily between the ages of 40 and 90 years with a peak at age 60 to 70 years. In one study, the prevalence of metabolic vitamin B12 deficiency was 24% in Dutch patients between the ages of 74 and 80 years (98).

Pathophysiology

The recommended daily allowance of vitamin B12 for adults is 2.4 µg per day. The median intake from food in the United States is 3.5 µg for women and 5 µg for men. Foods rich in the vitamin include meats, primarily game and organ, shellfish, eggs, and milk.

Vitamin B12 binds intrinsic factor in the stomach, and this complex is absorbed in the ileum. The liver takes up approximately 50% of the vitamin, and the rest is transported to tissues. Excess is excreted in the urine. Body stores of the vitamin are large at 2.5 mg, which explains why decreased dietary intake is rarely a cause for deficiency, and even in strict vegetarians, symptoms will not develop for about 2 to 5 years (99).

Vitamin B12 is a cofactor in the conversion of homocysteine to methionine, which is then adenosylated to form S-adenosylmethionine. Decreased production of S-adenosylmethionine in vitamin B12 deficiency leads to reduced myelin basic protein methylation and white matter vacuolization. Methionine also plays a key role in the formation of tetrahydrofolate, a precursor for purine and pyrimidine synthesis. Impaired DNA synthesis could interfere with oligodendrocyte growth and myelin production. It has also been suggested that increased myelinolytic tumor necrosis factor alpha and decreased epidermal growth factor and interleukin-6 may contribute to the neurologic manifestations of vitamin B12 deficiency.

Most patients with vitamin B12 deficiency have pernicious anemia, which results from a deficit of intrinsic factor, a metabolic component necessary for absorption of vitamin B12 (97). Several studies state that 70% of patients with pernicious anemia have antibodies against intrinsic factor (98, 100). Certain medications, such as acid reducers, like H2 blockers, and nitrous oxide, an inhalational anesthetic, can lead to deficiency. The latter precipitates symptoms relatively rapidly after use, either when used as a routine anesthetic or when abused as a recreational drug. Malabsorption may occur from structural problems, such as atrophic gastritis, which is common in elderly persons, or ileal resection from gastric bypass surgery. Infections leading to bacterial overgrowth or tropical sprue affect the ileum, and certain parasitic infections can block absorption of vitamin B12. Deficiency has also been described in patients with AIDS, although HIV itself is a known cause of myelopathy. Hereditary enzyme defects have also been described as an etiology. In juvenile megaloblastic anemia or Imerslund-Grasbeck disease, a qualitatively abnormal intrinsic factor is responsible for abnormal B12 absorption (101). Other causes of B12 deficiency include auto-antibodies against gastric parietal cells, gastrectomy, malnutrition, and infection from *Helicobacter pylori*.

Despite the name, pernicious anemia, anemia is often not seen in the setting of B12 deficiency. In a recent study, only 29% of patients with B12 deficiency had anemia, and only 64% had a mean corpuscular volume greater than 100 (98).

Pathology

The most severely affected regions of the spinal cord in B12 deficiency are the cervical and upper thoracic dorsal columns. When involved, the lateral columns are less affected. Rarely are anterior columns targeted. Microscopically, the white matter demonstrates spongiform changes, myelin loss, axonal degeneration, and gliosis.

Treatment

When normal absorption is present, oral administration of 3 to 5 µg daily is sufficient. In patients with food-bound B12 malabsorption from achlorhydria, 50 to 100 µg is necessary. Those with impaired absorption require parenteral therapy. A common regimen is 2 weeks of 100 µg intramuscularly daily or 1000 µg twice weekly followed by weekly injections of 1000 µg for 2 months and thereafter, 1000 µg intramuscular B12 monthly (102). Patients with B12 deficiency who will undergo anesthesia with nitrous oxide should be treated prophylactically.

Remission of symptoms is inversely related to time between symptom onset and initiation of therapy, which argues for early institution of treatment. Most symptomatic improvement occurs within the first 6 months. Methylmalonic acid and homocysteine levels will normalize after treatment, as will hematologic anomalies.

COPPER DEFICIENCY MYELOPATHY

Overview

The most common clinical manifestation of copper deficiency is a myelopathy or myeloneuropathy, which presents subacutely with a spastic gait and sensory ataxia. Patients complain of difficulty in walking and lower limb paresthesias. The symptoms and signs very closely resemble those of vitamin B12 deficiency and the 2 disorders may coexist (103–105). Other described features of copper deficiency include isolated peripheral neuropathy, central nervous system demyelination, myopathy, and optic neuritis (104).

Neurologic examination may demonstrate hyperreflexia with extensor plantar responses and clonus, but depressed or absent ankle reflexes may also be seen (105).

Differential diagnosis is broad when patients present with a myelopathy, particularly in the absence of spinal cord imaging abnormalities. Nutritional deficiencies (vitamin B12 and folate), infectious etiologies (HIV and HTLV-1), and autoimmune (Sjogren) and inflammatory processes (multiple sclerosis) are all possibilities (106).

Laboratory investigation includes serum copper, ceruloplasmin, and urinary copper excretion. Ceruloplasmin is an acute phase reactant and therefore is not as sensitive in diagnosing copper deficiency. Hematologic abnormalities are often, but not necessarily, present and usually involve anemia, neutropenia, and a left shift in granulocytic and erythroid maturation (107). Laboratory evaluation of copper deficiency myeloneuropathy includes electrophysiologic studies, which show varying degrees of axonal peripheral neuropathy. Magnetic resonance imaging of the spinal cord may reveal increased T2 signal in the paramedian dorsal column cervical cord; thoracic and lumbar segments are less commonly affected (103, 104, 106). Involvement of anterior segments of the cord and mild cord atrophy have also been reported in patients with copper deficiency myelopathy (106). The imaging findings often improve parallel to rising serum copper levels.

Pathophysiology

Copper is a prosthetic group in several metalloenzymes, which serve as oxidases. Many of these, including the copper/zinc superoxide dismutase, cytochrome c oxidase, dopamine B-monoxygenase, tyrosinase, and ferroxidase I and II, play a key role in maintaining the structure and function of the nervous system (103). The recommended daily allowance of copper for adults is 900 µg; median intake from foods is 1.0 to 1.6 mg per day. Foods rich in copper include organ meats, seafood, nuts, seeds, wheat bran cereals, whole grain products, and cocoa products (103). Copper absorption occurs primarily in the small intensine; copper is then bound to albumin and transported to the liver, after which it is released into the plasma and most of which is bound to ceruloplasmin. Excretion through the gastrointestinal tract is the main route through which copper toxicity is avoided (103).

Acquired copper deficiency secondary to low dietary intake is rare. Copper deficiency is often idiopathic. However, it is observed after gastric surgery and in malnourished or premature infants, in nephrotic syndrome, and in enteropathies associated with malabsorption. It can be a complication of inadequate copper supplementation in prolonged total parenteral nutrition or enteral feedings. Congenital copper deficiency is present in Menkes disease (103). Medications, including ascorbic acid and antacids, may interfere with copper bioavailability. Excessive ingestion of zinc and treatment with tetrathiomolybdate (in chemotherapeutic agents) can lead to copper deficiency (104).

Pathology

The typical distribution of lesions in copper deficiency is in the cervical cord; there is less severe involvement of the thoracic and lumbar regions. Wallerian degeneration and microcavitation of the white matter of the spinal cord and brainstem are seen (104).

Treatment

No studies have addressed the most appropriate dose, duration, route, and form of copper supplementation. Oral copper supplementation will typically lead to normal serum levels even when malabsorption is a concern. A proposed regimen is elemental copper, either copper gluconate or copper chloride, 6 mg per day for 1 week, followed by 4 mg per day for 1 week, and then 2 mg per day thereafter. Parenteral administration is occasionally used for initial therapy or because of a lack of improvement after prolonged oral therapy. In patients with zinc-induced copper deficiency, discontinuation of the offending agent may be sufficient (103).

Hematologic recovery is prompt. Complete neurologic recovery rarely occurs. Imaging studies can show reversal of signal abnormalities, but this improvement does not always predict symptomatic recovery (103). Treatment appears to stop progression of the disease; if improvement occurs, it more often affects sensory symptoms than motor. For this reason, early recognition and treatment can prevent significant neurologic morbidity.

References

1. Brooks BR, Miller RG, Swash M, Musat TL. World Federation of Neurology Research Group on Motor Neuron Diseases. El Escorial revisited: revised criteria for the diagnosis of amyotrophic lateral sclerosis. *Amyotroph Lateral Scler Other Motor Neuron Disord* 2000;(5):293–9.
2. Radunovic A, Mitsumoto H, Leigh PN. Clinical care of patients with amyotrophic lateral sclerosis. *Lancet Neurol* 2007;6:913–25.
3. Logroscino G, Traynor BJ, Hardiman O Chio' A Couratier P, Mitchell JD, Swingler RJ, Beghi E. Descriptive epidemiology of amyotrophic lateral sclerosis: new evidence and unresolved issues. *J Neurol Neurosurg Psychiatry* 2006; 79:6–11.
4. Valdmanis PN, Rouleau GA. Genetics of familial amyotrophic lateral scleorosis. *Neurology* 2008;7:144–152.
5. Kabashi E Valdmanis PN, Dion P Rouleau GA. Oxidized/misfolded superoxide dismutase-1: the cause of all amyotrophic lateral sclerosis? *Ann Neurol* 2007;62:553–559.
6. Cronin S, Hardiman O, Traynor BJ. Ethnic variation in the incidence of ALS. *Neurology* 2007;68:1002–1007.
7. Traynor, BJ, Bruijn, L Conwit, R Beal, F O'Neill, G Fagan, SC, Cudkowicz, M.E. Neuroprotective agents for clinical trials in ALS. *Neurology* 2006;7:20–27.
8. Choudry, RB, Cudkowicz, M. Clinical trials in amyotrophic lateral sclerosis: the tenuous past and the promising future. *J Clin Pharmacol* 2005;45:1334–1344.
9. Sheean, G. The pathophysiology of spasticity. *Eur J Neurol* 2002;9:3–9.
10. Katirji: *Neuromuscular disorders in clinical practice*, 1st ed. Copyright 2002. Butterworth-Heinemann.
11. Brown, P. Pathophysiology of spasticity. *J Neurol Neurosurg Psychiatry* 1994;57:773–7.
12. Kumar: Robbins and Cotran: *Pathologic basis of disease*, 7th ed. Copyright 2005. Saunders.
13. Bensimon G, Lacomblez L, Meininger V. (1994). A controlled trial of riluzole in amyotrophic lateral sclerosis. *NEJM* 1994;330:585–591.
14. Lacomblez L, Bensimon G, Leigh PN, Guillet P, Meininger V. (1996). Dose-ranging study of riluzole in amyotrophic lateral sclerosis. *Lancet* 347:1425–31.
15. Bensimon G, Lacomblez L, Delumeau JC, Bejuit R, Truffinet P, Meininger V. (2002). A study of riluzole in the treatment of advanced stage or elderly patients with amyotrophic lateral sclerosis. *J Neurol* 249:609–15.
16. Miller RG, Mitchell JD, Lyon M, Moore DH. Riluzole for amyotrophic lateral sclerosis (ALS)/motor neuron disease (MND).*Cochrane database of systematic reviews* 2007, Issue 1. Art. No.: CD001447. DOI: 10.1002/14651858.CD001447. pub2.
17. Miller RG, Moore D Young LA, Armon C Barohn RJ, Bromberg MB, Bryan WW, Gelinas DF, Mendoza MC, Neville HE, Parry GJ, Petajan JH, Ravits JM, Ringel SP, Ross MA, WALS Study Group. Placebo-controlled trial of gabapentin in patients with amyotrophic lateral sclerosis. *Neurology* 1996;47:1383–1388.
18. Miller RG, Moore DH, II, Gelinas DF, Dronsky V Mendoza M, Barohn RJ, Bryan W, Ravits J, Yuen E, Neville H, Ringel S, Bromberg M, Petajan J, Amato AA, Jackson C, Johnson W, Mandler R, Bosch P, Smith B, Graves M, Ross M, Sorenson EJ, Kelkar P, Parry G, Olney R, WALS Study Group. Phase III randomized trial of gabapentin in patients with amyotrophic lateral sclerosis. *Neurology* 2001;56:843–848.
19. Cudkowicz ME, Shefner JM, Shoenfield DA, Brown RH, Jr, Phil D, Johnson H, Qureshi M, Jacobs M, Rothstein JD, Appel SH, Pascuzzi RM, Heiman-Patterson TD, Donofrio PD, David WS, Russell JA, Tandan R, Pioro EP, Felice KJ, Rosenfeld J, Mandler RN, Sachs GM, Bradley WG, Raynor EM, Baquis GD, Belsh JM, Novella S, Goldstein J, Hulihan J, Northeast ALS Consortium. *Neurology* 2003;61:456–464.
20. Cudkowicz ME, Shefner JM, Shoenfield DA, Zhang H, Andreasson KI, Rothstein JD, Drachman DB. Trial of celecoxib in amyotrophic lateral sclerosis. *Arch Neurol* 2006;60:22–31.
21. Gordon PH, Moore DH, Gelinas DF, Qualls C, Meister ME, Werner J. Placebo-controlled phase I/II studies of minocycline in amyotrophic lateral sclerosis. *Neurology* 2004; 62:1845–1847.
22. Gordon PH, Moore DH, Miller RG, Florence JM, Verheijde JI, Doorish C, Hilton JF, Spitalny GM, MacArthur RB, Mitsumoto H, Neville HE, Boylan K, Mozaffar T, Belsh JM, Ravits J, Bedlock RS, Graves MC, McCluskey LF, Barohn RJ, Tandan R. Efficacy of minocycline in patients with amyotrophic lateral sclerosis: a phase III randomised trial. *Lancet Neurol* 2007;6:1045–53.
23. Desnuelle C, Dib M, Garrel C, Favier A. A double-blind, placebo-controlled randomized clinical trial of alpha-tocopherol (Vitamin E) in the treatment of amyotrophic lateral sclerosis. *Amyotroph Lateral Scler Other Motor Neuron Disord* 2001;2:9–18.
24. Graf M, Ecker D, Horowski R, Kramer B, Riederer P, Gerlach M, Hager C, Ludolph AC. High dose vitamin E therapy in amyotrophic lateral sclerosis as add-on therapy to riluzole: results of a placebo-controlled double-blind study. *J Neural Transm* 2005;112:649–660.
25. Groeneveld GJ, Veldink JH, van der Tweel I, Kalmijn S, Beijer C, de Visser M, Wokke JHJ, Franssen H, van den Berg LH. A randomized sequential trial of creatine in amyotrophic lateral sclerosis. *Ann Neurol* 2003;53:437–445.
26. Shefner JM, Cudkowicz ME, Schoenfeld D, Conrad T, Taft J, Chilton M, Urbinelli L, Qureshi M, Zhang H, Pestronk A, Caress J, Donofrio P, Sorenson E, Bradley W, Lomen-Hoerth C, Pioro E, Rezania K, Ross M, Pascuzzi R, Heiman-Patterson T, Tandan R, Mitsumoto H, Rothstein J, Smith-Palmer T, MacDonald D, Burke D. A clinical trial of creatine in ALS. *Neurology* 2004;63:1656–1661.
27. Miller RG, Petajan JH, Bryan WW, Armon C, Barohn RJ, Goodpasture JC, Hoagland RJ, Parry GJ, Ross MA, Stromatt SC, rhCNTF ALS Study Group. A placebo-controlled trial of recombinant ciliary neurotrophic (rhCNTF) factor in amyotrophic lateral sclerosis. *Ann Neurol* 1996;39: 256–260.
28. ALS CNTF Treatment Study Group. A double-blind placebo-controlled clinical trial of subcutaneous recombinant human ciliary neurotrophic factor (rhCNTF) in amyotrophic lateral sclerosis. *Neurology* 1996;46:1244–1249.
29. Bongioanni P, Reali C, Sogos V. Ciliary neurotrophic factor (CNTF) for amyotrophic lateral sclerosis or motor neuron disease. *Cochrane Database Syst Rev* 2004, Issue 3. Art. No.: CD004302. DOI: 10.1002/14651858.CD004302.pub2.
30. Mitchell JD, Wokke JHJ, Borasio GD. Recombinant human insulin-like growth factor I (rhIGF-I) for amyotrophic lateral sclerosis/motor neuron disease. *Cochrane Database Syst Rev* 2002, Issue 3. Art. No.: CD002064. DOI: 10.1002/14651858. CD002064.pub2.

31. Lai EC, Felice KJ, Festoff BW, Gawel MJ, Gelinas DF, Kratz R, Murphy MF, Natter HM, Norris FH, Rudnicki SA, North America ALS/IGF-1 Study Group. Effect of recombinant human insulin insulin-like growth factor-I on progression of ALS: a placebo-controlled study. *Neurology* 1997;49:1621–30.

32. Borasio GD, Robberecht W, Leigh PN, Emile J, Guiloff RJ, Jerusalem F, Silani V, Vos PE, Wokke JH, Dobbins T, European ALS/IGF-1 Study Group. A placebo-controlled trial of insulin-like growth factor-I in amyotrophic lateral sclerosis. *Neurology* 1998;51:583–586.

33. Mostad I, Dale I, Petlund CF, Sjaastad O. Plasma exchange in motor neuron disease: a controlled study. *J Neurol* 1979;221(1):59–66.

34. Silani V, Scarlato G, Valli G, Marconi M. Plasma exchange ineffective in amyotrophic lateral sclerosis. *Arch Neurol* 1980;37(8):511–3.

35. Simmons Z. Management strategies for patients with amyotrophic lateral sclerosis from diagnosis through death. *Neurologist* 2005;11:257–270.

36. Kita M, Goodkin DE. Drugs used to treat spasticity. *Drugs* 2000;59:487–495.

37. Abbruzzese G. The medical management of spasticity. *Eur J Neurol* 2002;9 (Suppl. 1):30–34.

38. Anderson, WS Jallo, GI. Intrathecal baclofen therapy and the treatment of spasticity. *Neurosurg Q* 2007;17:185–192.

39. Hsieh JC, Penn RD. Intrathecal baclofen in the treatment of adult spasticity. *Neurosurg Focus* 2006;21(2):1–6.

40. Marquardt G, Seifert V. Use of intrathecal baclofen for treatment of spasticity in amyotrophic lateral sclerosis. *J Neurol Neurosurg Psychiatry* 2002;72:275–6.

41. McClelland S, III, Bethoux FA, Boulis NM, Sutliff MH, Stough DK, Schwetz KM, Gogol DM, Harrison M, Pioro EP. Intrathecal baclofen for spasticity-related pain in amyotrophic lateral sclerosis: efficacy and factors associated with pain relief. *Muscle Nerve* 2008;37:396–398.

42. Lataste X, Emre M, Davis C, Groves L. Comparative profile of tizanidine in the management of spasticity. *Neurology* 1994;44(11 Suppl 9):553–9.

43. Wagstaff A, Bryson H. Tizanidine: a review of its pharmacology, clinical efficacy and tolerability in the management of spasticity associated with cerebral and spinal disorders. *Drugs* 1997;53(3):435–452.

44. Krause T, Gerbershagen M, Flege M, Wethorn R, Wappler F. Dantrolene—a review of its pharmacology, therapeutic use, and new developments. *Anesthesia* 2004;59(4):364–373.

45. Ward A, Chaffman M, Sorkin E. Dantrolene: a review of its pharmacodynamic and pharmacokinetic properties and therapeutic use in malignant hyperthermia, the neuroleptic malignant syndrome, and an update of its use in muscle spasticity. *Drugs* 1986;32(2):130–168.

46. Restivo DA, Lanza S, Marchese-Ragona R, et al. Improvement of masseter spasticity by botulinum toxin facilitates PEG placement in amyotrophic lateral sclerosis. *Gastroenterology* 2002;123:1749–1750.

47. Winterholler MG, Heckmann JG, Hecht M, Erguth FJ. Recurrent trismus and stridor in an ALS patient: successful treatment with botulinum toxin. *Neurology* 2002;58:502–503.

48. Drory VE, Goltsman E, Reznik JG, Mosek A, Korczyn AD. The value of muscle exercise in patients with amyotrophic lateral sclerosis. *J Neurol Sci* 2001;191:133–7.

49. Singer MA, Statland JM, Wolfe GI, Barohn RJ. Primary lateral sclerosis. *Muscle Nerve* 2007;35:291–302.

50. Becker A, Hardmeier M, Steck AJ, Czaplinski A. Primary lateral sclerosis presenting with isolated progressive pseudobulbar syndrome. *Eur J Neurol* 2007;14:63.

51. Peretti-Viton P, Azulay JP, Trefouret S, Brunel H, Daniel C, Viton JM, Flori A, Salazard B, Pouget J, Serratrice G, Salamon G. MRI of the intracranial corticospinal tracts in amyotrophic and primary lateral sclerosis. *Neuroradiology* 1999;41:744–749.

52. Tomik B, Zur KA, Szczudlik A. Pure primary lateral sclerosis-case reports. *Clin Neurol Neurosurg* 2008;110(4):387–391. Doi:10.1016/j.clineuro.2007.12.002.

53. Tartaglia MC, Rowe A, Findlater K, Orange JB, Grace G, Strong MJ. Differentiation between primary lateral sclerosis and amyotrophic lateral sclerosis. *Arch Neurol* 2007;64:232–36.

54. Pringle CE, Hudson AJ, Munoz DG, Kiernan JA, Brown WF, Ebers GC. Primary lateral sclerosis. *Brain* 1992; 115:495–520.

55. Gordon PH, Cheng B, Katz IB, Pinto M, Hays AP, Mitsumoto H, Rowland LP. The natural history of primary lateral sclerosis. *Neurology* 2006;66:647–653.

56. Swash M, Desai J, Mistra VP. What is primary lateral sclerosis? *J Neurol Sci* 1999;170:5–10.

57. Singer MA, Kojan S, Barohn RJ, Herbelin L, Nations SP, Trivedi JR, Jackson CE, Burns DK, Boyer PJ, Wolfe GI. Primary lateral sclerosis: clinical and laboratory features in 25 patients. *J Clin Neurosmuscul Dis* 2005;7:1–9.

58. Le Forestier N, Maisonobe T, Piquard A, Rivaud S, Creview-Buchman L, Salachas F, Pradat P-F, Lacomblez L, Meininger V. Does primary lateral sclerosis exist? A study of 20 patients and a review of the literature. *Brain* 2001;124:1989–99.

59. Kuipers-Upmeijer J, de Jager AE, Hew JM, Snoek JW, van Weerden TW. Primary lateral sclerosis: clinical, neurophysiological, and magnetic resonance findings. *J Neurol Neurosurg Psychiatry* 2001;71:615–20.

60. Le Forestier N, Maisonobe T, Spelle L, Lesort A, Salachas F, Lacomblez L, Samson Y, Bouche P, Meininger V. Primary lateral sclerosis: further clarification. *J Neurol Sci* 2001;185:95–100.

61. Sheean G. The pathophysiology of spasticity. *Eur J Neurol* 2002;9:3–9.

62. Katirji. *Neuromuscular disorders in clinical practice*, 1ˢᵗ ed. Copyright 2002. Butterworth-Heinemann.

63. Brown P. Pathophysiology of spasticity. *J Neurol Neurosurg Psychiatry* 1994;57:773–7.

64. Murray B, Mitsumoto H. Disorders of upper and lower motor neurons. Bradley: *Neurology in clinical practice*, 4ᵗʰ edition. Chapter 80, 2004.

65. Hudson AJ, Kiernan JA, Munoz DG, Pringle CE, Brown WF Ebers GC. Clinicopathologic features of primary lateral sclerosis are different from amyotrophic lateral sclerosis. *Brain Res Bull* 1993;30:359–364.

66. Milano JB, Neto MC, Hunhevicz SC, Arruda WO, Ramina R, Barros E, Jr. Intrathecal baclofen for spasticity in primary lateral sclerosis. *J Neurol* 2005;252:740–741.

67. Sadiq SA, Wang GC. Long-term intrathecal baclofen therapy in ambulatory patients with spasticity. *J Neurol* 2006;253:563–569.

68. McDermott CJ, White K, Bushby K, Shaw PJ. Hereditary spastic paraparesis: a review of new developments. *J Neurol Neurosurg Psychiatry* 2000;69:150–160.

69. Strong MJ, Gordon PH. Primary lateral sclerosis, hereditary spastic paraplegia and amyotrophic lateral sclerosis: discrete entities or spectrum? *Amyotroph Lateral Scler* 2005;6:8–16.

70. Singer MA, Statland JM, Wolfe GI, Barohn RJ. Primary lateral sclerosis. *Muscle Nerve* 2007;35:291–302.

71. Fink JK. Hereditary spastic paraplegia. *Neurol Clin N Am* 2002;20:711–726.

72. Fink JK. Advances in the hereditary spastic paraplegias. *Exp Neurol* 2003;184:S106–S110.

73. McDermott CJ, Burness CE, Kirby J, Cox LE, Rao DG, Hewamadduma C, Sharrack B, Hadjivassiliou M, Chinnery PF, Dalton A, Shaw PJ. Clinical features of hereditary spastic paraplegia due to spastin mutation. *Neurology* 2006;67:45–51.

74. Fink JK. Progressive spastic paraparesis: hereditary spastic paraplegia and its relation to primary and amyotrophic lateral sclerosis. *Semin Neurol* 2001;21:199–207.

75. Lambrecq V. Intrathecal baclofen in hereditary spastic paraparesis: benefits and limitations. *Ann Readapt Med Phys* 2007;50(7):577–81.

76. Meythaler JM, Steers WD, Tuel SM, Cross LL, Sesco DC, Haworth CS. Intrathecal baclofen in hereditary spastic paraparesis. *Arch Phys Med Rehabil* 1992;73(9):794–7.

77. Dan B, Bouillot E, Bengoetxea A, Cheron G. Effect of intrathecal baclofen on gait control in human hereditary spastic paraparesis. *Neurosci Lett* 2000;280:175–178.

78. Rousseaux M, Launay MJ, Kozlowski O, Daveluy W. Botulinum toxin injection in patients with hereditary spastic paraparesis. *Eur J Neurol* 2006;14:206–212.

79. Dunne JW, Heye N, Dunne SL. Treatment of chronic limb spasticity with botulinum toxin A. *J Neurol Neurosurg Psychiatry* 1995;58:232–235.

80. Harding AE. Friedreich's ataxia: a clinical and genetic study of 90 families with an analysis of early diagnostic criteria and intrafamilial clustering of clinical features. *Brain* 1981;104:589–620.

81. Pandolfo M. Friedreich ataxia. *Semin Pediatr Neurol* 2003;10(3):163–172.

82. Delatycki MB, Williamson R, Forrest SM. Friedreich ataxia: an overview. *J Med Genet* 37 2000;(1):1–8.

83. Lynch DR, Farmer JM, Balcer LJ, Wilson RB. Friedreich ataxia: effects of genetic understanding on clinical evaluation and therapy. *Arch Neurol* 2002;59:743–747.

84. Lhatoo SD, Rao DG, Kane NM, Ormerod IE. Very late onset Friedreich's presenting as spastic tetraparesis without ataxia or neuropathy. *Neurology* 2001;56:1776–7.

85. Castelnovo G, Biolsi B, Barbaud A, Labauge P. Isolated spastic paraparesis leading to diagnosis of Friedreich's ataxia. *J Neurol Neurosurg Psychiatry* 2000;69:693.

86. Bhidayasiri R, Perlman SL, Pulst S-M, Geschwind DH. Late-onset Friedreich ataxia. *Arch Neurol* 2005;62:1865–1869.

87. Gates PC, Paris D, Forrest SM, Williamson R, Mckinlay Gardner RJ. Friedreich's ataxia presenting as adult-onset spastic paraparesis. *Neurogenetics* 1998;1:297–299.

88. Fogel BL, Perlman S. Clinical features and molecular genetics of autosomal recessive cerebellar ataxias. *Lancet* 2007;6:245–257.

89. Campuzano V, Montermini L, Molto MD, Pianese L, Cossee M, Cavalcanti F, Monros E, Rodius F, Duclos F, Monticelli A, Zara F, Canizarea J, Koutnikova H, Bidichandani SI, Gellera C, Brice A, Trouillas P, de Michele G, Filla A, De Fruits R, Palau F, Patel PI, Di Donato S, Mandel J-L, Cocozza S, Koenig M, Pandolfo M. Friedreich ataxia: autosomal disease caused by an intronic GAA triplet repeat expansion. *Science* 1996;271:1423–1427.

90. Albin RL. Dominant ataxias and Friedreich ataxia: an update. *General Opinion in Neurology* 2003;16:507–514.

91. Buyse G, Mertens L, Di Salvo G, Matthijs I, Weidemann F, Eyskens B, Goossens W, Sutherland GR, Van Hove JLK. Idebenone treatment in Friedreich's ataxia: neurological, cardiac, and biochemical monitoring. *Neurology* 2003;60:1679–81.

92. Hausse AO, Aggoun Y, Bonnet D, Sidi D. Munnich A, Rotig A, Rustin P. Idebenone and reduced cardiac hypertrophy in Friedreich's ataxia. *Heart* 2002;87:346–49.

93. Mariotti C, Solari A, Torta D, Marano L, Fiorentini C, Di Donato S. Idebenone treatment in Friedreich patients: a one-year-long randomized placebo-controlled trial. *Neurology* 2003;60:1676–79.

94. Rustin P, von Kleist-Retzow JC, Chantrel-Goussard K, Sidi D, Munnich A, Rotig A. Effect of idebenone on cardiomyopathy in Friedreich's ataxia: a preliminary study. *Lancet* 1999;354:477–479.

95. Hart PE, Lodi R, Rajagopalan B, Bradley JL, Crilley JG Turner C, Blamire AM, Manners D, Styles P, Schapira AHV, Cooper JM. Antioxidant treatment of patients with Friedreich ataxia: four-year follow-up. *Arch Neurol* 2005;62:621–626.

96. Hemmer B, Glocker FX, Scumacher M, et al. Subacute combined degeneration: clinical, electrophysiological, and magnetic resonance imaging findings. *J Neurol Neurosurg Psychiatry* 1998;65: 822.

97. Pruthi RK, Tefferi A. Pernicious anemia revisted. *Mayo Clin Proc* 1994;69:144.

98. van Asselt DZ, de Groot LC, van Staveren WA, et al. Role of cobalamin intake and atrophic gastritis in mid cobalamin in older Dutch subjects. *Am J Clin Nutr* 1998;68:32

99. Green R, Kinsella LJ. Editorial: current concepts in the diagnosis of cobalamin deficiency. *Neurology* 1995;45:1435.

100. Carmel R. Prevalence of undiagnosed pernicious anemia in the elderly. *Arch Intern Med* 1996;156:1097.

101. Tanner SM, Li Z, Perko JD, et al. Hereditary juvenile cobalamin deficiency caused by mutations in the intrinsic factor gene. *Proc Natl Acad Sci U S A* 2005:102:4130.

102. Carmel R. How I treat cobalamin (vitamin B12) deficiency. *Blood* 2008;112:2214.

103. Kumar N. Nutritional neuropathies. *Neurol Clin* 2007;25:209–255.

104. Kumar N. Copper deficiency myelopathy (human swayback). *Mayo Clin Proc* 2006;81(10):1371–84.

105. Kumar N, Crum B, Petersen RC, Vernino SA, Ahlskog JE. Copper deficiency myelopathy. *Arch Neurol* 2004;61:762–66.

106. Kumar, N, Ahlskog, JE, Klein, CJ, Port, JD. Imaging features of copper deficiency myelopathy: a study of 25 cases. *Neuroradiology* 2006;48:78–83.

107. Kumar, N, Gross, JB, Ahlskog, JE. Copper deficiency myelopathy produces a clinical picture like subacute combined degeneration. *Neurology* 2004;63:33–39.

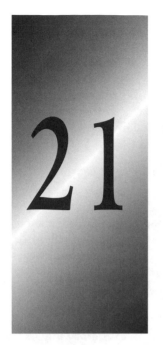

21

Spasticity Due to Disease of the Spinal Cord: Pathophysiology, Epidemiology, and Treatment

Heather W. Walker
Steven Kirshblum

Spasticity is a common sensorimotor symptom complex commonly experienced by individuals sustaining spinal cord injury (SCI) with upper motor neuron (UMN) involvement, that is, injury above the level of the conus medullaris. Although spasticity may occasionally contribute to improved function (ie, transfers, standing, ambulation, and assisting in activities of daily living [ADL]), it more often leads to various complications including contractures, pain, impaired function, and decreased quality of life (QOL). This chapter will discuss the presumed pathophysiology, causes, classification, and treatment options of this common problem in regard to the person with SCI.

DEFINITION AND SCOPE OF THE PROBLEM

Lance (1) classically described spasticity as "a motor disorder characterized by a velocity-dependent increase in tonic stretch reflexes (muscle tone) with exaggerated tendon jerks, resulting from hyperexcitability of the stretch reflex, as one component of the upper motor neuron syndrome" (UMNS). Others have proposed newer definitions to include the many dif-

ferent clinical signs and symptoms of spasticity (2–5). Spasticity is a component of the UMNS that is composed of positive and negative symptoms. The positive symptoms include hyperreflexia, clonus, spasms and postural abnormalities, and the negative symptoms include weakness, incoordination, fatigue, and pain (6). The positive symptoms are easier to see and treat, whereas the negative symptoms are more functionally limiting and may be more resistant to treatment. The components of spasticity may be further delineated into tonic and phasic spasticity; tonic spasticity manifests clinically as increased tone that is due to an exaggeration of the tonic component of the stretch reflex, whereas phasic spasticity can be observed clinically as hyperreflexia and clonus due to an exaggeration of the phasic component of the stretch reflex (2).

Spasticity is a common complication of SCI. The incidence in UMN-related SCI during rehabilitation is approximately 70%, with roughly half the patients requiring pharmacologic intervention (7, 8). At 1 year postdischarge, 78% of people have spasticity, with 49% requiring pharmacologic treatment (7). Spasticity occurs more frequently in persons with cervical and upper thoracic SCI than in those with lower thoracic and lumbosacral SCI and is usually more significant in persons with specific types of incomplete injuries, with persons with ASIA grades B and C having greater issues with spasticity than persons with grades A or D. In an analysis of 466 patients with traumatic SCI treated in model SCI centers over a 2-year period, Maynard et al. (7). reported a higher incidence of spasticity in individuals with SCI graded as Frankel B or C (50% and 52%) compared with those with Frankel A or D SCI (27% and 29%). Little et al. (9) found that individuals with motor incomplete SCI had a greater flexor withdrawal response and greater extensor spasms on examination than those individuals with complete SCI. In addition, these investigators reported that patients with Frankel C SCI had greater hypertonus and flexor withdrawal than those with Frankel D SCI. (Frankel scores were reported because this study was published before the ASIA Impairment Scale was available.) The authors explained that this finding may have been due to sparing of inhibitory descending spinal pathways in the patients with Frankel D SCI (9).

More recently, Skold et al. (10) published that patients with incomplete SCI reported a higher incidence of self-reported spasticity and possibly greater variability throughout the day as compared with individuals with complete SCI. This group also investigated the relationship between self-reported spasticity and objective evidence of spasticity and found that in patients reporting the presence of spasticity, only 60% had measurable spasticity on physical examination.

Although each of the components of the UMNS may have an impact on an individual's function (ie, fatigue, incoordination, cocontraction of antagonist muscles), QOL, pain, and other aspects of his or her life, this chapter will focus only on spasticity as one of the components of the UMNS.

PATHOPHYSIOLOGY

Immediately after SCI, there are depressed spinal reflexes during the state of spinal shock, followed by development of hyperreflexia and spasticity over the following weeks to months. The pathophysiology of spasticity is not completely understood; however, it is believed to arise primarily from loss of the effect of numerous descending inhibitory pathways. These include reciprocal Ia interneuronal inhibition, presynaptic inhibition, Renshaw-mediated recurrent inhibition, group II afferent inhibition, and the Golgi tendon organs (11). Axonal collateral sprouting and denervation supersensitivity are changes that may also play a role in the development of spasticity (12). In addition

to these changes that result in decreased input from descending inhibitory pathways, mechanical changes to the muscle after SCI may also play a role in the pathophysiology of spasticity (13). These mechanisms will be further explored individually.

NORMAL MOTOR CONTROL

To understand how loss of descending inhibition plays a role in spasticity, one must first understand the physiology of the monosynaptic stretch reflex arc. The muscle spindles are specialized intrafusal fibers that when stretched, send afferent impulses to the spinal cord by way of type Ia and type II afferent fibers, providing information about muscle length and position. Once activated, the Ia fibers make a monosynaptic connection with, and have an excitatory influence over, the alpha motor neurons supplying the extrafusal muscle fibers of both the agonist muscle and also the agonist's synergistic muscles, leading to contraction of these muscle groups. The Ia fibers also synapse on interneurons that inhibit antagonist muscle groups, thereby preventing contraction of these muscles during activation of the agonist muscle groups; this inhibitory pathway is referred to as reciprocal Ia inhibition and can be altered after SCI. Clinically, reciprocal inhibition can be grossly observed by eliciting monosynaptic muscle stretch reflexes: when the tendon is tapped, a stretch is applied to the target muscle, which is transmitted to the spinal cord through the Ia afferent fibers. The Ia afferent fibers exert an excitatory influence over the efferent alpha motor neurons that innervate the target muscle and an inhibitory influence to the interneurons that synapse on the alpha motor neurons that innervate the antagonist muscles. This reciprocal Ia inhibition allows contraction of the target muscle while inhibiting contraction of the antagonist muscles. Impairment of reciprocal inhibition after SCI may result in simultaneous coactivation of agonist and antagonist muscle groups, as is often seen in patients with spasticity (14).

Recurrent inhibition is mediated by Renshaw cells, which are inhibitory interneurons located in the ventral horn of the spinal cord. Axon collaterals from alpha motor neurons synapse on and activate the Renshaw cells, which in turn project inhibitory impulses back to these motor neurons, as well as to Ia inhibitory interneurons. Renshaw activity decreases the activity of the motor neurons that were previously active and also inhibits the Ia inhibitory interneurons. The level of recurrent inhibition has been explored in patients with UMN lesions, and these individuals have been noted to maintain normal recurrent inhibition at rest but impaired recurrent inhibition during voluntary movement; this may contribute to impaired motor function in these patients (12, 15). There is evidence for increased recurrent inhibition in the SCI population, which increases inhibition to the Ia interneurons (16). This ultimately allows for cocontraction of agonist and antagonist muscle groups due to the decreased Ia interneuron activity.

Reduction in presynaptic inhibition of Ia afferents is another potential contributor to the pathophysiology of spasticity in SCI. Reciprocal inhibition was described by Sherrington in 1906, and this process is responsible for relaxation of an antagonist muscle during contraction of the agonist (17). In the absence of reciprocal inhibition, cocontraction of agonist and antagonist muscle groups is seen simultaneously, interfering with intentional voluntary movement. GABA mediates spinal inhibition both presynaptically and postsynaptically. Presynaptic inhibition of Ia afferents occurs when the inhibitory amino acid GABA binds to receptors on the Ia terminals, which subsequently increases the amount of input required to activate the alpha motor neurons (18). The decreased excitatory input to the alpha motor neurons in turn depresses the monosynaptic stretch reflex. Postsynaptic activation of GABA-A receptors can decrease the activity of motor neurons and interneurons (18). After SCI, the decrease in presynaptic inhibition ultimately results in increased activity of the alpha motor neuron; this may contribute to the hyperreflexia and spasticity seen in these individuals (12). It is possible to modulate the presynaptic inhibition in individuals with SCI with the use of GABA-ergic medications including baclofen and diazepam, which will be discussed later in this chapter.

Nonreciprocal Ib inhibition is another mechanism that may play a role in the development of spasticity of supraspinal origin but does not appear to be involved in spasticity related to SCI. Golgi tendon organs, which are contraction-sensitive receptors, have group I afferents and Ib inhibitory interneurons that project to the spinal cord and are involved in preventing antagonist muscles from firing while the agonist is firing (19). There is evidence for replacement of Ib inhibition with facilitation in hemiplegic individuals with supraspinal lesions, leading to simultaneous cofiring of agonist and antagonist muscle groups (20); however, studies in individuals with SCI have shown that Ib inhibition is unaltered (Figure 21.1).

Two additional mechanisms that may play a role in the development of spasticity after SCI are axonal sprouting and denervation supersensitivity. Ditunno et al. (23) describe the transition from spinal shock immediately after SCI to the development of spasticity

and hyperreflexia 1 to 12 months later. In their proposed 4-phase model of spinal shock, there is observation of areflexia or hyporeflexia, as well as paralysis and muscle flaccidity for the initial 0 to 24 hours postinjury. These findings are due to loss of excitatory input from supraspinal pathways, including vestibulospinal and reticulospinal pathways, among others. Loss of descending inhibitory input to spinal inhibitory interneurons may cause further hyporeflexia. In the second phase of spinal shock, there is return of the tibial H reflex 1 to 3 days after injury, although muscle stretch reflexes are still absent. This is likely due to denervation supersensitivity, which causes increased neuronal firing in response to neurotransmitters and has been reported to occur in the brain and spinal cord. The denervation supersensitivity may be due to decreased reuptake of excitatory neurotransmitters, up-regulation of receptors on the postsynaptic membrane, or alteration of degradation and synthesis of receptors. Phases 3 and 4 of Ditunno's model describe early hyperreflexia and later development of spasticity in patients with SCI. The proposed physiologic mechanism for both phases is axonal regrowth. New synapses are formed by spinal afferents and interneurons, as well as spared supraspinal descending pathways (24). Axonal sprouting of spared descending motor tracts may result in motor recovery, whereas axonal sprouting of the neurons involved in segmental

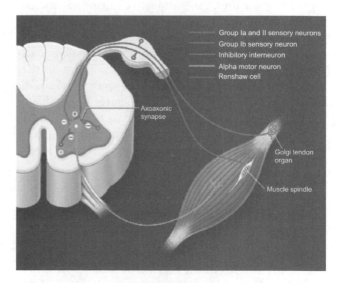

FIGURE 21.1

Potential spinal mechanisms involved in the development of spasticity. (Adapted from Satkunam LE. Rehabilitation medicine: 3. Management of adult spasticity. *CMAJ.* 2003;169:1175.)

reflexes may produce less desirable effects, such as the development of hyperreflexia and spasticity (25).

Intrinsic changes within the muscle may also play a role in the development of increased muscle tone. These mechanical changes may include loss of sarcomeres, increased stiffness of muscle fibers, altered muscle fiber size and distribution of fiber types, and changes in collagen tissue and tendons (22, 26). The work of Kamper et al. (27) in stroke patients demonstrated that muscle fiber played some part in the phenomenon of spasticity as decreasing the initial length of tested spastic metacarpophalangeal fibers reduced muscle stiffness suggesting that the biomechanical qualities of muscle fibers play some part in the development of spasticity. These changes in spastic muscle may be a result of the development of subclinical contracture rather than true reflex hyperexcitability (26) or be an intrinsic property of the changes in biomechanical properties of the muscle (27).

MEASURES

Although spasticity may seem simple to recognize clinically, it is difficult to quantify. Having tools available that objectively measure spasticity is important to evaluate and monitor response to treatment. Currently, there are a variety of different outcome measures available that can be used to quantify tone (28). These outcome measures can be categorized into subjective measures including clinical scales and self-reported measures, and objective measures including biomechanical techniques and electrophysiologic measurements. Extensive reviews have been published on the various subjective and objective spasticity measures (29–31); however, we will discuss the tools that are most commonly used to assess spasticity in individuals with SCI. A review of measures applicable in the clinical setting for persons with SCI has been undertaken that revealed 66 different measures found (5), of which only 6 had been tested psychometrically (32).

Clinical Measures

Ashworth Scale and Modified Ashworth Scale

The Ashworth Scale (AS) (33) (developed initially to assess hypertonicity in persons with multiple sclerosis [MS]) and the Modified Ashworth Scale (MAS) (34) (Table 21.1) are the most common clinical methods used to measure the degree of muscle tone or "the sensation of resistance felt as one manipulates a joint through a range of motion (ROM), with the subject

attempting to relax." (35) These tests are relatively quick and simple to perform and do not require any instrumentation. When performing these tests, the examiner passively moves the subject's joints through full ROM and judges the degree of tone felt during passive range on a 0-to-4 scale on the AS, with a score of 0 indicating that there is no increase in tone, and a score of 4 signifying that the affected part is rigid in flexion or extension. For the MAS, an additional grade was added (1+) to enhance sensitivity at the lower end of the scale. The amount of time allotted for passive movement of the joint through full ROM is not well specified, although several studies suggest 1 second. In regard to testing procedure, Pandyan (36) suggests that the examiner should limit the number of repetitions performed during the testing procedure because repetitive passive ROM will decrease the resistance of the muscle to passive stretch and may affect scoring on the AS and MAS. Skold et al. (37) likewise

---

TABLE 21.1
Clinical Measures of Spasticity

ASHWORTH SCALE

0	No increased tone
1	Slight increase in tone, giving a "catch" when affected part is moved in flexion or extension
2	More marked increase in tone, but affected part easily flexed
3	Considerable increase in tone; passive movement difficult
4	Affected part rigid in flexion or extension

MODIFIED ASHWORTH SCALE

0	No increased tone
1	*Slight increase in muscle tone, manifested by a catch and release or by minimal resistance at the end of the ROM when the affected part(s) is moved in flexion or extension*
1+	*Slight increase in muscle tone, manifested by a catch, followed by minimal resistance throughout the remainder (less than half) of the ROM*
2	More marked increase in tone, but affected part easily flexed
3	Considerable increase in tone; passive movement difficult
4	Affected part rigid in flexion or extension (Changes compared to the standard AS are italicized.)

reported a decrease in spasticity with repetitive passive movements.

A number of investigators have studied the interrater reliability of these scales when used to evaluate people with SCI. Haas et al. (38) found that the most commonly used scores were generally on the lower end of the scales, and interrater reliability was variable among muscle groups tested for both scales. Skold et al. investigated the relationship between the objective findings of spasticity rated using the MAS and patients' self-reported ratings of spasticity using a Visual Analogue Scale and found a significant correlation between these 2 measures (37). Lechner et al. (39) however reported a weak correlation between self-reported spasticity rated on the Visual Analogue Scale and clinical measures of spasticity according to the AS in 3 of 8 subjects with spasticity secondary to SCI and no correlation in the remaining 5 subjects.

Spasm Frequency Scales

Quantification of the frequency of spasm occurrence has also been described and is often used clinically. One of the most commonly used scales is the Penn spasm frequency scale (PSFS), which was created to measure the effectiveness of intrathecal baclofen (ITB) in the treatment of spasticity in subjects with spasticity of spinal origin (Table 21.2) (40). This scale measures the number of spasms experienced by patients within a 1-hour period. The PSFS measures an entity different from tone, as Priebe et al. found no correlation between it and the AS (40). The PSFS has been modified by Priebe et al. (41) and referred to as the modified PSFS. This consists of a second self-report 3-point scale only if the PSFS is greater than 1 and assesses severity of spasms from "1 = mild" to "3 = severe"; this provides a more comprehensive understanding of the individuals spasticity status. An alternative scale is the spasm frequency score, which measures the number of spasms per day (Table 21.2) (42).

Spinal Cord Assessment Tool for Spasticity

This scale was developed by Benz et al. (3) to measure spasticity in SCI. This easy-to-administer tool utilizes elements of the standard neurologic examination of the lower extremities (LE). The Spinal Cord Assessment Tool for Spasticity (SCATS) flexor spasms and clonus scores correlate well with AS scores, but only the SCATS clonus score correlated with the PSFS. This tool may provide additional information in comparison to the AS and MAS in assessing multijoint spas-

---

TABLE 21.2
Spasm Frequency Scales

PENN SPASM FREQUENCY SCORE (PSFS)

0	No spasms
1	Mild spasms induced by stimulation
2	Infrequent spasms occurring less than once per hour
3	Spasms occurring more than once per hour
4	Spasms occurring more than ten times per hour

MODIFIED PSFS: 2 PART

Part 1: spasm frequency score (as above)
Part 2: spasm severity scale

1	Mild
2	Moderate
3	Severe

SPASM FREQUENCY SCORE

0	No spasms
1	1 or fewer spasms per day
2	Between 1 and 5 spasms per day
3	5 to >10 spasms per day
4	10 or more spasms per day, or continuous contraction

---

ticity (3), although it has not as of yet been adopted widely (Table 21.3) (5).

Spinal Cord Injury Spasticity Evaluation Tool (SCI-SET)

Described by Adams et al. (43) the SCI-SET is a 35-item, 7-day recall self-report scale. This tool assesses the impact of spasticity on various ADL to issues of social participation, with a Likert scale of -3 (extremely problematic) to +3 (extremely helpful) in asking how spasticity affects their lives. It is a short survey that has shown test-retest reliability and construct validity (Table 21.4) (43).

Patient Reported Impact of Spasticity Measure

The Patient Reported Impact of Spasticity Measure is a new instrument that standardizes the collection of self-report information (both positive and negative impacts) relevant to the clinical assessment of spasticity (44). There are subscales that include social avoidance/anxiety, psychological agitation, daily activities, needs for assistance/positioning, needs for intervention, and social embarrassment from the spasticity.

TABLE 21.3
Spinal Cord Assessment Tool for Spastic Reflexes

SCATS: CLONUS

Clonus quantified in response to rapid dorsiflexion of the ankle.
- 0 No reaction
- 1 Mild, clonus maintained less than 3 seconds
- 2 Moderate, clonus persists 3–10 seconds
- 3 Severe, clonus persists >10 seconds

SCATS: FLEXOR SPASMS

Measurement of excursion of big toe into extension, ankle dorsiflexion, knee flexion, or hip flexion when pinprick stimulus applied to plantar surface of the foot.
- 0 No reaction to stimulus
- 1 Mild, <10°
- 2 Moderate, 10°–30°
- 3 Severe, ≥30°

SCATS: EXTENSOR SPASMS

Starting position with hip and knee placed at 90°–110° of flexion with contralateral limb extended. Hip and knee joints then simultaneously extended and duration of quadriceps muscle contraction is measured.
- 0 No reaction
- 1 Mild, contraction maintained <3 seconds
- 2 Moderate, contraction persists 3–10 seconds
- 3 Severe, contraction persists >10 seconds

(Summarized from Benz EN, Hornby TG, Bode RK, Scheidt RA, Schmit BD. A physiologically based clinical measure for spastic reflexes in spinal cord injury. *Arch Phys Med Rehabil.* 2005;86:52–59.)

Tardieu Scale

The Tardieu Scale was introduced in 1954 and has undergone some revisions. This scale has mostly been used in cerebral palsy and adult stroke but has some benefits over other scales. The key to this scale is that resistance to passive stretch may be from more than just spasticity (ie, soft tissue changes) and that there are "neural versus peripheral contributions" to the spasticity present. There are 3 key components to the testing: (1) velocity of stretch; (2) quality of muscle reaction, and (3) angle of muscle reaction. This can be used in SCI when serial casting is performed (see later). By varying the velocity of the stretch during testing, the Tardieu may be superior to the Ashworth in the assessment of true spasticity, which by definition has a velocity component.

Biomechanical Measures

Biomechanical techniques can be used to objectively quantify spasticity by evaluating resistance to passive movement at a joint. Commonly used techniques are the pendulum test and measurements using isokinetic dynamometers (45–49). The pendulum test was first described by Wartenberg (47) in 1951 and assesses spasticity in the hamstring and quadriceps muscles. To perform this test, the patient is in the seated or supine position with the examination table ending at the distal thigh of both legs; this allows passive flexion and extension at the knee joint without interference of movement from the examination table. The patient is asked to relax his lower limb, and the examiner passively extends the knee fully, then releases, allowing the limb to fall freely. Electrogoniometers may be used to evaluate the swing of the leg at the knee joint, and tachometers can assess the rate of movement. In the spastic limb, the degree of movement at the knee joint is decreased when compared to movement in the non-spastic limb. It is difficult to determine whether the dampening of movement is due to intrinsic changes within the spastic muscle, such as alterations in visco-elastic properties, or due to the other pathophysiologic changes after SCI that result in velocity-dependent resistance to movement (50). Although the pendulum test has its limitations, the test-retest variability and reliability have been evaluated, and this test has been shown to have a high correlation between measures on repeated trials using a commercially available isokinetic dynamometer (46). The pendulum test was one of the outcome variables used in the tizanidine trials for the management of spasticity in patients with SCI (51).

Electrophysiologic Measurements

There are a variety of electrophysiologic methods that can be used to objectively assess spasticity; however, these techniques are used primarily for research purposes. To understand the most commonly used methods, one must have a basic understanding of several electrophysiologic tests. Maximal electrical stimulation of a peripheral nerve results in the development of a compound motor action potential (CMAP), which can be recorded over a muscle innervated by the stimulated nerve; this is the M response. The Hoffman reflex, or H reflex, is a late response that can be obtained by delivering a submaximal electrical stimulus to the tibial nerve with the CMAP recorded over the soleus. The H reflex is an electrically elicited reflex comprised of an orthodromic sensory and an orthodromic motor response. The stimulus delivered to the

TABLE 21.4
SCI-SET

For each of the following, please choose the answer that best describes how your spasticity symptoms have affected that area of your life **during the past 7 years**. When I talk about "spasticity symptoms". I mean: A) uncontrolled, involuntary muscle contraction or movement (slow or rapid; short or prolonged), B) involuntary, repetitive, quick muscle movement (up and down; side to side), C) muscle tightness, and D) what you might describe as "spasms". Please let me know when a question is not applicable to you.

Extremely problematic	*Moderately problematic*	*Somewhat problematic*	*No effect*	*Somewhat helpful*	*Moderately helpful*	*Extremely helpful*
−3	−2	−1	0	+1	+2	+3

DURING **THE PAST 7 DAYS.** HOW HAVE YOUR SPASTICITY SYMPTOMS AFFECTED:

1. your showering?	−3	−2	−1	0	+1	+2	+3	N/A
2. your dressing/undressing?	−3	−2	−1	0	+1	+2	+3	N/A
3. your transfers (to and from bed, chair, vehicle, etc.)?	−3	−2	−1	0	+1	+2	+3	N/A
4. your sitting positioning (in your chair, etc.)?	−3	−2	−1	0	+1	+2	+3	N/A
5. the preparation of meals?	−3	−2	−1	0	+1	+2	+3	N/A
6. eating?	−3	−2	−1	0	+1	+2	+3	N/A
7. drinking?	−3	−2	−1	0	+1	+2	+3	N/A
8. your small hand movements (writing, use of computer, etc)?	−3	−2	−1	0	+1	+2	+3	N/A
9. your ability to perform household chores?	−3	−2	−1	0	+1	+2	+3	N/A
10. your hobbies/recreational activities?	−3	−2	−1	0	+1	+2	+3	N/A
11. your enjoyment of social outings?	−3	−2	−1	0	+1	+2	+3	N/A
12. your ability to stand/weight-bear?	−3	−2	−1	0	+1	+2	+3	N/A
13. your walking ability?	−3	−2	−1	0	+1	+2	+3	N/A
14. your stability/balance?	−3	−2	−1	0	+1	+2	+3	N/A
15. your muscle fatigue?	−3	−2	−1	0	+1	+2	+3	N/A
16. the flexibility of your joints?	−3	−2	−1	0	+1	+2	+3	N/A
17. your therapy/exercise routine?	−3	−2	−1	0	+1	+2	+3	N/A
18. your manual wheelchair use?	−3	−2	−1	0	+1	+2	+3	N/A
19. your power wheelchair use?	−3	−2	−1	0	+1	+2	+3	N/A
20. you lying position (in bed, etc.)?	−3	−2	−1	0	+1	+2	+3	N/A
21. your ability to change positions in bed?	−3	−2	−1	0	+1	+2	+3	N/A
22. your ability to get sleep?	−3	−2	−1	0	+1	+2	+3	N/A
23. the quality of your sleep?	−3	−2	−1	0	+1	+2	+3	N/A

(Continued)

TABLE 21.4
(Continued)

Extremely problematic	Moderately problematic	Somewhat problematic	No effect	Somewhat helpful	Moderately helpful	Extremely helpful
−3	−2	−1	0	+1	+2	+3

DURING **THE PAST 7 DAYS.** HOW HAVE YOUR SPASTICITY SYMPTOMS AFFECTED:

24. your sex life?	−3	−2	−1	0	+1	+2	+3	N/A
25. the feeling of being annoyed?	−3	−2	−1	0	+1	+2	+3	N/A
26. the feeling of being embarassed?	−3	−2	−1	0	+1	+2	+3	N/A
27. your feeling of comfort socially?	−3	−2	−1	0	+1	+2	+3	N/A
28. your feeling of comfort physically?	−3	−2	−1	0	+1	+2	+3	N/A
29. your pain?	−3	−2	−1	0	+1	+2	+3	N/A
30. your concern with falling?	−3	−2	−1	0	+1	+2	+3	N/A
31. your concern with getting injured?	−3	−2	−1	0	+1	+2	+3	N/A
32. your concern with accidentally injuring someone else?	−3	−2	−1	0	+1	+2	+3	N/A
33. your ability to concentrate?	−3	−2	−1	0	+1	+2	+3	N/A
34. your feelings of control over your body?	−3	−2	−1	0	+1	+2	+3	N/A
35. your need to ask for help?	−3	−2	−1	0	+1	+2	+3	N/A

Number of (+) items: _____   Negative score:_____
Number of (−) items: _____   Positive score:_____
Number of (0) items: _____   **Total score:**_____
                                     Applicable items (#):_____
                                     Average score:_____

tibial nerve travels up the large Ia afferents into the spinal cord, synapses with the alpha motor neurons after entering the spinal cord, and travels back down the alpha motor neurons innervating the soleus muscle, where the H reflex CMAP is ultimately recorded (52). The H reflex can be considered as the electrical equivalent of the Achilles reflex; however, the muscle spindle is bypassed (53).

The H(max)/M(max) ratio is the ratio of the maximal H reflex to the maximal M response and has been investigated in several studies of patients with SCI (54–56). The H(max)/M(max) ratio is used to determine the percentage of motor neurons that are acti-

vated reflexively (H reflex) compared to those that are directly activated (M response); this gives an estimation of motor neuron excitability at rest. Some studies have shown an increased H(max)/M(max) ratio in individuals with SCI; however, there is little correlation between severity of spasticity and H(max)/M(max) ratios (53). Similar results can be obtained by substituting T(max), the Achilles tendon jerk, for H(max). The T(max)/M(max) ratio is similar to the H(max)/M(max) ratio, with the exception that rather than activating the Ia afferent fibers electrically as with the H reflex, the fibers are activated with a mechanically induced stretch to the muscle fibers when the Achilles tendon is tapped. Similar to the H(max)/M(max) ratio, the T(max)/M(max) ratio reflects motor neuron excitability, and there is not a correlation between it and the severity of spasticity (51); however, unlike the H(max)/M(max) ratio, the T(max)/M(max) ratio is influenced by the gamma system (6).

F waves are another late response that, similar to the H-reflex, reflect proximal conduction along the peripheral nerves. The F wave is elicited by supramaximal electrical stimulation of a mixed nerve while recording over a distal muscle innervated by that nerve. The electrical stimulus travels antidromically along the motor nerve, and once it reaches the axon hillock, a small percentage of the motor neurons backfire, and the action potential then travels orthodromically back down the motor neurons; this causes a late response that can be recorded over the distal muscle (52). Some studies have shown increased amplitude and persistence of F waves in individuals with spasticity, and this may reflect excitability of the motor neuron pool (53).

Spasticity may also be evaluated using electromyography (EMG). Skold et al. evaluated lower extremity spasticity in patients with SCI by using surface EMG to record muscle activity of the quadriceps and hamstrings during passive flexion and extension at the knee joint, as well as using the MAS to clinically assess the presence of spasticity. These researchers found a correlation between spasticity ratings on the MAS and electrical activity on surface EMG recordings; in addition, they noted that with each increasing grade on the MAS, there was evidence of increased myoelectric activity on EMG recordings (57).

The difficulties with quantitative tests to measure spasticity are due to a number of reasons. These include difficulty using a static test for a dynamic process; spasticity changes based on time of day and with many other factors (ie, stress, infections); test position usually is not the position of function for the patient; different scales measure different aspects of spasticity; individual tools correlate weakly with each other (5); discrepancy between self-rated and clinical scores; and a decrease in a score does not necessarily correlate with improved function. There is still no accepted measure that addresses the specific impact of spasticity in limiting activity or participation. Priebe has suggested that spasticity is best measured by a battery of tests that assess the different variables and the patient's perspective (58).

TREATMENT

Spasticity is present in most individuals with SCI and may have a significant negative impact on QOL and functional activities. Little et al. (9) found that 59% of patients with traumatic SCI reported that spasticity interfered with transfers, and 65% claimed that it disrupted their sleep. Lundqvist et al. (59) noted that in patients with SCI, those with spasticity scored significantly worse on the Sickness Impact Profile for ambulation and feeding activities than those without. Other studies have not found a negative association between QOL and spasticity, and some have even reported a positive impact of spasticity. In a study by Skold et al., 40% of individuals with spasticity reported that it had a positive impact (10), and another study found that 23% reported the positive effects of spasticity outweighed the negative (44). Some individuals use their spasticity to assist with standing and positioning, as well as to aide them in ADL, such as assisting with lower body dressing by eliciting flexor spasms in the LE. Fifty-three percent of individuals with tetraplegia and 26% with paraplegia report that they elicit spasms to assist with repositioning, dressing, transfers, and pressure relief (9). Some individuals with SCI find spasticity useful because it can serve as a warning sign that there is a change in their normal physiologic state, including the presence of a distended bladder, urinary tract infection, or pressure ulcer (60). In addition, spasticity may help to preserve muscle bulk by preventing atrophy (61). Overall, it seems that spasticity more often than not can have a negative impact on a patient's life. Treatment should occur not because spasticity is present but rather because it interferes with specific activities and the treatment has the potential to address a passive or active functional goal. Because of the variable impact of spasticity on the QOL and functional status in individuals with SCI, it is important to determine the necessity of intervention, discuss treatment goals, and tailor treatment plans on an individual basis. Some of the most pertinent questions to ask include the following: Does the spasticity cause pain? Is it leading to contracture? Does it interfere with function or sleep? Does it affect QOL?

There are a variety of indications for treatment of spasticity, and the approach should be dictated by the patient's overall functional status and symptom severity. Some of the aspects that should be considered include the severity of the spasticity, the scope (ie, whether the spasticity is focal, regional, or generalized), what the medical and cognitive status of the patient is, and taking into account the side effects of treatments as well as the cost-benefit ratio. Treatment goals vary from patient to patient and may range from maximizing gait in a highly functional patients to goals of decreasing quantity of painful spasms or to improve the ease of care in patients who are dependent for their self-care needs (62).

Treatment of spasticity should be approached in a stepwise fashion, with initiation of noninvasive interventions including stretching and therapy programs before consideration of pharmacologic or surgical treatments (63). When increases in spasticity are noted in patients with a SCI that is stable, one must first consider potential causes of the change, such as presence of infection, bladder calculi, pressure ulcers, abdominal pathology, ingrown toenail, hemorrhoids, deep vein thrombosis, heterotopic ossification, or medication side effect, before initiating other interventions to treat the spasticity (6). Drug effects can serve as a source of newly increased spasticity, that is, selective serotonin reuptake inhibitors have been reported to increase spasticity (64). Changes in spasticity in an otherwise stable patient with a chronic SCI may also be an important presenting sign in syringomyelia (65). Spasticity-related interventions should be aimed at what matters most to the patient, improving comfort and function and allowing the individual to participate in life activities.

Nonpharmacologic Interventions

Initial treatment of spasticity typically involves nonpharmacologic, noninvasive measures. It is important to ensure that noxious stimuli are not contributing to the patient's spasticity. Prevention of pressure ulcers and complications related to the patient's neurogenic bowel and bladder by maintaining appropriate skin protocols and bowel and bladder management regimens will help to minimize noxious stimuli commonly encountered in this population. Positioning and stretching are also useful and necessary for decreasing spasticity and maintaining ROM at the affected joints and may even decrease long term spasticity (6, 66). The frequency, duration, and type of stretching that should be performed, as well as its long-term benefit, has been studied. A recent literature search on the effect of stretching showed that although there is some benefit to each stretching session, there is a wide diversity regarding its impact. Specifically, this review found that the available evidence on its clinical benefit is overall inconclusive (67). Tilt table standing reduces spasticity in individuals with SCI, most likely by providing a prolonged stretch on the ankle plantar flexors (68), and has demonstrated efficacy in reduction of extensor spasms (69). Posture and adequate low back support are also important factors for tone reduction. Adequate low back support in the wheelchair to maintain lumbar lordosis and a positive seat plane angle or "dump," with a reduction in seat-to-back angle, encourages proper upright posture and may reduce extensor tone.

Modalities

Other modalities and therapeutic interventions are available to therapists for the management of spasticity. Local cryotherapy has been reported to temporarily decrease spasticity, possibly due to temporary slowing of nerve conduction and reduction in the sensitivity of the muscle spindle fibers. The results obtained with local cooling typically diminish within 15 to 20 minutes after removal of the cold application (70). Electrical stimulation is another commonly used modality that is reported to decrease spasticity in individuals with SCI. Transcutaneous electrical nerve stimulation is one technique that has been utilized in the management of chronic pain using the gate control theory (71), and it may also play a role in the management of spasticity. Several studies have described a reduction in spasticity of the lower limbs in individuals with stroke or SCI receiving transcutaneous electrical nerve stimulation therapy over the spastic muscles or over corresponding spinal dermatomes (72–76). Functional electrical stimulation has been noted to have beneficial effects on cardiovascular function and circulation, reversal of muscle atrophy, and possible prevention of deep venous thrombosis and osteoporosis, and one study has shown that it may also be beneficial in reducing spasticity (77). In a crossover study comparing electrical stimulation to the LE in a small group of persons with SCI versus passive movement in an LE ergometer machine, spasticity as measured by the MAS and the pendulum test was significantly decreased (78). Electroejaculation using a rectal probe (79) as well as vibratory stimulation (80) have also shown to decrease spasticity in persons with SCI.

Orthotics

Tone-reducing orthotics are designed to improve gait patterns and decrease reflexive muscle activation in individuals with spasticity. There are several important design features of these orthotics that decrease spasticity in users, including the metatarsal pad and the great toe shelf that cause unloading of the metatarsal heads and extension of the great toe, delivery of constant pressure at the site gastrocnemius and soleus insertion into the calcaneous, joint stabilization, and full contact with the muscle bellies provided by the thermoplastic material (81). The use of tone-reducing orthotics has previously been described in individuals with spasticity due to stroke and cerebral palsy, and a recent study demonstrated efficacy when used in individuals with SCI. Nash et al. (81) demonstrated improvement in step length, gait velocity, and scores on the SCI-Functional Ambulation Inventory, as well as a reduction in abnormal EMG activity in the gastrocnemius in an individual with incomplete SCI and spasticity when using tone-reducing Ankle Foot Orthoses (AFO's) bilaterally.

Nontraditional Interventions

Other alternative interventions may play a role in the reduction of spasticity in individuals with SCI. Lechner et al. (82) reported a short-term decrease in spasticity as quantified by the Ashworth score in individuals with SCI after participation in hippotherapy sessions. The beneficial effects of hippotherapy on spasticity reduction are thought to be related to saddle position, which places the patient's LE into hip flexion, abduction, and external rotation; other benefits may be due to the effects of rhythmical trunk side flexion and extension produced during hippotherapy sessions. Acupuncture has been studied as a potential intervention in SCI-related conditions, including motor deficits, pain, and spasticity. Electroacupuncture and stimulation of acupoints may be beneficial in the reduction of spasticity related to SCI, but further studies are needed (83). Hydrotherapy has also been studied in persons with SCI. In a randomized control study of 20 patients, exercise in a 71°F pool, 3 times per week for 20 minutes, demonstrated an increase in Functional Independence Measure score, a decrease in spasm severity, and a decrease in oral baclofen dose intake (84).

Serial Casting

Serial casting involves a series of casts to reduce spasticity by stretching soft tissue and/or muscle lengthening. This can also be effective in stretching out a contracture. One can utilize the Tardieu Scale to know how much range one can achieve. The technique involves finding the end range, then slightly backing off to prevent tendonitis and improve tolerance to the cast. After 24 hours, the cast should be removed to check the skin. Subsequent casts can remain on for 2 to 3 days. The cast can be bivalved to allow for examination of the skin. Casting should continue until there is no improvement noted in 2 consecutive casts. To loosen the spasticity and improve the stretch, chemodenervation with localized injections can be administered first. Prolonged use of splints can be utilized in place of the casts.

Pharmacologic Interventions

A variety of pharmacologic agents with different mechanisms of action are available for the treatment of spasticity of spinal cord origin; however, only 4 are Food and Drug Administration (FDA)-approved for this use. These agents include baclofen, diazepam, dantrolene sodium, and tizanidine (85). A systematic review indicated that there is insufficient evidence to assist clinicians in a rational approach to antispasticity treatment in SCI (86), and therefore, some amount of trial-and-error is required. The person's age, comorbidities, and cognitive status should be carefully considered when choosing a medication for spasticity. Centrally acting agents typically suppress excitation or enhance inhibition within the central nervous system, whereas peripherally acting agents act directly at the neuromuscular sites (Table 21.5).

Baclofen (Lioresal®)

Baclofen is an antispasticity agent that is commonly used in the treatment of spasticity of spinal origin. Baclofen is considered by many to be the first-line of treatment, although there are no studies definitively supporting this approach (86). Baclofen is a derivative of the inhibitory neurotransmitter GABA. It binds presynaptically to the GABA-B receptors in the brain and spinal cord and is thought to decrease monosynaptic and polysynaptic reflexes. Binding of baclofen to the GABA-B receptors decreases calcium influx into the presynaptic terminal; this in turn decreases the release of excitatory neurotransmitters. The decreased release of excitatory neurotransmitters by the interneurons and afferent fibers is responsible for the diminution of reflex activity (87). Binding of baclofen to GABA-B receptors may also decrease gamma motor neuron activity, which may decrease muscle spindle activity (85).

The mean half-life of baclofen is approximately 3½ hours (range, 2–6 hours), necessitating dosing 3 to 4 times daily. Baclofen is excreted primarily by the kidney, although 15% is metabolized by the liver; therefore, caution must be exerted when using baclofen in patients with renal insufficiency, and liver function tests should be checked before initiation of treatment and periodically thereafter (85).

Baclofen can be administered orally and intrathecally; intrathecal dosing will be discussed later. Oral baclofen should be initiated at a dose of 5 mg 2 to 3 times daily and gradually titrated up to an appropriate dose based upon patient response and side effects. The Physician's Desk Reference recommends 80 mg as the maximum daily dose of baclofen; however, there are reports and clinical experience of using higher doses in SCI (88). A study by Aisen et al. (89) showed that higher doses of baclofen (up to 240 mg/d) may be used safely in patients with spasticity due to MS or SCI. We

TABLE 21.5
Oral Medications for Spasticity

Medication	Usual Dosage	Major Mechanism of Action	Common Side Effects
Baclofen	5 mg TID to 40 mg QID	Presynaptic inhibition of GABA-B receptors	Sedation, ataxia, muscle weakness. Abrupt withdrawal may result in seizures and hallucinations. May cause respiratory failure, seizures, coma and death in overdose.
Clonidine	0.05 mg BID to 0.2 mg BID (oral) 0.1–0.3 mg (transdermal)	Alpha-2 adrenergic agonist, increases presynaptic inhibition of motor neurons	Orthostasis, bradycardia dy mouth, constipation, ankle edema and drowsiness.
Diazepam	5 mg qday to 15 mg QID	Facilitates postsynaptic effects of GABA, increasing presynaptic inhibition	Sedation, impaired memory and attention, impaired motor coordination. May cause respiratory depression and coma in overdose.
Dantrolene	25 mg qday to 100 mg QID	Reduces calcium release, interfering with excitation contraction coupling in skeletal muscle	Nausea, vomiting, diarrhea, malaise, and generalized muscle weakness. May cause hepatotoxicity; therefore, liver enzymes should be monitored.
Tizanidine	2 mg qday to 36 mg/d in divided doses; better tolerated as a QID dosing	Alpha-2 adrenergic agonist, increases presynaptic inhibition of motor neurons	Dry mouth, sedation, dizziness, mild hypotension. May cause elevated liver enzymes, therefore must monitor.
Gabapentin	100 mg TID to 1200 mg QID	Unknown	Somnolence, dizziness, ataxia, tremor, dyspepsia and constipation.

(authors of this chapter) routinely titrate Lioresel up to 80 mg/d in divided doses (as long as there is continued benefit) and feel comfortable increasing to higher doses (monitoring for side effects), often adding a second agent between 80 and 160 mg/d.

Several open-label studies have demonstrated the effectiveness of baclofen. Baclofen has been shown to decrease spasticity in 70% to 87% of patients with SCI or MS, and it has also been shown to decrease flexor spasms in individuals with SCI (85–90), as well as to decrease pain in both animal and human studies (87). Baclofen appears to have an anxiolytic property as well, as has been demonstrated in the SCI population (91) as well as individuals with panic disorder and chronic schizophrenia (92, 93). Baclofen may also improve bladder function by decreasing outlet obstruction secondary to hyperreflexia of the external urethral sphincter (94). Baclofen has been compared to other antispasticity agents, and its effectiveness has been demonstrated to be equivalent to tizanidine in several studies; however, some studies showed more weakness in patients treated with baclofen compared to those treated with tizanadine. In studies comparing baclofen to diazepam, both were effective in decreasing spasticity; however, diazepam was more likely to cause sedation (90). As with many of the medications used for spasticity, although spasticity itself may be decreased, there is a paucity of literature documenting functional benefits. For this reason, dosages should be titrated based upon improvement noted by the patient in their daily routine.

Although baclofen is generally well tolerated, dose titration may be limited by side effects. Most commonly, baclofen can cause sedation and mental confusion, ataxia, hypotonia, muscle weakness, and constipation. Respiratory failure, seizures, coma, and death have been reported after significant overdose. Abrupt withdrawal of baclofen should be avoided because it can result in seizures, hallucinations, and potentially death. Clinicians need to be especially mindful of this fact after the placement of an ITB pump. Because the amount of medication that is needed for spasticity management is so low, there is a real risk for baclofen withdrawal if the oral dose is weaned too quickly.

Benzodiazepines

Diazepam (Valium®), a member of the benzodiazepine family, is one of the oldest antispasticity agents. Diazepam acts through the GABA system; however, its mechanism of action is different from baclofen in that it does not bind directly to the GABA receptor, rather it is presumed to bind near the GABA-A receptor to indirectly facilitate the binding of GABA to the GABA-A receptors, thereby increasing presynaptic inhibition and reducing monosynaptic and polysynaptic reflexes.

Diazepam displays good oral absorption; after oral administration, blood levels peak within 1 hour. It is one of the long-acting benzodiazepines, with a half-life of 20 to 80 hours. Diazepam is metabolized in the liver, so it may cause side effects in individuals with liver dysfunction. In addition, diazepam is 98% protein-bound so caution must be exercised when using this medication in individuals with low serum albumin (ie, acute SCI), as they may demonstrate increased susceptibility to side effects (85). Diazepam may be dosed starting at 5 mg when given at bedtime or 2 mg given during the daytime. Dosage should be gradually titrated up to a total daily dose of 40 to 60 mg (given in divided doses) as tolerated and required by the patient (6, 85).

Diazepam has been shown to be effective in treatment of spasticity; however, it was noted to be more sedating than baclofen in a comparison study (90). Benzodiazepines may affect cognitive performance measures such as attention, concentration, and memory and are not recommended in persons with concomitant brain injury. Diazepam may be less effective in treating spasticity in individuals with complete SCI compared to those with incomplete SCI, as it appears that the brainstem reticular formation is more sensitive to the effects of diazepam than other spinal pathways (95–97).

Diazepam produces depression of the central nervous system, which can decrease the level of arousal, can cause sedation and impaired motor coordination, impair memory and attention, and may cause respiratory depression and coma in overdose. Flumazenil is a benzodiazepine antagonist that may be effective if overdose occurs (98). Diazepam may cause physiologic addiction, and abrupt discontinuation may result in a withdrawal syndrome, with symptom onset typically occurring 2 to 4 days after discontinuation.

Typical withdrawal symptoms may include anxiety, agitation, nausea, and restlessness; however, severe cases can result in seizures and death (85). Because of the potential cognitive side effects associated with the use of diazepam, this medication should be avoided in those patients with SCI who have a concomitant brain injury.

Other benzodiazepine agents have been investigated for use in patients with spasticity. Ketazolam is a long-acting benzodiazepine given in a single daily dose of 30 to 60 mg. It has been studied in patients with spasticity secondary to MS, stroke, and brain injury and was noted to have equal efficacy and less sedating properties than diazepam (99, 100). Ketazolam is not FDA-approved in the United States but is available in Canada. Clonazepam (Klonopin®) is another benzodiazepine agent that may be considered for use in the treatment of spasticity and is typically used for painful nocturnal spasms. The half-life is 18 to 28 hours, and it is initiated at doses of 0.25 mg to 1 mg at night and titrated up to a total dose of 3 mg as tolerated and required. In a study comparing baclofen and clonazepam in the treatment of spasticity related to MS, clonazepam demonstrated similar efficacy to baclofen; however, sedation, fatigue, and confusion were more common with clonazepam use (101).

Dantrolene Sodium (Dantrium®)

Dantrolene sodium is the only antispasticity agent that acts peripherally within the muscle to decrease spasticity. It decreases the release of calcium from the sarcoplasmic reticulum within the skeletal muscle fibers, which results in decreased muscle contraction force generation due to partial excitation-contraction uncoupling (102, 103). Dantrolene sodium has little effect on cardiac and smooth muscles but acts on both intrafusal and extrafusal fibers in skeletal muscle. Dantrolene sodium is metabolized primarily in the liver and eliminated in the urine and bile. The blood concentration peaks in 3 to 8 hours after administration of an oral dose of 100 mg, and half-life is approximately 15 hours. Dantrolene sodium is initiated at 25 mg/d and slowly increased every 5 to 7 days to a maximal dosage of 100 mg given 4 times per day.

Dantrolene sodium has been used primarily in individuals with spasticity of cerebral origin. It has demonstrated efficacy in decreasing muscle tone, clonus, and tendon reflexes and improving ROM in this patient population (104, 105). Some studies have demonstrated efficacy of dantrolene sodium in the treatment of spasticity of spinal cord origin; however, it is usually considered a second-line medication (106). Dantrolene sodium may be considered as a first-line agent in individuals with SCI and concomitant cognitive dysfunction (6). Otherwise, dantrolene is not routinely used to treat spasticity in patients with SCI.

Common side effects of dantrolene sodium include nausea, vomiting, diarrhea, malaise, and dizziness. This medication has fewer cognitive side effects and is less likely to cause drowsiness than baclofen or diazepam. Dantrolene sodium may cause hepatotoxicity, which has been reported in 1% to 2% of patients, with fatal hepatitis occurring in up to 0.3%. The populations at greatest risk for hepatotoxicity are females more than 30 years of age, individuals taking other medications simultaneously that are processed through the liver, and those patients taking high-dose dantrolene sodium (300 mg or more per day) for more than 60 days (107). Because of this risk, baseline liver function tests should be obtained before initiation of treatment with dantrolene sodium, and liver function tests should be monitored intermittently thereafter. Concern also exists that dantrolene sodium may cause a slight decrease in maximal voluntary power; however, some studies show only modest reduction in strength, up to 93% of baseline (108). Other studies have shown functional loss of strength; Chyatte et al. (109) reported difficulty with stair-climbing ability in hemiplegic patients receiving dantrolene sodium for spasticity treatment. For patients with initial marginal strength, dantrolene may cause more obvious weakness and should be used cautiously.

Tizanidine (Zanaflex®)

Tizanadine is a centrally acting antispasticity agent that has been investigated for use in treatment of spasticity related to MS, SCI, stroke, and brain injury. The exact mechanism of action is not clearly understood, but tizanidine's antispastic effects are thought to be due primarily to its central alpha-2 agonist properties, although its ability to bind to the imidazole receptors may also play a role. Upon binding to the alpha-2 receptors, tizanidine prevents the release of the excitatory amino acids glutamate and aspartate presynaptically from spinal interneurons (110). Tizanidine may also enhance the release of the inhibitory neurotransmitter glycine, which may inhibit facilitatory coeruleospinal pathways (111, 112).

Tizanidine is well absorbed after oral administration and reaches peak plasma concentration and effect in 1 to 2 hours. It is a short-acting agent, with a half-life of 2 to 4 hours. Dosing recommendations suggest that tizanidine be given 2 to 3 times daily; however, due to its short half-life, it may be more effective when given in smaller doses at more frequent intervals (4 to 6 times daily) (113, 114). Treatment is initiated at

doses of 2 to 4 mg given initially at night, with gradual titration by 2 to 4 mg every 2 to 4 days, to a maximal daily dose of 36 mg/d, as tolerated and required (6). Tizanidine is metabolized in the liver by cytochrome P450 1A2 (115). It has recently been noted that CYP 1A2 inhibitors (including ciprofloxacin, fluvoxamine, rofecoxib, and certain oral contraceptives) may affect tizanidine kinetics, resulting in increased plasma levels and adverse effects of tizanidine (116–119). There does not appear to be a clinically significant interaction with coadministration of tizanidine with baclofen, (120) and they are frequently prescribed together.

In patients with SCI, tizanidine has been reported to significantly decrease muscle tone as determined on the AS, and with video motion analysis of the pendulum test, spasm frequency was reduced by 50%, and there were no significant decreases in strength noted in patients with SCI receiving tizanidine (50). Similarly, tizanidine has demonstrated efficacy in decreasing muscle tone in individuals with spasticity secondary to MS (121, 122), stroke (123), and acquired brain injury (traumatic brain injury versus stroke) (124), without adversely affecting muscle strength.

The most common side effects associated with tizanidine are dry mouth, drowsiness, and dizziness. Hallucinations have been reported in 3% of patients within the first several weeks of treatment, and elevated liver function tests have been noted in as many as 5% (113). For this reason, liver function tests should be monitored at baseline and at 1, 3, and 6 months after initiation of treatment with tizanidine (6). Because tizanidine is an alpha-2 agonist, some studies have indicated that tizanidine decreases blood pressure and heart rate in animals and humans (112); however, other studies do not support this finding (125, 126). Caution should be exercised when using tizanidine in conjunction with antihypertensive agents.

Tizanidine is available in a tablet or capsule formulation. A difference that the prescribers should be aware of is that while on an empty stomach, the time to peak plasma concentration is equal; however, if taken after a meal, the tablet is absorbed much faster than the capsule. Therefore, if the tablet is taken with food, the patient may experience increased adverse effects, including somnolence (127). In addition, if one opens the capsule, its absorption will be much faster.

Clonidine (Catapres®)

Clonidine is a well-known antihypertensive agent but has also demonstrated efficacy in the treatment of spasticity. Clonidine is a centrally acting agent that similar to tizanidine is an alpha-2 agonist. (Tizanidine has ~1/50th the antihypertensive effect of clonidine.)

Clonidine binds to alpha-2 receptors in the brain, brainstem, and dorsal horn of the spinal cord and is believed to exert its antispasticity effects through enhancement of presynaptic inhibition (128–130). Administration of yohimbine, an alpha-2 antagonist, has been shown to abolish the ability of clonidine to suppress spasticity (131).

Peak plasma concentration of clonidine occurs 3 to 5 hours after oral administration, and half-life is 5 to 19 hours in patients with normal renal function and up to 40 hours in those with impaired renal function. Approximately half of the dose is metabolized in the liver, and the remainder is excreted unchanged in the urine. Clonidine should be initiated at low doses and titrated cautiously to avoid adverse effects. Initial starting dose is 0.05 mg given twice daily; this can be increased to 0.1 mg twice daily after 3 days, then increases of 0.1 mg/d can be made on a weekly basis, with a maximal dosage of 0.4 mg/d (130). Studies have shown that oral clonidine is effective in decreasing spasticity in patients with SCI (128, 132). In addition, some patients were able to decrease baclofen dose requirements with the addition of clonidine to their medical regimen (130). Clonidine is available in a transdermal system (Catapres-TTS), and it is also available for intrathecal use. The transdermal Catapres® patch is available in 0.1 to 0.3 mg doses and is designed to deliver the designated dose of clonidine on a daily basis for 7 days. The transdermal Catapres® patch has demonstrated efficacy in the treatment of spasticity in patients with SCI with minimal side effects (133). Clonidine has also shown improvement in gait patterns (134) and walking speed (135) in patients with incomplete SCI. The most common side effects associated with the use of clonidine are orthostasis, bradycardia, dry mouth, constipation, ankle edema, and drowsiness (85).

Cyproheptadine (Periactin®)

Cyproheptadine is a medication with potent antihistamine activity, as well as antiserotonergic and mild anticholinergic properties. Its antispasticity effects are thought to be due to neutralization of serotonergic excitatory inputs at the spinal and supraspinal levels (136). Cyproheptadine has demonstrated efficacy in the reduction of clonus and spasms in patients with MS and SCI (136) and has also been shown to increase walking speed in individuals with spastic gait secondary to SCI (137, 138). When compared to baclofen and clonidine, cyproheptadine was noted to have efficacy superior to clonidine and similar to baclofen (139). The combined use of clonidine and cyproheptadine was shown to be more beneficial for improvement

of gait than treatment with either medication alone (135, 139, 140). Cyproheptadine can be initiated at doses of 4 mg given at bedtime, with dose increases of 4 mg every 3 to 4 days. The maximum recommended dose is 36 mg/d given in divided doses, although the most common effective dose is 16 to 24 mg/d. (6, 85) Side effects are generally related to the central nervous system depression and the anticholinergic activity of this medication, causing sedation and dry mouth. This medication will stimulate appetite and should be used with caution when weight gain will pose an impediment to activities.

Gabapentin (Neurontin®)

Gabapentin is an antiepileptic medication that is structurally similar to GABA and acts at the neocortex and hippocampus; it does not appear to bind to GABA-A, GABA-B, glycine, glutamate, benzodiazepine, or NMDA receptors (141). Gabapentin reaches peak plasma concentrations within 2 to 3 hours after oral administration. It is excreted unchanged in the urine, and literature has shown that doses up to 3600 mg/d are well tolerated (142), although higher doses are often used clinically when appropriate. In a crossover study by Priebe et al., gabapentin showed efficacy in decreasing spasticity in individuals with SCI, as demonstrated by a surface EMG technique designed to quantify spasticity. Only one individual demonstrated improvement of spasticity at doses of 400 mg 3 times daily; however, 5 subjects displayed reduced spasticity at doses up to 1200 mg 3 times daily in the open-label extension of the study (142). In another crossover study by Gruenthal et al. (143) 25 individuals with SCI received gabapentin at doses of 2400 mg given over 48 hours. These authors reported an 11% reduction in spasticity as measured by the AS and a 20% reduction in patient-reported spasticity severity as measured using a 6-point Likert scale. Gabapentin has also been investigated in a crossover study by Cutter et al. (144) as an antispasticity agent in the MS population. In doses titrated to 900 mg 3 times daily, gabapentin significantly improved spasticity compared to placebo as measured using the MAS and self-reported scales (144). The most common adverse effects associated with the use of gabapentin are somnolence, dizziness, ataxia, tremor, dyspepsia, and constipation (145).

Pregabalin (Lyrica®) is another antiepileptic agent that is used by some practitioners to treat pain associated with SCI and may be useful in the treatment of spasticity. The mechanism of action is not fully understood, but pregabalin is thought to increase GABA levels in the brain. It does not appear to bind to neurotransmitter receptors including GABA, glutamate, acetylcholine, or opiate receptors (146). In a retrospective study evaluating the effects of pregabalin in individuals with spasticity secondary to MS, brain injury, or cerebral palsy, more than half of the patients described positive effects of pregabalin on spasticity; however, one third reported side effects that limited the use of pregabalin (147). Further controlled studies investigating the role of pregabalin in the treatment of spasticity secondary to SCI are needed.

4-Aminopyridine (Fampridine®)

4-Aminopyridine is an agent that has a long history of various applications but most recently has gained interest due to evidence that it may restore neurologic function in individuals with SCI and MS (148). 4-Aminopyridine restores conduction along focally damaged axons by blocking the potassium channels, thereby increasing the safety factor and prolonging the action potential that allows for restoration of conduction across demyelinated internodes (149, 150). It also enhances transmission across spared neuronal tracts (148, 150). 4-Aminopyridine is available in an immediate-release formulation with peak plasma concentrations attained in approximately 1 hour, with half-life of 3.5 hours (148, 151). A sustained-release formulation of 4-aminopyridine (fampridine-SR) has been developed for investigational purposes to allow for less frequent dosing and to decrease side effects from high-peak serum levels that occur with the immediate-release formulation. Pharmacokinetic data from trials of fampridine-SR in patients with MS revealed peak plasma concentration at 5 hours, with mean serum half-life of 5.2 hours (152). Steady-state concentrations of fampridine-SR can be obtained with twice daily dosing after 5 days (153). Adverse events associated with fampridine in doses less than 80 mg/d include dizziness, headache, paresthesias, insomnia, and nausea (154). Seizures have been reported in overdoses with fampridine (150, 154). The immediate-release formulation of 4-aminopyridine can be obtained from compounding pharmacies; however, the sustained release formulation is not available in the United States.

Several small randomized controlled trials have been conducted to investigate the safety and efficacy of the use of fampridine-SR in SCI (155–160). These studies indicate that the use of fampridine may enhance neurologic recovery after SCI, as noted by improvement in motor and sensory function, pulmonary function, and reductions in spasticity, and sexual dysfunction; however, the magnitude of gains noted in most studies was generally small. Phase 2 randomized controlled trials investigating the efficacy of fampridine-SR in individuals with chronic incomplete SCI have been completed. These studies showed benefits including reduction in spasticity as measured by the Ashworth score, as well as improvement in motor and sensory scores and patient satisfaction measures in the groups receiving fampridine-SR (154, 161). In 2004, Acorda therapeutics completed 2 large phase 3 randomized controlled trials evaluating fampridine-SR for the management of spasticity in individuals with chronic SCI. These studies did not reach statistical significance in the primary end point (reduction of spasticity as measured by the AS) in those individuals receiving fampridine-SR (162). However, positive results from phase 3 clinical trials have shown that fampridine-SR can improve walking speed and lower extremity strength in patients with MS and may be on the path for approval (152).

Cannabinoids (Marinol®, Cesamet®)

Although it is not approved for clinical use in the treatment of spasticity secondary to SCI, marijuana (cannabis) is often used by individuals with SCI to prevent or relieve spasticity (60). The active chemical in marijuana, Δ9-tetrahydrocannabinol (THC), was investigated in a double-blind, placebo-controlled trial in individuals with spasticity from central origin, including patients with MS or SCI. Clinical measures of spasticity and EMG activity were noted to be decreased in the study group receiving THC (163). Hagenbach et al. (164) performed a 3-phase study evaluating the effect of treatment with THC on spasticity in patients with SCI. In the initial open-label phases, subjects received either oral or rectal THC in escalating doses. During the third phase, which was a randomized controlled study, subjects received oral THC or placebo. The investigators reported that THC was safe and effective for the treatment of spasticity in doses of 15 to 20 mg/d. There were a relatively high number of dropouts in this study secondary to exacerbation of pain and adverse psychological effects in some subjects with the use of THC (164).

Opiates exhibit potent antispasticity activity (165) by suppressing polysynaptic reflexes to a greater extent than monosynaptic reflexes but are not considered a primary treatment option for SCI-related spasticity.

Intrathecal Baclofen

Intrathecal baclofen may be an option for spasticity management in patients who benefit from oral baclofen but cannot tolerate side effects. Oral baclofen has poor lipid solubility and does not cross the blood-brain barrier well, so relatively high doses are necessary to achieve therapeutic benefit. Unlike oral baclofen, ITB is delivered directly to the central nervous system, thereby avoiding the blood-brain barrier. Therapeutic effects are achieved with ITB using only 1% of the total dose that would be required orally to produce similar effects (166). This allows for delivery of much higher concentrations of baclofen to the intrathecal space at doses that are much lower than required with oral delivery of baclofen, which simultaneously improves spasticity control and reduces side effects. Intrathecal baclofen is FDA-approved for spasticity management in SCI, and in multiple studies, it has been proven efficacious in reducing spasticity, (39, 166) improving sleep (167), decreasing caregiver burden, and improving ADL (168).

Intrathecal baclofen is delivered by an electronic pump and catheter system. The most commonly used pump is an electronic programmable pump. The SynchroMed-EL® and the SynchroMed-II® are 2 programmable pumps that are commonly used for delivery of ITB. The original Synchromed-EL® pump has an 18-mL reservoir, whereas the newer SynchroMed-II® pump has a 40-mL medication reservoir, allowing for less frequent pump refills. Pump refills can be performed in an outpatient setting. The pump reservoir is accessed through a central access port; the medication remaining in the pump reservoir at time of refill is removed, and the new drug is subsequently injected into the reservoir. The pump is reprogrammed with updated information including reservoir volume, drug concentration, dosing regimen, and alarm dates using an external programming device that communicates with the computer chip in the pump via radio-telemetry.

The pump is approximately 8 cm in diameter and is placed subcutaneously or subfascially into the anterior abdominal wall. The catheter is tunneled subcutaneously to the low lumbar area where the catheter tip is subsequently inserted into the spinal canal by paramedian approach at the L1 level and is then threaded to the appropriate level into the subarachnoid space. Historically, the catheter tip has been threaded to the low thoracic or high lumbar area; however, more recently, some clinicians have placed the catheter tip higher in an attempt to influence spasticity in the upper extremities. Positioning of the catheter tip affects the site of action of the medication, as the ITB concentration is highest at the catheter tip and does not tend to diffuse cranially within the spinal canal. Upon injection of baclofen intrathecally at L1, concentrations gradients are 4:1 when comparing the lumbar and cervical regions (169); therefore, control of spasticity is more effective in the LE than the upper extremities. Currently, there is no standard protocol for catheter tip placement; however, Vender et al. (170) report positive outcomes when using their protocol of catheter tip placement between T6–T10 for spastic diplegia, T1-T2 for spastic tetraplegia, and in the mid cervical region for dystonia. Another study reported the importance of catheter tip level (at T6) in obtaining good upper extremity relief of spasticity (171).

Appropriate patient selection is important to avoid complications and maximize benefits of ITB. The patient should be free from any infections and should not have any active pressure ulcers, unless the spasticity is the source of the pressure ulcer (85). In addition, the patient should have good social support and demonstrate compliance with medical recommendations because the patient will be required to return to the clinic approximately every 3 to 6 months for pump refills. Penn et al. (40) propose that appropriate candidates for ITB therapy should have severe spasticity lasting for at least 6 months, with a spasticity rating of at least 3 on the AS or a Penn spasm frequency score of at least 2 during screening. In addition, the patient should have failed or shown intolerance to maximal doses of oral antispasticity agents (172). During the screening trial, a lumbar puncture is performed, and an initial test dose of 50 µg is delivered. Onset of action is 30 to 60 minutes, with peak effect achieved at 4 hours (6). Patient response to the ITB is closely monitored every 2 hours after drug administration through measurements of spasticity using the Modified Ashworth Score, frequency of spasms, and other functional tests including the timed up and go test (173) or other timed walking tests if appropriate. If the patient does not demonstrate an appropriate response to the initial test dose (reduction in objectively measured spasticity, spasm frequency, or improvement in functional tasks), a second test dose of 75 µg may be given 24 hours later. Occasionally, a third test dose of 100 µg is required.

Following implantation of the pump, patients are started on a continuous infusion of ITB. If the patient initially demonstrated improvement in symptoms for greater than 12 hours with the test dose, then the pump is programmed to give that dose over 24 hours; if the effects lasted less than 12 hours, a dose equal to double the initial test dose is used. A maintenance dose is eventually reached with titration of the daily dose in 10% to 20% increments, with increases performed no more often than every 24 hours. Normally, dosing ranges from 200 to 1000 µg per day but can be as high as 1500 µg in some patients (174), and a dosing plateau is usually reached by 6 months postimplantation (85). More complex programmable dosing schedules may be used in patients with specific needs, such as bolus dosing to better control spasticity at certain times of the day to assist with sleep or functional activities. If patients are noted to require continually escalating doses of ITB and are not showing improvement in spasticity, one must consider possible device malfunction.

Complications from ITB can include hypotonia, headaches, dizziness, sedation, seizures, and weakness; (6) these adverse effects can usually be reversed by decreasing the total daily dose of ITB by 10% to 20%. Intrathecal baclofen can also impair sexual function (in males and females), including affecting erection and ejaculation in some patients. Clinicians should be aware of this risk and inform patients of this possibility. This effect is reversible (175, 176). In cases of ITB overdose, patients should be admitted to the hospital for supportive measures, as reversible coma and respiratory depression may occur (85). Physostigmine has been used in overdose with ITB (177); however, this should be considered with caution because it may induce cardiac arrythmias and seizures.

Complications may also arise due to withdrawal from ITB due to failure of drug delivery. Symptoms may include seizures, auditory and visual hallucinations, dyskinesia, rebound spasticity, hyperthermia, and death (178). Intrathecal baclofen withdrawal can occur if the patient fails to return for pump refills, or it may be a result of device malfunction, including pump or catheter failure. Plassat et al. (179) reported that 63% of patients receiving ITB had at least one episode of pump malfunction, of which 90% required surgical intervention, whereas Gooch et al. (180) reported a complication rate of 24% in the pediatric population, most commonly as a result of proximal catheter disconnection (9%) or dislodgement from the intrathecal space (8%). In cases of baclofen withdrawal due to device failure, symptoms usually present over a course of 1 to 3 days. Multiple regimens have been presented for treatment and include oral baclofen and benzodiazepines, as well as other medications such as propranolol, cyproheptadine, dantrolene, and opiates in addition to supportive care. Oral baclofen dosage is typically 10 to 30 mg, given every 4 to 8 hours, and improvement may not be seen for several hours after administration. Intravenous benzodiazepines (or even intramuscular) can also be given. Alternatively, a lumbar puncture may be performed with direct administration of a bolus dose of baclofen into the intrathecal space. After initiation of ITB, symptoms should resolve within 30 minutes, with maximal benefit in 4 to 6 hours. When withdrawal is associated with severe hyperthermia, dantrolene is recommended (181).

Other medications may be given intrathecally for the management of spasticity. Intrathecal clonidine may also be effective either alone (182) or in combination with baclofen (183), although this is not FDA-approved.

Chemoneurolysis

Several options are available for management of focal spasticity with chemical neurolysis. Diagnostic and therapeutic peripheral nerve blocks can be performed using anesthetic agents or alcohol and phenol. Other potential options for treatment of focal spasticity include botulinum toxin injections into spastic muscle, as well as motor point blocks. These injections techniques should be utilized when focal management of spasticity will allow improvement in functional tasks, decrease pain, prevent or delay musculoskeletal complications, reduce disfigurement, or ease caregiver burden.

Peripheral Nerve Blocks

Temporary peripheral nerve blocks can be performed using anesthetic agents such as lidocaine or bupivicaine, whereas phenol and alcohol are utilized for more permanent nerve blocks. Temporary nerve blocks can help delineate which muscles are most involved in the spastic positioning, differentiate between severe spasticity and contracture, and can also help determine if a more permanent nerve block will potentially help to meet treatment goals (6). Target nerves are localized using landmarks and electrical stimulation. When using electrical stimulation for nerve localization, the injector attempts to elicit a marked clinical contraction of the muscles innervated by the target nerve with decreasing level of current. The goal is to produce a maximal muscle contraction with 1.0 mA or less of current being used; this indicates that the tip of the monopolar needle electrode is situated near the target nerve. Specific landmarks and descriptions of techniques used for various peripheral nerve injections are discussed elsewhere (184). When performing temporary diagnostic nerve blocks, the injector may use 1 to 5 mL of 0.5% to 2% lidocaine, which has onset of action within 3 minutes and can last up to 2 hours. An alternative anesthetic agent that is often used is 1 to 5 mL of 0.25% to 0.5% bupivicaine, which may last up to 7 hours (6).

Therapeutic nerve blocks can be accomplished using longer-acting agents, such as alcohol or phenol. The same injection technique is used as described above. The use of phenol in concentrations as low as 2% has been shown to damage the microcirculation around peripheral nerves, whereas higher concentrations of phenol (5% phenol in saline) cause protein denaturation and coagulation of peripheral nerves at the site of injection (185). Dilutions of 5% to 7% phenol are most frequently used for chemoneurolysis in volumes up to 10 cc per nerve. In the weeks after the perineural injection of phenol, Wallerian degeneration occurs; however, axonal regrowth eventually occurs. It is for this reason that the effects of chemoneurolysis with phenol are not permanent, and typically, the results last approximately 6 months (184). The maximum dose of 5% phenol is 20 mL (1 g/d) (6). Side effects associated with the use of phenol include painful paresthesias and dysesthesias, which may occur in 10% to 32% of patients (186–188). The risk for development of these symptoms appears higher with sensorimotor blocks than with pure motor blocks. Symptom onset is usually within days to weeks of injection and may last for several weeks or longer (189). These painful dysesthesias and paresthesias are likely due to incomplete block or axonal regrowth of sensory nerves. Treatment options include desensitization techniques, compressive garments, antidepressants, or membrane-stabilizing anticonvulsant agents (184). Repeat nerve block may also be an effective way to treat these symptoms, as has been described by Petrillo et al. (190) If this is not effective, surgical neurolysis is an option (191).

Ethyl alcohol has been used in the treatment of spasticity since the early 1900s (184) and has been used in individuals with spasticity secondary to cerebral palsy, MS, multifocal leukoencephalopathy, and SCI (192). Ethyl alcohol may be used (usually in concentrations of 40% to 49%) at doses of 2 to 5 mL per site (6). Currently, its use is limited in the United States despite the fact that it appears to be a relatively safe, effective means for treatment of spasticity. There have been few reports of adverse events associated with the use of ethyl alcohol, especially in comparison to phenol. It is unclear whether this is due to a safer side effect profile associated with the use of alcohol or just due to more frequent use of phenol (189). Complications associated with the use of alcohol include skin ulceration at sites of superficial injections, paresthesias, vascular phlebitis, and vasovagal attacks (193, 194).

Motor Point Blocks

Motor point blocks are another option for the management of focal spasticity. With this technique, phenol or alcohol solutions are injected using electrical stimulation guidance to localize the greatest concentration of motor end plates within the target muscle

(6). The technique is similar to that described above for peripheral nerve injections; however, different landmarks are utilized to localize the motor. This is followed by needle localization using electrical stimulation guidance. A smaller quantity of phenol or alcohol is used for motor point blocks in comparison to nerve blocks, typically 0.5 to 1.5 mL per site (6). Potential complications include phlebitis, muscle necrosis, nerve palsy, and systemic effects (189). Therapeutic effects can last from 3 to 8 months (6).

Botulinum Toxin Injections

Botulinum toxin injections are another therapeutic intervention that clinicians have available for the treatment of focal spasticity in individuals with SCI. Botulinum toxin was initially introduced for clinical use in the 1980s, at which time it was used in the treatment of strabismus (195). Botulinum toxin has since gained wider use in the management of other disorders including dystonias and spasticity secondary to the ease of use and the effectiveness of this treatment, although the use of botulinum toxin in the treatment of spasticity is not FDA-approved.

Seven serotypes of the potent botulinum toxin produced by the bacterium *Clostridium botulinum* have been identified (A through G). The toxin is comprised of light and heavy chains that are joined by a disulfide bond. Botulinum toxin ultimately inhibits muscular contraction by blocking the release of acetylcholine from presynaptic nerve terminals into the neuromuscular junction, thereby uncoupling excitation contraction. Botulinum toxin's paralytic effects are dependent on a 3-step process, including internalization of the toxin, molecule cleavage, and inhibition of neurotransmitter release. The intact botulinum toxin molecule is initially taken up into the nerve terminal by receptor-mediated endocytosis (196). After internalization, the disulfide bond is cleaved, allowing separation of the light and heavy chains; the light chain subsequently interrupts the binding of synaptosomal vesicles, preventing the release of acetylcholine from the nerve terminal. Vesicles containing acetylcholine normally bind to the inner membrane of the nerve terminal with the assistance of a complex of docking proteins including synaptosomal-associated protein (SNAP-25), vesicle-associated membrane protein, and syntaxin. Botulinum toxins A and E cleave SNAP-25; botulinum toxins B, D, F, and G have been noted to cleave vesicle-associated membrane protein; and botulinum toxin C cleaves syntaxin and SNAP-25 (197, 198). Although the mechanism of action differs for each of these serotypes, they all prevent the docking and fusion of the synaptic vesicles containing acetylcholine to the nerve membrane, thereby inhibiting the release of acetylcholine from the nerve terminal.

OnabotulinumtoxinA (Botox®), abobotulinumtoxinA (Dysport®), and rimabotulinumtoxinB (Myobloc®) are the only serotypes that are available for clinical use. AbobotulinumtoxinA has recently been approved by the FDA and will soon be available for clinical use in the United States. OnabotulinumtoxinA is currently FDA-approved for the treatment of blepharospasm, strabismus, cervical dystonia, axillary hyperhydrosis, and glabeller lines. RimabotulinumtoxinB is approved for the treatment of cervical dystonia. There is typically a 24- to 72-hour delay between injection of the botulinum toxin into spastic muscles and onset of clinical effect, although some individuals report immediate benefits. Peak action is noted at 2 to 6 weeks, and clinical effects last for approximately 3 to 5 months (6). Basic science and clinical studies indicate that the duration of action is slightly longer for onabotulinumtoxinA than rimabotulinumtoxinB (14 vs 12 weeks) (199). The use of rimabotulinumtoxinB may potentially result in a higher incidence of antibody-mediated nonresponsiveness to botulinum toxin, as indicated by several studies using onabotulinumtoxinA and rimabotulinumtoxinB in the treatment of cervical dystoni (199). There are also more anticholinergic side effects noted with rimabotulinumtoxinB. Long-term exposure to the botulinum toxin results in reversible denervation atrophy, with reinnervation occurring through noncollateral sprouting (196).

OnabotulinumtoxinA is available in 100-U vials that must be kept frozen until used. The onabotulinumtoxinA is reconstituted by injecting sterile preservative-free normal saline into the vial, which is then gently swirled rather than shaken to prevent protein denaturation (201). No study in SCI has definitively determined if there is a benefit to higher versus lower dilutions; however, there is some evidence that high-volume dilution (20 U/mL) may be superior to lower-volume dilutions (100 U/mL) in management of spasticity in the biceps brachii (202). Once onabotulinumtoxinA is reconstituted, it should be used within 24 hours. RimabotulinumtoxinB is available in an injectable solution and does not require reconstitution. It is available in vials containing dosage of 2500, 5000, and 10,000 U. The maximum dose of onabotulinumtoxinA used per patient per injection session varies among clinicians; however, most feel that it is safe and efficacious to use doses as high as 400 to 600 U per session, with some individuals using as much as 1200 U per session (203). There is however a potentially higher risk of the development of antibody-mediated resistance to the botulinum toxin due to the higher protein load. The maximum recommended dose of onabotulinumtoxinA per injection site is 50 U, 200 U for abobotulinumtoxinA, or 2500 U of rimabotulinumtoxinB, although the total dose recommended per muscle group varies depending on the size of the muscle. The maximum dose recommendations for Dysport® and Myobloc® are 1500 and 10,000 U per session, respectively (Table 21.6) (203).

There are several techniques that are commonly used for injection of botulinum toxin into spastic muscles, including utilization of anatomic landmarks, electrical stimulation, and EMG guidance. More recently, ultrasound guidance for localization for spasticity management has been suggested as being a superior way to identify sites for injection (204). Botulinum toxin has a great propensity to seek the neuromuscular junction, and placing the toxin as near as practical to them may achieve better results. This may possibly allow a smaller dose to achieve the same clinical outcome (205). The use of EMG guidance or electrical stimulation may not be necessary for large, easily isolated muscles (although recommended); however, it is preferable to use these methods for localizing smaller, deep muscles. Muscles that are commonly injected with the assistance of EMG guidance include the wrist and finger flexors and extensors, hand intrinsics, hip flexors, and lower leg muscles including posterior tibialis and extensor hallucis longus (206). When using EMG guidance for localization, a hollow Teflon-coated EMG needle with a port for syringe attachment is used. The goal is to position the needle tip near the motor end plate to produce the most effective results. If the injection is positioned 0.5 cm away from the motor endplate, there may be as much as a 50% decrease in the paralysis of the target muscle (207). With the use of EMG guidance, the clinician should note either crisp sounding motor unit potential on auditory evaluation or motor unit potentials with a sharp rise time (<500 microseconds) on visual analysis. The accurate localization of the motor end plate may decrease the required dose of botulinum toxin, helping to control cost as well as decreasing the potential for development of antibody-mediated nonresponsiveness to the botulinum toxin, which may be associated with repetitive injections in high doses (205). Motor point stimulation using electrical stimulation can also be useful for botulinum toxin administration but is typically more time-consuming than EMG guidance. This technique is also performed using a Teflon-coated needle as described for the EMG guidance procedure. The needle is inserted into the target muscle, and an electrical stimulus is delivered in an attempt to produce a muscular contraction in the target muscle. The injector will attempt to continue

TABLE 21.6
Botulinum Toxin Dosing Guidelines

Muscle	OnabotulinumtoxinA Dose (u)	AbobotulinumtoxinA Dose (u)	RimabotulinumtoxinB Dose (u)
Pectoralis	75–150		2500–5000
Biceps	50–200	100–400	2500–5000
Triceps	50–200		
Flexor carpi radialis	25–100	150	1000–3000
Flexor carpi ulnaris	20–70	100–150	1000–3000
Flexor digitorum superficialis	20–60	150–300	1000–3000
Flexor digitorum profundus	20–60	150–200	1000–3000
Hip adductors	200–400	500–1000	5000–10,000
Quadriceps	50–200		5000–7500
Gastrocnemius	50–250	250–1000	3000–7500
Posterior tibialis	50–150	200–500	3000–7500
Anterior tibialis	50–150		2500–5000

Dosing table summarized from Francisco GE. Botulinum toxin: dosing and dilution. *Am J Phys Med Rehabil.* 2004;83:S30–S37 and www.mdvu.org; Gracies JM. Impact of botulinum toxin type A (BTX-A) dilution and ENdplate targeting technique in upper limb spasticity. *Ann Neurol* 2002;52:S87; Chambers FG, Koshy SS, Saidi RF, Clark DP, Moore RD, Sears CL. Bacteroides fragilis toxin exhibits polar activity on monolayers of human intestinal epithelial cells (T84 cells) in vitro. *Infect Immun* 1997;65:3561–70.

to elicit the desired muscular contraction using sequentially lower levels of current with the electrical stimulation device, with the ultimate goal being elicitation of muscular contraction using 1.0 mA or less of current; this indicates that the tip of the needle is situated near the target motor point. This is particularly useful for muscles like the flexor digitiorum profundus and extensor digitorum communis, which are organized in similar fascicles supplying each digit. Correct placement of the needle can allow a more accurate result (205).

Botulinum toxin has been shown to be effective in the treatment of focal spasticity in the upper and LE resulting from diverse etiologies, including stroke, trauma, and MS by reducing muscle tone and improving function (208). Although there are no randomized controlled trials evaluating the efficacy of botulinum toxin injections in the treatment of spasticity secondary to SCI, Marciniak et al. (209) published a retrospective study addressing this issue. These investigators reviewed the charts of 28 patients receiving their first injections of botulinum toxin type A for spasticity management, and they found improvement in upper extremity function, hygiene, and pain after botulinum toxin type A injections in individuals with spasticity secondary to SCI (209). The effectiveness of botulinum toxin injections may be enhanced with the use of adjunct therapeutic techniques after injection, including gait training, stretching, positioning, and use of modalities such as taping, serial casting, and electrical stimulation (203, 205, 210). Botulinum toxin injections have also shown benefit before serial casting in relieving the spasticity and pain (221). Botulinum toxin injections have also been investigated for the management of detrusor overactivity due to various disease processes including MS, stroke, Parkinson disease, and SCI. Results from a systematic review suggest that botulinum toxin injections may be an effective treatment option for neurogenic bladder in individuals with SCI or MS (212).

The use of botulinum toxin is contraindicated in patients who have neuromuscular disorders, are taking aminoglycoside antibiotics, or are pregnant or lactating. Botulinum toxin injections are well tolerated, although some patients may experience discomfort at the injection site, including bruising and hematoma formation. Other reported side effects include weakness of nontarget muscles due to toxin spread or inadvertent injection of nontarget muscles, generalized weakness, flu-like symptoms, and dysphagia (213). Dysphagia most commonly occurs after the treatment of cervical dystonia due to spread of toxin from injection sites in the sternocleidomastoid, scalene, or other anterior neck muscles (214, 215); however, onset of dysphagia after botulinum toxin injections into the extremities has also been reported (216).

Surgical Interventions

Surgical interventions for the control of spasticity may be necessary in some individuals with SCI who have failed other less invasive measures. The goal of the various surgical procedures is to decrease spasms and spasticity without having a detrimental effect on the patient's motor, sensory, or bowel and bladder function. Neurotomies may be performed in the peripheral nervous system to obtain more permanent results than what can be accomplished with phenol or alcohol nerve blocks. During this surgical procedure, the target nerve is selectively exposed and transected. Obturator neurotomy for adductor spasticity is the most common of these procedures to be performed; however, neurotomy of the tibial nerve for foot spasticity and selective neurotomy of the sciatic branches for knee flexor spasms have been described (217). Neurotomies may be combined with tendon-lengthening procedures (218).

Ventral (anterior) and dorsal (posterior) root rhizotomies have been described for spasticity management. In these procedures, the nerve rootlets are severed as they enter the spinal cord. Anterior rhizotomies have been performed in individuals with complete SCI; this procedure abolishes voluntary and involuntary movement in the muscles innervated by the ablated nerve rootlets. Anterior rhizotomies may provide complete resolution of spasticity; however, side effects include muscle atrophy and flaccidity, making this procedure less popular at present (217). Dorsal rhizotomy involves sectioning of the dorsal rootlets as they enter the spinal cord. Sectioning of these roots disrupts the afferent limb of the reflex arc, resulting in decreased spasticity without adversely affecting muscle bulk. Sensory function may be diminished depending on the extent of rootlet ablation (217). Bowel and bladder reflexes usually are not altered, as long as rootlets at or below S1 are not sectioned. Selective dorsal rhizotomy may provide similar results with less risk of hypoesthesia. During this procedure, individual rootlets are stimulated to evaluate for an abnormal EMG response with stimulation; if so, an abnormal response is noted, the nerve root is cut. Usually 25% to 50% of the tested rootlets are cut. Sensory deficit is usually limited due to the selective nature of this procedure and the overlapping innervation within adjacent dermatomes (219, 220).

CONCLUSION

Spasticity is a very common condition resulting from SCI that can have an adverse effect on some individuals resulting in pain and impaired functional status and may have a negative impact on overall QOL. It is important to recognize spasticity clinically, but it is also important to appreciate that a significant number of individuals with SCI who experience painful spasms and spasticity may not always demonstrate measurable increases in tone on physical examination. As described above, there are a variety of treatment options available; before initiation of treatment, it is important to establish realistic goals with the patient. Therapeutic interventions should begin with the least invasive options and progress to pharmacologic and invasive interventions only when necessary.

References

1. Lance JW. The control of muscle tone, reflexes, and movement: Robert Wartenberg lecture. *Neurology* 1980;30: 1303–13.
2. Decq P. [Pathophysiology of spasticity]. *Neurochirurgie* 2003;49:163–84.
3. Benz EN, Hornby TG, Bode RK, Scheidt RA, Schmit BD. A physiologically based clinical measure for spastic reflexes in spinal cord injury. *Arch Phys Med Rehabil* 2005;86: 52–9.
4. Pandyan AD, Gregoric M, Barnes MP, et al. Spasticity: clinical perceptions, neurological realities and meaningful measurement. *Disabil Rehabil* 2005;27:2–6.
5. Hsieh JT, Wolfe DL, Miller WC, Curt A. Spasticity outcome measures in spinal cord injury: psychometric properties and clinical utility. *Spinal Cord* 2008;46:86–95.
6. Kirshblum S. Treatment alternatives for spinal cord injury related spasticity. *J Spinal Cord Med* 1999;22:199–217.
7. Maynard FM, Karunas RS, Waring WP, 3rd. Epidemiology of spasticity following traumatic spinal cord injury. *Arch Phys Med Rehabil* 1990;71:566–9.
8. Levi R, Hultling C, Seiger A. The Stockholm spinal cord injury study: 2. Associations between clinical patient characteristics and post-acute medical problems. *Paraplegia* 1995;33:585–94.
9. Little JW, Micklesen P, Umlauf R, Britell C. Lower extremity manifestations of spasticity in chronic spinal cord injury. *Am J Phys Med Rehabil* 1989;68:32–6.
10. Skold C, Levi R, Seiger A. Spasticity after traumatic spinal cord injury: nature, severity, and location. *Arch Phys Med Rehabil* 1999;80:1548–57.
11. Smyth MD, Peacock WJ. The surgical treatment of spasticity. *Muscle Nerve* 2000;23:153–63.
12. Nielsen JB, Crone C, Hultborn H. The spinal pathophysiology of spasticity—from a basic science point of view. *Acta Physiol (Oxf)* 2007;189:171–80.
13. Foran JR, Steinman S, Barash I, Chambers IIG, Lieber RL. Structural and mechanical alterations in spastic skeletal muscle. *Dev Med Child Neurol* 2005;47:713–7.
14. Myklebust BM, Gottlieb GL, Penn RD, Agarwal GC. Reciprocal excitation of antagonistic muscles as a differentiating feature in spasticity. *Ann Neurol* 1982;12:367–74.
15. Katz R, Pierrot-Deseilligny E. Recurrent inhibition in humans. *Prog Neurobiol* 1999;57:325–55.
16. Shefner JM, Berman SA, Sarkarati M, Young RR. Recurrent inhibition is increased in patients with spinal cord injury. *Neurology* 1992;42:2162–8.
17. Ivanhoe CB, Reistetter TA. Spasticity: the misunderstood part of the upper motor neuron syndrome. *Am J Phys Med Rehabil* 2004;83:S3–9.
18. Oertel WH. Distribution of synaptic transmitters in motor centers with reference to spasticity. In: Emre M, Benecke R, eds. *Spasticity: the current status of research and treatment* Park Ridge, NJ: Parthenon Publishing Group; 1989.
19. Gracies JM. Pathophysiology of spastic paresis. II: emergence of muscle overactivity. *Muscle Nerve* 2005;31:552–71.

20. Delwaide PJ, Oliver E. Short-latency autogenic inhibition (IB inhibition) in human spasticity. *J Neurol Neurosurg Psychiatry* 1988;51:1546–50.

21. Downes L, Ashby P, Bugaresti J. Reflex effects from Golgi tendon organ (Ib) afferents are unchanged after spinal cord lesions in humans. *Neurology* 1995;45:1720–4.

22. Young RR. Physiology and pharmacology of spasticity. In: Gelber DA, Jeffrey DR, eds. Clinical evaluation and management of spasticity. Totowa, N.J.: *Humana Press*; 2002: 3–12.

23. Ditunno JF, Little JW, Tessler A, Burns AS. Spinal shock revisited: a four-phase model. *Spinal Cord* 2004;42:383–95.

24. Murray M, Goldberger ME. Restitution of function and collateral sprouting in the cat spinal cord: the partially hemisected animal. *J Comp Neurol* 1974;158:19–36.

25. Little JW, Ditunno JF, Jr., Stiens SA, Harris RM. Incomplete spinal cord injury: neuronal mechanisms of motor recovery and hyperreflexia. *Arch Phys Med Rehabil* 1999;80:587–99.

26. Dietz V, Sinkjaer T. Spastic movement disorder: impaired reflex function and altered muscle mechanics. *Lancet Neurol* 2007;6:725–33.

27. Kamper DG, Schmit BD, Rymer WZ. Effect of muscle biomechanics on the quantification of spasticity. *Ann Biomed Eng* 2001; 29(12):1122–1134.

28. Pierson SH. Outcome measures in spasticity management. *Muscle Nerve Suppl* 1997;6:S36–60.

29. Platz T, Eickhof C, Nuyens G, Vuadens P. Clinical scales for the assessment of spasticity, associated phenomena, and function: a systematic review of the literature. *Disabil Rehabil* 2005;27:7–18.

30. Voerman GE, Gregoric M, Hermens HJ. Neurophysiological methods for the assessment of spasticity: the Hoffmann reflex, the tendon reflex, and the stretch reflex. *Disabil Rehabil* 2005;27:33–68.

31. Wood DE, Burridge JH, van Wijck FM, et al. Biomechanical approaches applied to the lower and upper limb for the measurement of spasticity: a systematic review of the literature. *Disabil Rehabil* 2005;27:19–32.

32. SCIRE Team. SCIRE: Spinal Cord Injury Rehabilitation Evidence 2006. (Accessed 1/10/09, 2009, at http://www.icord. org/scire/.)

33. Ashworth B. Preliminary trial of carisoprodol in multiple sclerosis. *Practitioner* 1964;192:540–2.

34. Bohannon RW, Smith MB. Interrater reliability of a Modified Ashworth Scale of muscle spasticity. *Phys Ther* 1987;67: 206–7.

35. Lance JW. Disordered muscle tone and movement. *Clin Exp Neurol* 1981;18:27–35.

36. Pandyan AD, Johnson GR, Price CI, Curless RH, Barnes MP, Rodgers H. A review of the properties and limitations of the Ashworth and Modified Ashworth Scales as measures of spasticity. *Clin Rehabil* 1999;13:373–83.

37. Skold C. Spasticity in spinal cord injury: self- and clinically rated intrinsic fluctuations and intervention-induced changes. *Arch Phys Med Rehabil* 2000;81:144–9.

38. Haas BM, Bergstrom E, Jamous A, Bennie A. The inter rater reliability of the original and of the Modified Ashworth Scale for the assessment of spasticity in patients with spinal cord injury. *Spinal Cord* 1996;34:560–4.

39. Lechner HE, Frotzler A, Eser P. Relationship between self- and clinically rated spasticity in spinal cord injury. *Arch Phys Med Rehabil* 2006;87:15–9.

40. Penn RD, Savoy SM, Corcos D, et al. Intrathecal baclofen for severe spinal spasticity. *N Engl J Med* 1989;320:1517–21.

41. Priebe MM, Sherwood AM, Thornby JI, Kharas NF, Markowski J. Clinical assessment of spasticity in spinal cord injury: a multidimensional problem. *Arch Phys Med Rehabil* 1996;77:713–6.

42. Snow BJ, Tsui JK, Bhatt MH, Varelas M, Hashimoto SA, Calne DB. Treatment of spasticity with botulinum toxin: a double-blind study. *Ann Neurol* 1990;28:512–5.

43. Adams MM, Ginis KA, Hicks AL. The spinal cord injury spasticity evaluation tool: development and evaluation. *Arch Phys Med Rehabil* 2007;88:1185–92.

44. Cook KF, Teal CR, Engebretson JC, et al. Development and validation of Patient Reported Impact of Spasticity Measure (PRISM). *J Rehabil Res Dev* 2007;44:363–72.

45. Perell K, Scremin A, Scremin O, Kunkel C. Quantifying muscle tone in spinal cord injury patients using isokinetic dynamometric techniques. *Paraplegia* 1996;34:46–53.

46. Bohannon RW. Variability and reliability of the pendulum test for spasticity using a Cybex II isokinetic dynamometer. *Phys Ther* 1987;67:659–61.

47. Wartenberg R. Pendulousness of the legs as a diagnostic test. *Neurology* 1951;1:18–24.

48. Firoozbakhsh KK, Kunkel CF, Scremin AM, Moneim MS. Isokinetic dynamometric technique for spasticity assessment. *Am J Phys Med Rehabil* 1993;72:379–85.

49. Bajd T, Vodovnik L. Pendulum testing of spasticity. *J Biomed Eng* 1984;6:9–16.

50. Biering-Sorensen F, Nielsen JB, Klinge K. Spasticity-assessment: a review. *Spinal Cord* 2006;44:708–22.

51. Nance PW, Bugaresti J, Shellenberger K, Sheremata W, Martinez-Arizala A. Efficacy and safety of tizanidine in the treatment of spasticity in patients with spinal cord injury. North American Tizanidine Study Group. *Neurology* 1994;44: S44–51; discussion S-2.

52. Dumitru D, Zwarts M. Special nerve conduction techniques. In: Dumitru D, Amato A, Zwarts M, eds. *Electrodiagnostic medicine*. Philadelphia: Hanley & Belfus, INC.; 2002:225–56.

53. Katz RT, Rymer WZ. Spastic hypertonia: mechanisms and measurement. *Arch Phys Med Rehabil* 1989;70:144–55.

54. Schindler-Ivens SM, Shields RK. Soleus H-reflex recruitment is not altered in persons with chronic spinal cord injury. *Arch Phys Med Rehabil* 2004;85:840–7.

55. Shemesh Y, Rozin R, Ohry A. Electrodiagnostic investigation of motor neuron and spinal reflex arch (H-reflex) in spinal cord injury. *Paraplegia* 1977;15:238–44.

56. Little JW, Halar EM. H-reflex changes following spinal cord injury. *Arch Phys Med Rehabil* 1985;66:19–22.

57. Skold C, Harms-Ringdahl K, Hultling C, Levi R, Seiger A. Simultaneous Ashworth measurements and electromyographic recordings in tetraplegic patients. *Arch Phys Med Rehabil* 1998;79:959–65.

58. Priebe M. Assessment of spinal cord injury spasticity in clinical trials. *Top Spinal Cord Inj Rehabil* 2006;11:69–77.

59. Lundqvist C, Siosteen A, Blomstrand C, Lind B, Sullivan M. Spinal cord injuries. Clinical, functional, and emotional status. *Spine* 1991;16:78–83.

60. Mahoney JS, Engebretson JC, Cook KF, Hart KA, Robinson-Whelen S, Sherwood AM. Spasticity experience domains in persons with spinal cord injury. *Arch Phys Med Rehabil* 2007;88:287–94.

61. Gorgey AS, Dudley GA. Spasticity may defend skeletal muscle size and composition after incomplete spinal cord injury. *Spinal Cord* 2008;46:96–102.

62. Satkunam LE. Rehabilitation medicine: 3. Management of adult spasticity. *CMAJ* 2003;169:1173–9.

63. Merritt JL. Management of spasticity in spinal cord injury. *Mayo Clin Proc* 1981;56:614–22.

64. Stolp-Smith KA, Wainberg MC. Antidepressant exacerbation of spasticity. *Arch Phys Med Rehabil* 1999;80:339–42.

65. Schurch B, Wichmann W, Rossier AB. Post-traumatic syringomyelia (cystic myelopathy): a prospective study of 449 patients with spinal cord injury. *J Neurol Neurosurg Psychiatry* 1996;60:61–7.

66. Odeen I. Reduction of muscular hypertonus by long-term muscle stretch. *Scand J Rehabil Med* 1981;13:93–9.

67. Bovend'Eerdt TJ, Newman M, Barker K, Dawes H, Minelli C, Wade DT. The effects of stretching in spasticity: a systematic review. *Arch Phys Med Rehabil* 2008;89:1395–406.

68. Kunkel CF, Scremin AM, Eisenberg B, Garcia JF, Roberts S, Martinez S. Effect of "standing" on spasticity, contracture, and osteoporosis in paralyzed males. *Arch Phys Med Rehabil* 1993;74:73–8.

69. Bohannon RW. Tilt table standing for reducing spasticity after spinal cord injury. *Arch Phys Med Rehabil* 1993;74:1121–2.

70. Gracies JM. Physical modalities other than stretch in spastic hypertonia. *Phys Med Rehabil Clin N Am* 2001;12:769–92, vi.

71. Melzack R, Wall PD. Pain mechanisms: a new theory. *Science* 1965;150:971–9.

72. Bajd T, Gregoric M, Vodovnik L, Benko H. Electrical stimulation in treating spasticity resulting from spinal cord injury. *Arch Phys Med Rehabil* 1985;66:515–7.

73. Goulet C, Arsenault AB, Bourbonnais D, Laramee MT, Lepage Y. Effects of transcutaneous electrical nerve stimulation on H-reflex and spinal spasticity. *Scand J Rehabil Med* 1996;28:169–76.

74. Joodaki MR, Olyaei GR, Bagheri H. The effects of electrical nerve stimulation of the lower extremity on H-reflex and F-wave parameters. *Electromyogr Clin Neurophysiol* 2001;41:23–8.

75. Potisk KP, Gregoric M, Vodovnik L. Effects of transcutaneous electrical nerve stimulation (TENS) on spasticity in patients with hemiplegia. *Scand J Rehabil Med* 1995;27:169–74.

76. Wang RY, Chan RC, Tsai MW. Effects of thoraco-lumbar electric sensory stimulation on knee extensor spasticity of persons who survived cerebrovascular accident (CVA). *J Rehabil Res Dev* 2000;37:73–9.

77. Creasey GH, Ho CH, Triolo RJ, et al. Clinical applications of electrical stimulation after spinal cord injury. *J Spinal Cord Med* 2004;27:365–75.

78. Krause P, Szecsi J, Straube A. Changes in spastic muscle tone increase in patients with spinal cord injury using functional electrical stimulation and passive leg movements. *Clin Rehabil* 2008;22:627–34.

79. Halstead LS, Seager SW, Houston JM, Whitesell K, Dennis M, Nance PW. Relief of spasticity in SCI men and women using rectal probe electrostimulation. *Paraplegia* 1993;31:715–21.

80. Alaca R, Goktepe AS, Yildiz N, Yilmaz B, Gunduz S. Effect of penile vibratory stimulation on spasticity in men with spinal cord injury. *Am J Phys Med Rehabil* 2005;84:875–9.

81. Nash B, Roller JM, Parker MG. The effects of tone-reducing orthotics on walking of an individual after incomplete spinal cord injury. *J Neurol Phys Ther* 2008;32:39–47.

82. Lechner HE, Feldhaus S, Gudmundsen L, et al. The short-term effect of hippotherapy on spasticity in patients with spinal cord injury. *Spinal Cord* 2003;41:502–5.

83. Paola FA, Arnold M. Acupuncture and spinal cord medicine. *J Spinal Cord Med* 2003;26:12–20.

84. Kesiktas N, Paker N, Erdogan N, Gulsen G, Bicki D, Yilmaz H. The use of hydrotherapy for the management of spasticity. *Neurorehabil Neural Repair* 2004;18:268–73.

85. Gracies JM, Nance P, Elovic E, McGuire J, Simpson DM. Traditional pharmacological treatments for spasticity. Part II: general and regional treatments. *Muscle Nerve Suppl* 1997;6: S92–120.

86. Taricco M, Pagliacci MC, Telaro E, Adone R. Pharmacological interventions for spasticity following spinal cord injury: results of a Cochrane systematic review. *Eura Medicophys* 2006;42:5–15.

87. Davidoff RA. Antispasticity drugs: mechanisms of action. *Ann Neurol* 1985;17:107–16.

88. Kirkland LR. Baclofen dosage: a suggestion. *Arch Phys Med Rehabil* 1984;65:214.

89. Aisen ML, Dietz MA, Rossi P, Cedarbaum JM, Kutt H. Clinical and pharmacokinetic aspects of high dose oral baclofen therapy. *J Am Paraplegia Soc* 1992;15:211–6.

90. Dario A, Tomei G. A benefit-risk assessment of baclofen in severe spinal spasticity. *Drug Saf* 2004;27:799–818.

91. Hinderer SR. The supraspinal anxiolytic effect of baclofen for spasticity reduction. *Am J Phys Med Rehabil* 1990;69:254–8.

92. Breslow MF, Fankhauser MP, Potter RL, Meredith KE, Misiaszek J, Hope DG, Jr. Role of gamma-aminobutyric acid in antipanic drug efficacy. *Am J Psychiatry* 1989;146:353–6.

93. Gulmann NC, Bahr B, Andersen B, Eliassen HM. A double-blind trial of baclofen against placebo in the treatment of schizophrenia. *Acta Psychiatr Scand* 1976;54:287–93.

94. From A, Heltberg A. A double-blind trial with baclofen (Lioresal) and diazepam in spasticity due to multiple sclerosis. *Acta Neurol Scand* 1975;51:158–66.

95. Tseng TC, Wang SC. Locus of action of centrally acting muscle relaxants, diazepam and tybamate. *J Pharmacol Exp Ther* 1971;178:350–60.

96. Cook JB, Nathan PW. On the site of action of diazepam in spasticity in man. *J Neurol Sci* 1967;5:33–7.

97. Verrier M, Ashby P, MacLeod S. Diazepam effect on reflex activity in patients with complete spinal lesions and in those with other causes of spasticity. *Arch Phys Med Rehabil* 1977;58:148–53.

98. Stahl MM, Saldeen P, Vinge E. Reversal of fetal benzodiazepine intoxication using flumazenil. *Br J Obstet Gynaecol* 1993;100:185–8.

99. Basmajian JV, Shankardass K, Russell D. Ketazolam once daily for spasticity: double-blind cross-over study. *Arch Phys Med Rehabil* 1986;67:556–7.

100. Basmajian JV, Shankardass K, Russell D, Yucel V. Ketazolam treatment for spasticity: double-blind study of a new drug. *Arch Phys Med Rehabil* 1984;65:698–701.

101. Cendrowski W, Sobczyk W. Clonazepam, baclofen and placebo in the treatment of spasticity. *Eur Neurol* 1977;16:257–62.

102. Herman R, Mayer N, Mccomber SA. Clinical pharmaco-physiology of dantrolene sodium. *Am J Phys Med* 1972;51:296–311.

103. Ward A, Chaffman MO, Sorkin EM. Dantrolene. A review of its pharmacodynamic and pharmacokinetic properties and therapeutic use in malignant hyperthermia, the neuroleptic malignant syndrome and an update of its use in muscle spasticity. *Drugs* 1986;32:130–68.

104. Pinder RM, Brogden RN, Speight TM, Avery GS. Dantrolene sodium: a review of its pharmacological properties and therapeutic efficacy in spasticity. *Drugs* 1977;13:3–23.

105. Katrak PH, Cole AM, Poulos CJ, McCauley JC. Objective assessment of spasticity, strength, and function with early exhibition of dantrolene sodium after cerebrovascular accident: a randomized double-blind study. *Arch Phys Med Rehabil* 1992;73:4–9.

106. Weiser R, Terenty T, Hudgson P, Weightman D. Dantrolene sodium in the treatment of spasticity in chronic spinal cord disease. *Practitioner* 1978;221:123–7.

107. Utili R, Boitnott JK, Zimmerman HJ. Dantrolene-associated hepatic injury. Incidence and character. *Gastroenterology* 1977;72:610–6.

108. Mai J, Pedersen E. Mode of action of dantrolene sodium in spasticity. *Acta Neurol Scand* 1979;59:309–16.

109. Chyatte SB, Birdsong JH, Bergman BA. The effects of dantrolene sodium on spasticity and motor performance in hemiplegia. *South Med J* 1971;64:180–5.

110. Davies J. Selective depression of synaptic transmission of spinal neurones in the cat by a new centrally acting muscle relaxant, 5-chloro-4-(2-imidazolin-2-yl-amino)-2, 1, 3-benzothiodazole (DS103-282). *Br J Pharmacol* 1982;76:473–81.

111. Coward DM. Tizanidine: neuropharmacology and mechanism of action. *Neurology* 1994;44:S6–10; discussion S-1.

112. Kamen L, Henney HR, 3rd, Runyan JD. A practical overview of tizanidine use for spasticity secondary to multiple sclerosis, stroke, and spinal cord injury. *Curr Med Res Opin* 2008;24:425–39.

113. Wallace JD. Summary of combined clinical analysis of controlled clinical trials with tizanidine. *Neurology* 1994;44: S60–8; discussion S8–9.

114. van Oosten BW, Truyen L, Barkhof F, Polman CH. Multiple sclerosis therapy. A practical guide. *Drugs* 1995;49:200–12.

115. Granfors MT, Backman JT, Laitila J, Neuvonen PJ. Tizanidine is mainly metabolized by cytochrome p450 1A2 in vitro. *Br J Clin Pharmacol* 2004;57:349–53.

116. Granfors MT, Backman JT, Laitila J, Neuvonen PJ. Oral contraceptives containing ethinyl estradiol and gestodene markedly increase plasma concentrations and effects of tizanidine by inhibiting cytochrome P450 1A2. *Clin Pharmacol Ther* 2005;78:400–11.

117. Granfors MT, Backman JT, Neuvonen M, Ahonen J, Neuvonen PJ. Fluvoxamine drastically increases concentrations and effects of tizanidine: a potentially hazardous interaction. *Clin Pharmacol Ther* 2004;75:331–41.

118. Granfors MT, Backman JT, Neuvonen M, Neuvonen PJ. Ciprofloxacin greatly increases concentrations and hypotensive effect of tizanidine by inhibiting its cytochrome P450 1A2-mediated presystemic metabolism. *Clin Pharmacol Ther* 2004;76:598–606.

119. Backman JT, Karjalainen MJ, Neuvonen M, Laitila J, Neuvonen PJ. Rofecoxib is a potent inhibitor of cytochrome P450 1A2: studies with tizanidine and caffeine in healthy subjects. *Br J Clin Pharmacol* 2006;62:345–57.

120. Shellenberger MK, Groves L, Shah J, Novack GD. A controlled pharmacokinetic evaluation of tizanidine and baclofen at steady state. *Drug Metab Dispos* 1999;27:201–4.

121. Nance PW, Sheremata WA, Lynch SG, et al. Relationship of the antispasticity effect of tizanidine to plasma concentration in patients with multiple sclerosis. *Arch Neurol* 1997;54: 731–6.

122. Smith C, Birnbaum G, Carter JL, Greenstein J, Lublin FD. Tizanidine treatment of spasticity caused by multiple sclerosis: results of a double-blind, placebo-controlled trial. US Tizanidine Study Group. *Neurology* 1994;44:S34–42; discussion S-3.

123. Gelber DA, Good DC, Dromerick A, Sergay S, Richardson M. Open-label dose-titration safety and efficacy study of tizanidine hydrochloride in the treatment of spasticity associated with chronic stroke. *Stroke* 2001;32:1841–6.

124. Meythaler JM, Guin-Renfroe S, Johnson A, Brunner RM. Prospective assessment of tizanidine for spasticity due to acquired brain injury. *Arch Phys Med Rehabil* 2001;82:1155–63.

125. A double-blind, placebo-controlled trial of tizanidine in the treatment of spasticity caused by multiple sclerosis. United Kingdom Tizanidine Trial Group. *Neurology* 1994;44:S70–8.

126. Knutsson E, Martensson A, Gransberg L. Antiparetic and antispastic effects induced by tizanidine in patients with spastic paresis. *J Neurol Sci* 1982;53:187–204.

127. Shah J, Wesnes KA, Kovelesky RA, Henney HR, 3rd. Effects of food on the single-dose pharmacokinetics/pharmacodynamics of tizanidine capsules and tablets in healthy volunteers. *Clin Ther* 2006;28:1308–17.

128. Nance PW, Shears AH, Nance DM. Clonidine in spinal cord injury. *Can Med Assoc J* 1985;133:41–2.

129. Nance PW, Shears AH, Nance DM. Reflex changes induced by clonidine in spinal cord injured patients. *Paraplegia* 1989;27:296–301.

130. Donovan WH, Carter RE, Rossi CD, Wilkerson MA. Clonidine effect on spasticity: a clinical trial. *Arch Phys Med Rehabil* 1988;69:193–4.

131. Unnerstall JR, Kopajtic TA, Kuhar MJ. Distribution of alpha 2 agonist binding sites in the rat and human central nervous system: analysis of some functional, anatomic correlates of the pharmacologic effects of clonidine and related adrenergic agents. *Brain Res* 1984;319:69–101.

132. Maynard FM. Early clinical experience with clonidine in spinal spasticity. *Paraplegia* 1986;24:175–82.

133. Yablon SA, Sipski ML. Effect of transdermal clonidine on spinal spasticity. A case series. *Am J Phys Med Rehabil* 1993;72:154–7.

134. Stewart JE, Barbeau H, Gauthier S. Modulation of locomotor patterns and spasticity with clonidine in spinal cord injured patients. *Can J Neurol Sci* 1991;18:321–32.

135. Norman KE, Pepin A, Barbeau H. Effects of drugs on walking after spinal cord injury. *Spinal Cord* 1998;36:699–715.

136. Barbeau H, Richards CL, Bedard PJ. Action of cyproheptadine in spastic paraparetic patients. *J Neurol Neurosurg Psychiatry* 1982;45:923–6.

137. Wainberg M, Barbeau H, Gauthier S. The effects of cyproheptadine on locomotion and on spasticity in patients with spinal cord injuries. *J Neurol Neurosurg Psychiatry* 1990;53:754–63.

138. Wainberg M, Barbeau H, Gauthier S. Quantitative assessment of the effect of cyproheptadine on spastic paretic gait: a preliminary study. *J Neurol* 1986;233:311–4.

139. Nance PW. A comparison of clonidine, cyproheptadine and baclofen in spastic spinal cord injured patients. *J Am Paraplegia Soc* 1994;17:150–6.

140. Fung J, Stewart JE, Barbeau H. The combined effects of clonidine and cyproheptadine with interactive training on the modulation of locomotion in spinal cord injured subjects. *J Neurol Sci* 1990;100:85–93.

141. Kita M, Goodkin DE. Drugs used to treat spasticity. *Drugs* 2000;59:487–95.

142. Priebe MM, Sherwood AM, Graves DE, Mueller M, Olson WH. Effectiveness of gabapentin in controlling spasticity: a quantitative study. *Spinal Cord* 1997;35:171–5.

143. Gruenthal M, Mueller M, Olson WL, Priebe MM, Sherwood AM, Olson WH. Gabapentin for the treatment of spasticity in patients with spinal cord injury. *Spinal Cord* 1997;35:686–9.

144. Cutter NC, Scott DD, Johnson JC, Whiteneck G. Gabapentin effect on spasticity in multiple sclerosis: a placebo-controlled, randomized trial. *Arch Phys Med Rehabil* 2000;81:164–9.

145. Dougherty JA, Rhoney DH. Gabapentin: a unique antiepileptic agent. *Neurol Res* 2001;23:821–9.

146. Selak I. Pregabalin (Pfizer). *Curr Opin Investig Drugs* 2001; 2:828–34.

147. Bradley LJ, Kirker GB. Pregabalin in the treatment of spasticity: a restrospective case series. *Disabil Rehabil* 2008; 30:1230–2.

148. Hayes KC, Potter PJ, Hsieh JT, Katz MA, Blight AR, Cohen R. Pharmacokinetics and safety of multiple oral doses of sustained-release 4-aminopyridine (Fampridine-SR) in subjects with chronic, incomplete spinal cord injury. *Arch Phys Med Rehabil* 2004;85:29–34.

149. Blight AR. Effect of 4-aminopyridine on axonal conduction-block in chronic spinal cord injury. *Brain Res Bull* 1989;22:47–52.

150. Hayes KC. The use of 4-aminopyridine (fampridine) in demyelinating disorders. *CNS Drug Rev* 2004;10:295–316.

151. Evenhuis J, Agoston S, Salt PJ, de Lange AR, Wouthuyzen W, Erdmann W. Pharmacokinetics of 4-aminopyridine in human volunteers. A preliminary study using a new GLC method for its estimation. *Br J Anaesth* 1981;53:567–70.

152. Korenke AR, Rivey MP, Allington DR. Sustained-release fampridine for symptomatic treatment of multiple sclerosis. *Ann Pharmacother* 2008;42:1458–65.

153. Hayes KC, Potter PJ, Hansebout RR, et al. Pharmacokinetic studies of single and multiple oral doses of fampridine-SR (sustained-release 4-aminopyridine) in patients with chronic spinal cord injury. *Clin Neuropharmacol* 2003;26:185–92.

154. Cardenas DD, Ditunno J, Graziani V, et al. Phase 2 trial of sustained-release fampridine in chronic spinal cord injury. *Spinal Cord* 2007;45:158–68.

155. Grijalva I, Guizar-Sahagun G, Castaneda-Hernandez G, et al. Efficacy and safety of 4-aminopyridine in patients with long-term spinal cord injury: a randomized, double-blind, placebo-controlled trial. *Pharmacotherapy* 2003;23:823–34.

156. Hansebout RR, Blight AR, Fawcett S, Reddy K. 4-Amino-pyridine in chronic spinal cord injury: a controlled, double-blind, crossover study in eight patients. *J Neurotrauma* 1993;10:1–18.

157. Segal JL, Pathak MS, Hernandez JP, Himber PL, Brunnemann SR, Charter RS. Safety and efficacy of 4-aminopyridine in humans with spinal cord injury: a long-term, controlled trial. *Pharmacotherapy* 1999;19:713–23.

158. van der Bruggen MA, Huisman HB, Beckerman H, Bertelsmann FW, Polman CH, Lankhorst GJ. Randomized trial of 4-aminopyridine in patients with chronic incomplete spinal cord injury. *J Neurol* 2001;248:665–71.

159. Isoda WC, Segal JL. Effects of 4-aminopyridine on cardiac repolarization, PR interval, and heart rate in patients with spinal cord injury. *Pharmacotherapy* 2003;23:133–6.

160. Wolfe DL, Hayes KC, Hsieh JT, Potter PJ. Effects of 4-amino-pyridine on motor evoked potentials in patients with spinal cord injury: a double-blinded, placebo-controlled crossover trial. *J Neurotrauma* 2001;18:757–71.

161. Potter PJ, Hayes KC, Segal JL, et al. Randomized double-blind crossover trial of fampridine-SR (sustained release 4-aminopyridine) in patients with incomplete spinal cord injury. *J Neurotrauma* 1998;15:837–49.

162. http://www.acorda.com/pipeline_fampridine_sci1.asp. (Accessed 12/12/2008, at

163. Petro DJ, Ellenberger C, Jr. Treatment of human spasticity with delta 9-tetrahydrocannabinol. *J Clin Pharmacol* 1981;21:413S–6S.

164. Hagenbach U, Luz S, Ghafoor N, et al. The treatment of spasticity with Delta9-tetrahydrocannabinol in persons with spinal cord injury. *Spinal Cord* 2007;45:551–62.

165. Advokat C, Mosser H, Hutchinson K. Morphine and dextrorphan lose antinociceptive activity but exhibit an antispastic action in chronic spinal rats. *Physiol Behav* 1997;62:799–804.

166. Penn RD, Kroin JS. Continuous intrathecal baclofen for severe spasticity. *Lancet* 1985;2:125–7.

167. Parke B, Penn RD, Savoy SM, Corcos D. Functional outcome after delivery of intrathecal baclofen. *Arch Phys Med Rehabil* 1989;70:30–2.

168. Loubser PG, Narayan RK, Sandin KJ, Donovan WH, Russell KD. Continuous infusion of intrathecal baclofen: long-term effects on spasticity in spinal cord injury. *Paraplegia* 1991;29:48–64.

169. Kroin JS, Ali A, York M, Penn RD. The distribution of medication along the spinal canal after chronic intrathecal administration. *Neurosurgery* 1993;33:226–30; discussion 30.

170. Vender JR, Hester S, Waller JL, Rekito A, Lee MR. Identification and management of intrathecal baclofen pump complications: a comparison of pediatric and adult patients. *J Neurosurg* 2006;104:9–15.

171. Burns AS, Meythaler JM. Intrathecal baclofen in tetraplegia of spinal origin: efficacy for upper extremity hypertonia. *Spinal Cord* 2001;39:413–9.

172. Brennan PM, Whittle IR. Intrathecal baclofen therapy for neurological disorders: a sound knowledge base but many challenges remain. *Br J Neurosurg* 2008;22:508–19.

173. Podsiadlo D, Richardson S. The timed "up & go": a test of basic functional mobility for frail elderly persons. *J Am Geriatr Soc* 1991;39:142–8.

174. Nance P, Schryvers O, Schmidt B, Dubo H, Loveridge B, Fewer D. Intrathecal baclofen therapy for adults with spinal spasticity: therapeutic efficacy and effect on hospital admissions. *Can J Neurol Sci* 1995;22:22–9.

175. Saval A, Chiodo AE. Sexual dysfunction associated with intrathecal baclofen use: a report of two cases. *J Spinal Cord Med* 2008;31:103–5.

176. Denys P, Mane M, Azouvi P, Chartier-Kastler E, Thiebaut JB, Bussel B. Side effects of chronic intrathecal baclofen on erection and ejaculation in patients with spinal cord lesions. *Arch Phys Med Rehabil* 1998;79:494–6.

177. Muller-Schwefe G, Penn RD. Physostigmine in the treatment of intrathecal baclofen overdose. Report of three cases. *J Neurosurg* 1989;71:273–5.

178. Green LB, Nelson VS. Death after acute withdrawal of intrathecal baclofen: case report and literature review. *Arch Phys Med Rehabil* 1999;80:1600–4.

179. Plassat R, Perrouin Verbe B, Menei P, Menegalli D, Mathe JF, Richard I. Treatment of spasticity with intrathecal Baclofen administration: long-term follow-up, review of 40 patients. *Spinal Cord* 2004;42:686–93.

180. Gooch JL, Oberg WA, Grams B, Ward LA, Walker ML. Complications of intrathecal baclofen pumps in children. *Pediatr Neurosurg* 2003;39:1–6.

181. Reeves RK, Stolp-Smith KA, Christopherson MW. Hyperthermia, rhabdomyolysis, and disseminated intravascular coagulation associated with baclofen pump catheter failure. *Arch Phys Med Rehabil* 1998;79:353–6.

182. Remy-Neris O, Barbeau H, Daniel O, Boiteau F, Bussel B. Effects of intrathecal clonidine injection on spinal reflexes and human locomotion in incomplete paraplegic subjects. *Exp Brain Res* 1999;129:433–40.

183. Middleton JW, Siddall PJ, Walker S, Molloy AR, Rutkowski SB. Intrathecal clonidine and baclofen in the management of spasticity and neuropathic pain following spinal cord injury: a case study. *Arch Phys Med Rehabil* 1996;77:824–6.

184. Zafonte RD, Munin MC. Phenol and alcohol blocks for the treatment of spasticity. *Phys Med Rehabil Clin N Am* 2001;12:817–32, vii.

185. Okazaki A. The effects of two and five percent aqueous phenol on the cat tibial nerve in situ–II: effect on the circulation of the tibial nerve. *Masui* 1993;42:819–25.

186. Khalili AA, Betts HB. Peripheral nerve block with phenol in the management of spasticity. Indications and complications. *JAMA* 1967;200:1155–7.

187. Spira R. Management of spasticity in cerebral palsied children by peripheral nerve block with phenol. *Dev Med Child Neurol* 1971;13:164–73.

188. Moritz U. Phenol block of peripheral nerves. *Scand J Rehabil Med* 1973;5:160–3.

189. Gracies JM, Elovic E, McGuire J, Simpson DM. Traditional pharmacological treatments for spasticity. Part I: local treatments. *Muscle Nerve Suppl* 1997;6:S61–91.

190. Petrillo CR, Knoploch S. Phenol block of the tibial nerve for spasticity: a long-term follow-up study. *Int Disabil Stud* 1988;10:97–100.

191. Braun RM, Hoffer MM, Mooney V, McKeever J, Roper B. Phenol nerve block in the treatment of acquired spastic hemiplegia in the upper limb. *J Bone Joint Surg Am* 1973;55:580–5.

192. Asensi V, Asensi JM, Carton JA, Maradona JA, Ona M, Arechaga C. Successful intrathecal ethanol block for intractable spasticity of AIDS-related progressive multifocal leukoencephalopathy. *Spinal Cord* 1999;37:450–2.

193. O'Hanlan JT, Galford HR, Bosley J. The use of 45 percent alcohol to control spasticity. *Va Med Mon (1918)* 1969;96:429–36.

194. Carpenter EB, Seitz DG. Intramuscular alcohol as an aid in management of spastic cerebral palsy. *Dev Med Child Neurol* 1980;22:497–501.

195. Scott AB. Botulinum toxin injection into extraocular muscles as an alternative to strabismus surgery. *Ophthalmology* 1980;87:1044–9.

196. Brin MF. Botulinum toxin: chemistry, pharmacology, toxicity, and immunology. *Muscle Nerve Suppl* 1997;6:S146–68.

197. Simpson LL. Identification of the major steps in botulinum toxin action. *Annu Rev Pharmacol Toxicol* 2004;44:167–93.

198. Humeau Y, Doussau F, Grant NJ, Poulain B. How botulinum and tetanus neurotoxins block neurotransmitter release. *Biochimie* 2000;82:427–46.

199. Comella CL, Jankovic J, Shannon KM, et al. Comparison of botulinum toxin serotypes A and B for the treatment of cervical dystonia. *Neurology* 2005;65:1423–9.

200. Mueller J. Re: Botulinum toxin type B vs. type a in toxin-naive patients with cervical dystonia: randomized, double-blind, noninferiority trial. *Mov Disord* 2008;23:510–517.
201. Brin MF. Dosing, administration, and a treatment algorithm for use of botulinum toxin A for adult-onset spasticity. Spasticity Study Group. *Muscle Nerve Suppl* 1997;6:S208–20.
202. Gracies JM. Impact of botulinum toxin type A (BTX-A) dilution and ENdplate targeting technique in upper limb spasticity. *Ann Neurol* 2002;52:S87.
203. Francisco GE. Botulinum toxin: dosing and dilution. *Am J Phys Med Rehabil* 2004;83:S30–7.
204. Py AG, Zein Addeen G, Perrier Y, Carlier RY, Picard A. Evaluation of the effectiveness of botulinum toxin injections in the lower limb muscles of children with cerebral palsy. Preliminary prospective study of the advantages of ultrasound guidance. *Ann Phys Rehabil Med* 2009;52:215–23.
205. Ward AB. Spasticity treatment with botulinum toxins. *J Neural Transm* 2008;115:607–16.
206. O'Brien CF. Injection techniques for botulinum toxin using electromyography and electrical stimulation. *Muscle Nerve Suppl* 1997;6:S176–80.
207. Shaari CM, Sanders I. Quantifying how location and dose of botulinum toxin injections affect muscle paralysis. *Muscle Nerve* 1993;16:964–9.
208. Simpson DM, Gracies JM, Graham HK, et al. Assessment: botulinum neurotoxin for the treatment of spasticity (an evidence-based review): report of the Therapeutics and Technology Assessment Subcommittee of the American Academy of Neurology. *Neurology* 2008;70:1691–8.
209. Marciniak C, Rader L, Gagnon C. The use of botulinum toxin for spasticity after spinal cord injury. *Am J Phys Med Rehabil* 2008;87:312–7; quiz 8–20, 29.
210. Albany K. Physical and occupational therapy considerations in adult patients receiving botulinum toxin injections for spasticity. *Muscle Nerve Suppl* 1997;6:S221–31.
211. Newman CJ, Kennedy A, Walsh M, O'Brien T, Lynch B, Hensey O. A pilot study of delayed versus immediate serial casting after botulinum toxin injection for partially reducible spastic equinus. *J Pediatr Orthop* 2007;27:882–5.
212. MacDonald R, Monga M, Fink HA, Wilt TJ. Neurotoxin treatments for urinary incontinence in subjects with spinal cord injury or multiple sclerosis: a systematic review of effectiveness and adverse effects. *J Spinal Cord Med* 2008;31:157–65.
213. Cote TR, Mohan AK, Polder JA, Walton MK, Braun MM. Botulinum toxin type A injections: adverse events reported to the US Food and Drug Administration in therapeutic and cosmetic cases. *J Am Acad Dermatol* 2005;53:407–15.
214. Brin MF, Lew MF, Adler CH, et al. Safety and efficacy of NeuroBloc (botulinum toxin type B) in type A-resistant cervical dystonia. *Neurology* 1999;53:1431–8.
215. Comella CL, Tanner CM, DeFoor-Hill L, Smith C. Dysphagia after botulinum toxin injections for spasmodic torticollis: clinical and radiologic findings. *Neurology* 1992;42:1307–10.
216. Rossi RP, Strax TE, Di Rocco A. Severe dysphagia after botulinum toxin B injection to the lower limbs and lumbar paraspinal muscles. *Am J Phys Med Rehabil* 2006;85:1011–3.
217. Barolat G. Surgical management of spasticity and spasms in spinal cord injury: an overview. *J Am Paraplegia Soc* 1988;11:9–13.
218. Chambers HG. The surgical treatment of spasticity. *Muscle Nerve Suppl* 1997;6:S121–8.
219. Chambers FG, Koshy SS, Saidi RF, Clark DP, Moore RD, Sears CL. Bacteroides fragilis toxin exhibits polar activity on monolayers of human intestinal epithelial cells (T84 cells) in vitro. *Infect Immun* 1997;65:3561–70.
220. MDVU-BTX-B (Myobloc) Adult Dosing Guidelines. (Accessed 10/17/2006, at www.mdvu.org/library/dosingtables/btxb_adg.html.)

Spasticity Due to Multiple Sclerosis: Epidemiology, Pathophysiology and Treatment

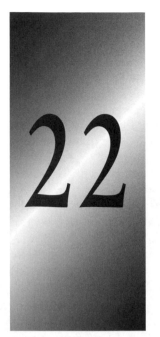

Anjali Shah
Ian Maitin

SPASTICITY IN MULTIPLE SCLEROSIS

Multiple sclerosis (MS) is a chronic, debilitating, inflammatory disease of the central nervous system. There is no cure for the disease, and management of it includes use of disease-modifying therapies and symptomatic agents to reduce and/or prevent relapses and disease progression. Multiple sclerosis affects approximately 350,000 persons in the United States (1, 2), with an estimated prevalence of 1 in 1000 individuals in North America and is one of the most common causes of disability in young adults. The symptoms of MS are numerous and include weakness, paresthesias, visual changes, fatigue, cognitive dysfunction, ataxia, and spasticity. Patients with MS report that their spasticity has a significant detrimental effect on their lives. A survey of 1554 self-reporting people with MS residing in the United Kingdom demonstrated that 82% experience spasticity and 54% classified the impact of spasticity as "high" or "moderate." (3) Greater than 80% of patients with MS report some degree of spasticity, with one third of these modifying or eliminating daily activities as a result of it (4).

Spasticity is a disorder of increased resistance of a muscle, or group of muscles, to an externally imposed stretch, with more resistance to rapid stretch (5, 6). What differentiates spasticity from other components of the upper motor neuron (UMN) syndrome is its relationship to the velocity of movement. A rigid muscle displays the same mechanical properties whether it is stretched slowly or quickly. Spasticity in the patient with MS ultimately leads to a detrimental increase in disability resulting in increased energy requirement for daily activities and decreased quality of life (7, 8).

Treating spasticity in the person with MS poses some unique challenges. By definition, MS is a progressive disease, and it is common for a patient's symptoms to fluctuate daily and is highly dependent on temperature, time of day, and fatigue. Patients with MS-related spasticity frequently present clinically similar to patients with stroke, traumatic brain injury (TBI), or spinal cord injury (SCI) secondary to the distribution of plaque in the brain and spinal cord. However, unlike those patients who have static injuries, MS-related symptoms vacillate frequently by nature of the disease process. This logic extends to include spasticity. The clinician and the patient must be aware of this to allow for varying dosage of medications or treatments at different points in the disease.

It is important for the clinician to be aware of the profound effect fatigue and cognitive dysfunction have on people with MS. Patients will frequently forego spasticity treatment options if their fatigue or cognitive function is compromised. It is vital for the clinician to treat spasticity adequately without worsening other symptoms.

The goal of this chapter is to review the etiology, pathophysiology, diagnosis, and evaluation of spasticity in this patient population. In addition, treatment and management strategies of MS-associated spasticity will be reviewed with emphasis on those items that are unique to this clinical population.

EPIDEMIOLOGY

About 1 in 1000 persons is affected with MS in North America (1, 2), with a worldwide prevalence of more than 1,000,000 persons. Females are affected about twice as frequently as males; diagnosis typically occurs between ages 20 and 40 years, and first-degree relatives of a person with MS have approximately 2% to 5% risk of being diagnosed with MS (9). The advent of magnetic resonance imaging has allowed for earlier diagnosis. Multiple sclerosis was originally deemed a disease of Northern European descents and more prevalent in populations further from the equator; however, MS now affects persons of all races and ethnicity and the latitude gradient of MS are believed to be decreasing (10, 11). Whites remain the most commonly affected group.

There are 4 main types of MS (see Figure 22.1):

- Relapsing-Remitting—This is the most common form of MS and affects approximately 85% of patients. Individuals have relapses or exacerbations with remissions during which time some or all of their disability recovers to their baseline. Females are affected twice as frequently as males in this form.
- Secondary Progressive—These individuals experienced relapsing-remitting MS initially and then

begin to have increasing amounts of disability accumulation or progression with no remission. All relapsing-remitting patients will convert to this form at some stage of their disease.

- Primary Progressive—This subtype is characterized by increasing disability accumulation over time without periods of relapses or remissions. The course and severity vary between individuals. Currently, there are no disease-modifying agents for this type of MS. Males and females are equally affected, and about 10% of MS patients have primary progressive MS.
- Progressive Relapsing—This is the most aggressive and rarest type of MS. Approximately 5% of patients are affected. The disease course is characterized by rapid accumulation of disability with or without periods of remission.

The North American Research Committee on Multiple Sclerosis conducted a survey studying the prevalence of spasticity as well as its relationship to functional activity. The survey results reported that 84% of patients reported some degree of spasticity ranging from mild to completely incapacitating (4). In addition, patients with higher levels of spasticity were more likely to be male, disabled, and unemployed compared to those with reduced amounts of spasticity. The study found a linear correlation in the amount of spasticity and degree of disability ranging from ambulatory to bed-bound.

PATHOPHYSIOLOGY

Normal muscle does not display resistance to passive movement, nor does it exhibit electromyographic activity. A spastic muscle will have abnormal muscle activity with slow or fast stretch movements (12). Spasticity is a component of the UMN syndrome, which also includes increased spinal reflexes, muscle hyperactivity, flexor spasms, and disordered control. Although the pathophysiology remains a subject of debate, spasticity appears to occur as a result of spinal, supraspinal, and/or cerebral dysfunction. The result is an imbalance between classic inhibitory (dorsal reticulospinal) and excitatory (mostly bulbopontine tegmentum) pathways that leads to abnormal proprioceptive input in the spinal cord (12–15). The clinical presentation is largely dependent on the anatomic site of injury or insult.

In MS, spasticity can be due to lesions in the brain, spinal cord, or both (5), with lower limb spasticity almost twice as prevalent as upper limb spasticity (97% vs 50%) (7). One of the most common questions asked by a person who is newly diagnosed with

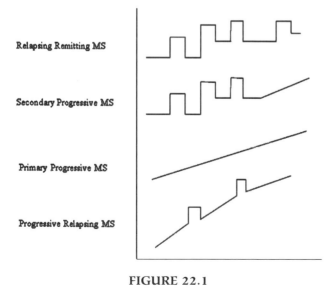

Relapsing Remitting MS

Secondary Progressive MS

Primary Progressive MS

Progressive Relapsing MS

FIGURE 22.1

Four main subtypes of MS.

MS is if their ability to ambulate will be affected and how quickly they will be in a wheelchair. Adequate assessment and timely treatment of spasticity can help ensure long-term ambulatory and functional ability of the patient with MS.

In addition to receiving input from the muscle spindle, motor units receive information and are influenced by proprioceptive, enteroceptive, and suprasegmental pathways. Noxious stimuli, such as pain, distended bladder, renal calculi, constipation, ingrown toenail, infection, or pressure ulcers, as well as nonnoxious stimuli (yawning, transferring), can trigger exacerbation of spasticity or other components of the UMN syndrome. Patients who complain of sudden worsening should be screened for the presence of above noxious stimuli before making more aggressive changes to their treatment.

NEGATIVE EFFECTS OF SPASTICITY AND REASONS TO TREAT

Spasticity can have deleterious effects on the performance of numerous tasks that are important to one's daily living. When compared to healthy subjects, patients with gait abnormalities secondary to MS-related spasticity demonstrated increased cost of walking in the 10-meter walking test (7). The increased cost of walking, coupled with a population with decreased cardiorespiratory systems, frequently results in diminished endurance for ambulation or other activities.

The involvement of spasticity in one or more limbs can lead to immobility and/or inactivity. The long-term effects of immobility have been well characterized in several studies involving prolonged bed rest (16, 17). Prolonged periods of bed rest have been reported to be detrimental and could potentially lead to further complications to multiple body systems (18). Immobility can lead to disuse atrophy and loss of strength and endurance in the musculoskeletal system. This is commonly seen in the patient with muscle atrophy in the involved spastic limb(s). People who are on bed rest may lose 10% to 15% of their muscle mass in 1 week and the time required to regain this bulk is frequently 2 to 3 times the duration of their bed rest (19). Daily isometric exercises focusing on the gastrocnemius, soleus, and tibialis anterior muscles should be encouraged to maintain muscle mass. Lower limb exercises should be performed regularly because these muscles lose significantly more muscle mass with inactivity compared to the upper limbs.

Collagen comprises 20% of total body mass and is the most abundant protein in the body (20). During periods of inactivity or immobility, the connective tissue properties of tendons and ligaments change drastically and affect the collagen and proteoglycan properties of soft tissue. This can lead to decreased gliding and lubrication of tendons and ligaments resulting in myogenic and soft tissue contractures. This can profoundly compromise one's independence and may necessitate assistance for transfers, toileting, bathing, and dressing. Patients should be encouraged to stretch daily for 15 minutes with focus on the spastic limbs (21). Patients who are bed-bound would benefit from active and passive range of motion (ROM) exercises. They may require hospital beds that are equipped with side rails and an overhead trapeze so that they can conduct some position changes independently.

Bone mineral status is affected by immobility (22, 23). Repeated loading will increase bone mass, whereas decreased loading will negatively affect the mass. In addition, patients with MS are frequently treated with intravenous or oral steroids for exacerbations or maintenance therapy, which adds additional risk for bone mineral decline. Glucocorticoids are the most common form of drug-related osteoporosis. They should be counseled to perform weight-bearing exercises (standing daily for 15–20 minutes either alone or with assistance of a walker, tilt table, or standing frame). For those who are unable to stand, isometric exercise and supplementation with calcium, vitamin D, and bisphosphonate therapy is strongly recommended.

Immobility due to spasticity will also compromise cardiovascular and pulmonary status. Periods of prolonged immobility can increase heart rate by 1 beat/min every 2 days (24). Patients may acquire immobilization tachycardia and reduced exercise tolerance. Stroke volume and maximal oxygen uptake by the heart and skeletal muscles decrease in as little as 2 to 3 weeks of inactivity (25).

Adequate and timely treatment of spasticity can prevent compromise of the cardiovascular, pulmonary, and musculoskeletal systems. In addition, preservation of bone mineral density status is maintained. Finally, through the above preventative measures, prevention of long-term complications of inactivity such as pressure ulcers, contractures, and deep venous thrombosis formation secondary to spasticity can occur.

EVALUATING SPASTICITY

Although spasticity is generally recognized as a symptom of MS, it is frequently not adequately controlled or assessed in routine office visits (5). A study of people with MS in England reported that about 50% of patients were either on a suboptimal dosage of their oral antispasmodic medication or not treated at all (7). Only 32% of the group reportedly had adequate treatment of their spasticity. Clinicians are encouraged to question and assess the presence of increased muscle tone of patients with MS at their office visits.

The Consortium of Multiple Sclerosis Centers recommends that spasticity be screened as part of routine visits for patients with MS. In addition to evaluating a patient's strength, ROM, deep tendon reflexes, and muscle tone with the patient seated on the examination table, the patient should be examined in a dynamic setting such as observing their gait pattern and how their hand intrinsics flex and extend while picking up an object and looking for evidence of cocontraction. The patient may also report difficulty falling or staying asleep due to increased muscle spasticity at night.

In addition to the clinical examination, spasticity can be assessed based on clinical scales, neurophysiologic testing, or biomechanical techniques (26). No single measurement has demonstrated superiority over the other, as the evaluation and assessment of spasticity can focus on several areas including ROM, resistance, and speed, which can be subjective or objective evaluations. The varying number of scales available for spasticity make study comparison challenging, as it is not unusual to see different scales used in papers dealing with the evaluation and management of spasticity.

Multiple Sclerosis Spasticity Scale

The Multiple Sclerosis Spasticity Scale is an 88-item self-reported questionnaire (26). It was generated through a series of 2 postal surveys, face-to-face interviews with people with MS, and focus groups of MS specialists, patients, and other health professionals involved in the care of this treatment population. The questionnaire is designed to provide information about the *impact* of spasticity on a patient's mobility, pain, activities of daily living (ADL), emotions, and social functioning. It consists of 8 subscales that can be used alone or in conjunction with each other. The Multiple Sclerosis Spasticity Scale is unique in providing information about the multiple ways spasticity can affect a patient. It can be used to complement clinical scales (summarized below) that clinicians frequently use to score the level of spasticity involvement.

Ashworth and Modified Ashworth Scale

Spasticity assessment is most commonly performed using the Ashworth (Table 22.1) and the Modified Ash-

worth Scale (MAS) (Table 22.2) (27). The Ashworth Scale (AS) was developed in 1964 (28). The MAS was developed in 1987 in response to concerns by the authors that the "Ashworth grade of '1' was indiscrete." (29). Both scales are ordinal scales with scores ranging from 0 to 4. The MAS has an additional value of 1+ and has demonstrated interrater reliability of 86.7% in assessment of elbow flexor muscle spasticity. Both scales have been criticized for their lack of sensitivity to subtle changes in spasticity and therefore exhibit challenges in demonstrating clinical effect in trials.

Tardieu Scale

The Tardieu Scale evaluates muscle response to velocity and movement quality (29). It adds the response to muscle moved at 3 different speeds. The original scale was developed in 1954 and has undergone several revisions. The following 3 factors are involved in the Tardieu Scale when assessing spasticity: (1) strength and duration of the stretch reflex (2), angle at which the stretch reflex is activated, and (3) the speed necessary to trigger the stretch reflex (30). It is also an ordinal scale that is graded from 0 to 4. The patient should be seated for upper limb evaluation, whereas supine position is recommended for lower limb testing (31).

Penn Spasm Frequency Scale and Spasm Frequency Scale

The Penn spasm frequency scale is a self-reported scale that was developed to assess spasticity in patients with MS and SCI after insertion of an intrathecal baclofen (ITB) pump (Table 22.3) (32). The scale ranks the occurrence of spasms by scoring as follows: 0, no spasm; 1, mild spasm induced by stimulation; 2, infrequent full spasms occurring less than 1 per hour; 3, spasms occurring more than once per hour; and 4, spasms occurring more than 10 times per hour (15). A variation to the Penn spasm frequency scale is the spasm fre-

---

TABLE 22.1
Ashworth Scale

0	Normal tone
1	Slight hypertonus, a "catch" when limb is moved
2	Mild hypertonus, limb moves easily
3	Moderate hypertonus, passive limb movement difficult
4	Severe hypertonus, limb rigid

Ashworth B. Preliminary trial of carisoprodol in multiple sclerosis. *Practitioner* 1964;192:540–2.

TABLE 22.2
Modified Ashworth Scale

0	No increase in tone
1	Slight increase in tone, manifested by a catch and release or by minimal resistance at the end of the ROM when the affected part(s) is moved in flexion or extension
1+	Slight increase in muscle tone, manifested by a catch, followed by minimal resistance throughout the remainder (less than half) of the ROM
2	More marked increase in muscle tone through most of the ROM, but affected part(s) easily moved
3	Considerable increase in muscle tone, passive movement difficult
4	Affected part(s) rigid in flexion or extension

Bohannon RW, Smith MB. Interrater reliability of a Modified Ashworth Scale of muscle spasticity. *Phys Ther* 1987;67:206–7.

quency scale that ranks the number of spasms occurring by day instead of by the hour (33).

Timed Up and Go Test

The timed up and go test is a functional assessment that requires a person to stand from a chair, walk 3 m, turn around, walk back to the chair, and return to a seated position (34). The patient performs the test at a comfortable pace and may use any required assistive device. Timing of the test commences as the patient stands and is complete with a return to the chair. The normal duration of the timed up and go test is 7 to 10 seconds. Patients requiring greater than 20 seconds are considered to have functional mobility problems. The test is validated, reliable, and correlated with the Berg Balance Scale.

TABLE 22.3
Penn Spasm Frequency Scale

Score	
0	No spasm
1	Mild spasm at stimulation
2	Irregular strong spasms less occurring <1 per hour
3	Spasms occurring >1 per hour
4	Spasms occurring >10 per hour

Penn RD, Savoy SM, Corcos D, et al. Intrathecal baclofen for severe spinal spasticity. *N Engl J Med* 1989;320:1517–21.

Ambulation Index

The Ambulation Index (AI) was developed for patients with MS. It assesses a patient's ability to walk a 25-ft distance rapidly and safely (35). The time required to complete the AI and assistive device used are documented. Scores range from 0, which indicates an independent ambulator, to 10, which indicates a bedridden patient. Similar to the AS and MAS, the AI is not always sensitive to changes in focal spasticity.

Berg Balance Scale

The Berg Balance Scale is a 14-item scale that assesses balance by means of a series of tasks, which require a patient to hold postures for a given duration (36). It is a 5-point ordinal scale, with 0 the lowest and 4 the highest score. Points are deducted for patients who cannot hold a position for the required time, as well for patients who lose their balance and require assistance. The test takes approximately 10 minutes to administer. Scores are stratified according to fall risk as follows: 41 to 56, low fall risk; 21 to 40, medium fall risk; 0 to 20, high fall risk. A score of 45/56 is considered the cutoff for safe independent ambulation.

Expanded Disability Status Scale

The Expanded Disability Status Scale (EDSS) is an ordinal scale ranging from 0 to 10 that is utilized in assessment of disability in people with MS (37). A score of 0 indicates no disability, and a score of 10 is death due to MS. There are 8 functional systems (FS) included in the EDSS: visual, pyramidal, cerebellar, brainstem, sensory, bowel and bladder function, cognition, mental, and other. In addition to assessing the 8 FS, a patient's ambulation ability and reliance on an assistive device are assessed. A patient's score on each FS is evaluated in conjunction with their ambulatory ability for their score. In general, scores of 0 to 4.0 mean patients can ambulate with no assistance and the FS score has greater influence over the overall scale. An EDSS score of 4.0 to 7.5 indicates dependence on an assistive device with limited ambulation distance. A score of 6.0 or greater indicates reliance on at least a single point cane. Scores of 7.5 to 10.0 are determined by the patient's ability to transfer from a wheelchair to bed.

TREATMENT

Prevention

People with MS and their caregivers should receive an education about the risk of developing spasticity and suggested methods to prevent the onset of spasticity. Suggested factors that could negatively affect spasticity are listed in Table 22.4. It is recommended that patients stretch frequently, even before the onset of spasticity, to prevent or delay the onset of changes in muscle tone or weakness. For patients with limited mobility, caregivers are encouraged to perform passive stretches of commonly affected muscles on a daily basis because this patient population is at greater risk of contracture and decubitus ulcer formation. There are several online resources available that demonstrate stretches and exercises for patients with MS. Interestingly, there is no research study of the effects of exercise on the ramifications of spasticity in this population.

Rehabilitative Strategies

There are several rehabilitative interventions available for spasticity management. The Consortium of Multiple Sclerosis Centers panel on spasticity recommends the use of skilled rehabilitation strategies for its management. A summary of possible therapeutic interventions is listed below.

Range of Motion and Stretching. Muscles that cross 2 joints (e.g., lumbricals, gastrocnemius, iliopsoas, hamstring) are most at risk for the development of spasticity. Daily stretching to maintain full

TABLE 22.4
Potential Spasticity Precipitating Factors in Patients With MS

Noxious stimuli
MS exacerbation
MS pseudo-exacerbation
MS disease progression
Urinary tract infection
Kidney Stone
Heat/Cold
Fatigue
Menses
Pain
Distended bladder or bowel
Pressure ulcer
Infection
Stool impaction
Fracture

Haselkorn JK, Balsdon Richer C, Fry Welch D, et al. Overview of spasticity management in multiple sclerosis. Evidence-based management strategies for spasticity treatment in multiple sclerosis. *J Spinal Cord Med* 2005;28:167–99.

ROM of these muscles is suggested. The lower limbs are more frequently involved and stretching of the heel cord and hamstrings with Thera-bands is encouraged (7). Stretches should be sustained for at least 30 seconds and done multiple times in each leg.

Strengthening. The development of spasticity can lead to decreased activity and muscle weakness. Although no specific recommendations exist for people with MS, therapies should be prescribed based on a person's abilities and can include isometric exercises, progressive resistance exercises, endurance exercises, and core body strengthening. No specific type of exercise has been proven superior in this population.

Stroking. One small pilot study that included 10 people with MS-related plantar flexor spasticity evaluated the effects of "slow stroking" over the lower limbs for the management of their spasticity (38). H reflex activity was measured prestroking, immediate poststroking, and 30 minutes poststroking. There was a 30% decrease in H reflex amplitude from baseline, reflecting reduced spasticity. Light pressure may facilitate decreases in spasticity; however, larger studies are necessary.

Heat Therapy. Approximately 80% of patients with MS exhibit heat insensitivity, which can lead to the temporary development of new symptoms or worsening of current symptoms (39). In general for people with MS, function generally deteriorates with heat and improves with cold (40). As a result, heating modalities are generally not recommended as a treatment in this population (5).

Cold Therapy. Muscle cooling has been found to reduce muscle stretch activity and clonus (41). Cooling demyelinated nerves can reduce conduction block and transiently improve nerve conduction (42), as well as reduce fatigue in patients with MS. Fifteen minutes of muscle cooling before engaging in heavy physical activity is recommended to reduce spasmodic activity (43); however, it should be noted that the immediate effect of cooling is transient increase in muscle tone. The use of cooling suits can reduce core body temperature by 0.2°F to 1.8°F (44). In addition to the traditional cooling vest, other cooling devices such as hats, bandanas, seats, and pillows are also commercially available. Aquatic therapy in swimming pools that are approximately 80°F to 82°F is recommended to stretch spastic muscles and for cardiovascular and muscle-strengthening therapeutic interventions (5). Swimming pools maintained at a temperature greater than 85°F should be avoided at all times. It is critical that therapists should be cautioned to ensure that the patient's sensory system is intact before engaging in heating or cooling applications.

Transcutaneous Electrical Stimulation. Transcutaneous electrical stimulation (TENS) is used to control pain in several disorders, and the utility of TENS units demonstrated spasticity reduction in spasticity secondary to stroke and SCI (45, 46). Armutlu et al. (47) reported significant reduction in plantar flexor spasticity in 10 patients with MS using high-frequency (100 Hz) TENS unit for 20 minutes daily for 4 weeks. Reduction was noted on MAS, electrophysiologic measurements, and the AI (35). Long-term effects on spasticity after discontinuation of TENS application was not commented on in this study.

Another study assessed the utility of TENS for management of spasticity using a crossover design. Thirty-two subjects were divided and received either 60 minutes or 8 hours of high-frequency (100 Hz) TENS treatment daily for 2 weeks (48). No reduction in spasticity was found in either group. Despite the lack of significant reduction in spasticity, 87.5% of participants noted reduction in spasms, 73.3% reported pain reduction, and 73.3% had reduced stiffness. Follow-up of the subjects ranged from 8 to 20 months, and the authors reported that most subjects were still using TENS units on an as needed basis.

The use of TENS units is recommended in the skilled rehabilitation setting under the guidance of a trained therapist. If the patient demonstrated clinical improvement, recommendation for purchase is appropriate and indicated.

There is some evidence to suggest that functional electrical stimulation may result in a reduction of spasticity. Szecsi et al. (49) found a significant short-term reduction in spasticity in patients with MS who engaged in functional electrical stimulation–assisted cycling for 2 weeks. In addition, there are currently 2 Functional Neuromuscular Electrical Stimulation devices, the BioNess L300 and the Walkaide, that are being used clinically to manage MS-related foot drops. Although there has been significant marketing and media hype regarding the efficacy of these devices on safety, gait quality and speed, ambulation distance, and overall strengthening, there is currently a paucity of research documenting the manufactures' claims.

Orthotics. Various bracing devices are frequently prescribed to assist patients with weakness or joint instability secondary to spasticity. There are conflicting reports on the benefit of orthotics such as the hip flexion assist orthosis, static ankle foot orthosis, and dynamic ankle foot orthosis in terms of improved ambulation (50–52). It is postulated that the use of assistive devices such as orthotics may reduce energy expenditure by assisting mobility and improving balance. However, there are no published studies on the effects of orthotics in reducing spasticity.

Serial Casting. This modality is utilized to correct deformity, lengthen contractures, and reduce spasticity through the repeated application and removal of casts (53). The precise mechanism of serial casting is unknown. Muscles immobilized in a shortened state usually lose sarcomeres. It has been theorized that serial casting may reduce excitation of the alpha or gamma motor neurons in the spinal cord and increase the length and number of sarcomeres in the targeted muscle (54, 55). Serial casting is noninvasive and strong enough to counteract joints with increased tone that may not be amenable to dynamic casts. In addition, serial casting can be done as an adjunctive agent to oral agents, as well as nerve blocks. The disadvantage of casting is the time required to apply and change the cast. It can be difficult for caregivers, as the cast cannot get wet and is heavy, making assistance with transferring challenging. Skin ulcers or breakdown are uncommon but can occur with improperly placed casts. Contraindications to casting include open wounds, unhealed fractures, impaired sensation or circulation, and uncontrolled hypertension.

Oral Medications

Oral agents are frequently used in the management of spasticity for people with MS. The choice of the most appropriate agent is dependent on the characteristics of the person and their muscle overactivity, distribution (focal vs. diffuse), time of presentation (all day vs. nighttime), presence of other medical conditions, and cognitive status. There are also factors that are agent-specific, such as the side effect profile and cost of each agent. Three agents are approved for use in the treatment of spasticity: baclofen, dantrolene, and tizanidine (56). Although only these agents have an approval for the management of spasticity, there are several other oral medications that are commonly used. It has been reported that most patients with MS are inadequately treated with oral medications due to clinician's concern about sedation and fatigue (7). The discussion that follows contains a summary of the agents most commonly used in this population.

Baclofen. Baclofen is believed to mediate its activity at the GABA receptors. Through its binding to GABA-B receptors, it reduces spasticity, specifically flexor-type spasticity. Baclofen is well tolerated in the MS patient population and is dosed between 5 and 120 mg daily (57–60). It is a typical first-line oral agent for spasticity management. Renal, hepatic, and hematopoietic safety has been demonstrated in patients with MS taking the medication for more than 3 years (61). Treatment is more effective when begun at earlier stages of spasticity. Typically, initial dosing is recommended at night and titrated gradually to TID dosing. Common side effects include somnolence, fatigue, constipation, nausea, and vomiting. Liver function testing is recommended every 6 months.

Dantrolene Sodium. Dantrolene inhibits calcium release from the sarcoplasmic reticulum and thereby reduces the strength of muscle contraction (62). The recommended dosage is 25 to 400 mg daily with a slow titration. Doses higher than this can result in severe hepatotoxicity (63). The half-life of dantrolene is approximately 15 hours. Although dantrolene had reduced muscle tone and increased ROM, its most profound effect is reduction in clonus. Because of its effect at the skeletal muscle level, it usually does not affect cognitive functioning. However, because of dantrolene's site of action at the skeletal muscle level, one of its main side effects is muscle weakness. This effect severely limits its use in the MS patient population (64, 65).

Tizanidine. Tizanidine modulates the release of glycine and excitatory neurotransmitters and is an alpha-2 central agonist (63). Several studies investigated its efficacy in the management of spasticity for people with MS (66–69). It is available in capsule and tablet formulation. It is recommended to begin dosing at 2 mg and gradually titrate up to 36 mg daily as tolerated. Comparative studies between tizanidine, baclofen, and dantrolene demonstrate increased to equivalent efficacy with tizanidine and baclofen. The side effect profile for tizanidine includes sedation, dizziness, dry mouth, and asthenia, which has limited its usefulness in this population due to poor tolerability. It is suggested that liver function testings be monitored every 3 to 6 months to ensure patient safety. Hepatic transaminase levels of 3 times the upper limit of normal has been reported in 5% of patients who participated in postmarketing surveillance studies (56). Patients are typically asymptomatic, and a return to normal transaminase levels usually occurs after withdrawal of tizanidine therapy.

Benzodiazepines. Diazepam and clonazepam are commonly used for spasticity management in patients with MS. Diazepam is a GABA-A agonist, and animal studies have found that it increases presynaptic inhibition of polysynaptic and monosynaptic reflexes (70). Past work has demonstrated the efficacy of diazepam in the management of spasticity associated with MS (71–73). The recommended dosage for diazepam is between 4 and 40 mg daily and should be given in 2 to 4 divided doses. The side effect profile is significant and includes sedation and memory impairment. Although comparative studies between diazepam, dantrolene sodium, and baclofen showed no significant difference in therapeutic effects, diazepam's side ef-

fect profile has limited patient tolerance. Overdosage can lead to somnolence, coma, and death, and abrupt withdrawal can lead to insomnia, anxiety, seizures, psychosis, and even death (63).

When compared to baclofen, clonazepam has demonstrated equivalent clinical efficacy in the management of spasticity overall and superior efficacy with spasticity secondary to cerebral origin (74). It is frequently used to treat phasic limb spasticity in people with MS.

Cannabis. Cannabis has been used as an agent to treat spasticity and pain that is found in patients with MS. It also demonstrated reduced central nervous system neurodegeneration in animal models of MS (75). The active component of marijuana is 9-tetrahydrocannibinol (9-THC) (76), and it is believed that most of the effects of cannabinoids occur through binding to CB1 and CB2 receptors. CB1 receptors are present throughout the nervous system, and CB2 receptors are located mainly on immune cells (63, 77, 78).

Cannabis is available as synthetic THC agents in 2 tablet forms, dronabinol and nabilone. Both agents are approved for chemotherapy-induced nausea, human immunodeficiency virus–related wasting, and glaucoma (63). Dronabinol is marketed under the trade name Marinol® and is available in 2.5-, 5-, and 10-mg capsules, with a maximum daily dosage of 20 mg. Nabilone is marketed under the name Cesamet®. It is available in 1-mg capsules with a recommended maximum dose of 6 mg per 24 hours. Sativex® is an 9-THC containing oral-mucosal spray currently available in Canada, where it is approved for the treatment of MS-related pain (79).

The literature concerning the use of cannabis on MS-related spasticity has been mixed. Zajicek et al. (77) conducted a randomized, double-blind, placebo-controlled trial evaluating the effects of cannabinoids on spasticity in 611 patients and found that the use of cannabis did not result in significant change in spasticity scores. They did note subjective improvement in spasm and sleep quality as well as a decrease in hospitalizations for exacerbation in the treatment group. The authors hypothesized that their inability to detect changes in spasticity may have been due to the inadequacy of the metric used (AS) to detect subtle changes. In addition, the patient sample consisted of a very impaired population as demonstrated by the fact that the EDSS of almost all the participants was greater than 6.0. It is possible that similar to the other oral antispasmodic medications, a greater benefit occurs when interventions are implemented earlier in the MS disease course. A 12-month follow-up study was conducted on the same patient group (80). Eighty percent of the original participants were followed up and they remained on active or placebo treatment. No significant improvement in spasticity scores was noticed in the active or placebo group. Another randomized, double-blind, placebo-controlled trial of 160 patients with MS demonstrated statistically significant reduction of spasticity with active cannabis compound over placebo (81). Both studies reported good tolerance of the medication. Common reported side effects of oral THC included increased appetite, dry mouth, somnolence, and bowel disturbance.

The potential clinical benefit of cannabis for people with MS remains unclear. In a survey of 14 patients with MS, each subject was asked a series of questions regarding the perceived benefit of marijuana (82). The participants reported improvement and reduction in spasms, pain, tremors, nausea, numbness, and bladder and bowel symptoms. Some negative effects reported by patients included decreased ability to concentrate as well as ataxia and fatigue. All participants used medical marijuana. Smoking marijuana for medical purposes is currently legal in 12 states; however, the federal government's authority can override a state's position.

Other Oral Medications. Threonine is a naturally occurring amino acid that is believed to have effects on the motor reflex arc and was reported to increase glycine levels in animal studies (83). Glycine is released from the interneurons in the gray matter of the spinal cord and Renshaw cells and is believed to inhibit excessive motor reflexes. Threonine is believed to further enhance glycinergic postsynaptic inhibition and thereby reduce increased motor activity or spasticity. A double-blind, placebo-controlled crossover trial in 26 ambulatory patients with MS was conducted to evaluate the effects of 7.5 mg/d of threonine on objective and subjective measures of spasticity (83). Threonine failed to demonstrate improvement in Ashworth scores or in the Patient Spasticity Scale or elevated glycine levels despite demonstration of elevated threonine levels in the cerebrospinal fluid and plasma. There was also no improvement in neurophysiologic studies. Another double-blind, placebo-controlled crossover study in patients with MS and SCI showed modest benefit in AS spasticity scores (84). This study by Lee et al suggested greater benefit in patients with spinal cord involvement. Both studies reported little if any sedative or confusion as side effects during the administration of threonine.

Gabapentin is approved for use as an anticonvulsant for partial seizures and for treatment of postherpetic neuralgia; however, its mechanism of action for spasticity is unknown (85). The literature is limited, with Dunevsky and Perel (86) reporting on its effectiveness on the spasticity of 2 people with MS-related

spasticity. A double-blind, placebo-controlled trial evaluated the utility of gabapentin as a primary and an adjunctive treatment for the management of spasticity (85). Gabapentin was noted to be superior as an adjunctive agent than as a primary antispasmodic therapy. It is generally well tolerated but can cause somnolence and fatigue in some patients and required no laboratory monitoring for safety.

Cyproheptadine is another drug that has been studied for its antispasmodic effects in this population (87). It is also indicated for the treatment of allergic symptoms as well as appetite stimulation (63). Interestingly, it has also been studied as a treatment for baclofen withdrawal symptoms (88). It functions as a serotonergic antagonist that modulates spinal reflexes to reduce spasticity. The recommended dosing is 4 mg qhs with gradual titration to 16 mg. Doses of 12 to 24 mg of cyproheptadine were studied in people with or SCI-related spasticity over 4 to 24 months and found effective as a primary and adjunctive antispasmodic agent (87).

Another drug studied for its antispasmodic effects is progabide, a GABA-A and GABA-B agonist (89). A randomized, double-blind, placebo-controlled crossover trial was conducted with this agent but failed to demonstrate functional changes. There was also issues with tolerability due to its side effects of drowsiness, dizziness, and nausea. In addition, elevation of transaminase levels required discontinuations in some people.

Carisoprodol, a derivative of the muscle relaxant meprobamate, is used for the treatment of skeletal muscle pain and frequently used to treat low back pain and fibromyalgia (28). Meprobamate functions through GABAergic neurotransmitter pathways and inhibits polysynaptic spinal reflexes. Carisoprodol was beneficial in patients with MS at 350 mg, BID. Its overall tolerability was good, with drowsiness and confusion as the main side effects.

All of the above agents can be used alone or in combination with each other as well as in combination with other modalities including therapy, chemodenervation, ITB pump, and surgery. Gradual titration is recommended for all of the antispasmodic medications to minimize side effects severity. Conversely, when discontinuing an agent, gradual titration is also recommended, as abruptly stopping the medication can trigger the onset of seizures and withdrawal symptoms.

Chemical Denervation

Spasticity that is focal or segmental can be effectively managed with chemical denervation (CD). Many of the systemic treatments for MS can cause sedation and fatigue confusion or negatively affect cognition. One of the biggest advantages of CD over oral medications is the lack of these side effects, which may make it much more appealing to patients. Unfortunately, none of the agents are permanent remedies, and people will have to return for reinjection. Chemical denervation is used to alleviate spasticity or flexor synergy patterns caused by UMN lesions. It can also be used before orthopedic procedures to determine if a joint has intra-articular contracture. If no improvement in spasticity or ROM is achieved through CD, then surgical intervention is usually recommended. As previously stated, spasticity can lead to inactivity, decreased joint ROM, and possibly contractures. Contractures can lead to skin breakdown and increased difficulty for the individual or caregiver to perform ADL. Another benefit of CD is ease in caregiving and reduced risk of contracture, ulcer, and inactivity. Agents commonly used for CD include lidocaine, bupivacaine, phenol, and botulinum toxin (BT).

Phenol/Ethanol/Alcohol. The first use of phenol for the treatment of spasticity was in 1965 by Nathan et al. (90) Concentrations of 5% to 7% of phenol are recommended for optimal effect and minimal side effects. Concentrations lower than 5% are usually ineffective, whereas concentrations greater than 7% can cause significant side effects including dysesthias, fibrosis, cellular damage, and cardiovascular complications. Phenol mixed with glycerin will form a more viscous solution that can reduce medication spread and minimize nerve injury and side effects (91). Phenol is indicated in patients with upper and lower limb spasticity who have demonstrated little to no functional benefit from other interventions including therapy, oral medications, and possibly BT injections. The effect of ethanol on spasticity in patients with MS is unknown. Phenol treatment has demonstrated improved personal hygiene care, transfers, ADL management, and decrease in skin ulcer formation in patients with MS (92, 93). It has also resulted in improved gait pattern with decreased scissoring in patients who underwent obturator nerve blocks (94).

Ethanol concentrations between 45% and 100% are recommended for CD. It has demonstrated benefit in poststroke knee flexor spasticity, elbow flexor spasticity, ankle spasticity, and adductor spasticity secondary to stroke or TBI (95–99). The advantages of both phenol and ethanol include immediate onset of action, duration of action spanning 3 to 9 months, and low cost. Both phenol and ethanol are indicated for relief of spasticity in ambulatory and bed-bound patients.

The potential adverse effects of phenol and ethanol injections includes paresthesias, dysesthesias, and pain and are more likely if sensory fibers are affected. Peripheral edema and muscle necrosis are also possible.

Botulinum Toxin. There are 7 immunological types of BT available with only types A and B approved for clinical use in the United States. (100) Although all 7 serotypes work through inhibition of acetylcholine release from the neuromuscular junction, they differ in their specific site of action. The toxin works selectively at peripheral cholinergic endings that lead to binding, internalization, and toxin activation at the neuromuscular junction resulting in CD. The inhibition of acetylcholine release causes muscle weakness. The effects of the toxin last approximately 60 to 90 days, depending on the serotype injected (101).

The efficacy of BT type A in the management of MS-related spasticity has been demonstrated in several studies (33, 102, 103). There are 2 important points that should be noted when using BTs for the management of spasticity. First is that the Food and Drug Administration has not approved the use of toxin in the management of spasticity, and therefore, one is using it off-label (104). Second, there is now a black box warning because of the relatively minimal risk of distal spread of toxin from the site that was injected. Dosing recommendations often do not reflect clinical practice. Allergan has suggested a starting dose of 400 U for their toxin Botox®, and Ipsen has suggested a starting dose of 1000 U for their toxin Dysport® in the treatment of arm spasticity, whereas published data showed safety using 1500 U of Dysport® (103). Experienced clinicians have often pushed to levels substantially higher than these (104), but this may require reevaluation with the new Food and Drug Administration black box warning. Patients with MS may be more prone to fatigue at higher doses. It is recommended to begin chemodenervation at low doses and undergo a gradual titration that balances positive effect while limiting fatigue or excessive flaccidity.

The advantages of BT for MS-associated spasticity are numerous. It can be used for focal or segmental areas of involvement and serve as a substitute for oral medications. The duration of effect of BT injections is usually several weeks to months, and the effects are reversible (105). The injections are usually well tolerated and do not cause sedation or negative cognitive effects and only rarely do people report fatigue. Injection site pain or discomfort is common and transient. Caution for aspiration pneumonia or dysphagia is necessary if cervical muscles are targeted. In addition, it is safe if used as an adjunctive treatment. Botulinum toxin injections localizations are normally done with electromyographic guidance or with neurostimulation. Some injection sites may require ultrasound or fluoroscopic guidance. The injector must be knowledgeable about the anatomy, innervations, kinesiology, and function of the muscles that are targeted. Although surface palpation can be used, the accuracy of injecting the targeted muscle declines as the muscle size diminishes (106–108). The disadvantages of BT injection are cost and the need for repeat injection (100). The use of BT for spasticity is an off-label use in the United States and therefore is not always covered by insurance plans.

In patients with MS-related spasticity, BT injection is indicated for equinovarus deformity, striatal toe, elbow flexor, or extensor spasticity, as well as hand involvement. Botulinum toxin injections have demonstrated benefit in patients with MS with adductor spasticity. Snow et al. (33) conducted the first double-blind, placebo-controlled crossover study in 9 wheelchair or bed-bound MS subjects with adductor spasticity. Each subject underwent injection of 400 U of BT type A (Dysport®) into the adductor brevis (2 sites of 50 U), adductor longus (100 U), and adductor magnus (100 U) through palpation-guided injection technique. A significant reduction in spasticity and improvement of hygiene were noted at 6 weeks in the active group compared to the placebo injection. No adverse events were reported.

A similar but larger dose-response, double-blind, placebo-controlled study was conducted by Hyman et al. (103) Seventy-four patients with MS with EDSS scores 7 or higher (rely on assistive device for ambulation) completed the trial with 4 study groups: placebo, 500 U, 1000 U, and 1500 U of BT type A (Dysport®). The medication was injected by palpation-guided technique targeting the adductors. Any oral antispasmodic medication or therapy the patient was taking or participating in before study initiation was continued. The study reported decrease in hip adductor spasticity in all groups, including the placebo group, with the greatest benefit and longest duration of action in the 1500 U dose group. Reduction in muscle tone was unique to the Dysport group. No statistically significant reduction was reported at any dose. Adverse events were similar across all groups except for muscle weakness, which was dose-dependent.

Physical and occupational therapy after injection of BT is frequently indicated and recommended. This allows for the subject's muscle to undergo "retraining" as well as to assist with improving ROM, gait, positioning, and performance of ADL. The use of BT injections combined with physical therapy to treat upper and lower limb spasticity in patients with MS has been studied and demonstrated benefit over BT alone (109).

Intrathecal Medications

The most common intrathecal drug used for spasticity treatment is baclofen. This is indicated in patients whose spasticity is so profound or diffuse that oral medications alone, or in combination with chemodenervation, are not sufficient to optimally manage spasms. An ITB pump allows for direct infusion of baclofen into the spinal fluid. Through this, the patient receives a dose that is 4 times the strength of oral dosages with 1/100 the systemic dose and 1/100 the plasma dose. Patients should undergo a trial before ITB pump implantation. The ITB pump trial involves injection of approximately 50 to 100 µg of baclofen injected into the intrathecal space, and the patient's response to the drug is monitored over several hours. This helps discern between increased muscle tone and contracture, as well as to give the patient and their family an idea of how their spasticity can be controlled with an ITB pump. The infusion of the drug occurs in a 4:1 lumbar-to-cervical spine ratio, meaning that significantly more drug will be delivered to the lower limbs compared to the upper limbs.

The benefit of ITB is reduced cognitive or fatiguing effects as compared to systemic agents (110). In addition, there is also no respiratory depression or adverse effect on sleep reported in patients with MS (111). Postimplantation, it generally takes about 6 months for stabilization and optimal dosing of the ITB pump. The additional challenge in MS as compared to other conditions (stroke, TBI, cerebral palsy [CP]) is the disease variability and its vulnerability to heat and fatigue. It normally requires several months for ITB pump optimization to obtain maximum function and comfort (112).

In the population with MS, the use of ITB pumps has resulted in improvements in spasticity, quality of life, sleep quality, bowel and bladder performance, skin integrity, and ambulation in numerous studies (32, 112–116). Potential complications include pump failure, infection, and catheter kinking, dislodgement, or occlusion. The complication rate has also declined over the past several years. Catheter problems remain one of the most common complications (112). A 10-year retrospective analysis of 50 patients who had MS (n = 19), TBI (n = 28), or CP (n = 13) was conducted. The patients with MS who underwent ITB pump implantation reported increase in comfort, ease of care, improved safety on transfers, increased independence, and better communication (117). Seventy-eight percent of subjects self-reported that their long-term goals were achieved with pump implantation. The average ITB dosage for the patient with MS was 238 compared to 535 and 908 µg/d for CP and TBI patients, respectively.

Intrathecal phenol in concentration of 5% to 8% has been administered in 25 patients with MS whose EDSS is 8.0 or higher, with significant lower limb spasticity, and who did not have any noticeable benefit from other treatments (oral medication, therapies CD) (91). After a diagnostic trial was done with bupivacaine, those patients that responded positively received 1.5 to 2.5 mL of intrathecal phenol at the L2-3 or L3-4 space. All patients had significant decreases in Ashworth spasticity scales in all tested muscle groups with specific decreases in flexor, extensor, and dorsiflexor tone in both lower limbs. Pain was not affected but also did not increase from the phenol injections. Adverse effects included transient bowel dysfunction. Bladder and sexual function were not affected. The positive study results suggest another intervention option to ITB in patients who may not have positive benefit from the trial, are not suitable candidates, or cannot afford the procedure.

Surgical Interventions

Surgical interventions in the patient with MS can be for diagnostic or therapeutic reasons (118). Symptomatic surgical interventions for spasticity primarily involve dorsal rhizotomy, which is believed to alleviate the imbalance in the sensory input affecting motor control. Other surgical procedures, including myelotomy and cordectomy, are no longer commonly performed. A retrospective study of 154 patients (52 patients with MS) who underwent posterior rhizotomy reported improved spasticity in all patients, an 86% improvement in ROM, and an 80% reduction in pain (119). Adverse reactions included transient bladder incontinence and wound infection.

SUMMARY

A multimodal and dynamic approach to managing spasticity in the MS population is crucial for best results (120). In contrast to the previously preferred stepwise approach to therapies, the combination of various modalities, therapies, and interventions is now recommended. Establishing clear short-term and long-term goals with the patient and caregivers is crucial. A person's MS can cause neurologic change from day to day, even hour to hour, so it is important that patients are aware of their body and be attuned to possible relapses, infection, or disease progression. Accordingly, professionals treating patients with MS must be aware that spasticity in MS can change rapidly and should be prepared to adjust treatments as needed to accommodate the patient's condition.

Short-term and long-term goal-setting is crucial in the process. Input from the patient, clinician, and care providers should be taken into consideration when forming goals. Additional factors to consider include the time since onset of spasticity, the severity of any deformity, and its functional effects. The cognitive status of the patient will help determine if compliance is anticipated. Finally, cost and adherence to therapy are important, especially when considering procedures that require regular follow-up, such as serial casting or ITB placement.

Spasticity in MS does not have to be a significant barrier to function and well-being. Creative planning and intervention with an armamentarium of treatments can result in minimization of the negative effects of spasticity with preservation of function and comfort for the patient.

References

1. Anderson DW, Ellenberg JH, Leventhal CM, Reingold SC, Rodriguez M, Silberberg DH. Revised estimate of the prevalence of multiple sclerosis in the United States. *Ann Neurol* 1992;31:333–6.
2. Hirtz D, Thurman DJ, Gwinn-Hardy K, Mohamed M, Chaudhuri AR, Zalutsky R. How common are the "common" neurologic disorders? *Neurology* 2007;68:326–37.
3. Hemmett L, Holmes J, Barnes M, Russell N. What drives quality of life in multiple sclerosis? *QJM* 2004;97:671–6.
4. Rizzo MA, Hadjimichael OC, Preiningerova J, Vollmer TL. Prevalence and treatment of spasticity reported by multiple sclerosis patients. *Mult Scler* 2004;10:589–95.
5. Haselkorn JK, Balsdon Richer C, Fry Welch D, et al. Overview of spasticity management in multiple sclerosis. Evidence-based management strategies for spasticity treatment in multiple sclerosis. *J Spinal Cord Med* 2005;28:167–99.
6. Lance JW. The control of muscle tone, reflexes, and movement: Robert Wartenberg lecture. *Neurology* 1980;30:1303–13.
7. Barnes MP, Kent RM, Semlyen JK, McMullen KM. Spasticity in multiple sclerosis. *Neurorehabil Neural Repair* 2003;17:66–70.
8. Olgiati R, Burgunder JM, Mumenthaler M. Increased energy cost of walking in multiple sclerosis: effect of spasticity, ataxia, and weakness. *Arch Phys Med Rehabil* 1988;69:846–9.
9. Weinshenker BG. Epidemiology of multiple sclerosis. *Neurol Clin* 1996;14:291–308.
10. Alonso A, Hernan MA. Temporal trends in the incidence of multiple sclerosis: a systematic review. *Neurology* 2008;71:129–35.
11. Rosati G. The prevalence of multiple sclerosis in the world: an update. *Neurol Sci* 2001;22:117–39.
12. Sheean G. The pathophysiology of spasticity. *Eur J Neurol* 2002;9 Suppl 1:3-9; dicussion 53–61.
13. Satkunam LE. Rehabilitation medicine: 3. Management of adult spasticity. *CMAJ* 2003;169:1173–9.

14. Nielsen JB, Crone C, Hultborn H. The spinal pathophysiology of spasticity—from a basic science point of view. *Acta Physiol (Oxf)* 2007;189:171–80.

15. Ivanhoe CB, Reistetter TA. Spasticity: the misunderstood part of the upper motor neuron syndrome. *Am J Phys Med Rehabil* 2004;83:S3–9.

16. Haus JM, Carrithers JA, Carroll CC, Tesch PA, Trappe TA. Contractile and connective tissue protein content of human skeletal muscle: effects of 35 and 90 days of simulated microgravity and exercise countermeasures. *Am J Physiol Regul Integr Comp Physiol* 2007;293:R1722–7.

17. LeBlanc AD, Spector ER, Evans HJ, Sibonga JD. Skeletal responses to space flight and the bed rest analog: a review. *J Musculoskelet Neuronal Interact* 2007;7:33–47.

18. Allen C, Glasziou P, Del Mar C. Bed rest: a potentially harmful treatment needing more careful evaluation. *Lancet* 1999;354:1229–33.

19. Berg HE, Dudley GA, Haggmark T, Ohlsen H, Tesch PA. Effects of lower limb unloading on skeletal muscle mass and function in humans. *J Appl Physiol* 1991;70:1882–5.

20. Braddom R. *Physical medicine and rehabilitation.* Third ed. Philadelphia: WB Saunders; 2005.

21. Hidler JM, Harvey RL, Rymer WZ. Frequency response characteristics of ankle plantar flexors in humans following spinal cord injury: relation to degree of spasticity. *Ann Biomed Eng* 2002;30:969–81.

22. Kelsey JL. Risk factors for osteoporosis and associated fractures. *Public Health Rep* 1989;104 Suppl:14–20.

23. Statement NC. Osteoporosis prevention, diagnosis, and therapy. *NIH Consens Statement* 2000;17:1–45.

24. Taylor ML. The effects of rest in bed and of exercise on cardiovascular function. *Circulation* 1968;38:1016–7.

25. Dorfman TA, Levine BD, Tillery T, et al. Cardiac atrophy in women following bed rest. *J Appl Physiol* 2007;103:8–16.

26. Hobart J, Lamping D, Fitzpatrick R, Riazi A, Thompson A. The Multiple Sclerosis Impact Scale (MSIS-29): a new patient-based outcome measure. *Brain* 2001;124:962–73.

27. van Wijck FM, Pandyan AD, Johnson GR, Barnes MP. Assessing motor deficits in neurological rehabilitation: patterns of instrument usage. *Neurorehabil Neural Repair* 2001;15:23–30.

28. Ashworth B. Preliminary trial of carisoprodol in multiple sclerosis. *Practitioner* 1964;192:540–2.

29. Bohannon RW, Smith MB. Interrater reliability of a Modified Ashworth Scale of muscle spasticity. *Phys Ther* 1987;67:206–7.

30. Held JP. The reeducation of paraplegics. *Cah Coll Med Hop Paris* 1967;8:679–86.

31. Haugh AB, Pandyan AD, Johnson GR. A systematic review of the Tardieu Scale for the measurement of spasticity. *Disabil Rehabil* 2006;28:899–907.

32. Penn RD, Savoy SM, Corcos D, et al. Intrathecal baclofen for severe spinal spasticity. *N Engl J Med* 1989;320:1517–21.

33. Snow BJ, Tsui JK, Bhatt MH, Varelas M, Hashimoto SA, Calne DB. Treatment of spasticity with botulinum toxin: a double-blind study. *Ann Neurol* 1990;28:512–5.

34. Podsiadlo D, Richardson S. The timed "up & go": a test of basic functional mobility for frail elderly persons. *J Am Geriatr Soc* 1991;39:142–8.

35. Hauser SL, Dawson DM, Lehrich JR, et al. Intensive immunosuppression in progressive multiple sclerosis. A randomized, three-arm study of high-dose intravenous cyclophosphamide, plasma exchange, and ACTH. *N Engl J Med* 1983;308:173–80.

36. Berg KO, Wood-Dauphinee SL, Williams JI, Maki B. Measuring balance in the elderly: validation of an instrument. *Can J Public Health* 1992;83 Suppl 2:S7–11.

37. Kurtzke JF. Rating neurologic impairment in multiple sclerosis: an Expanded Disability Status Scale (EDSS). *Neurology* 1983;33:1444–52.

38. Brouwer B, de Andrade V. The effects of slow stroking on spasticity in patients with multiple sclerosis: a pilot study. *Physiother Theory Pract* 1995;11:13–21.

39. Beenakker EA, Oparina TI, Hartgring A, Teelken A, Arutjunyan AV, De Keyser J. Cooling garment treatment in MS: clinical improvement and decrease in leukocyte NO production. *Neurology* 2001;57:892–4.

40. Chiara T, Carlos J, Jr., Martin D, Miller R, Nadeau S. Cold effect on oxygen uptake, perceived exertion, and spasticity in patients with multiple sclerosis. *Arch Phys Med Rehabil* 1998;79:523–8.

41. Hartviksen K. Ice therapy in spasticity. *Acta Neurol Scand* 1962;38 (suppl):79–84.

42. Schwid SR, Petrie MD, Murray R, et al. A randomized controlled study of the acute and chronic effects of cooling therapy for MS. *Neurology* 2003;60:1955–60.

43. Little JW, Massagli TL. *Spasticity and associated abnormalities of muscle tone.* 3 ed. Philadelphia: Lippincott-Raven; 1998.

44. Flensner G, Lindencrona C. The cooling-suit: a study of ten multiple sclerosis patients' experiences in daily life. *J Adv Nurs* 1999;29:1444–53.

45. Tekeoglu Y, Adak B, Goksoy T. Effect of transcutaneous electrical nerve stimulation (TENS) on Barthel Activities of Daily Living (ADL) index score following stroke. *Clin Rehabil* 1998;12:277–80.

46. Goulet C, Arsenault AB, Bourbonnais D, Laramee MT, Lepage Y. Effects of transcutaneous electrical nerve stimulation on H-reflex and spinal spasticity. *Scand J Rehabil Med* 1996;28:169–76.

47. Armutlu K, Meric A, Kirdi N, Yakut E, Karabudak R. The effect of transcutaneous electrical nerve stimulation on spasticity in multiple sclerosis patients: a pilot study. *Neurorehabil Neural Repair* 2003;17:79–82.

48. Miller L, Mattison P, Paul L, Wood L. The effects of transcutaneous electrical nerve stimulation (TENS) on spasticity in multiple sclerosis. *Mult Scler* 2007;13:527–33.

49. Szecsi J, Schlick C, Schiller M, Pollmann W, Koenig N, Straube A. Functional electrical stimulation–assisted cycling of patients with multiple sclerosis: biomechanical and functional outcome—a pilot study. *J Rehabil Med* 2009; 41(8):674–680.

50. Sheffler LR, Hennessey MT, Knutson JS, Naples GG, Chae J. Functional effect of an ankle foot orthosis on gait in multiple sclerosis: a pilot study. *Am J Phys Med Rehabil* 2008;87:26–32.

51. Sutliff MH, Naft JM, Stough DK, Lee JC, Arrigain SS, Bethoux FA. Efficacy and safety of a hip flexion assist orthosis in ambulatory multiple sclerosis patients. *Arch Phys Med Rehabil* 2008;89:1611–7.

52. Cattaneo D, Marazzini F, Crippa A, Cardini R. Do static or dynamic AFOs improve balance? *Clin Rehabil* 2002;16:894–9.

53. Stoeckmann T. Casting for the person with spasticity. *Top Stroke Rehabil* 2001;8:27–35.

54. Kay RM, Rethlefsen SA, Fern-Buneo A, Wren TA, Skaggs DL. Botulinum toxin as an adjunct to serial casting treatment in children with cerebral palsy. *J Bone Joint Surg Am* 2004;86-A:2377–84.

55. Robichaud JA, Agostinucci J. Air-splint pressure effect on soleus muscle alpha motoneuron reflex excitability in subjects with spinal cord injury. *Arch Phys Med Rehabil* 1996;77:778–82.

56. Chou R, Peterson K, Helfand M. Comparative efficacy and safety of skeletal muscle relaxants for spasticity and musculoskeletal conditions: a systematic review. *J Pain Symptom Manage* 2004;28:140–75.

57. Basmajian JV. Lioresal (baclofen) treatment of spasticity in multiple sclerosis. *Am J Phys Med* 1975 Aug;54:175–177.

58. From A, Heltberg A. A double-blind trial with baclofen (Lioresal) and diazepam in spasticity due to multiple sclerosis. *Acta Neurol Scand* 1975 Feb;51:158–166.

59. Hedley DW, Maroun JA, Espir ML. Evaluation of baclofen (Lioresal) for spasticity in multiple sclerosis. *Postgrad Med J* 1975 Sep;51:615–618.

60. Orsnes GB, Sorensen PS, Larsen TK, Ravnborg M. Effect of baclofen on gait in spastic MS patients. *Acta Neurol Scand* 2000 Apr;101:244–248.

61. Feldman RG, Kelly-Hayes M, Conomy JP, Foley JM. Baclofen for spasticity in multiple sclerosis. Double-blind crossover and three-year study. *Neurology* 1978;28:1094–8.

62. Ward A, Chaffman MO, Sorkin EM. Dantrolene. A review of its pharmacodynamic and pharmacokinetic properties and therapeutic use in malignant hyperthermia, the neuroleptic malignant syndrome and an update of its use in muscle spasticity. *Drugs* 1986;32:130–68.

63. Zafonte R, Lombard L, Elovic E. Antispasticity medications: uses and limitations of enteral therapy. *Am J Phys Med Rehabil* 2004;83:S50–8.

64. Chyatte SB, Birdsong JH, Bergman BA. The effects of dantrolene sodium on spasticity and motor performance in hemiplegia. *South Med J* 1971 Feb;64:180–185.

65. Tolosa ES, Soll RW, Loewenson RB. Letter: treatment of spasticity in multiple sclerosis with dantrolene. *JAMA* 1975 Sep 8;233:1046.

66. Nance PW, Sheremata WA, Lynch SG, et al. Relationship of the antispasticity effect of tizanidine to plasma concentration in patients with multiple sclerosis. *Arch Neurol* 1997;54:731–6.

67. A double-blind, placebo-controlled trial of tizanidine in the treatment of spasticity caused by multiple sclerosis. United Kingdom Tizanidine Trial Group. *Neurology* 1994;44:S70–8.

68. Bass B, Weinshenker B, Rice GP, et al. Tizanidine versus baclofen in the treatment of spasticity in patients with multiple sclerosis. *Can J Neurol Sci* 1988;15:15–9.

69. Lapierre Y, Bouchard S, Tansey C, Gendron D, Barkas WJ, Francis GS. Treatment of spasticity with tizanidine in multiple sclerosis. *Can J Neurol Sci* 1987;14:513–7.

70. Naftchi NE, Schlosser W, Horst WD. Correlation of changes in the GABA-ergic system with the development of spasticity in paraplegic cats. *Adv Exp Med Biol* 1979;123:431–50.

71. Cartlidge NE, Hudgson P, Weightman D. A comparison of baclofen and diazepam in the treatment of spasticity. *J Neurol Sci* 1974;23:17–24.

72. Verrier M, Ashby P, MacLeod S. Diazepam effect on reflex activity in patients with complete spinal lesions and in those with other causes of spasticity. *Arch Phys Med Rehabil* 1977;58:148–53.

73. Schmidt RT, Lee RH, Spehlmann R. Comparison of dantrolene sodium and diazepam in the treatment of spasticity. *J Neurol Neurosurg Psychiatry* 1976;39:350–6.

74. Cendrowski W, Sobczyk W. Clonazepam, baclofen and placebo in the treatment of spasticity. *Eur Neurol* 1977;16:257–62.

75. Pryce G, Ahmed Z, Hankey DJ, et al. Cannabinoids inhibit neurodegeneration in models of multiple sclerosis. *Brain* 2003;126:2191–202.

76. Wade DT, Makela P, Robson P, House H, Bateman C. Do cannabis-based medicinal extracts have general or specific effects on symptoms in multiple sclerosis? A double-blind, randomized, placebo-controlled study on 160 patients. *Mult Scler* 2004;10:434–41.

77. Zajicek J, Fox P, Sanders H, et al. Cannabinoids for treatment of spasticity and other symptoms related to multiple sclerosis (CAMS study): multicentre randomised placebo-controlled trial. *Lancet* 2003;362:1517–26.

78. Ben Amar M. Cannabinoids in medicine: a review of their therapeutic potential. *J Ethnopharmacol* 2006;105:1–25.

79. Barnes MP. Sativex: clinical efficacy and tolerability in the treatment of symptoms of multiple sclerosis and neuropathic pain. *Expert Opin Pharmacother* 2006;7:607–15.

80. Zajicek JP, Sanders HP, Wright DE, et al. Cannabinoids in multiple sclerosis (CAMS) study: safety and efficacy data for 12 months follow up. *J Neurol Neurosurg Psychiatry* 2005;76:1664–9.

81. Collin C, Davies P, Mutiboko IK, Ratcliffe S. Randomized controlled trial of cannabis-based medicine in spasticity caused by multiple sclerosis. *Eur J Neurol* 2007;14:290–6.

82. Page SA, Verhoef MJ. Medicinal marijuana use: experiences of people with multiple sclerosis. *Can Fam Physician* 2006;52:64–5.

83. Hauser SL, Doolittle TH, Lopez-Bresnahan M, et al. An antispasticity effect of threonine in multiple sclerosis. *Arch Neurol* 1992;49:923–6.

84. Lee A, Patterson V. A double-blind study of L-threonine in patients with spinal spasticity. *Acta Neurol Scand* 1993;88: 334–8.

85. Mueller ME, Gruenthal M, Olson WL, Olson WH. Gabapentin for relief of upper motor neuron symptoms in multiple sclerosis. *Arch Phys Med Rehabil* 1997;78:521–4.

86. Dunevsky A, Perel AB. Gabapentin for relief of spasticity associated with multiple sclerosis. *Am J Phys Med Rehabil* 1998;77:451–4.

87. Barbeau H, Richards C, Bedard P. Action of cyrohepatadine in spastic paraparetic patients. *J Neurol Neurosurg Psychiatry* 1982;45:923–6.

88. Meythaler JM, Roper JF, Brunner RC. Cyproheptadine for intrathecal baclofen withdrawal. *Arch Phys Med Rehabil* 2003;84:638–42.

89. Rudick RA, Breton D, Krall RL. The GABA-agonist progabide for spasticity in multiple sclerosis. *Arch Neurol* 1987;44:1033–6.

90. Nathan PW, Sears TA, Smith MC. Effects of phenol solutions on the nerve roots of the cat: an electrophysiological and histological study. *J Neurol Sci* 1965;2:7–29.

91. Jarrett L, Nandi P, Thompson AJ. Managing severe lower limb spasticity in multiple sclerosis: does intrathecal phenol have a role? *J Neurol Neurosurg Psychiatry* 2002;73: 705–9.

92. Awad EA. Phenol block for control of hip flexor and adductor spasticity. *Arch Phys Med Rehabil* 1972;53:554–7.

93. Copp EP, Harris R, Keenan J. Peripheral nerve block and motor point block with phenol in the management of spasticity. *Proc R Soc Med* 1970;63:937–8.

94. Wassef MR. Interadductor approach to obturator nerve blockade for spastic conditions of adductor thigh muscles. *Reg Anesth* 1993;18:13–7.

95. Chua KS, Kong KH. Clinical and functional outcome after alcohol neurolysis of the tibial nerve for ankle-foot spasticity. *Brain Inj* 2001;15:733–9.

96. Chua KS, Kong KH. Alcohol neurolysis of the sciatic nerve in the treatment of hemiplegic knee flexor spasticity: clinical outcomes. *Arch Phys Med Rehabil* 2000;81:1432–5.

97. Kong KH, Chua KS. Neurolysis of the musculocutaneous nerve with alcohol to treat poststroke elbow flexor spasticity. *Arch Phys Med Rehabil* 1999;80:1234–6.

98. Jang SH, Ahn SH, Park SM, Kim SH, Lee KH, Lee ZI. Alcohol neurolysis of tibial nerve motor branches to the gastrocnemius muscle to treat ankle spasticity in patients with hemiplegic stroke. *Arch Phys Med Rehabil* 2004;85: 506–8.

99. Viel EJ, Perennou D, Ripart J, Pelissier J, Eledjam JJ. Neurolytic blockade of the obturator nerve for intractable spasticity of adductor thigh muscles. *Eur J Pain* 2002;6:97–104.

100. Davis EC, Barnes MP. Botulinum toxin and spasticity. *J Neurol Neurosurg Psychiatry* 2000;69:143–7.

101. Ramachandran M, Eastwood DM. Botulinum toxin and its orthopaedic applications. *J Bone Joint Surg Br* 2006;88:981–7.

102. Giovannelli M, Borriello G, Castri P, Prosperini L, Pozzilli C. Early physiotherapy after injection of botulinum toxin increases the beneficial effects on spasticity in patients with multiple sclerosis. *Clin Rehabil* 2007; 21(4):331–337.

103. Hyman N, Barnes M, Bhakta B et al. Botulinum toxin (Dysport) treatment of hip adductor spasticity in multiple sclerosis: a prospective, randomised, double blind, placebo controlled, dose ranging study. *J Neurol Neurosurg Psychiatry* 2000; 68(6):707–712.

104. Elovic,EP, Eisenberg, ME, Jasey,N.N. *Spasticity and muscle overactivity as components of the upper motor neuron syndrome in physical medicine and rehabilitation: principles and practice* 5th Edition; Lippincott Williams & Wilkins (Publishers) Editors Frontera. Philadelphia in press

105. Jost WH. Botulinum toxin in multiple sclerosis. *J Neurol* 2006;253 Suppl 1:I16–20.

106. Kinnett D. Botulinum toxin A injections in children: technique and dosing issues. *Am J Phys Med Rehabil* 2004;83:S59–64.

107. Chin TY, Nattrass GR, Selber P, Graham HK. Accuracy of intramuscular injection of botulinum toxin A in juvenile cerebral palsy: a comparison between manual needle placement and placement guided by electrical stimulation. *J Pediatr Orthop* 2005;25:286–91.

108. Molloy FM, Shill HA, Kaelin-Lang A, Karp BI. Accuracy of muscle localization without EMG: implications for treatment of limb dystonia. *Neurology* 2002;58:805–7.

109. Giovannelli M, Borriello G, Castri P, Prosperini L, Pozzilli C. Early physiotherapy after injection of botulinum toxin increases the beneficial effects on spasticity in patients with multiple sclerosis. *Clin Rehabil* 2007;21:331–7.

110. Zierski J, Muller H, Dralle D, Wurdinger T. Implanted pump systems for treatment of spasticity. *Acta Neurochir Suppl* (Wien) 1988;43:94–9.

111. Bensmail D, Quera Salva MA, Roche N, et al. Effect of intrathecal baclofen on sleep and respiratory function in patients with spasticity. *Neurology* 2006;67:1432–6.

112. Sadiq SA, Wang GC. Long-term intrathecal baclofen therapy in ambulatory patients with spasticity. *J Neurol* 2006;253:563–9.

113. Coffey JR, Cahill D, Steers W, et al. Intrathecal baclofen for intractable spasticity of spinal origin: results of a long-term multicenter study. *J Neurosurg* 1993;78:226–32.

114. Ben Smail D, Peskine A, Roche N, Mailhan L, Thiebaut I, Bussel B. Intrathecal baclofen for treatment of spasticity of multiple sclerosis patients. *Mult Scler* 2006;12:101–3.

115. Parke B, Penn RD, Savoy SM, Corcos D. Functional outcome after delivery of intrathecal baclofen. *Arch Phys Med Rehabil* 1989;70:30–2.

116. Zahavi A, Geertzen JH, Middel B, Staal M, Rietman JS. Long term effect (more than five years) of intrathecal baclofen on impairment, disability, and quality of life in patients with severe spasticity of spinal origin. *J Neurol Neurosurg Psychiatry* 2004;75:1553–7.

117. Rawlins PK. Intrathecal baclofen therapy over 10 years. *J Neurosci Nurs* 2004;36:322–7.

118. Patwardhan RV, Minagar A, Kelley RE, Nanda A. Neurosurgical treatment of multiple sclerosis. *Neurol Res* 2006;28:320–5.

119. Salame K, Ouaknine GE, Rochkind S, Constantini S, Razon N. Surgical treatment of spasticity by selective posterior rhizotomy: 30 years experience. *Isr Med Assoc J* 2003;5:543–6.

120. Kabus C, Hecht M, Japp G, et al. Botulinum toxin in patients with multiple sclerosis. *J Neurol* 2006;253 Suppl 1:I26–8.

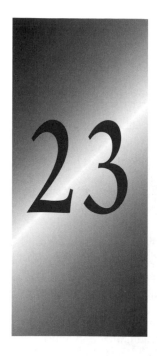

Spasticity Due to Stroke Pathophysiology

23

Anthony B. Ward
Surendra Bandi

What is spasticity and why is it so important to manage it effectively? This chapter will address these 2 questions to assist the reader to recognize, assess, and treat people with this impairment. Spasticity is a physiological consequence of an insult to the brain or spinal cord, which can lead to life-threatening, disabling, and costly consequences. It is a common but not an inevitable outcome of the upper motor neuron (UMN) syndrome—typically occurring after a stroke, brain injury (whether due to trauma or other causes, eg, hypoxia, infections, or postsurgery), spinal cord injury, multiple sclerosis, cerebral palsy, and other disabling neurologic disorders. It is characterized by muscle overactivity and high tone spasms, which, if left untreated, will lead to muscle and soft tissue contracture (1). It is a complex problem, which can cause profound disability, alone or in combination with the other features of the UMN syndrome and can give rise to significant difficulties during the process of rehabilitation.

DEFINITION OF SPASTICITY

Over time there have been many different attempts to define spasticity (2). The difficulty in defining spasticity reflects the complex features of the syndrome. Lance's (3) definition since 1980 is still relevant and is widely accepted. Lance states, "Spasticity is a motor disorder characterized by a velocity-dependent increase in tonic stretch reflexes (muscle tone) with exaggerated tendon jerks, resulting from hyper-excitability of the stretch reflex, as one component of the upper motor neuron syndrome."

More recently, this definition was broadened to include other signs of the UMN syndrome and described spasticity as "a motor disorder characterized by a velocity dependent increase in tonic stretch reflexes that results from abnormal intra-spinal processing of primary afferent input." (4)

Applying Lance's definition to patients in clinical settings has been difficult because UMN lesions produce an array of responses. The pattern depends on the age and onset of the lesion and its location and size. Patients with diffuse lesions produce, for instance, different characteristics to those with localized pathology, and the speed of onset changes this again (3). The Support Programme for Assembly of Database for Spasticity Measurement (SPASM) consortium has attempted to adapt the accepted definition to a more practical base and make it more relevant to clinical practice and to clinical research (2). Its definition is thus as follows in Table 23.1.

The epidemiology put in terms of a 250,000 population (9) thus equates to:

- 320 new first time strokes with a prevalence of 1675 people

357

TABLE 23.1
SPASM Principles

DOMAIN	DESCRIPTION
Etiology	Typically occurs in patients after any dysfunction to the UMN, such as stroke, brain injury (trauma and other causes, e.g., anoxia, postneurosurgery), spinal cord injury, multiple sclerosis, and other disabling neurologic diseases and cerebral palsy (5, 6).
Classification	Frequently classified by its presentation, and differences exist between the clinical features seen after a spinal cause as opposed to a cerebral cause. It is not always harmful but can create problems, which may be: –generalized, and/or –regional, and/or –focal problems
Epidemiology	Figures for prevalence of spasticity in different conditions are variable (5–7). This may be due to the presence of many patients with mild spasticity for whom little or no treatment is required for their condition. However, it is estimated that 38% of patients after stroke develop a degree of spasticity. Of which about 16% require pharmacologic treatment. Of these, about one third (5% of total) will benefit from BoNT injection (8). In addition, 18% of patients with severe traumatic brain injury and 60% of patients moderately severely and severely disabled by multiple sclerosis (30% of the total population of patients with multiple sclerosis) require specific treatment along with smaller numbers of people with cerebral palsy, spinal cord injury, and other cerebral and spinal cord pathologies.

SPASM definition. *Disabil Rehabil.* 2006;28 (Suppl. 1).

- 48 people with severe traumatic brain injury with a prevalence of 260 people
- 500 people with multiple sclerosis, of whom 100 are severely disabled
- 31 adults with cerebral palsy
- plus other conditions affecting the UMN.

About 500 patients require spasticity treatment at some point time.

PATHOPHYSIOLOGY OF SPASTICITY

Overview

Spasticity is one feature of the UMN syndrome—historically been described as a collection of positive and negative features. Positive features include muscle overactivity, hyperactive tendon reflexes, clonus, brisk reflexes, cutaneous reflexes (the most familiar of which is the Babinski sign), flexor and extensor spasms, spastic dystonia, and mass synergy patterns. The negative phenomena are paresis, loss of dexterity and fine control, fatigability, and early hypotonia (4).

Pathophysiology

The pathophysiology of the UMN syndrome and its associated features are complex and are described in the appendix of this chapter for those wishing for a more detailed account. This addresses and distinguishes spasticity itself from spinal reflexes, hypertonia, clasp-knife response, associated reactions and mass reflex action, flexor muscle spasms, disordered control of movement, thixotropy, and muscle contractures and as one consequence of an injury to the UMN and results in several physiological scenarios, including muscle overactivity.

WHY TREAT SPASTICITY?

The consequences of not treating spasticity adequately are listed in Table 23.2. The misery of painful spasms or of tendon traction on bones is well known, and the complications will prevent patients from achieving their optimal functioning (9). Deconditioning from ill health and pain will also have a negative effect, which will reduce quality of life for patients and their carers. There are therefore very good clinical, humanis-

TABLE 23.2
Some Consequences of Inadequate Spasticity Treatment

DOMAIN	CONSEQUENCE
Impairment	Muscle shortening
	Stiff, painful joints
	Joint subluxation
	Contractures
	Limb deformity and disfigurement
	Pain—muscle spasms, enthesopathy, bone (osteoporosis)
	Loading on pressure points and pressure sores
	Mood problems
Activity	Loss of mobility, dexterity
	Self-care problems
	Loss of sexual functioning
Participation	Need for special wheelchairs and seating and pressure-relieving equipment
	Inability to participate in rehabilitation
	Increased care
Quality of Life	Altered body image

TABLE 23.3
Goals for Treatment

INDICATION	EXAMPLE
Functional improvement	Mobility: enhance speed, quality or endurance of gait or wheelchair propulsion
	Improve transfers
	Improve dexterity and reaching
	Ease sexual functioning
Symptom relief	Relieve pain and muscle spasms
	Allow wearing of splints and orthoses
	Promote hygiene
	Prevent contractures
Postural improvement	Enhance body image
Decrease carer burden	Help with dressing
	Improve care and hygiene
	Positioning for feeding, etc
Enhance service activity	Prevent need for unnecessary medication & other treatments
	Facilitate therapy
	Delay or prevent surgery

tic, and economic reasons to treat it effectively and judiciously.

PRINCIPLES OF SPASTICITY TREATMENT

Aims of Management

The main goals for therapy are the following:

- To increase functional capacity, where it is possible to do so
- To relieve symptoms
- To improve posture, appearance, and body image
- To decrease carer burden
- To prevent complications, facilitate therapy, and enhance effect of other treatments.

Some goals are listed in Table 23.3 but should be consistent with the overall rehabilitation goals agreed between the patient, family/carers, and rehabilitation professionals (10). All those involved require to be clear on the treatment goal(s), and patient expectations need to be managed in some cases.

Successful treatment strategies have now been developed, and there is good evidence of treatment effectiveness (Figure 23.1). Physical management (good nursing care, physiotherapy, occupational therapy) through postural management, exercise, stretching and

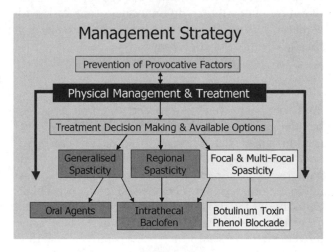

FIGURE 23.1

Management strategy in a patient with spasticity.

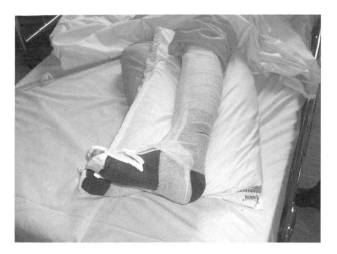

FIGURE 23.2

A patient with lower extremity spasticity undergoing casting.

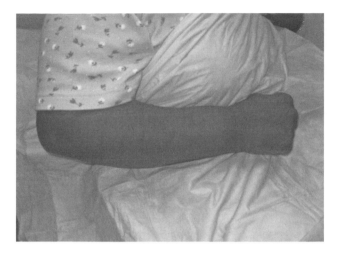

FIGURE 23.3

Focal spasticity of the hand and wrist.

strengthening of limbs, splinting, and pain relief is the basis of spasticity management (9). Figure 23.2 demonstrates early casting for spasticity management. The aim of treatment in all cases is to reduce abnormal sensory inputs in order to decrease excessive α-motor neuron activity (11). A program of physical treatment should thus be in place before, during, and after any pharmacologic, medical, or surgical intervention, but there is little evidence on the ideal prescription for this (12). All pharmacologic interventions are adjunctive to a program of physical intervention. Stretching plays an important part in physical management but needs to be applied for several hours per day (13, 14). This is of course impossible to do on a one-to-one basis with a therapist, and limb casting has been developed in this field to provide a prolonged stretch (14).

Patient Assessment

Spasticity is a movement disorder, and patients cannot be adequately assessed unless they are observed during movement and function (10). All the team members contribute to the clinical evaluation, but some patients with complex movement patterns need assessing in a gait laboratory. The assessment process highlights the differences in patterns of limb posture and movement after a UMN lesion. Where there is no movement, the assessment process is fairly straightforward, but where there is loss of motor control rather than a spastic dystonia, one has to attempt to identify the different aspects of motor impairment. Patients with long-standing problems also develop compen-

satory movements, which may or may not require treatment, and the clinician has to be clear about the underlying pathophysiological processes.

It is important to identify how function is impaired and whether the generalized, focal, or regional problem is due to spasticity. Figures 23.3 and 23.4 demonstrate examples of focal and generalized spasticity. This will then point to the options for treatment. The indication for pharmacologic treatment therefore is when spasticity is causing the patient harm. Some patients early on in their rehabilitation after a stroke or brain injury use their spasticity to walk on, when their weakness would otherwise not allow it (10). Clearly, treating the spasticity here would not be helpful and

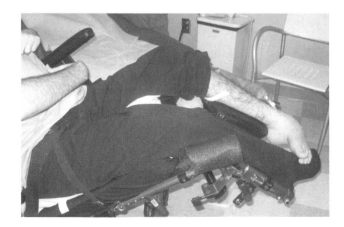

FIGURE 23.4

Diffuse spasticity of the lower extremities, commonly seen in patients with more generalized spasticity.

TABLE 23.4
Prevention of Provocative Factors

- Avoidance of noxious stimuli
  - pressure ulcers
  - urinary retention
  - constipation
  - infection
  - pain

- Patient and carer education
  - proper positioning
  - regular skin inspection
  - good management of bladder and bowel,
  - Proper positioning

- Daily stretching to maintain range of motion

- Splinting and serial casting, if necessary

- Functional electrical stimulation, motor reeducation, and biofeedback

physical measures to utilize the developing movement patterns would be the treatment of choice, but where the spasticity gives rise to problems for either the patient or the carer, then treatment is required.

It is sometimes quite difficult to distinguish between severe spasticity and contracture formation, but it is important to do so and to know what antispastic treatment can or cannot achieve so that there are realistic expectations. Limb contracture occurs through shortening of muscles and tendons in inadequately treated patients (14). If a contracture is fixed, it will require serial splinting or surgery to correct it, but before it becomes fixed and is dynamic, treating the underlying spasticity may allow easier treatment of the contracture. Although one way to do this is through examination under intravenous sedation (12), it is advisable to use a general anesthetic for children. This relaxes spastic muscles and allows the range of passive joint movement to be assessed.

Management

Preventing spasticity from causing problems is very important in initial management. See Table 23.4 for a list of provocative factors involved in spasticity.

Medical

All medical interventions are an adjunct to a program of physical treatment, removal of exacerbating stimuli, and patient and carer education.

Oral Medication

Oral agents are useful in treating mild to moderate spasticity. The use of baclofen and dantrolene sodium has not changed much over the years (15, 16), but some newer products have emerged. Forty percent of patients are unable either to tolerate oral agents because of side effects or are unable to produce an adequate antispastic effect before side effects occur (17). See Table 23.5 for a short synopsis of these treatments.

Intrathecal Treatments

Intrathecal Baclofen

This consists of fitting a programmable electronic pump in the anterior abdominal wall with a subcutaneous catheter tunnelled around the trunk and inserted into the spine canal. The catheter is placed at about the L2/3 level with its tip at a level between D8 and D10. This allows baclofen to be delivered at higher concentrations at its site of action than would be possible with oral administration and without the expected central nervous system side effects (44).

The main indication is for people with significant disability. It is usually used in people with regional problems from spasticity, such as those with tetraplegia and paraplegia, who are unable to tolerate or respond adequately to oral antispastic drugs (45–47). It is particularly useful in both brain-injured and spinal cord–injured patients who do not have residual functioning, but the pump settings can also deliver doses in a highly specific manner to allow ambulant people to balance the weakening effect of baclofen against the spasticity required for weight support and joint mobility (47).

Intrathecal Phenol

Five percent intrathecal phenol in glycerine is given on infrequent occasions for the management of people with very severe spasticity (48). This is only indicated for people with progressive disease who are refractory to other antispastic treatments, who have no ambulatory function, and who are incontinent (eg, terminally ill patients with multiple sclerosis). The block is usually painless, as the phenol exerts a local anesthetic effect, and the procedure can be repeated as required.

Chemodenervation

Perineural injection of motor nerves using 3% to 6% phenol in aqueous solution blocks groups of muscles. This provides an initial local anesthetic effect, which

TABLE 23.5
Treatments for Spasticity

DRUG	PROPERTIES
Baclofen	– Structural analogue of GABA – Binds to GABA-B receptors both pre- and postsynaptically (18, 19) – Used as an antispastic drug for more than 30 years – Used as first-line treatment for cerebral and spinal cord spasticity – Effective in reducing spasticity and for sudden painful flexor spasms (20)
Dantrolene sodium	– Acts peripherally on muscle fibers by suppressing release of Ca2+ ions from sarcoplasmic reticulum – Dissociates excitation-contraction coupling and diminishes force of muscle contraction (21) – Generally preferred for spasticity due to supraspinal lesions (22, 23) – Reported that patients with SCI also responded well to dantrolene (23) but was somewhat less effective in patients with MS (24, 25) – Associated with idiosyncratic symptomatic hepatitis (fatal in 0.1%–0.2% patients (26, 27)) – Three monthly liver function tests required
Tizanidine	– Imidazoline derivative with agonistic action at central alpha-2 adrenergic receptor sites – Beneficial in spasticity due to MS and SCI, but definite functional improvements have not been shown (28–30) – Comparable to baclofen in efficacy in MS and SCI patients (31–34) – Efficacious compared to diazepam in hemiplegia due to stroke and traumatic brain injury and allowed significantly better walking distance ability (34) – Favorable adverse effects profile, although sedation remained a prominent side effect (35, 36) – Visual hallucinations and liver function test abnormalities in 5%–7% of patients (37) – Liver function tests recommended before starting tizanidine and after 1 month of treatment
Benzodiazepines	– Antispastic effect mediated via GABA receptors – Diazepam earliest antispasticity drug—rarely used now because of sedation – Effective and compares well to baclofen in MS and SCI patients (38) – Clonazepam used in epilepsy—comparable in effect to baclofen (39) – Found to be equally effective as diazepam, but less well tolerated due to sedation, confusion, and fatigue resulting in more frequent discontinuation of the drug – Thus used mainly for suppression of nocturnal painful spasms
Gabapentin (40) and pregabalin (41)	– Useful when there is pain (particularly in cortical dysesthesia) giving rise to abnormal sensory inputs (40, 41) – Gaining in popularity as an adjunct in combination to other anti-spastic treatments – Poorly tolerated in a significant proportion of patients and therefore limited use
Cannabinoids	– No real evidence of efficacy in MS (42) but anecdotal evidence of help in spasticity – CAMS study compared oral cannabis extract and delta 9-tetrahydrocannabinol with placebo in 667 patients (43) – 1o outcome measure was a change the Ashworth Scale – No beneficial effect on spasticity but evidence of a treatment effect on patient-reported spasticity and pain (43)

Abbreviations: GABA, gamma-amiobutyric acid; MS, multiple sclerosis; SCI, spinal cord.

is later followed by blockade 1 hour later, as protein coagulation and inflammation occur (49). Wallerian degeneration occurs later on before healing by fibrosis. This leaves the nerve with about 25% less function than before but does not disadvantage people with little or no residual function, as a mild progressive denervation can be beneficial in reducing spasticity (49). The effect can last for 4 to 6 months, and the renewal of muscle overactivity is probably due to nerve regeneration (50). The indications for use are as an alternative to botulinum toxin (BoNT) or surgery in the treatment of focal problems (51). Its disadvantages are that it takes relatively more time to perform the injection and can cause dysesthesia if the phenol is placed in proximity to sensory nerve fibers.

Neuromuscular Blockade

Botulinum toxin is injected into the overactive target muscles, which are responsible for the clinical picture. It is a potent neurotoxin that inhibits the release of neurotransmitter chemicals by disrupting the functioning of the SNARE complex required for exocytosis of synaptic vesicles (52–54). It is suitable for long-term blocking of neuromuscular transmission through the inhibition of release of acetyl choline. This leads to muscle paralysis over 3 to 4 months, but this can be extended by a program of physical activity (55). The toxin will cross about 4 to 5 sarcomeres to get to the neuromuscular junction and can be seen there after about 12 hours. The toxin's clinical effect is seen at about 4 days and is certainly working at 7 days. It works optimally at 1 month and will go to produce a clinical effect for 3 to 4 months. The end effect is weakening and relaxation of muscle overactivity in people experiencing the effects of the UMN syndrome. This results in a biomechanical change in the muscle's function and makes it amenable to stretching and lengthening. In addition, the weakening allows an opportunity to strengthening of antagonist muscles, and thereby, it is possible to restore some of the balance between the two. Electromyographic (EMG) guidance can be used to locate the smaller muscles precisely. Contraindications for BoNT injection include known sensitivity to BoNT, concurrent aminoglycoside antibiotics, myasthenia gravis, Lambert-Eaton syndrome, motor neuron diseases, and upper eyelid apraxia (56, 57).

OUTCOME MEASURES

Outcome measurement in spasticity is controversial because of the lack of a uniform measure, which is applicable across all the domains of the International Classification of Functioning, Disability and Health (58–60). As a result, a large of number of tools are used in an attempt to reflect change after the treatment process. Most clinicians do not actually measure the outcomes of their interventions in terms of the change to the neurogenic component of the UMN lesion. They more often measure the change in either the biomechanical consequence of the spastic limb (at impairment level) or the functional change (activity) of the goal of treatment. The main problem here is that the accepted measure of spasticity, the Ash-

worth score, does not actually measure what it purports to do. It does not follow Lance's definition and measures limb stiffness rather than velocity-dependent resistance (61). The Tardieu Scale (62) and the Wartenberg pendulum test (63), on the other hand, do a better job but are more unwieldy to use in clinical practice.

In clinical practice, measures of disability are the most useful to quantify and relate to the patient's rehabilitation aims. Spasticity is but one component that has to be dealt with, and the outcomes of rehabilitation depend on issues relating to other impairments, to activity, and to participation. An easy-to-measure tool is needed, whereas in research, a standardized testing protocol is required to follow the definition of the condition as closely as possible. The Ashworth Scale fails in this and to measure clinically important changes in spasticity but remains a useful bedside clinical measure. For research purposes, the Wartenberg pendulum test follows the definition and gets round the complex variables that occur in the α-motor neurons of agonist and antagonist muscles during passive movements (63). Katz et al. (64) conclude, however, that biomechanical measures correlate most closely with the clinical state, as extending a limb against passive resistance may be related more to the viscoelastic properties of the soft tissues than to spasticity. The EMG activity and the motor unit magnitude correlate well with the torque and ramp and hold displacement around the elbow (65).

Functional aspects are important to measure, but one of the problems is that functional change with treatment may be dependent on factors other than the spasticity. Few studies have shown a global correlation with the Ashworth score and the measurement of function, as in the Rivermead or the Fugl-Meyer Motor Assessment scores (66, 67) is best correlated with other impairment measures, like the spasm frequency score, adductor tone, pain score, and so on. Therein lies the dilemma. We will probably have to keep on using the Ashworth Scale in the clinical setting but realize its limitations and always combine management of the patient with a functional outcome measure in relation to the rehabilitation goal.

Other measures have a particular use in physiotherapy practice and contribute to the overall picture of change after treatment. The walking speed (measured by a 10-meter walking time), the stride length, and the joint goniometry are useful in measuring change in hip and thigh spasticity in spastic diplegics (67). Pain has been addressed above, and the Jebsen Taylor Hand test demonstrates improvement in dexterity and isolated finger movement (68), whereas the Berg Balance Scale evaluates what it suggests (69). The final

TABLE 23.6
Outcome Measures

ASHWORTH SCALE (61)

- The measure against which all other measures are compared
- Based on assessment of resistance to stretch when a limb passively moved
- Originally validated in patients with Multiple Sclerosis (61) and in lower limbs (70)
- Good interrater and intrarater reliability (71)
- Measures multiple aspects of limb stretch, but generally used as a screening tool for spasticity assessment
- Limitation
  - Grade 0 is not a floppy limb
  - No reference to normality
  - Reliability questioned by observer subjectivity during test (11)
  - Does not distinguish between spasticity and mechanical limb stiffness

SCORE	ASHWORTH (61)	MODIFIED ASHWORTH (72)
0	No increase in tone	No increase in tone
1	Slight increase in tone giving a catch when the limb is moved in flexion/extension	Slight increase in tone giving a catch, release and minimal resistance at the end of range of motion ROM when the limb is moved in flexion/extension
1+		Slight increase in tone giving a catch, release and minimal resistance throughout the remainder (less than half) of ROM
2	More marked increase in tone, but the limb is easily moved through its full ROM	More marked increased in tone through most of the ROM, but limb is easily moved
3	Considerable increase in tone—passive movement difficult and ROM decreased	Considerable increase in tone—passive movement difficult
4	Limb rigid in flexion and extension	Limb rigid in flexion and extension

TARDIEU SCALE (62)

- Note angle of catch at point of resistance by stretching a limb passively
  - During as slow a movement as possible (V1)
  - Under gravitational pull (V2)
  - At a fast rate (V3)
- Good interrater and intrarater reliability (62)
- Training required to achieve this

STRETCH VELOCITY	Y ANGLE (DYNAMIC RANGE OF MOTION)	QUALITY OF MUSCLE REACTION COURSE OF PASSIVE MOVEMENT
V1 Slow as possible	R2 Slow velocity passive joint range of motion or muscle length	0 No resistance
V2 Speed of limb falling under gravity	R1 Fast velocity movement through full range of motion	1 Slight resistance 2 Clear catch at precise angle, then release 3 Fatigable clonus at precise angle 4 Unfatigable clonus at precise angle 5 Rigid limb and joint
V3 fast as possible		

TABLE 23.6 (*Continued*)
WARTENBERG PENDULUM TEST (63)
Leg moves under gravity Observer measures pendular activity of a spastic limb as it relaxes Only reliable in lower limb
OTHER METHODS
Clinical Muscle grading, deep tendon reflexes, range of joint motion, adductor tone, Visual Analogue Scale, spasm frequency score, torque devices Neurophysiological Dynamic multichannel EMG, tonic vibratory reflexes Tests related to the H reflex, H reflex/M wave ratio and T wave.
Note: Most are time-consuming, expensive, require specialized equipment, and are used mainly in research.

thought is that clinicians tend to measure what they feel is the most relevant aspect of treatment. Just as we need to ask the patient and family their views of the treatment goal, we should involve them more in the measurement process too. Patient satisfaction scores are useful in identifying whether patents feel they are meeting their targets, so long as there are clear realistic expectations of outcome. Patient and physician global scores can thus address this aspect (Table 23.6).

APPENDIX

PATHOPHYSIOLOGY OF THE FEATURES OF THE UMN SYNDROME (INCLUDING SPASTICITY)

Damage to pyramidal tracts alone does not result in spasticity. It occurs only when lesion involves premotor and supplementary motor areas. It arises because of hyperexcitability of segmental central nervous system processing of sensory feedback from the periphery, and they depend on the location, size, and age of the lesion. Spasticity is not the only result of a damaged UMN. Muscle overactivity occurs in 2 scenarios. The first involves high-stretch sensitivity when excessive motor unit recruitment occurs with recruitment of stretch receptors and forms the stretch-sensitive forms of muscle overactivity, which includes spasticity itself, spastic dystonia, and cocontraction. These are distinguished by their primary triggering factor, that is, phasic muscle stretch, tonic muscle stretch, or volitional command. The second scenario is found in muscles that are not particularly stretch-sensitive. They include

associated reactions when there is extrasegmental co-contraction due to cutaneous or nociceptive stimuli or inappropriate muscle recruitment during autonomic or reflex activities, such as yawning (73).

Spasticity is associated with hyperexcitable tonic stretch reflexes. It can be distinguished from hypertonia by its dependence on the speed of the muscle stretch (74, 75). A UMN lesion disturbs the balance of supraspinal inhibitory and excitatory inputs, which leads to net disinhibition of the spinal reflexes.

Hyperactive spinal reflexes appear to mediate most of the positive phenomena associated with the UMN syndrome, whereas abnormal efferent drives and disordered control of voluntary movements account for the other positive features of the syndrome.

- Spinal reflexes rely on afferent sensory feedback from the periphery, for example, muscle stretch, pain, or cutaneous stimulation.
- Stretch reflexes are proprioceptive and can be either tonic (from sustained stretch, as in resting muscle tone) or phasic (from a short stretch, as in deep tendon reflexes). Exaggerated tendon jerks cause clonus.
- Flexor and extensor spasms are nociceptive reflexes, whereas the Babinski sign is the most familiar cutaneous reflex (74).

Lesions of the UMN present a number of patterns, such as muscle overactivity in the absence of a volitional command (1). Spastic dystonia is a tonic muscle contraction in the absence of a phasic stretch or volitional command (5). It is primarily due to abnormal supraspinal descending drive, which causes a failure of muscle relaxation (despite efforts to do so) and is sensitive to the degree of tonic stretch imposed on that muscle (76). There is inappropriate recruitment of antagonist muscles in spastic cocontraction upon triggering of the agonist under volitional command. This occurs in the absence of phasic stretch and is sensitive to the degree of tonic stretch of the cocontracting antagonist (76). The excitability of the spinal reflexes is under supraspinal control, both inhibitory and excitatory, by the UMNs. The UMN fibers descend to the spinal cord to exert a balanced control on spinal reflex activity. Both positive and negative features of the UMN syndrome are largely due to dysfunction of the parapyramidal fibers and to a lesser extent the pyramidal fibers. It has been suggested that isolated pyramidal tract lesions do not cause spasticity or other forms of muscle overactivity. They may, on the other hand, cause some weakness with an initial depression followed by some exaggeration of deep tendon reflexes and a Babinski sign.

The main tract that inhibits the spinal reflex activity is the dorsal reticulospinal tract, which originates in the ventromedial reticular formation. The excitatory fibers come down in the medial reticulospinal tract, arising in the bulbopontine tegmentum in the brainstem. The vestibulospinal fibers also have an excitatory effect on spinal reflexes (77).

Most of the important UMNs controlling spinal reflex activity arise in the brainstem. However, the ventromedial reticular formation, from which the dorsal reticulospinal tract (main supraspinal inhibitory tract) originates, is under cortical control (77).

The cortical motor areas augment the inhibitory drive down to the spinal cord through corticobulbar fibers. A lesion of these fibers (either in the cortex or in the internal capsule) will mildly reduce inhibitory drive and excitation of spinal reflex activity, as cortical facilitation of inhibitory pathways is suppressed and the resultant positive UMN features are less severe than those resulting from a lesion of the dorsal reticulospinal tract. This explains why the degree of spasticity, hyperreflexia, and possibly clonus resulting from a cortical/supraspinal lesion is less severe than that produced by a spinal cord lesion (78).

A partial lesion of the spinal cord, which damages inhibitory pathways but preserves the excitatory fibers, would leave a strongly unopposed excitatory drive to the spinal reflexes and causes severe spasticity, hyperreflexia, and flexor and extensor spasms. With a complete spinal cord lesion, spinal reflexes lose both inhibitory and excitatory supraspinal control and ultimately become hyperactive (6).

Immediately after injury, a period of neuronal shock occurs and spinal reflexes are lost, which include stretch reflexes. A flaccid weakness in seen, but even during this, the positive features of hypertonia can start to be seen. Limbs are not sufficiently stretched and may be immobilized in shortened positions. Rheological changes occur within muscles in the form of loss of proteins and sarcomeres and accumulation of connective tissue and fibroblasts (77). Unless treated, tendon and soft tissue contracture and limb deformity are established. Altered sensory inputs such as pain, recurrent infection, and poor posture maintain a further stimulus to lead to yet further shortening, and this cycle is difficult to break (8).

Spasticity appears later on, as plastic rearrangement occurs within the brain, spinal cord, and muscles. This attempt at restoration of function through new neuronal circuitry creates movement patterns based on existing damaged pathways. Neuronal sprouting occurs at many levels with interneuronal endings moving into unconnected circuits from decreased supraspinal command through the vestibular, rubrospinal, and reticulospinal tracts (79). The end effect is muscle overactivity and exaggerated reflex responses to peripheral stimulation (80). This process occurs at anytime but is usually seen between 1 and 6 weeks after the insult. Muscle overactivity declines over time, and the following are suggested as possible causes:

- Structural and functional changes due to plastic rearrangement
- Axonal sprouting
- Increased receptor density.

In reality, biomechanical stiffness takes over and tends to diminish exaggerated α-motor neuronal activity.

Spinal Reflexes

The hyperactive spinal reflexes seen in the positive phenomena of the UMN syndrome can be explained in 3 ways.

1. There is disinhibition of the existing normal reflex activity. One type is the proprioceptive phasic stretch reflex, known as deep tendon reflexes. This reflex activity becomes disinhibited causing clonus, which is an abnormally exaggerated phasic stretch reflex after a UMN lesion. Another form of a normally existing reflex that becomes disinhibited is the flexor withdrawal reflex. This nociceptive reflex occurs in response to sudden pain, for example, standing on a sharp object, which produces a swift ankle dorsiflexion, hip flexion, and knee flexion to withdraw the limb from the stimulus. An exaggerated flexor withdrawal re-

flex, as happens in the UMN syndrome, leads to flexor spasms.

2. There is release of primitive reflexes, which are normally present at birth and later disappear with development, such as the Babinski sign and the positive support reaction.

3. An active tonic stretch reflex appears to enhance spasticity. This does not normally exist at rest because reflex activity is not detectable in response to muscle stretch at the rates used clinically to test for muscle tone. So in this context, spasticity may not be considered the result of disinhibition of a normally existing reflex but rather due to a new reflex activity.

Hypertonia

Among its various definitions, spasticity has been described as hypertonia with one or both of the following features present:

1. resistance to externally imposed movement that increases with increasing the speed of stretch and varies with direction of the joint movement
2. resistance to externally imposed movement that increases above a threshold speed or joint angle (6, 81).

It is important to remember that spasticity is a hyperexcitable tonic stretch reflex and that it is mediated by afferents predominantly in the muscle spindle. The latter gets excited by passive muscle stretch and sends sensory input to the spinal cord through mono-, oligo-, and polysynaptic reflexes, which in turn send efferent impulse to the muscle to cause it to contract. In spastic patients, the excitability of the reflex is increased centrally within the spinal cord. This is contrary to what was thought initially, that the greater reflex output was due to the muscle spindles becoming more sensitive to muscle stretch, feeding back a larger impulse to the spinal cord and causing a greater muscle contraction.

Hence, spasticity should be considered a spinal phenomenon and not a peripheral one (82). The excitability of the tonic stretch reflex depends upon the length of the muscle at which it is stretched. The shorter the muscle, the greater the tonic stretch response, and so spasticity is length-dependent. Classically, spasticity is considered as a dynamic phenomenon; a stretched muscle should stop contracting if the movement is stopped and the muscle is held stretched. It has been demonstrated, however, that if the stretch is maintained, the stretch reflex activity continues, thereby maintaining muscle contraction for some time. On this basis, there may also be a static component to spasticity.

The increased resistance to imposed passive movements is velocity-dependent. Muscle activity increases with the speed of linear stretch. If the muscle is stretched at low speed, tone may feel relatively normal, but if the stretch is done at high speed, there will be clear resistance. However, this is not exclusive to spasticity (5, 80), and the velocity-dependent change in stiffness is a characteristic response of the viscoelastic properties of soft tissues (muscles, tendons, ligaments, etc) (83–85). It is also argued that spasticity may not be a pure motor disorder, as other afferents (eg, cutaneous and proprioceptive pathways) have been shown to be implicated in stretch reflex activity (75) and that there is insufficient evidence to support the theory that the abnormal muscle activity observed in spasticity results exclusively from hyperexcitability of the stretch reflex. The SPASM group concluded that Lance's definition was too restrictive and proposed an updated definition based on the available evidence (6). It could be redefined as a "disordered sensori-motor control, resulting from an upper motor neurone lesion, presenting as intermittent or sustained involuntary activation of muscles." Under this definition, the term spasticity can be used collectively to describe the whole range of signs and symptoms that constitute the positive features of the UMN syndrome, but it narrows the term sufficiently to exclude the negative features and the pure biomechanical changes in the soft tissue and joints.

Pandyan et al. (80) suggested that this new definition does not express a causal relationship between spasticity and other impairments (eg, contractures), activity limitations, participation restrictions, and pain and that if links do exist, then they should be independently demonstrated. A number of different UMN syndromes may thus present, of which spasticity is but one of a number of features.

Clasp-Knife Response

The clasp-knife is an initial resistance to stretch, which then suddenly gives way. It is another manifestation of the tonic stretch reflex underlying spasticity, modified by flexor reflex afferents (78). Because the tonic stretch reflex is greater when the muscle is short, stretch will eventually lead to a point at which the resistance to stretch is inhibited. This is important to consider when looking at interventions such as casting and chemical denervation (8).

This is exemplified by the stretch applied to a muscle when a limb is flexed. There comes a point where the resistance to stretch disappears and where the combination of length dependence and velocity dependence leads to a point where the muscle length is so long and the stretch so slow that the excitability of the tonic stretch reflex is subthreshold, causing the resistance to disappear (86).

Associated Reactions and Mass Reflex

Associated reactions are sudden responses due to the abnormal spread of motor activity. They have been likened to a form of spastic dystonia (85) and are exemplified by the abducted arm on walking, yawning, coughing, and so on. The patient with stroke may demonstrate increasing synergy patterns with increasing effort. These patterns are movements that occur with other activities that are not necessary. Synergy and associated reactions may be due to radiation or overflow of excitation from the cortex or the spinal cord during volitional tasks. Associated reactions may interfere with dynamic balance but are not valid indicators of spasticity after stroke (83). Successful treatment of associated reactions in ambulatory stroke patients with BoNT may result in a more symmetrical gait and increased walking speed.

Another reflex response associated with spasticity is the mass reflex. Here, the spinal cord suddenly becomes active in response to nociceptive stimuli, producing excitation of large areas of the cord. Clinically, this usually occurs in patients with long-standing spastic paraplegia and presents with urinary and fecal incontinence, diaphoresis, elevations in blood pressure, and frequently painful muscle spasms.

Flexor Spasms

Flexor spasms are simply disinhibited normal flexor withdrawal reflexes. They occur normally in a painful limb withdrawal, but in the UMN syndrome, they are pathophysiologically independent of spasticity, deep tendon jerks, and clonus. Possible mechanisms are increased excitability in the flexor reflex afferents, decreased presynaptic inhibition, increased α-motor neuron excitability, altered reciprocal inhibition, and decreased recurrent inhibition (76, 87). In complete spinal cord transaction, all the supraspinal inhibitory influences are abolished causing intense flexor spasms.

Disordered Control of Movement

A phenomenon often confused with synergies and associated reactions is cocontraction. It is an example of disordered control of voluntary movement, which is encountered as one of the positive features of the UMN syndrome. Cocontraction refers to the simultaneous firing of agonist and antagonist muscle groups. Sherrington (88), in 1906, described reciprocal innervation as the process that controls agonist and antagonist muscle actions. One muscle group (agonists) must relax to allow another group (antagonists) to contract. This is called reciprocal inhibition. Normally, agonist and antagonist muscle groups cocontract to stabilize a joint during a strenuous activity. The UMN syndrome interferes with normal movement and function with reciprocal innervation occurring at both cortical and spinal levels to allow for appropriate cocontraction. It may present as either of the following:

1. reduced leading to impaired cocontraction—for example, in attempting to extend the elbow, there may be cocontraction of both elbow extensors and flexors. Instead of the elbow extensors inhibiting the flexors to allow the movement, they oppose the movement. Thus, elbow flexor activity is a combination of a tonic stretch reflex (elbow extension stretches the flexors) and simultaneous UMN activation of the elbow flexors and extensors (11).
2. excessive inhibition preventing weakened muscles from demonstrating their underlying strength.

Thixotropy and Muscle Contractures

Not every "tight" muscle is spastic. Thixotropy is the property of some gels to turn into liquids under certain conditions. There is a small degree of stiffness in the normal resting muscle that disappears on voluntary movement or passive muscle stretch. Thixotropy is the physiological term used to describe this component of muscle tone. The stiffness is determined by the length of the muscle fiber in the resting state immediately before the muscle contracts (89) and reduces as the fiber length of the contractile unit changes. In healthy individuals, the contribution of thixotropy to muscle tone is negligible, but when spastic muscles are held for a prolonged time, secondary biochemical changes occur causing an increase in the thixotropic component of muscle stiffness and eventually leading to contracture. Fixed contractures develop when the muscle fiber is maintained in a shortened state by immobilization or sustained muscle activity. The latter is the hallmark of spasticity and is the main factor predisposing to the development of contractures in patients with UMN lesions.

The contractures are usually aggravated by the reduced mobility and poor postures, which are often seen in these patient (90–92). Both stiffness and contracture cause a reduced range of movement and impaired function.

References

1. Sheean G. Botulinum toxin should be first-line treatment for post-stroke spasticity. J Neurol Neurosurg Psychiatry. 2009; 80 (4):359.
2. SPASM definition. Disabil Rehabil. 2006;28 (Suppl. 1)
3. Lance JW. Symposium synopsis: pp 485–494. In Feldman RG, Young RR, Koella WP. Eds. Spasticity: disordered control. Chicago. 1980. Yearbook Medical.
4. Young RR. Spasticity: a review. Neurology. 1994;44:512–520.
5. Mayer NH. Clinicophysiologic concepts of spasticity and motor dysfunction in adults with an upper motoneuron lesion pp. 1-10. In Spasticity: etiology, evaluation, management and the role of botulinum toxin. 2002. New York. We Move.
6. A European thematic network to develop standardised measures of spasticity (SPASM). CREST—Centre for Rehabilitation and Engineering Studies, University of Newcastle, Stephenson Building, Claremont Road, Newcastle upon Tyne, NE1 7RU, UK. 2006;28 (Suppl. 1).
7. Sommerfeld DK, Eek EU, Svensson AK, Holmqvist LW, von Arbin MH. Spasticity after stroke: its occurrence and association with motor impairments and activity limitations. Stroke. 2004;35 (1):134–9.
8. Verplancke D, Snape S, Salisbury CF, Jones PW, Ward AB. A randomised controlled trial of the management of early lower limb spasticity following acute acquired severe brain injury. Clin Rehabil. 2005;19 (2):117–125.
9. Ward AB (Chairman) et al. Working party report on the management of adult spasticity using botulinum toxin type A—a guide to clinical practice. 2001. Radius Healthcare, Byfleet.
10. Ward AB. Botulinum toxin in spasticity management. British Journal of Therapy & Rehabilitation. 1999;6(7):26–34.
11. Barnes M.P, et al. (Chairman) Neurological rehabilitation—a working party report of the British Society of Rehabilitation Medicine and the Neurological Alliance. 1992. London. British Society of Rehabilitation Medicine.
12. Ward AB. Use of botulinum toxin type A in spastic diplegia resulting from cerebral palsy. Eur J Neurol. 1999;6 (Suppl 4): S46–S48.
13. Gracies JM, Wilson L, Gandevia SC, Burke. Stretched position of spastic muscle aggravates their co-contraction in hemiplegic patients. Ann Neurol. 1997a;42 (30):438–438.
14. Tardieu C, Lespargot A, Tabary C, Bret MD. For how long must the soleus muscle be stretched each day to prevent contracture? Dev Med Child Neurol. 1988;30;3–10.
15. Gracies JM, Elovic E, McGuire JR, Simpson DM. Traditional pharmacological treatments for spasticity. Part I: local treatments. pp. 44–64. In Spasticity: etiology, evaluation, management and the role of botulinum toxin. 2002. New York. We Move.
16. Pinder RM, Brogden RN, Speight TM, Avery GS. Dantrolene sodium: a review of its pharmacological properties and therapeutic efficacy in spasticity. Drugs 1977;13:3–23.
17. Ward AB. A summary of spasticity management—a treatment algorithm. Eur J Neurol 2002;9 (Suppl 1):48–52.
18. Hwang AS, Wilcox GL. Baclofen, gamma-aminobutyric acid B receptors and substance P in the mouse spinal cord. J Pharmacol Exp Ther. 1989;248:1026–33.
19. Price GW, Wilkin GP, Turnbull MJ, Bowery NG. Are baclofen-sensitive GABA-B receptors present on primary afferent terminals of the spinal cord? Nature. 1984;307:71–3.
20. Hudgson P, Weightman D. Baclofen in the treatment of spasticity. Br Med J. 1971;4:155–157.
21. Chyatte SB, Birdsong JH, Bergman BA. The effects of dantrolene sodium on spasticity and motor performance in hemiplegia. South Med J. 1971;64(2):180–5.
22. Ketel WB, Kolb ME. Long-term treatment with dantrolene sodium of stroke patients with spasticity limiting the return of function. Curr Med Res Opin. 1984;9 (3):161–8.
23. Weiser R, Terenty T, Hudgson P, et al. Dantrolene sodium in the treatment of spasticity in chronic spinal cord disease. Practitioner. 1978;221:123–7.
24. Gelenberg AJ, Poskanzer DC. The effect of dantrolene sodium on spasticity in multiple sclerosis. Neurology. 1973; 23: 1313–5.
25. Tolosa ES, Soll RW, Loewenson. Treatment of spasticity in multiple sclerosis with dantrolene. JAMA. 1975;233(10): 1046.
26. Utili R, Boitnott JK, Zimmerman HJ. Dantrolene-associated hepatic injury: incidence and character. Gastroenterology. 1977;72:610–6.
27. Wilkinson SP, Portmann B, Williams R. Hepatitis from dantrolene sodium. Gut 1979;20:33–6.
28. Smith C, Birnbaum G, Carter JL, et al. Tizanidine treatment of spasticity caused by multiple sclerosis: results of a double-blind, placebo-controlled trial. Neurology 1994;44(Suppl 9): S34–S43.
29. Nance PW, Bugaresti J, Shellengerger K, et al. Efficacy and safety of tizanidine in the treatment of spasticity in patients with spinal cord injury. Neurology. 1994;44 (Suppl 9):S44–S52.
30. The United Kingdom Tizanidine Trial Group. A double-blind, placebo-controlled trial of tizanidine in the treatment of spasticity caused by multiple sclerosis. Neurology. 1994;44:(Suppl 9):S70–S78.
31. Hassan N, McLellan DL. Double-blind comparison of single doses of DS103-282, baclofen, and placebo for suppression of spasticity. J Neurol Neurosurg Psychiatry. 1980;43: 1132–6.
32. Smolenski C, Muff S, Smolenski-Kautz S. A double-blind comparative trial of a new muscle relaxant, tizanidine and baclofen in the treatment of chronic spasticity in multiple sclerosis. Curr Med Res Opin. 1981;7:374–83.
33. Newman PM, Nogues M, Newman PK, et al. Tizanidine in the treatment of spasticity. Eur J Clin Pharmacol. 1982;23: 31–5.
34. Stein R, Nordal HJ, Oftedal SI, Slettebo M. The treatment of spasticity in multiple sclerosis: a double-blind clinical trial of a new anti-spasticity drug tizanidine compared with baclofen. Acta Neurol Scand. 1987;75:190–4.
35. Bes A, Eyssette M, Pierrot-Deseilligny E, et al. A multi-centre, double-blind trial of tizanidine, a new antispastic agent, in spasticity associated with hemiplegia. Curr Med Res Opin. 1988;10:709–18.
36. Wagstaff AJ, Bryson HM. Tizanidine: a review of its pharmacology, clinical efficacy and tolerability in the management of spasticity associated with cerebral and spinal disorders. Drugs. 1997;53(3):435–52.
37. Wallace JD. Summary of combined clinical analysis of controlled clinical trial with tizanidine. Neurology. 1994;44 (Suppl 9):S60–8.
38. Ketelaer CJ, Ketelaer P. The use of Lioresal in the treatment of muscular hypertonia due to multiple sclerosis: spasticity: a topical survey, in Birkmayer (Ed): An international symposium, Vienna 1971. Vienna, Huber. 1972;128–31.
39. Cendrowski W, Sobczyk W. Clonazepam, baclofen and placebo in the treatment of spasticity. Eur J Neurol. 1977;16: 257–62.
40. Francisco, G E. Kothari, S. Huls, C. GABA agonists and gabapentin for spastic hypertonia. Phys Med Rehabil Clin N. Am 2001;12 (4):875–88.
41. Pollmann W. Feneberg W. Current management of pain associated with multiple sclerosis. CNS Drugs. 2008;22(4): 291–324.
42. Zajicek J. Fox P. Sanders H. Wright D. Vickery J. Nunn A. Thompson A. UK MS Research Group. Cannabinoids for treatment of spasticity and other symptoms related to multiple sclerosis (CAMS study). Lancet. 2003;362 (9395):1517–26.
43. Killestein J. Uitdehaag BM. Polman CH. Cannabinoids in multiple sclerosis: do they have a therapeutic role? Drugs. 2004:64 (1):1–11.
44. Francisco GE. Latorre JM. Ivanhoe CB. Intrathecal baclofen therapy for spastic hypertonia in chronic traumatic brain injury. Brain Inj. 2007;21(3):335–8.
45. Albright AL. Gilmartin R. Swift D. Krach LE. Ivanhoe CB. McLaughlin JF. Long-term intrathecal baclofen therapy for severe spasticity of cerebral origin. J Neurosurg. 2003;98(2): 291–5.

46. Guillaume D. Van Havenbergh A. Vloeberghs M. Vidal J. Roeste G. A clinical study of intrathecal baclofen using a programmable pump for intractable spasticity. *Arch Phys Med Rehabil.* 2005;86(11):2165–71.

47. Ben Smail D. Peskine A. Roche N. Mailhan L. Thiebaut I. Bussel B. Intrathecal baclofen for treatment of spasticity of multiple sclerosis patients. *Mult Scler.* 2006;12 (1):101–3.

48. Kelly RE, Gautier-Smith PC. Intrathecal phenol in the treatment of reflex spasms and spasticity. *Lancet.* 1959;ii:1102–1105.

49. Burkel WE, McPhee M. Effect of phenol injection on peripheral nerve of rat: electron microscope studies. *Arch Phys Med Rehabil.* 1970;51:391–397.

50. Bodine-Fowler SC, Allsing S, Botte MJ. Time course of muscle atrophy and recovery following a phenol-induced nerve block. *Muscle Nerve.* 1996;19 (4):497–504.

51. Kirazli Y, On AY, Kismali B, Aksit R. Comparison of phenol block and botulinum toxin type A in the treatment of spastic foot after stroke: a randomized double-blind trial. *Am J Phys Med Rehabil.* 1998;77 (6):510–515.

52. Pellizzari R. Rossetto O. Schiavo G. Montecucco C. Tetanus and botulinum neurotoxins: mechanism of action and therapeutic uses. *Philos Trans R Soc Lond B Biol Sci.* 1999;354 (1381):259–68.

53. Dolly O. Synaptic transmission: inhibition of neurotransmitter release by botulinum toxins. *Headache.* 2003;43 (Suppl 1): S16–S24.

54. Dolly JO, Aoki K. The structure and mode of action of botulinum toxins. *Eur J Neurol.* 2006;13 (Suppl 4):1–9.

55. Giovannelli M, Borriello G, Castri P, et al. Early physiotherapy after injection of botulinum toxin increases the beneficial effects on spasticity in patients with multiple sclerosis. *Clin Rehabil.* 2007;21 (4):331–337.

56. Bakheit AMO, Thilmann AF, Ward AB, *et al.* A randomized, double-blind, placebo-controlled, dose-ranging study to compare the efficacy and safety of three doses of botulinum toxin type A (Dysport) with placebo in upper limb spasticity after stroke. *Stroke.* 2000;31(10):2402–2406.

57. Moore A, Naumann M. General and clinical aspects of treatment with botulinum toxin. Moore A, Naumann N. *Handbook of botulinum toxin treatment.* 2nd edition. Oxford: Blackwell Science. 2003:28–75.

58. World Health Organisation. International classification of functioning, disability and health: ICF: Geneva: WHO; 2001.

59. Turner-Stokes (Chair) et al. Working Party on Guidelines for the management of spasticity in adults: management using botulinum toxin—national guidelines. In press 2009.

60. Tardieu G, Shentoub S, Delarue R. A la recherche d'une technique de mesure de la spasticité. *Rev Neurol. (Paris)* 1954;91: 143–144.

61. Ashworth B. Preliminary trial of carisprodal in multiple sclerosis. *Practitioner.* 1964;192:540–542.

62. Gracies JM. Evaluation de la spasticité. Apport de l'echelle de Tardieu. *Motricité Cérébrale.* 2001;22:1–16.

63. Wartenburg R. Pendulousness of the legs as a diagnostic test. *Neurology.* 1951;1:18–24.

64. Katz RT, Rovai GP, Brait C, Rymer WZ. Objective quantification of spastic hypertonia: correlation with clinical findings. *Arch Phys Med Rehabil.* 1994;73 (4):339–347.

65. Nathan P: Some comments on spasticity and rigidity. In: *New developments in electromyography and clinical neurophysiology.* Desmedt JE (Ed.). Basel, Karger, 1973;13–14.

66. Wade DT. *Measurement in neurological rehabilitation* 1992. Oxford. Oxford University Press.

67. Roden-Jullig A. Britton M. Gustafsson C. Fugl-Meyer A. Validation of four scales for the acute stage of stroke. *J Intern Med.* 1994;236(2):125–36.

68. Jebsen RH. Taylor N. Trieschmann RB. Trotter MJ. Howard LA. An objective and standardized test of hand function. *Arch Phys Med Rehabil.* 1969;50(6):311–9.

69. Bogle Thorbahn LD. Newton RA. Use of the Berg balance test to predict falls in elderly persons.[see comment]. [Journal Article] *Phys Ther.* 2006;76 (6):576–83.

70. Pandyan AD, Johnson GR, Price CIM, Curless RH, Barnes MP, Rodgers H. A review of the properties and limitations of the Ashworth and Modified Ashworth Scales as measures of spasticity. *Clin Rehabil.* 1999;13:373–383.

71. Lee K, Carson L, Kinnin E, Patterson V. The Ashworth Scale: a reliable and reproducible method of measuring spasticity. *J Neurol Rehabil.* 1989;3:205–208.

72. Bohannon RW, Smith MB. Inter-rater reliability of a modified Ashworth Scale of muscle spasticity. *Phys Ther.* 1987;67: 206–27.

73. Pfister AA, Roberts AG, Taylor HM, Noel-Spaudling S, Damian MM, Charles PD. Spasticity in adults living in a developmental center. *Arch Phys Med Rehabil.* 2003;84(12):1808–12.

74. Ivanhoe CB, Reistetter TA: Spasticity: the misunderstood part of the upper motor neurone syndrome. *Am J Phys Med Rehabil.* 2004;83 (suppl):S3–S9.

75. Sheean G: The pathophysiology of spasticity. *Eur J Neurol.* 2002;9 (suppl.1):3–10.

76. Denny-Brown D. *The cerebral control of movement.* pp. 124–143. 1966. Liverpool. Liverpool University Press.

77. Sheean G. Neurophysiology of spasticity. In Barnes MP and Johnson GR, Eds. *Upper motor neurone syndrome and spasticity: clinical management and neurophysiology.* Cambridge: Cambridge University Press; 2001. pp. 12–78.

78. Krenz NR, Weaver LC. Sprouting of primary afferent fibres after spinal cord transection in the rat. *Neuroscience* 1998;85: 443–458.

79. Farmer SE, Harrison LM, Ingram DA, Stephens JA. Plasticity of central motor pathways in children with hemiplegic cerebral palsy. *Neurology.* 1991;15045–1510.

80. Pandyan AD, Gregoric M, Barnes MP, Wood D, Van Wijck F, Burridge J, Hermens H, Johnson GR. Spasticity: clinical perceptions, neurological realities and meaningful measurement. *Disabil Rehabil.* 2005;27 (1/2):2–6.

81. Dewald JPA, Given JD. Electrical stimulation and spasticity reduction. Fact or fiction? *Physical Medicine & Rehabilitation: State of the Art Reviews.* 1994;8:507–522.

82. Hufschmidt A, Mauritz K. Chronic transformation of muscle in spasticity: a peripheral contribution to increased tone. *J Neurol Neurosurg Psychiatry.* 1985;48:676–685.

83. Singer BJ, Dunne JW, Singer KP, Allison GT. Velocity dependant passive plantar flexor resistive torque in patients with acquired brain injury. *Clin Biomech.* 2003;18:157–165.

84. Rothwell J. *Control of human voluntary movement.* 2nd ed. London: Chapman & Hall; 1994.

85. Ada L, O'Dwyer N: Do associated reactions in the upper limb after stroke contribute to contracture formation? *Clin Rehabil.* 2001;15:186–94.

86. Burke D. Spasticity as an adaptation to pyramidal tract injury. *Adv Neurol.* 1988;47:401–422.

87. Bennett DJ, Li Y, Harvey PJ, Gorassini M. Evidence for plateau potentials in the tail motor neurons of awake chronic spinal rats with spasticity. *J Neurophysiol.* 2001;86:1979–1982.

88. Sherrington CS (1906). *The integrative action of the nervous system.* Yale University Press, New Haven.

89. Axelson, H W. Hagbarth, K E. Human motor control consequences of thixotropic changes in muscular short-range stiffness. *J Physiol.* 2001;535 (Pt 1):279–88.

90. Bakheit AM. Muscle spasticity and its management. In: *Botulinum toxin: treatment of muscle spasticity.* Blackhall Publishing, 2001.

91. Knutsson E, Martensson A. Dynamic motor capacity in spastic paresis and its relation to prime mover dysfunction, spastic reflexes and agonist co-activation. *Scand J Rehabil Med.* 1980; 12:93–106.

92. Sahrmann SA, Norton BJ. The relationship of voluntary movement to spasticity in the upper motor neurone syndrome. *Trans Am Neurol Assoc.* 1977;102:108–111.

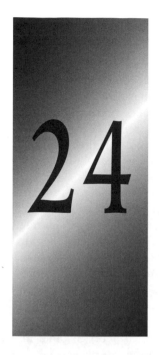

Spasticity in Traumatic Brain Injury

Ross Zafonte
Stephanie Co
Anath Srikrishnan

Spasticity remains among the most vexing problems after severe traumatic brain injury (TBI). Because of the often diffuse nature of TBI and its association with other forms of polytrauma (eg, limb-based injury) and hypoxic ischemic injury, patterns of spasticity with TBI can be more complicated and certainly more diffuse (1). Spasticity can be the source of lost function, pain, contracture, frustration, and behavioral disturbance. To avoid replications with other sections in this text, this chapter will focus on the issues most applicable to those with TBI throughout the continuum of care. Because of limited data in this population, in some cases, specific reference is made to data from parallel populations.

EPIDEMIOLOGY

Although there are varying accounts of incidence of spasticity and more research is required in this area, 1 study found that 25% of TBI patients in an inpatient setting develop spasticity (2). A comparable value was found in a study in Turkey consisting of 30 TBI patients, where 23.4% of patients developed spasticity as a complication (3). Most of these patients (73%) were severely injured, with Glasgow COMA Scale (GCS) scores between 3 and 8, and with 63.3% of the patients with spasticity having an Ashworth score of 1, 16.7% with 2, and only 6.7% with 3. Ten percent of these patients had contractures, and this may be increased in more severe injured brain injury patients. The national guidelines for the management of spasticity using botulinum toxin (BoNT) by the Royal College of Physicians estimated that 75% of patients with severe TBI would develop spasticity requiring treatment, compared to 33.3% of patients with stroke and 60% of patients with severe multiple sclerosis (4).

A study by Singer et al. showed that spasticity in the plantar flexor and invertor muscles was present in 13.3% of patients with moderate to severe brain injury admitted to an inpatient unit in Western Australia (5). In a retrospective cohort study of patients with severe acquired brain injury, predictors of spasticity at 1 year postinjury were low Functional Independence Measure score at admission ($P < .001$), longer length of stay ($P < .036$), and lower age ($P = .01$) (6). Spasticity was more frequent in patients with brainstem injury compared to those with other types of severe brain injury in a retrospective clinical study (7). Immobilization, motor weakness, hypoxic ischemic injury, spinal cord injury (SCI), and age are risk factors associated with early spasticity. (8, 9) Exacerbating factors in spasticity include occult injury, infection, Heterotopic Ossification (HO), and pain (10). One study found that severe brain injuries accompanying SCI, hypoxic ischemic injury, and autonomic dysfunction are associated with earlier and more severe spasticity (11).

PATHOPHYSIOLOGY AND UNIQUE ASPECTS OF TBI

Spasticity has been defined by Lance as a motor disorder characterized by a velocity-dependent increase in the tonic stretch reflexes (muscle tone) with exaggerated tendon jerks, resulting from hyperexcitability of the stretch reflex as 1 component of the upper motor syndrome (12, 13). In addition to inhibitory influences arising from the brain, there are also nonreciprocal Ib inhibition (from Golgi tendon organ receptors in tendons), presynaptic inhibition of the Ia terminal (at the axoaxonic synapse between 2 axons), reciprocal Ia inhibition (inhibition of antagonistic muscles), and recurrent Renshaw inhibition (inhibitory feedback of the alpha motor neuron cell body by the inhibitory interneuron) (14). In brain injury, multiple excitatory and inhibitory influences on the stretch reflex are affected, leading to imbalance that presents as spasticity.

Decorticate posturing may be seen in association with spasticity, presenting with arms in flexion and legs in extension. Flexion in the arms is the result of disinhibition of the red nucleus, leading to the facilitation of the rubrospinal tract. This tract facilitates motor neurons in the cervical spinal cord that innervate flexor muscles in the upper extremities. The rubrospinal tract originates in the ipsilateral motor cortex and projects to the red nucleus in the midbrain, where the fibers decussate in the midbrain and descend in the lateral brainstem and spinal cord, intermixed with the lateral corticospinal tract. Brain lesions often occur in conjunction with the corticospinal tract in the internal capsule and cerebral peduncle, resulting in contralateral spastic hemiplegia.

The rubrospinal tract and the medullary reticulospinal tract favor flexion and overpower the medial and lateral vestibulospinal and pontine reticulospinal tracts, which favor extension. The lateral vestibulospinal tract originates in the lateral vestibular nucleus and connects to ipsilateral lower motor neurons involved in extensor movements, especially proximal. Inhibitory connections from the red nucleus and cerebellum hold this powerful extensor movement in check, preventing extensor hypertonia. The medial vestibulospinal tract originates from the medial vestibular nucleus to inhibit lower motor neurons involving neck and axial muscles.

The reticulospinal has pontine and medullary origins. The pontine tract originates in the medial pontine reticular formation and descends ipsilaterally and medially in the spinal cord and terminates directly and indirectly on lower motor neurons. It works in conjunction with the lateral vestibulospinal tract with extensor influence. It is not influenced strongly by cerebral inputs, but from trigeminal and somatosensory inputs. The medullary reticulospinal tract originates in the medial medullary Reticular Formation (RF) and ends bilaterally and directly and indirectly on lower motor neurons at all levels. It has flexor influence along with the corticospinal and reticulospinal tracts and receives input from cortex, especially motor and premotor/supplemental motor cortices. They regulate basic tone and posture and are not organized somatotopically. In the lower extremities, extension is the result of the disruption of the lateral corticospinal tract, which facilitates motor neurons in the lower spinal cord supplying flexor muscles of the lower extremities. Because the corticospinal tract is interrupted, the pontine reticulospinal and the medial and lateral vestibulospinal-biased extension tracts overwhelm the medullary reticulospinal tract.

The effect on these 2 tracts (corticospinal and rubrospinal) by lesions above the red nucleus is what leads to the characteristic flexion posturing of the upper extremities and extensor posturing of the lower extremities. Decorticate posturing indicates that there may be damage to areas including the cerebral hemispheres, the internal capsule, and the thalamus. It may also indicate damage to the midbrain. Lesions above the red nucleus lead to decorticate posturing, whereas lesions at or below the level of the red nucleus, in the midbrain or cerebellum, lead to decerebrate posturing. Decerebrate posturing presents with arms and legs in extension, and the head may arch back as well. Such postures are typically seen in those with severe brain stem disruption and associated hypoxic injury.

CONFOUNDING CAUSES AND ASSESSMENT

As one evaluates those patients with TBI, it is important to note that in both acute and postacute settings, spasticity can be influenced by superimposed intracranial, metabolic, and infectious problems. In this chapter, we will not discuss patterns of spasticity because these patterns and treatment paradigms are discussed elsewhere in this text.

ACUTE MANAGEMENT OF POST-TBI SPASTICITY

It is important to initiate management and treatment of spasticity in the acute care setting to prevent and manage the secondary effects of spasticity, especially loss of range of motion (ROM), before they become severe. Although the patient is in a bed-bound, unconscious state, it requires particular attention and vigilance to these issues that may otherwise only be noted later when the patient improves from a low-level state. Early occurring spasticity, which is associated with SCI, hypoxic ischemic injury, and autonomic dysfunction, also tends to be more severe. Hinderer et al. (15) has proposed that patients be evaluated in the following areas: clinical history, stretch examination, passive motion examination, active motion examination, and functional examination. Clinical history should note risk factors, such as immobilization, motor dysfunction, hypoxic ischemic injury, SCI, and age, as well as prior functional history and any previous neurological dysfunction. Zafonte et al. (16) also suggest using an objective measurement of tone such as the Ashworth Scale and to assess at multiple times of the day as the tone may be affected by medications, procedures, and other stimuli. One must evaluate for any compounding factors, such as occult injury, hydrocephalus or central nervous system lesion, infection, heterotopic ossification, and pain. Attention should be given to several medications in the acute care setting that may affect tone. Neuroparalytic agents can eliminate tone, opioids and benzodiazepines can decrease tone, and propofol, a short-acting sedative, may also decrease tone.

Physical modalities can be the first line of treatment, without the risk of systemic side effects seen in other treatments. Passive stretching with flexion and extension of the elbow has been shown to be effective in reducing tone in patients with brain injury (17). Stretching may be performed 1 to 2 times a day. Family members can also be involved in this care. Cryotherapy also helps reduce spasticity and provide analgesia (5). Treatment should not exceed 20 minutes so as to avoid potential injury to sensitive, possibly insensate skin in patients with decreased consciousness. Cryotherapy efficacy, however, is limited to about half an hour.

Splinting and serial casting may also be used in the acute care setting. Singer et al. (18) found that in patients with brain injury with spastic equinovarus deformity, serial casting for 5 weeks significantly increased muscle extensibility of the triceps surae in 9 patients and decreased passive torque in 8 patients. There was a median improvement in ankle dorsiflexion of 30° with knees flexed and 15° with knees extended (18). Mortenson and Eng (19) wrote a review on 13 studies on the use of casts in patients with brain injury. Of these, 2 studies were rated level II.

Moseley (9) conducted a randomized crossover in 1997 on 9 patients with acute brain injury. Casting plus stretching was compared to stretching alone. Torque-controlled passive range of motion (PROM)

was significantly increased by a mean difference of 15.4° ($P < .5$) in the casted group. In a double randomized crossover by Hill in 1994 on 15 patients after acute TBI, serial casting applied to the elbow or wrist 4 to 6 times over 1 month was compared to traditional therapy alone. (20) Outcome measures included (1) PROM using goniometer, (2) 3-point functional scale, and (3) spasticity as determined by (a) the angle when stretch reflex was elicited and (b) timed rapid alternating movements. There was a significant increase in PROM in the casting group ($P = .014$), improved spasticity only in the group casted first, and no effect on function. In the process, staff must be alert to avoid pressure sores.

A case comparison study by Pohl has shown that duration of 1 to 4 days is as effective as 5 to 7 days (21). This was a retrospective study of 2 historic groups (1997–1998 for 5–7 days and 1999–2001 for 1–4 days) of 105 patients with serial casting of elbows, wrists, knees, and ankles, which showed improvement in PROM in both groups ($P < .001$) with no significant difference between groups ($P = .71$) and less complications in the shorter-duration group. Casting may also reduce spasticity in areas beyond the specific area being treated. Barnard et al. (22) showed a reduction in tone throughout the patient after 10 days of casting the ankles of a comatose patient 10 days postinjury. In the acute setting, clinicians should be cautious regarding increases in Intra Cranial Pressure (ICP) due to casting, however, in patients who are at risk.

Mills (23) showed significant increases in ROM of extension in the elbows, wrists, and ankles of patients with brain injury with flexion posturing with splinting. The results did not show any increased electromyography (EMG) activity during splinting for 2 hours, which the authors interpreted as accommodation of the muscles without any increase in tone with splinting. Lai et al. (24) studied the efficacy of dynamic splinting on stroke patients with elbow flexion spasticity. Thirty patients were randomized to control or experimental groups. Both groups received uniform doses of botox-A to biceps (150 U), brachialis (75 U), and brachioradialis (75 U) muscles and occupational, manual therapy weekly for 16 weeks. Protocol for therapy included moist heat, patient education, joint mobilization, passive and active ROM, proprioneural facilitation to retrain sensorimotor deficits, and therapeutic exercise. The experimental group received this treatment as well as dynamic splinting with the elbow extension Dynasplint, worn 6 to 8 hours at night, and increasing tension every 2 weeks, as tolerated by the patients. The percentage of change in active ROM in elbow extension after 14 weeks was greater for the experimental than for the control subjects (33.5%

vs 18.7%). The Modified Ashworth Scale (extension) scores showed comparable changes of a mean 9.3% improvement for experimental versus 8.6% for the control subjects. A randomized controlled study by Lannin et al. (25) showed that static palmar hand splints in the resting functional position worn for up to 12 hours overnight in patients with TBI within 6 months from injury who had no active wrist extension did not show any significant improvement in wrist and finger flexor muscle length, hand function, or pain compared to patients who received motor training and stretching alone (25). Spasticity itself was not used as an outcome measure. Custom dynamic splints are better tolerated than noncustomized.

Electrical stimulation applied to muscles, motor nerves, and sensory dermatomes has also shown to produce reduction of tone in patients with brain injury. This may be due to fatiguing or inhibition of spastic muscles and activation of antagonist muscles. It generally lasts a few hours but has been shown to last up to 24 hours by Seib et al (26). They showed a significant decrease in ankle tone in 9 of 10 patients with TBI and SCI after electrical stimulation to the tibialis anterior muscle and no significant change after a sham procedure.

POSTACUTE AND PHARMACOLOGIC MANAGEMENT

Tizanidine

Tizanidine has also been used effectively in the treatment of spasticity. Its mechanism of action is a central alpha-2-adrenoreceptor agonist, and its side effect profile is considerably better than some of the other drugs that are typically used for spasticity, such as baclofen and diazepam. Although its structure (and possibly its mechanism of action) is similar to clonidine, tizanidine, when tested on animals, has a far smaller incidence of bradycardia or hypotension than clonidine. It works at both the spinal level and the supraspinal level. Despite the facts stated above, the precise mechanism of action of tizanidine has not yet been fully elucidated. It has both alpha-2 adrenergic and imidazoline-binding properties, and whereas the majority of its impact is believed to be due to the former, the latter may also have a significant role.

Tizanidine mainly acts at the presynaptic level, decreasing the release of neurotransmitters aspartate and glutamate from interneurons in the spinal cord. However, the drug also exerts an impact on neurotransmitter receptors in the postsynapse. Postsynaptically, the impact is again exerted on excitatory amino acid neurotransmitters. In addition to these effects on excitatory neurotransmitters, tizanidine may also potentiate the activity of the inhibitory amino acid neurotransmitter glycine, which, in turn, inhibits pathways traveling from the coeruleus to the spine. Unlike other drugs in this chapter, tizanidine does not have any GABA-ergic or GABA-inhibitory properties, nor does it affect opioid or dopamine systems.

Tizanidine is metabolized in the liver by cytochrome P450 1A2. Therefore, the clinician must be aware of whether he or she is coadministering known inhibitors of this enzyme, such as rofecoxib. Notably, baclofen and acetaminophen can be coadministered without any adverse effects, at least according to the current state of the literature.

The major adverse effects of tizanidine were summarized by a review article: "dry mouth, somnolence, asthenia, and dizziness," along with transient and reversible elevation in liver function tests. Although rare, visual hallucinations have been noted. A recent study by Gelber showed that somnolence was the most frequently noted side effect (62%), followed by dizziness (32%) and asthenia (30%). A notable finding of the study, however, is that only 21% of patients tolerated their dose of the medicine being increased to the maximum level of 36 mg (27).

Tizanidine has been used for spasticity that is caused by a number of different diseases, including (i) SCI, (ii) multiple sclerosis, (iii) stroke, and (iv) TBI. Its effectiveness with regard to all of these diseases has been studied. In spinal cord patients, a double-blind, placebo-controlled, parallel, randomized, multicenter trial was conducted on 118 patients (28). The Ashworth Scale and the pendulum test were used as a metric for spasticity (29, 30). Both measures of spasticity declined in a statistically significant way in the tizanidine-treated group. In addition, when asked about the frequency of their daytime spasms, the patients treated with tizanidine gave a number that was one half as large as their previous baseline level. Finally, with respect to adverse effects, the tizanidine-treated group did not experience any adverse changes to vital signs or muscle strength (nor did the placebo group).

Multiple studies have been conducted investigating the efficacy of tizanidine for use in multiple sclerosis. Nance et al. (31) in 1997 showed in a multicenter, placebo-controlled study involving 142 patients that tizanidine reduced spasticity in a dose-dependent manner. Adverse effects, such as hypotension, were also dose-dependent.

A multicenter, placebo-controlled, randomized study undertaken by the US Tizanidine Study Group yielded more ambiguous results. Based on Ashworth score comparisons, there was no difference between the drug and the placebo groups. Why did this occur? There was an anomalous decrease of –2.84 on the Ashworth Scale of the placebo group toward the end of the study; this effect is believed to have caused the lack of difference between the 2 groups. However, when the investigators reanalyzed the data to look at the change in Ashworth score 3 hours after administration of the drug, they found that a significantly larger decrease in the Ashworth Scale occurred during that 3-hour period (but not after). This rather atypical pattern of data means that this study, although valuable, is of uncertain significance.

Another similar study was done by the United Kingdom Tizanidine Trial Group. The sample size was 187 patients. The duration of the study was 12 weeks, with 9 of those weeks consisting of optimal dosing. As measured by the Ashworth score, the patients taking tizanidine had a notably greater decrease in spasticity than the placebo group. The patient-reported impression of effectiveness was also greater for tizanidine. Unlike other studies, the frequency of patient-reported spasms was not affected by the choice of drug versus placebo (32).

A study of patients with either TBI or stroke and refractory spastic hypertonia was treated with tizanidine or placebo in a double-blind, placebo-controlled, crossover, randomized study. Spasticity was preferentially reduced by tizanidine, as measured by both Ashworth score and motor tone. Spasm was reduced, but only in the lower extremities. Unlike other studies of tizanidine, muscle strength also increased, however, only by a small amount (33). Other studies have also yield similar results (34).

Baclofen

The mechanism of action of baclofen consists of GABA-ergic activity at both presynaptic and postsynaptic receptors. This effect influences both monosynaptic and polysynaptic reflex responses. The exact neurophysiological mechanism by which the GABA-ergic activity occurs is not known. The pharmacological structure of baclofen is similar to that of GABA, and thus baclofen may directly potentiate the GABA receptor. The overall effect of baclofen is to increase the amount of presynaptic inhibition while simultaneously decreasing the amount of excitatory neurotransmitters that are emitted. In addition to its GABA-related effects, it has been postulated that baclofen has antidopaminergic effects centered around the mesolimbic and nigrostriatal pathways (or possibly via antagonist effects on substance P) (35). Baclofen is given intrathecally and enterically, as will be discussed below.

Enteral Baclofen

The literature regarding enteral baclofen is limited. (A PubMed study using the search term *enteral baclofen* yields only 4 citations. In comparison, a search for *intrathecal baclofen* yielded more than 800 results.) Although baclofen is frequently given to patients as a treatment for spasticity secondary to spinal disease, there have been very few studies demonstrating its efficacy in this regard for either enteric or intrathecal mode of administration. A recent review (2000) pointed out that one study (the only article on this topic mentioned in the review) involving enteric baclofen for spine-caused spasticity was comprised of only 6 patients (36).

An important distinction in the treatment of spasticity with enteral baclofen (and, indeed, with all pharmacological agents) is that between symptomatic amelioration of spasticity versus improvement of functional outcomes (eg, ability to ambulate, ability to perform activities of daily living). As discussed below, baclofen has shown more efficacy in the former than in the latter.

A significant, and one of the earliest, investigations concerning enteral baclofen was performed in 1974 by Basmaijan and Yucel (37).

The inclusion criteria for this study was (i) having spasticity for at least 90 days before onset of study, (ii) absence of diseases that might negatively affect joint function (peripheral vascular disease, arthritis, etc), and (iii) absence of serious renal, liver, gastrointestinal, or hemorrhagic disease. The structure of the study was a double-blind, randomized, crossover study of 5-week duration (with a 1-week "washout" period).

Two principal measurements of spasticity were "patellar reflex force" and quadricep "myoelectrical activity." Spasticity was assessed clinically involving a combination of objective tests, subjective patient interviews, and functional assessment.

The study, overall, concluded the following: "Ba-34647 was shown . . . to successfully control spasticity in patients with SCI, but it was less impressive with MS patients." (38)

Although there is a fair amount of evidence that baclofen improves spasticity, there is far less evidence that baclofen improves functional outcomes. According to one review article, a study has noted that muscle strength is actually reduced in patients who are on baclofen treatment (39). One potential reason for this has been discussed in a paper by Nielsen et al. The authors argue that the peripheral effects of baclofen operate at cross purposes to its central effects. In addition, there may be an underlying muscle weakness that is concealed by spasticity and that then becomes significant when the spasticity is treated (36).

TABLE 24.1
Spasticity – Pharmacotherapy For TBI – Study Table

Study	Type	Drug/ Intervention	Population	No.	Metric	Findings/ Results
Nance et al. 1994	Multicenter (all tertiary centers), double-blind, placebo-controlled, randomized study	Tizanidine	Patients with spasticity secondary to MS with no pharmacological treatment that might impede the study	142	Ashworth Scale, pendulum test	Tizanidine significantly decreases spasticity in MS in a dose-dependent manner
Nance et al. 1994	Multicenter, placebo-controlled	Tizanidine	Patients who have had a spinal cord injury for 12+ months	124	Ashworth Scale, pendulum test	Both pendulum-test performance and Ashworth score underwent a positive change in the tizanidine population
Smith et al. 1994	Multicenter, placebo-controlled, double-blind, randomized, with stratification	Tizanidine	Patients with spasticity caused by MS	N = 220 (111 tizanidine-treated + 109 placebo-treated)	Ashworth Scale, patient self-reporting, physician clinical assessment	"Patient and physician perception of improvement demonstrated more consistent differences between groups than did the Ashworth scale, perhaps because of inexperience with this measure or failure to consider time between drug administration and assessment."
The United Kingdom Tizanidine Trial Group, 1994	Prospective study, placebo-controlled, randomized, double-blind trial	Tizanidine	Patients with MS	187	Patient self-reporting	"Approximately 75% of patients, with all degrees of spasticity, reported subjective movement without an increase in muscle weakness, but there was no improvement in activities of daily living dependent on movement."

Study	Study design	Intervention	N	Patient population	Outcome measures	Results
Meythaler et al. 2001	Prospective, crossover study, double-blind, placebo-controlled, randomized	Tizanidine	17. (8 TBI, 9 stroke)	Patients with stroke and/or TBI, with 6 months of spasticity ("intractable spastic hyperonia")	Ashworth score for rigidity; assessment of motor strength, spasm, and deep tendon reflexes	Upper extremity: decrease (ie, improvement) in Ashworth score; no statistically significant change in reflex, spasm. Lower extremity: decrease in Ashworth score; decrease spasm score; reflex score unchanged; reduction in motor tone; enhancement of motor strength
Gelber et al. 2001	Multi-center, open label	Tizanidine	47	Patient with stroke occurring 6+ months ago; and, spasticity	Modified Ashworth Scale Pain and Functional Spasticity Questionnaires Assessment of muscle strength Assessment of functional improvement	Decrease in upper extremity modified Ashworth score Amelioration of pain intensity Improvement in quality of life as assessed by physician Improvement of disability as assessed by physician Strength unchanged
Penn et al. 1989	Crossover study. Randomized, double-blind. Followed by open-label long-term study	Intrathecal baclofen by programmable pump	10	Patients with spasticity secondary to MS or spinal cord injury intractable to oral baclofen	Ashworth Scale Assessment of spasms Assessment of whether baclofen being administered	Improvement in muscle tone and decrease in spasms to a level that does not impede activities of daily living; both of which are sustained through long-term investigation
Hugenholts et al. 1992. (abstract only)	Double-blind, crossover study	Intrathecal baclofen injections	6	Patients with intractable spasticity of the spinal cord	A number of objective and subjective tests of clinical state and physiological state	Baclofen patients showed reduction of spasticity in lower extremities, as well as improvements in passive range of motion of joints, number of spasms, muscle tone, and hyperreflexia

(Continued)

TABLE 24.1
Spasticity – Pharmacotherapy For TBI – Study Table (Continued)

STUDY	TYPE	DRUG/ INTERVENTION	POPULATION	No.	METRIC	FINDINGS/ RESULTS
Gruenthal et al. 1997	Crossover, prospective study, unicenter, double-blind, placebo controlled	Oral gabapentin	Patients with spasticity secondary to MS	22	Patient self-reporting: "spasm frequency scale, spasm severity scale, interference with function scale, painful spasm scale, and gobal assessment scale". Physician assessment: "Modified Ashworth Scale, clonus scale, deep tendon reflexes, plantar stimulation, and Kurtzke Expanded Disability status scale."	Gabapentin reduces spasticity and the difficulties caused thereby, according to both patient self-reporting and physician assessments such as Ashworth Scale. Side effects such as impairment of concentration and fatigue were not prominently noted
Schmidt et al. 1976	Crossover study	Comparison of dantrolene sodium and diazepam	Patients with spasticity secondary to MS	42	i. Kurtzke disability scale ii. Quantitative assessment of spasticity and other physical function variables iii. Patient self-reporting and surveys	Dantrolene reduces spasticity more than diazepam, as per both physician assessments and patient self-reporting
Nogen et al. 1976. (Abstract only).	Double-blind, 2-segment, comparison study	Comparison between dantrolene sodium and diazepam	Patients with spasticity secondary to cerebral palsy	22	NA	Dantrium more effective in 9/22 patients; valium more effective in 7/22 patients; the 2 drugs were equally beneficial in 4 patients. Combination yielded greatest benefit in 8 patients, particularly in upper limbs and hip

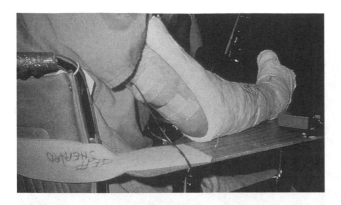

FIGURE 24.1

Electrotherapy (with antagonist stimulation) and casting for a spastic upper extremity.

Another study assessed the "effect of baclofen on gait in spastic MS patients." This double-blind, placebo-controlled, crossover study was performed on 14 patients with spastic multiple sclerosis; the patients had a median Ashworth composite score of 0.8. The authors measured several outcomes, but the most relevant for our purposes are (i) spasticity and (ii) improvements in gait that may or may not have been caused by a decrease in spasticity. A computer-associated treadmill device was used to evaluate gait, and a "computer-assisted force plate" was used to evaluate postural stability.

The authors found that baclofen did not exert any significant ameliorative effect on gait and postural stability in patients with multiple sclerosis. They concluded that there are only valid reasons to use baclofen for "painful spasms, flexor spasms, frequently occurring mass reflexes, and co-contractions." (40)

Another double-blind, placebo-controlled, crossover study performed in children with cerebral palsy showed that baclofen reduced spasticity. (This study was only available in abstract form.) Thus, both adult and pediatric populations can be treated for spasticity with baclofen (41).

Intrathecal Baclofen

A study conducted in 1989 by Penn et al. (42) tested the efficacy of intrathecal baclofen on patients with spasticity from SCI (along with others with multiple sclerosis). This was a double-blind, randomized, crossover study. All of the patients suffered from spasticity that could not be appropriately treated with an oral antispastic pharmaceutical agent. The outcomes were measured by 2 separate metrics. First, the Ashworth score declined by 2.8 points on average, specifically from a level of 4 to 1.2. Second, a spasm index was

used, and this also reduced by an average of 2.9 points. The patients were then subsequently observed for 19 months on average, and the outcome persisted during this time (42).

A follow-up to the Penn study was conducted by Kravitz. Six of the patients who participated in the Penn trial participated in this study. These patients were given electromyograms, and the results from those were analyzed. Four patients had altered EMGs; specifically, their "phasic EMG activity" had decreased since they started taking baclofen (43).

A study by Hugenholz, involving 6 patients, was conducted in a double-blind, placebo, randomized, cross-over fashion to investigate intrathecal baclofen. This involved patients with spasticity due to multiple sclerosis or SCI. The study was an open-observation, double-blind, crossover, randomized study. The main outcome measurements were self-reported symptoms and physical examination. All of the patients reported a decreased amount of muscle tone and spasms in their lower limbs. Most patients described a greater capacity to perform activities of daily living (ADL) and lower limb PROM. The upper limb joints did not display an increased PROM. Of 6 patients, 5 underwent a reduction in their disability index. The 2 principal side effects reported were (i) drowsiness and (ii) lumbar catheter repositioning (44).

A study by Burke utilized a different structure. It involved patients treated with diazepam who were now treated with baclofen. The major metrics were the following: decrease in spasticity (5/6 patients), reduction in frequency of spasms (3/6), reduction in the length of time for ankle clonus (2/6), and finally, stretch reflex. All 6 patients displayed a decrease in

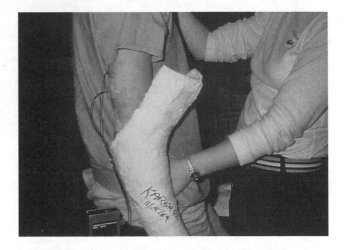

FIGURE 24.2

Resultant improvement in range of motion at the elbow from electrotherapy and casting.

FIGURE 24.3

Severe bridging HO (Heterotopic Os-sification) at the elbows. Arrows note bridging HO.

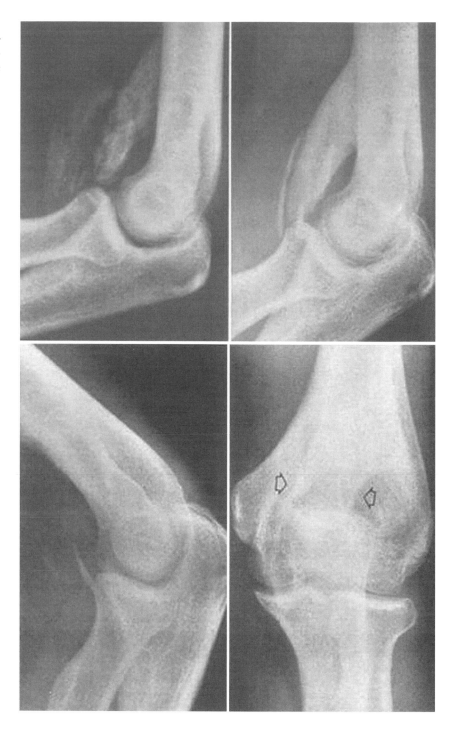

stretch reflex at a velocity of 200°/s. Tendon reflexes were unchanged (45).

In summary, then, baclofen may be said to be a drug with strengths and clear limitations. It can treat spasticity; however, it is primarily effective on spasticity of spinal origin. There is not much evidence for its effectiveness in spasticity of cerebral origin. Second, although it can ameliorate the symptom of spasticity, it

has much less of an improved impact on ambulation, muscle strength, ability to perform activities of daily living, and functional outcomes (Table 24.1) (39, 46).

Gabapentin

Gruenthal et al. performed a double-blind, random-ized, placebo-controlled crossover trial (N = 25), and

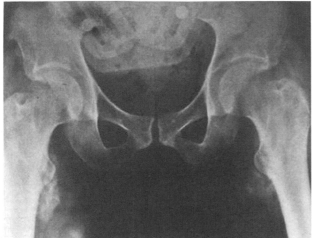

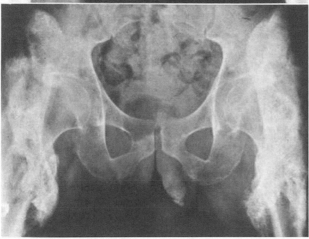

FIGURE 24.4

Severe HO at the hips with resultant no range of motion.

the patients all had SCI. The 2 metrics used were the Ashworth Scale and the Likert scale. The Ashworth Scale was found to have been decreased by 11%, and the Likert scale was decreased by 20%. One potential flaw in this study is that some of the necessary biostatistical data, such as 95% confidence intervals, were not described in the study (47).

Valium

Another study was conducted comparing Valium and Amytal to a placebo. Unlike other studies, in this randomized, double-blind study, the metric used was an independent clinical observation. The study was conducted on 22 patients with SCI. (This is due to the fact that this study was conducted prior to the development of the Ashworth Scale.) The doctors (and 1

patient) who observed the patients in the study rated them on a scale of 1 to 4. The patients with Valium showed an improvement of $c^2 = 7.091$. (Figure 24.1) (48).

(See below for additional studies involving a comparison between Valium and dantrolene.)

Dantrolene

Dantrolene mechanism of action differs from most of the other drugs in this chapter. It acts directly on the sarcoplasmic reticuli of the skeletal muscle, inhibiting the efflux of calcium therefrom. An important adverse effect of dantrolene is hepatotoxicity; therefore, it has been recommended that patients taking this drug should undergo monitoring of liver enzymes (49).

A study comparing the efficacy of dantrolene and diazepam was performed by Schmidt in 1976 (50). All of the patients had spasticity due to multiple sclerosis, and a total of 46 patients participated in the study. This was a single-center, double-blind, controlled study. The metric used was a neurologist's evaluation of the patient's spasticity, clonus, and reflexes, as measured in a 6-point scale (not the Ashworth Scale). The study also evaluated the patient's functional status using methodology and parameters that are delineated in the ACTH Cooperative Study (51, 52).

The results of this study showed that both dantrolene and diazepam reduced spasticity in a dose-dependent manner; moreover, the magnitude of reduction was approximately equal between the 2 drugs. With respect to adverse effects, the principal ones seen were drowsiness, weakness, and feelings of light-headedness. Weakness predominated in Dantrium, and drowsiness, unsurprisingly, was more often seen in diazepam. Another study was conducted by Glass and Hannah (53) in 1974. The study involved patients with spasticity and did not find any notable distinction between the efficacy of dantrolene or diazepam (n = 16) for this study.

A third study involved 22 pediatric patients with spasticity due to cerebral palsy (54). (This study was only reviewed in abstract form.) In this study, as well, there was not a large disparity found between the effectiveness of dantrolene versus diazepam. The authors reported that 7 patients saw more of a benefit with diazepam, 9 patients saw more of a benefit from Dantrium, and 4 patients appeared to experience an equal benefit. However, 8 patients seemed to undergo the greatest benefit from a combination of the 2 drugs. The authors concluded that "the combination of peripherally and centrally acting agents is more beneficial than either medication alone." (54)

TABLE 24.2
Spasticity – Interventional Therapy for TBI – Study Table

Study	Type	Drug/Intervention	Population	No.	Metric	Findings/Results
Guettard et al. (1)	Prospective study	Botulinum toxin A injections	Pediatric patients with spasticity, dystonia, and other neurologic abnormalities secondary to acquired brain injury	25	Ashworth Scale; muscle testing/Zancolli I/II scale; 4-level functional assessment scale; interviews of patients, parents, and caregivers	Spasticity "dramatically reduced" via Ashworth Scale; lower limb, equinus is the most commonly observed difficulty; in upper limb Zancolli changed from class III to class I. "In conclusion, these results suggest that a combination of BTX-A and rehabilitation to treat spasticity and dystonia. . . is a good option."
Simpson et al. (2)	Mulitcenter, placebo-controlled, randomized, interventional, double-blind, parallel group investigation	Botulinum toxin vs. tizanidine	Patients with upper limb spasticity secondary to stroke or TBI	60	Ashworth disability scale, disability assessment scale, (both at multiple joints); side effects/adverse effects	BoNT caused a greater reduction in muscle tone in both wrist and finger flexors, compared to tizanidine and placebo BoNT had a lower number of adverse effects than tizanidine or placebo; most common adverse effect in all three was somnolence; no liver function test abnormalities noted with BoNT, unlike tizanidine
Chang et al. 2009 (3)	Prospective cohort investigation, conducted in outpatient clinic	Botulinum toxin A injections; subsequently, patients given 1.5 months of therapy	Patients who have spastic hemiparesis	23	Motor Activity Log-28, Motor Activity Log items. Secondarily, Motor Activity Log Self-Report Action Research Arm Test, and Modified Ashworth Scale	Higher degree of change on Motor Activity Log-28 for high functioning group; both high and low functioning group showed ameliorated hand function and decrease spasticity
Francisco et al. 2002 (4)	Controlled, randomized, blinded trial	Botulinum toxin A injections in either a high-volume or low-volume preparation	Patients with spasticity in wrist flexor or finger flexor, caused by acquired brain injury	13	Patients divided into high-volume injection group, and low-volume injection group. Spasticity measured by Modified Ashworth Scale	Both high-volume and low-volume injected patients experienced an important reduction in spasticity. However, the magnitude of said reduction was approximately equal in both groups
Keenan 1988 (abstract only) (5)	"Management of the spastic upper extremity in the neurologically impaired adult"	Phenol	NA	NA	NA	NA

Study	Study type	Intervention	N	Population	Methods	Results
Keenan MA et al. 1990 (abstract only) (6)	Prospective study	Phenol	17	Adults with traumatic brain injury and spasticity	Patients injected with percutaneous phenol blocks; range of motion, resting position measured	93% of extremities improved after the initial injection; effect lasted 5 months on average. No significant adverse effects noted. "This study indicates that percutaneous phenol injection of the musculocutaneous nerve provides reliable, temporary relief of spasticity...."
Wissel et al. 1999 (abstract only; article in German) (7)	Interventional	Single-dose botulinum toxin A	204	Adults with acute or chronic spasticity secondary to traumatic brain injury, stroke, and spinal cord injury	Patients injected with botulinum toxin A in approximately 3 muscles. Results measured using Rating of response to Btx	~93% of patients showed amelioration; none worsened. Severity decreased and functional improvement was noted. 5.9% had temporary side effects; none had permanent side or adverse effects
Pavesi et al. 1998 (8)	Open-labeled investigation	Botulinum toxin type A	6	Patients with severe traumatic brain injury and spasticity	Botulinum toxin A administered by electromyography-guided injection. Assessed by physiatrist and neurologist; metrics included Modified Ashworth Scale; goniometry-assessed range of motion; clinical assessment of posture, voluntary motion, and functional outcomes	Improvements in Ashworth scale, improved functional activity of upper limb, reduced spasticity. "These preliminary data show that BTX-A treatment is effective in reducing spasticity in selected patients with focal upper limb muscular tone disorders secondary to traumatic brain injuries."

1. Guettard E, et al. Management of spasticity and dystonia in children with acquired brain injury with rehabilitation and botulinum toxin A. *Developmental Neurorehabilitation.* 2009;12(3):128–138.
2. Simpson. Botulinum neurotoxicity versus tizanidine in upper limb spasticity: a placebo-controlled study. *J Neurol Neurosurg Psychiatry.* 2008;80:380–385.
3. Chang Chia-Lin, et al. Effect of Baseline Spastic Hemiparesis on Recovery of Upper-Limb Function Following Botulinum Toxin Type A Injections and Postinjection Therapy. *Arch Phys Med Rehabil.* 2009;90:1462–1468.
4. Francisco GE, et al. Botulinum Toxin in Upper Limb Spasticity After Acquired Brain Injury: A Randomized Trial Comparing Dilution Techniques. *Am J Phys Med Rehabil.* 2002;81(5):355–363.
5. Keenan M. Management of the spastic upper extremity in the neurologically impaired adult. *Clin Orthop Relat Res.* 1988;233:116–125.
6. Keenan M, et al. Percutaneous Phenol Block of the musculocutaneous nerve to control elbow flexor spasticity. *Hand Surg Am.* 1990;15(2):340–346.
7. Wissel J, et al.[Safety and Tolerance of Single-dose botulinum toxin Type A treatment in 204 patients with spasticity and localized associated symptoms, Austrian and German botulinum toxin A spasticity study group]. *Wien Klin Wochenschr.* 1999;111(20):637–642.
8. Pavesi G, et al. Botulinum toxin type A in the treatment of upper limb spasticity among patients with traumatic brain injury. *J Neurol Neurosurg Psychiatry.* 1998;64(3):419–420.

INJECTION GUIDED THERAPY

Phenol

One possible method of treating spasticity secondary to TBI is the use of phenol injections. There are not many recent studies of this therapeutic method because it has largely been supplanted (as is discussed elsewhere in this text) by more effective methodologies, such as BoNT injections and tizanidine. A 1990 prospective study of 17 patients focused on adult patients who had spasticity secondary to TBI. (Available to the author in abstract form only.) The patients were subjected to percutaneous phenol injections and evaluated for mean resting position, elbow ROM, and adverse effects. The authors reported that "93% of extremities improved after the initial injection," with no adverse effects noted (Figures 24.2 and 24.3) (55).

In general, a significant adverse effect of phenol is dysesthesia. Other side effects include fibrosis of the soft tissues. The procedural exigencies of injecting phenol are significant as well, which means that the effectiveness of phenol injections is contingent on operator skill. A review article by Elovic et al lists the advantages and disadvantages of phenol and alcohol as follows. The advantages are the following: "less costly than BoNT; rapid onset of action; facilitation of serial casting; potency; its effect on sensory fibers can further decrease spasticity reflex arc; potency for large muscle groups (hip adductors); less injection sites; more spastic regions can be treated at one time than BoNT; less storage requirements; can reinject or booster in less than 3 months." The disadvantages are the following: " risk of dysesthesias; muscle fibrosis; need for patient sedation; scarring; risk of granuloma formation; reduce contraction during voluntary movement; edema can develop after infection; greater patient discomfort during procedure; procedure requires more time to perform; procedure requires more skill to perform than toxin[.]" (Figure 24.4, Table 24.2) (56).

Botulinum Toxin

The treatment of focal spastic hypertonia has been greatly advanced by the introduction of BoNT as a therapeutic modality. Several studies have demonstrated the effectiveness of BoNT in this regard. Many of these investigations are discussed below (Figure 24.5) (57).

Guettard et al. (58) studied the effect of BoNT injections on pediatric patients with spasticity or dystonia secondary to TBI. Assessments were done with Zancolli scale, Ashworth Scale, and clinical interviews of patients and their families. The basic finding was that spasticity was "dramatically reduced," as measured by the Ashworth Scale. In the patients' upper

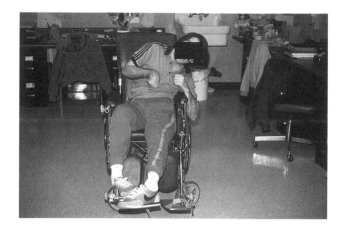

FIGURE 24.5

Severe spasticity with contracture and poor seating posture.

limbs, the Zancolli scale changed from class III to class I. The most common negative effect in the lower limbs was equinus. In summary, the authors conclude that ". . . these results suggest that a combination of BTX-A and rehabilitation to treat spasticity and dystonia . . . is a good option" (58).

Chang et al. (59) performed a prospective cohort investigation conducted in an outpatient clinic. Twenty-three patients who have spastic hemiparesis were given BoNT-A injections; subsequently, they received 1.5 months of therapy. Their response was assessed using Motor Activity Log-28, Motor Activity Log items. Secondarily, Motor Activity Log Self Report Action Research Arm Test, and Modified Ashworth Scale. The results revealed a higher degree of change on Motor Activity Log-28 for the high functioning group; both high and low functioning patients showed an amelioration of hand function and a reduction in spasticity (59).

Simpson et al. (60) conducted a multicenter, placebo-controlled, randomized, interventional, double-blind, parallel group investigation that compared BoNT and tizanidine. The target population was patients with upper limb spasticity secondary to stroke or TBI. Sixty patients in total were studied. The metrics used were the Ashworth Disability Scale (assessed at multiple joints), the Disability Assessment Scale (again at multiple joints), and, finally, a measurement of side effects/adverse effects. The results were as follows. Botulinum toxin caused a greater reduction in muscle tone in both wrist and finger flexors compared to tizanidine and placebo. Second, BoNT had a lower number of adverse effects than tizanidine or placebo. The most common adverse effect in all 3 was somnolence; no liver function test abnormalities were noted with BoNT, unlike tizanidine (60).

Francisco et al. (61) conducted a controlled, randomized, blinded trial. Thirteen patients with spasticity in the wrist flexor or finger flexor, caused by acquired brain injury, were given BoNT-A injections in either high-volume or low-volume preparation. Spasticity was measured by the Modified Ashworth Scale. Both high-volume and low-volume injected patients experienced an important reduction in spasticity. However, the magnitude of this reduction was approximately equal in both groups (61).

Wissel et al. (62) conducted an interventional study involving single-dose BoNT-A. (Unfortunately, this study was published in German and only the abstract was available to the author of this review.) The patient population consisted of 204 adults with acute or chronic spasticity secondary to TBI, stroke, and SCI. Patients were injected with BoNT-A in approximately 3 muscles. Results measured using Rating of Response to BoNT. The results showed that ~93% of patients showed an amelioration of their spasticity; none showed a worsening thereof. In addition, functional improvement was noted; 5.9% of patients had temporary side effects; none had permanent side or adverse effects (62).

Pavesi et al. (63) published an open-labeled investigation involving the use of BoNT type A on 6 patients with severe TBI and spasticity. Botulinum toxin type A was administered by EMG-guided injection. Its effects were assessed by physiatrists and neurologists. The metrics used included the Modified Ashworth Scale, goniometry-assessed ROM, clinical assessment of posture, voluntary motion, and functional outcomes.

Beneficial effects were seen, including improvements in Ashworth Scale, improved functional activity of the upper limb, and reduced spasticity. The authors concluded: "These preliminary data show that BTX-A treatment is effective in reducing spasticity in selected patients with focal upper limb muscular tone disorders secondary to traumatic brain injuries." (63)

Although further studies need to be performed, it is clear that BoNT can be of great benefit in patients who are experiencing spasticity and dystonia. The efficacy of BoNT is greater than phenol, and its side effects are less deleterious. However, further research needs to be done with respect to the ability of BoNT to improve functional outcomes; the evidence here is less than clear (57).

SUMMARY

The physiology of spasticity after acquired brain injury is complex and influenced by multiple factors. Studies examining treatment paradigms in the acute and post-acute setting have been limited and have often contained methodologic flaws. Enteral pharmacotherapy has limitations based on limited impact and potential cognitive side effects. Interventional therapies hold the promise of more targeted therapies, yet their impact on functional status and performance of activities of daily living needs to be further appreciated.

References

1. Zafonte R, Elovic EP, Lombard L. Acute care management of post-TBI spasticity. *J Head Trauma Rehabil.* 2004;19: 89–100.
2. Hinderer SR, Dixon K. Physiologic and clinical monitoring of spastic hypertonia. *Phys Med Rehabil Clin N Am.* 2001;12:733–746.
3. Zafonte R, Elovic EP, Lombard L. Acute care management of post-TBI spasticity. *J Head Trauma Rehabil.* 2004;19:89–100.
4. Starring DT, Gossman MR, Nicholson GG, Jr., Lemons J. Comparison of cyclic and sustained passive stretching using a mechanical device to increase resting length of hamstring muscles. *Phys Ther.* 1988;68:314–320.
5. Knutsson E. Topical cryotherapy in spasticity. *Scand J Rehabil Med.* 1970;2:159–163.
6. Singer BJ, Jegasothy GM, Singer KP, Allison GT. Evaluation of serial casting to correct equinovarus deformity of the ankle after acquired brain injury in adults. *Arch Phys Med Rehabil.* 2003;84:483–491.
7. Mortenson PA, Eng JJ. The use of casts in the management of joint mobility and hypertonia following brain injury in adults: a systematic review. *Phys Ther.* 2003;83:648–658.
8. Hill J. The effects of casting on upper extremity motor disorders after brain injury. *Am J Occup Ther.* 1994;48:219–224.
9. Moseley AM. The effect of a regimen of casting and prolonged stretching on passive ankle dorsiflexion in traumatic head-injured adults. *Physiother Theory Pract.* 1993;9:215–221.
10. Pohl M, Ruckriem S, Mehrholz J, Ritschel C, Strik H, Pause MR. Effectiveness of serial casting in patients with severe cerebral spasticity: a comparison study. *Arch Phys Med Rehabil.* 2002;83:784–790.
11. Barnard P, Dill H, Eldredge P, Held JM, Judd DL, Nalette E. Reduction of hypertonicity by early casting in a comatose head-injured individual. A case report. *Phys Ther.* 1984;64: 1540–1542.
12. Mills VM. Electromyographic results of inhibitory splinting. *Phys Ther.* 1984;64:190–193.
13. Lai JM, Francisco GE, Willis FB. Dynamic splinting after treatment with botulinum toxin type-A: a randomized controlled pilot study. *Adv Ther.* 2009;26:241–248.
14. Lannin NA, Horsley SA, Herbert R, McCluskey A, Cusick A. Splinting the hand in the functional position after brain impairment: a randomized, controlled trial. *Arch Phys Med Rehabil.* 2003;84:297–302.
15. Hinderer SR, Dixon K. Physiologic and clinical monitoring of spastic hypertonia. *Phys Med Rehabil Clin N Am.* 2001;12:733–746.
16. Zafonte R, Elovic EP, Lombard L. Acute care management of post–TBI spasticity. *J Head Trauma Rehabil.* 2004;19: 89–100.
17. Starring DT, Gossman MR, Nicholson GG, Jr., Lemons J. Comparison of cyclic and sustained passive stretching using a mechanical device to increase resting length of hamstring muscles. *Phys Ther.* 1988;68:314–320.
18. Singer BJ, Jegasothy GM, Singer KP, Allison GT. Evaluation of serial casting to correct equinovarus deformity of the ankle after acquired brain injury in adults. *Arch Phys Med Rehabil.* 2003;84:483–491.

19. Mortenson PA, Eng JJ. The use of casts in the management of joint mobility and hypertonia following brain injury in adults: a systematic review. *Phys Ther.* 2003;83:648–658.

20. Hill J. The effects of casting on upper extremity motor disorders after brain injury. *Am J Occup Ther.* 1994;48:219–224.

21. Pohl M, Ruckriem S, Mehrholz J, Ritschel C, Strik H, Pause MR. Effectiveness of serial casting in patients with severe cerebral spasticity: a comparison study. *Arch Phys Med Rehabil.* 2002;83:784–790.

22. Barnard P, Dill H, Eldredge P, Held JM, Judd DL, Nalette E. Reduction of hypertonicity by early casting in a comatose head–injured individual. A case report. *Phys Ther.* 1984;64:1540–1542.

23. Mills VM. Electromyographic results of inhibitory splinting. *Phys Ther.* 1984;64:190–193.

24. Lai JM, Francisco GE, Willis FB. Dynamic splinting after treatment with botulinum toxin type-A: a randomized controlled pilot study. *Adv Ther.* 2009;26:241–248.

25. Lannin NA, Horsley SA, Herbert R, McCluskey A, Cusick A. Splinting the hand in the functional position after brain impairment: a randomized, controlled trial. *Arch Phys Med Rehabil.* 2003;84:297–302.

26. Seib TP, Price R, Reyes MR, Lehmann JF. The quantitative measurement of spasticity: effect of cutaneous electrical stimulation. *Arch Phys Med Rehabil.* 1994;75:746–750.

27. Gelber DA, Good DC, Dromerick A, Sergay S, Richardson M. Open-label dose-titration safety and efficacy study of tizanidine hydrochloride in the treatment of spasticity associated with chronic stroke. *Stroke.* 2001;32:1841–1846.

28. Nance PW, Bugaresti J, Shellenberger K, Sheremata W, Martinez–Arizala A. Efficacy and safety of tizanidine in the treatment of spasticity in patients with spinal cord injury. North American Tizanidine Study Group. *Neurology.* 1994;44:S44–S51.

29. Ashworth B. Preliminary trial of carisoprodol in multiple sclerosis. *Practitioner.* 1964;192:540–542.

30. Wartenberg R. Pendulousness of the legs as a diagnostic test. *Neurology.* 1951;1:18–24.

31. Nance PW, Sheremata WA, Lynch SG et al. Relationship of the antispasticity effect of tizanidine to plasma concentration in patients with multiple sclerosis. *Arch Neurol.* 1997;54:731–736.

32. A double-blind, placebo-controlled trial of tizanidine in the treatment of spasticity caused by multiple sclerosis. United Kingdom Tizanidine Trial Group. *Neurology.* 1994;44:S70–S78.

33. Meythaler JM, Guin-Renfroe S, Johnson A, Brunner RM. Prospective assessment of tizanidine for spasticity due to acquired brain injury. *Arch Phys Med Rehabil.* 2001;82:1155–1163.

34. Gelber DA, Good DC, Dromerick A, Sergay S, Richardson M. Open–label dose–titration safety and efficacy study of tizanidine hydrochloride in the treatment of spasticity associated with chronic stroke. *Stroke.* 2001;32:1841–1846.

35. Mohammed I, Hussain A. Intrathecal baclofen withdrawal syndrome- a life-threatening complication of baclofen pump: a case report. *BMC Clin Pharmacol.* 2004;4:6.

36. Taricco M, Adone R, Pagliacci C, Telaro E. Pharmacological interventions for spasticity following spinal cord injury. *Cochrane Database Syst Rev.* 2000;(2) CD001131.

37. Basmajian JV, Yucel V. Effects of a GABA–derivative (BA–34647) on spasticity. Preliminary report of a double–blind cross–over study. *Am J Phys Med.* 1974;53:223–228.

38. Basmajian JV, Yucel V. Effects of a GABA—derivative (BA–34647) on spasticity. Preliminary report of a double–blind cross–over study. *Am J Phys Med.* 1974;53:223–228.

39. Gracies JM, Nance P, Elovic E, McGuire J, Simpson DM. Traditional pharmacological treatments for spasticity. Part II: General and regional treatments. *Muscle Nerve Suppl.* 1997;6:S92–120.

40. Orsnes GB, Sorensen PS, Larsen TK, Ravnborg M. Effect of baclofen on gait in spastic MS patients. *Acta Neurol Scand.* 2000;101:244–248.

41. Milla PJ, Jackson AD. A controlled trial of baclofen in children with cerebral palsy. *J Int Med Res.* 1977;5:398–404.

42. Penn RD, Savoy SM, Corcos D et al. Intrathecal baclofen for severe spinal spasticity. *N Engl J Med.* 1989;320:1517–1521.

43. Kravitz HM, Corcos DM, Hansen G, Penn RD, Cartwright RD, Gianino J. Intrathecal baclofen. Effects on nocturnal leg muscle spasticity. *Am J Phys Med Rehabil.* 1992;71:48–52.

44. Hugenholtz H, Nelson RF, Dehoux E, Bickerton R. Intrathecal baclofen for intractable spinal spasticity—a double-blind cross-over comparison with placebo in 6 patients. *Can J Neurol Sci.* 1992;19:188–195.

45. Burke D, Gillies JD, Lance JW. An objective assessment of a gamma aminobutyric acid derivative in the control of spasticity. *Proc Aust Assoc Neurol.* 1971;8:131–134.

46. Zafonte R, Lombard L, Elovic E. Antispasticity medications: uses and limitations of enteral therapy. *Am J Phys Med Rehabil.* 2004;83:S50–S58.

47. Gruenthal M, Mueller M, Olson WL, Priebe MM, Sherwood AM, Olson WH. Gabapentin for the treatment of spasticity in patients with spinal cord injury. *Spinal Cord.* 1997;35:686–689.

48. Corbett M, Frankel HL, Michaelis L. A double blind, crossover trial of valium in the treatment of spasticity. *Paraplegia.* 1972;10:19–22.

49. Satkunam LE. Rehabilitation medicine: 3. Management of adult spasticity. *CMAJ.* 2003;169:1173–1179.

50. Schmidt RT, Lee RH, Spehlmann R. Comparison of dantrolene sodium and diazepam in the treatment of spasticity. *J Neurol Neurosurg Psychiatry.* 1976;39:350–356.

51. Rose AS, Kuzma JW, Kurtzke JF, Sibley WA, Tourtellotte WW. Cooperative study in the evaluation of therapy in multiple sclerosis; ACTH vs placebo in acute exacerbations. Preliminary report. *Neurology.* 1968;18:Suppl-10.

52. Rose AS, Kuzma JW, Kurtzke JF, Namerow NS, Sibley WA, Tourtellotte WW. Cooperative study in the evaluation of therapy in multiple sclerosis. ACTH vs. placebo—final report. *Neurology.* 1970;20:1–59.

53. Glass A, Hannah A. A comparison of dantrolene sodium and diazepam in the treatment of spasticity. *Paraplegia.* 1974;12:170–174.

54. Nogen AG. Medical treatment for spasticity in children with cerebral palsy. *Childs Brain.* 1976;2:304–308.

55. Keenan M, Tomas E, Stone L, Gersten L. Percutaneous phenol block of the musculocutaneous nerve to control elbow flexor spasticity. *J Hand Surg Am.* 1990;15:340–346.

56. Elovic E, Esquenazi A, Alter A, Lin J, Alfaro A, Kaelin D. Chemodenervation and nerve blocks in the diagnosis and management of spasticity and muscle overactivity. *PMR.* 2009;1:842–851.

57. Botulinum neurotoxin intramuscular chemodenervation. Role in the management of spastic hypertonia and related motor disorders. *Phys Med Rehabil Clin N Am.* 2001;12:833–874.

58. Guettard E. management of spasticity and dystonia in children with acquired brain injury with rehabilitation and botulinum toxin A. *Dev Neurorehabil.* 2009;12(3):128–138.

59. Chang Chia Lin Effect of baseline spastic hemiparesis on recovery of upper limb function following botulinum toxin type A injections and postinjection therapy. *Arch Phys Med Rehabil.* 2009;90:1462–1468.

60. Simpson D Botulinum neurotoxicity versus tizanidine in upper limb spasticity: a placebo controlled study. *J Neurol Neurosurg Psychiatry.* 2008;80:380–385.

61. Francisco G. Botulinum toxin in the upper limb spasticity after acquired brain injury: a randomized trial comparing dilution techniques. *Am J Phys Med Rehabil.* 2002;81:355–363.

62. Wissel J. Safety and tolerance of single dose botulinum toxin type A in 204 patients with spasticity and localized associated symptoms (Austrian and German botulinum toxin A spasticity study group. *Wien Klin Wochenschr.* 1999;111(20):637–642.

63. Pavesi G Botulinum toxin type A in the treatment of upper limb spasticity among patients with traumatic brain injury. *J Neurol Neurosurg Psychiatry.* 1998;64(3):419–420.

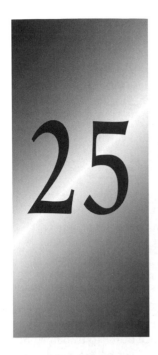

25 Evaluation, Treatment Planning, and Nonsurgical Treatment of Cerebral Palsy

Ann Tilton

DEFINITION OF CEREBRAL PALSY

Cerebral palsy (CP) is a clinical syndrome rather than a specific disease. Although older definitions focused exclusively on the motor disorder, the newest definition from the Executive Committee for the Definition of Cerebral Palsy from the American Academy for Cerebral Palsy and Developmental Medicine broadens the focus to include accompanying disorders:

"Cerebral palsy (CP) describes a group of disorders of the development of movement and posture, causing activity limitation, that are attributed to non-progressive disturbances that occurred in the developing fetal or infant brain. The motor disorders of cerebral palsy are often accompanied by disturbances of sensation, cognition, communication, perception, and/or behaviour, and/or by a seizure disorder." (1)

Thus, the label of CP does not imply anything specific about etiology, and the child with CP may or may not have significant impairments of other systems beyond the motor system. This chapter primarily focuses on the motor aspects of CP and their nonsurgical treatment.

ETIOLOGY AND EPIDEMIOLOGY

The incidence of CP is approximately 3 in 1000 live births, making it the most common cause of physical disability in children in developed countries. Prenatal disturbances including infection, clotting disorders, and inflammation are the most common cause of CP and are often the most difficult to diagnose. Perinatal asphyxia is no longer considered a leading cause of CP, likely accounting for less than 10% of cases (2).

Although the brain injury causing CP is static, the consequences for the child often are not due to developmental changes. Spastic posturing and muscle contracture, for instance, may become more severe as the child grows.

CLINICAL PRESENTATIONS OF CP

The movement disorders of CP may be classified based on their distribution and the types of movements present, as indicated in Table 25.1. The classification may be used to help guide therapy decisions, as discussed in more detail below.

The motor symptoms of CP can also be grouped into 4 categories based on their functional consequences, which makes their therapeutic implications clear (3).

1. Loss of selective motor control, which impairs the development of sequential motor skills, due to difficulty in individuation and coordination of movements. There are no

TABLE 25.1
Clinically Based Classification Systems of CP

Movement disorder
    Spastic
    Dystonic
    Mixed
    Athetoid
    Ataxic
Topographical distribution
    Unilateral
        Monoplegia
        Hemiplegia
    Bilateral
        Diplegia
        Triplegia
        Quadriplegia

TABLE 25.2
The Modified Ashworth Scale

0 = No increase in muscle tone
1 = Slight increase in tone with a catch and release
    or minimal resistance at end of range
1+ = As 1 but with minimal resistance through range
    following catch
2 = More marked increase tone through range of
    motion
3 = Considerable increase in tone, passive move-
    ment difficult
4 = Affected part rigid

Bohannon RW, Smith MB. Interrater reliability of a Modi-fied Ashworth Scale of muscle spasticity. *Phys Ther* 1987; 67(2):206–207.

effective treatments to overcome loss of selective control.

2. Abnormal muscle tone influenced by abnormal posture. Hypertonia interferes with normal movement and may lead to pain, contracture, and other complications. Medical treatments for hypertonia are discussed in detail below. Surgery is also an important option.

3. Imbalance between muscle agonists and antagonists, which decreases motor control and may lead to contracture. Selective weakening of overactive muscles, and strengthening of weak ones, may address this problem.

4. Impaired balance, which interferes with mobility. Orthotics and mobility devices may be used to address impaired balance.

EVALUATION

A comprehensive evaluation of the child with CP is the cornerstone of treatment planning. Although we confine ourselves here to motor evaluation, it is of paramount importance that the child be fully evaluated in all realms, including sensory, language, social, family, school, and recreational activities. The entire treatment team—physicians, allied health therapists, nurses, and caregivers, as well as surgeons and other professionals as needed—should have input into the evaluation process.

Evaluation of muscle tone is typically done using the Modified Ashworth Scale (4) (Table 25.2). This clinically useful scale grades tone from 0 to 5, as indicated in Table 25.2. Of note, it does not measure function. The goal of measuring excess tone is not simply to document its presence but also to determine if it is interfering with some aspect of function, care, comfort, or cosmesis. If it is, treatment may be warranted. If it is not, or if reducing tone would present new problems (such as increased difficulty with transfers) that outweigh the benefits, then a specific treatment should not proceed.

Evaluation should also include determining the child's level of function, which is often done using the Gross Motor Function Classification System (5), as shown in Table 25.3. Other useful scales include the Functional Independence Measure (6) and the Barthel Index (7). In each case, the goal is to document the child's functional status as it changes over time and in response to therapy. When choosing a measure to use for longitudinal evaluation, it is critical that it be relatively easy to administer, in order that it be used routinely during clinical visits.

TREATMENT PLANNING

Once the decision to treat has been made, multiple considerations come into play in determining the choice

TABLE 25.3
Gross Motor Function Classification System

Level I	Walks and runs independently
Level II	Walks independently
Level III	Walks with assistance
Level IV	Stands for transfers
Level V	Absent head control and sitting balance

Palisano R, Rosenbaum P, Walter S, Russell D, Wood E, Galuppi B. Development and reliability of a system to classify gross motor function in children with cerebral palsy. *Dev Med Child Neurol* 1997;39(4):214–223.

and timing of treatment. The goals in all cases are to maximize the functional independence of the child and to facilitate efforts by the family to aid in the goal. For example, the therapeutic program for the school-aged child should be tailored to maximizing the child's ability to participate in school activities—sitting in class, taking part in play, carrying out fine motor activities such as writing, and especially communicating with others.

Factors to consider in choosing therapy include the age of the child; any comorbidities including ophthalmologic, cognitive, or seizure disorders; distribution of excess tone; existing or potential spasticity-related complications (eg, contracture); mobility; and recreational activities that may be incorporated into the therapeutic program. In addition, financial and transportation concerns may impact the decision on the most appropriate treatments.

Depending on the child, treatment goals may include the following:

- reduce pain
- decrease decubiti and contracture formation
- promote safe and comfortable seating
- promote plantegrade foot under the pelvis for gait and plantegrade hand under the shoulder for weight-bearing
- promote motor control development
- minimize cost, invasiveness, and required maintenance of treatment.

Treatment options include the following:

- physical and occupational therapy
- orthotics and casting
- oral medications
- nerve and motor point blocks
- botulinum toxin
- selective dorsal rhizotomy
- intrathecal baclofen
- orthopedic interventions.

PHYSICAL TREATMENTS

Stretching is an essential part of any treatment program for muscle overactivity in CP. Spasticity leads to adoption of fixed postures, setting the stage for muscle contracture. Stretching counteracts contracture development by maintaining the full range of motion of affected muscles. The normal or adapted activities of play of an active child can often provide a significant portion of the needed range of motion and stretch. Special attention must be given to those joints limited by muscle overactivity.

Physical therapy (PT) goes far beyond stretching, however. Programs include motor retraining, sensory integration, and strengthening, and the physical therapist aids in the selection and modification of orthotics and mobility aids, such as walkers or wheelchairs. The PT program may also include activities such as horseback riding, hydrotherapy, and modalities including biofeedback and electrical stimulation. Bower et al. (8) have shown that intensive therapy (1 hour per day, 5 days per week) was not more effective in improving function than routine amounts of therapy.

An ankle-foot orthosis is often used to treat dynamic equinus in CP and has been shown to reduce ankle excursion and increase dorsiflexion at foot strike, along with other biomechanical benefits (9). For preambulatory children whose ability to stand is impaired by equinus, an ankle-foot orthosis can also aid the sit-to-stand transition (10).

Children with balance difficulties are often aided with a walker or crutches. In patients with spastic diplegia, posterior balance is usually the major limitation to mobility; a posterior walker or crutches may allow the child to ambulate independently.

When stretching is inadequate to regain full range of motion in a tight joint, serial casting or prolonged splinting may be indicated. The cast is typically applied at a fraction of the desired final angle, and then reapplied at an increased angle every 4 to 7 days. Once the desired joint range of motion is achieved, an orthosis may be fabricated to use as a splint to maintain the desired angle. Although there is debate as to the optimal technique, serial casting is often used in combination with botulinum toxin (BoNT) injections, with the toxin first weakening the overactive muscle and the cast used to apply prolonged stretch. In comparative trials, toxin injection alone has been shown to be as effective as casting alone (11, 12). The 2 treatments together have been shown superior to either alone in one trial (13), but other trials have not supported this (14, 15). This important issue is reviewed in more detail by Logan and Gaebler-Spira elsewhere (16).

Recently, interest in constraint-induced therapy (CIT) has undergone a renaissance based on increased understanding of the brain's inherent capacity for "rewiring," known as plasticity. The underlying idea is to prevent the patient from using his or her "good" limb, forcing the brain to strengthen firing patterns that work around the damaged motor control region to activate and control the impaired limb. Taub et al. (17) studied 18 children with hemiparesis, with ages 7 months to 8 years, randomly assigned to CIT or conventional PT. Constraint was applied for 21 days, 6 hours per day (17). The CIT-treated children acquired significantly more new classes of motor skills

(9 vs 2) and used the affected limb more and with better-quality movements. These benefits were sustained at 6 months, suggesting the occurrence of true plasticity-dependent brain changes. Similar beneficial results have been seen in other recent trials (18, 19). However, a CIT program may be a significant burden to the child and the family, and more research is needed to define the least intrusive and most effective regimen.

ORAL MEDICATIONS

Oral medications can effectively reduce muscle overactivity in the child with CP but often at the expense of significant adverse effects, especially sedation. For this reason, their role is not as large as that of other treatment options. They also reduce tone globally, which, for many children with focal spasticity, is not desirable. Thus, oral medications may be most appropriate for those with widespread spasticity for whom some sedation is not a contraindication. Relatively few double-blind trials of oral medications have been conducted in children. In addition, older studies measured technical measures such as tone but did not address functional gains.

Diazepam is the most commonly used benzodiazepine for spasticity. Trials of diazepam in CP have shown its ability to reduce spasticity, especially in younger children and those with athetosis (20–24). One trial suggests that a combination with dantrolene may be superior to either agent alone (25). Side effects including excessive somnolence, dizziness, mild weakness, and withdrawal syndrome may limit its use (26).

Baclofen is a GABA-B agonist. It is commonly prescribed in CP despite the limited evidence from clinical trials supporting its efficacy. One trial indicated it was superior to placebo in reducing spasticity and improving passive and active limb movements (27). It is not Food and Drug Administration (FDA)-approved for use in CP.

Dantrolene acts peripherally, inhibiting calcium release in muscle, thereby reducing contractility and weakening the muscle. A series of clinical trials 3 decades ago established its efficacy in CP (28, 29). Sedation does occur despite the peripheral site of action. The small risk of hepatotoxicity necessitates frequent monitoring of liver functions.

Tizanidine is an alpha-2 agonist, inhibiting the release of excitatory amino acids and facilitating the action of the inhibitory neurotransmitter glycine both spinally and supraspinally. Tizanidine is approved only in adults, where it has been well studied. It has

not been studied in pediatric patients with CP. It has a very short duration of action so frequent dosing is required. Adverse effects include sedation, hypotension, and dry mouth. Clinically, the sedation and short action become assets when the medication is used at night for the initiation of sleep. It offers tone improvement with sedation, and the effects are concluded upon awakening.

CHEMODENERVATION

The use of BoNT for chemodenervation of overactive muscle in CP is now widespread, but FDA approval has not been achieved. Its use has largely replaced the use of phenol or ethyl alcohol injection for the same purpose. Nonetheless, these agents continue to be an important option in some cases. The comparative advantages of BoNT include ease of administration and highly predictable and repeatable clinical benefits with minimal side effects, whereas the advantages of phenol or alcohol include low cost and low antigenicity.

The most appropriate candidate for chemodenervation is the patient with focal muscle overactivity for whom weakening those muscles may potentially provide a meaningful improvement in active function, comfort, care, or cosmesis. Patients with widespread muscle overactivity may nonetheless benefit from this

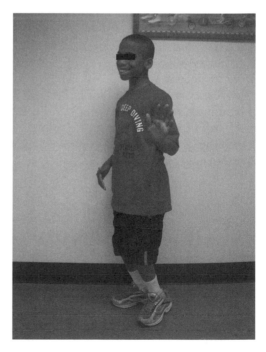

FIGURE 25.1

A 10-year old boy diagnosed with spastic diplegia.

focal treatment, as long as the treatment of a subset of muscles has the potential to lead to benefit. Chemodenervation therapy may be used with other treatments, including oral medications, intrathecal baclofen (ITB), and rhizotomy, which may provide a more global reduction of hypertonia, whereas chemodenervation provides focal tone reduction.

Case Study

John is a 10-year-old boy who was born at 27 weeks of gestation and had a 3-month neonatal intensive care unit stay. Complications during his hospitalization included respiratory difficulties and apnea. Neuroimaging revealed periventricular leukomalacia.

He is now entering fifth grade in regular classes. He receives PT for spastic diplegia and has bilateral ankle foot orthoses. The therapists report that although he has been compliant with an aggressive therapy program, his gait is deteriorating with significant toe walking, and his heels are very difficult to secure in his braces.

It was decided to deliver BoNT-A (as BOTOX) to the gastrocsoleus complex bilaterally. He received 60 U per side. His toe walking improved substantially as did his brace wear, comfort, and speed of walking. He has had subsequent injections 6 months later in response to his growth spurt. Quantitative and functional measures have documented improvement (Figure 25.1).

Botulinum Toxin

Of the 7 serotypes of BoNT produced by clostridium botulinum, 2—A and B—are available for commercial use and are approved by the United States Food and Drug Agency, as well as European regulatory agencies. Botulinum toxin type A is marketed in the United States as Botox®, and BoNT-B as Myobloc® (Neurobloc® in Europe). Two other BoNT-A formulations, Dysport® and Xeomin®, are available outside the United States but are not FDA-approved as of late 2008. Neither Botox nor Myobloc has FDA approval for treatment of spasticity, although each has been widely used for that purpose as an off-label use.

In our experience, younger children respond more fully and for longer periods than do older children, possibly due to progression from dynamic posturing to fixed contracture in the older child. Children with spastic hemiplegia and spastic diplegia can be safely injected as early as age 18 months. Treatment should be in the context of a global tone management program including the use of orthoses, serial casting, and PT. Physical function begins to plateau

in later childhood, and by age 6 to 10 years, many children no longer require injection therapy. Fixed contracture may have developed by this time and is typically managed by casting and orthopedic surgical procedures.

Muscles selected for injection may be localized either with palpation or with an assisted guidance technique such as electromyography, electrical stimulation, or ultrasonography. Because these techniques may increase the anxiety of the child, they are usually best left for injections of those muscles that are difficult to palpate, such as the psoas. Initial clinical benefit is seen within several days of injection, and the effect peaks at around 3 to 4 weeks. Waning of benefit occurs thereafter, with reinjection usually considered at 3 to 4 months. Injections at more frequent intervals than 3 months are not recommended, to minimize the potential for development of neutralizing antibodies. For the same reason, guidelines for Botox have been developed addressing maximum dose, number of injection sites, and other parameters (3). Recommendations from expert injectors suggest a maximum of 16 U Botox per kilogram or 400 U total, whichever is less, at each injection session (3). Muscle bulk, degree of spasticity, and injector experience all ultimately influence the dosing. Each commercial BoNT product has its own profile of side effects, duration of effect, and antigenicity, and dose recommendations for one product cannot be used to determine the proper dose of another.

Botulinum toxin type A has been evaluated in more than 3 dozen clinical trials in CP, and its ability to reduce spasticity in both upper and lower limbs has been demonstrated conclusively (11–14, 30–36). More recently, trials have attempted to demonstrate functional gains from injection, but this has proven more difficult. This is likely due in part to the outcome measures typically used to evaluate function in CP. The Gross Motor Functional Measure, for instance, evaluates the whole child and is not designed to capture the focal improvements in function—better control of a utensil, for instance—that are commonly seen by clinicians treating with BoNT. Nonetheless, some trials have shown functional improvements (13, 32, 34, 36). For example, Steenbeek et al. (34) showed that injection of BoNT-A in the lower limbs promoted significant improvement on 18 of 33 individually set goals in 9 of 11 subjects. Fehlings et al. (32) showed that upper limb injection plus PT was superior in promoting self-care to PT alone.

Botulinum toxin treatment may also provide an alternative to orthopedic surgery in selected patients. Recent data support that BoNT-A is equal in efficacy to soft tissue surgery in the prevention of progressive hip subluxation or dislocation (37).

A controversial issue is the long-term benefit of chemodenervation. A recent article called into question the long-term effects of BoNT but did recognize the limitations of the instrument to measure improvement (38). Further trials of BoNT with measures that are designed to evaluate focal improvements are likely to strengthen the impression from clinical practice that BoNT is a valuable treatment for improving function in this population.

Both serotypes of BoNT have a favorable safety profile when used as directed. The most common side effects are short-term injection-site soreness and bruising. Botulinum toxin type B may cause stinging upon injection. Although systemic spread of either agent is minimal, there have been occasional reports of incontinence and dysphagia after injection. Although both resolve quickly, dysphagia may lead to aspiration and respiratory infection. Children with spastic quadriplegia with pseudobulbar palsy seem to be much more sensitive to systemic spread after focal injection of BoNT, and treatment may be relatively contraindicated in this group for this reason (39).

Phenol and Ethyl Alcohol

Before the introduction of BoNT, phenol and ethyl alcohol were the major choices available for focal tone reduction. Botulinum toxin has largely replaced these 2 agents (and significantly expanded the use of chemodenervation as a whole). Both medications can still be useful in some situations, including when treatment of multiple powerful muscles with BoNT would exceed dose recommendations, when cost is an issue, or when the patient has developed antibody-based resistance to BoNT therapy.

Both phenol and ethyl alcohol are injected in close proximity to a motor nerve near where it enters a muscle (called a motor nerve block) or within the muscle near the nerve terminals (motor point block) (40). Both techniques require considerable clinical skill, obtained only through experience with repeated injections. Even with best practices, both agents may cause significant adverse effects, including dysesthesias, pain, vascular complications, and muscle necrosis. Kolaski et al. (41) recently reported encouraging results from a review of 336 children (90% CP) treated with both BoNT and phenol. The overall complication rate was 6.8%, with 1.2% anesthesia-related and 6.3% injection-related. Most injection-related complications were localized and of short duration, and dysesthesias from phenol treatment were seen in only 0.4% of cases (41).

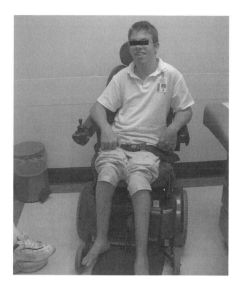

FIGURE 25.2

A 15-year old boy who developed meningitis 3 weeks after birth resulting in spasticity affecting his upper and lower extremities.

Few trials of either agent have been conducted in children. Wong et al. (42) compared BoNT-A to phenol in 27 ambulatory children with lower limb spasticity and gait dysfunction. Sixteen received BoNT-A, and 11 received phenol motor point blocks. Gait analysis at 1 week before and 2 months after treatment showed superior results for BoNT-A, with fewer adverse effects. In a retrospective study of 68 patients, most of whom had CP, Gooch et al. (43) showed that adverse effects from either treatment were infrequent and that using them in combination allowed many more muscles to be injected.

Case Study

Ben is a 15-year-old young man who was a full-term infant who developed meningitis 3 weeks after birth. He had a 1-month hospitalization. He displayed spasticity and delayed motor milestones from that point forward. He has been able to successfully advance in school with special education resources.

His spasticity currently involves his upper and lower extremities. Functionally, it limits his ability to accurately operate his power chair and independently achieve several of his dressing and computer skills. In his lower extremities, the hypertonia interferes with tub and chair transfers due to clonus and extensor tone.

After a successful ITB trial, a pump was placed with the catheter tip at the T2 level. He has had a significant reduction in his generalized tone and clonus. His transfers now require less support. In addition, dressing, either by him or assisted by caregivers, is much improved. He is more active with friends and in school activities (Figure 25.2).

Intrathecal Baclofen

Delivery of baclofen to the intrathecal space provides the medication to the central nervous system in a much more effective manner and dramatically lowers the amount of baclofen required compared to oral administration. Thus, the cognitive side effects that limit the utility of oral antispasmodics are significantly reduced (44). Baclofen is delivered to the intrathecal space by the Synchromed® infusion system, consisting of a pump and drug reservoir implanted subcutaneously in the abdomen, and a catheter. Originally, the catheter was most commonly inserted at the T11–T12 level, but now, it is common practice to advance it to the mid to upper thoracic area to more effectively provide medication to the upper extremities. An exception would be in the patient with significant truncal weakness or minimal involvement of the upper extremities.

The pump is programmable via a telemetry device that communicates with the pump's computer chip. The pump reservoir, which contains an alarm indicating low drug level, is refilled percutaneously, usually every 12 to 24 weeks, depending on pump size and medication demands.

Appropriate candidates for ITB therapy are patients with severe spasticity due to multiple causes including multiple sclerosis, CP, brain injury, stroke, or spinal cord injury. In addition, patients must have sufficient body mass to support the programmable implantable infusion system and typically have a lower extremity spasticity of 3 or greater on the Ashworth Scale, indicating significant muscle overactivity. The following groups of pediatric patients are often considered as potential candidates for ITB therapy: patients with their gait impeded by spasticity and poor strength; older patients with lower extremity spasticity; quadriplegic patients for whom tome reduction may improve activities of daily living; patients without active function but for whom spasticity reduction may improve care and comfort.

Because bolus infusion is frequently used as a screening tool, with a decrease in one unit on the Ashworth Scale being the standard for proceeding to implantation in most centers. In the bolus trials, the medication is delivered via spinal tap and the patient is evaluated systematically over the next several hours to determine if there is an adequate response. The initial dose is 50 µg, and if the response is not adequate, the dose is advanced to 75 and 100 µg on consecutive days. If after the final dose the patient does not have an acceptable response, then they are not considered an eligible candidate.

Clinical trials of ITB indicate that the medication is capable of reducing muscle overactivity and providing an improvement in function over prolonged treatment periods (44–47). Potential benefits include reduced spasticity, easier care giving, and reduced pain. The effects on ambulation may be unpredictable, ranging from improvement to worsening (48). Gerszten et al. (49) published data showing that ITB may reduce the need for orthopedic surgeries to the lower limbs. In the 48 patients studied who had received pumps, 28 had been recommended for but had not yet received orthopedic intervention. In 18 of the 28, surgery was not deemed necessary after the pump implantation due to reduction in lower extremity muscle overactivity.

There have been considerable concerns raised about the possibility of an increased risk of scoliosis after ITB pump placement. Senaran et al. (50) demonstrated in a retrospective review of matched controls that ITB had no significant effect on curve progression, pelvic obliquity, or the incidence of scoliosis when compared with spastic CP without ITB. In addition, on a comprehensive review of the cost-effectiveness based on mathematical modeling of incremental cost, this modality was found to offer good value for the investment (51).

Intrathecal baclofen therapy does carry the risk for significant complications. Infection, pump malfunction, programming errors, and catheter kinking are all important concerns (52). These issues are discussed more fully elsewhere in this volume by Koman. Life-threatening drug overdose and withdrawal are real possibilities, and families must be educated on how to recognize its symptoms and how to respond quickly to this medical emergency (53, 54).

References

1. Bax M, Goldstein M, Rosenbaum P et al. Proposed definition and classification of cerebral palsy, April 2005. *Dev Med Child Neurol* 2005;47(8):571–576.
2. Nelson KB, Grether JK. Causes of cerebral palsy. *Curr Opin Pediatr* 1999;11(6):487–491.
3. Russman BS, Gormley ME, Jr., Tilton A. Cerebral palsy: a rational approach to a treatment protocol, and the role of botulinum toxin in treatment. In: Brashear A, Mayer NH, editors.

Spasticity and other forms of muscle overactivity in the upper motor neuron syndrome: etiology, evaluation, management, and the role of botulinum toxin. New York: WE MOVE, 2008:179–192.

4. Bohannon RW, Smith MB. Interrater reliability of a Modified Ashworth Scale of muscle spasticity. *Phys Ther* 1987; 67(2):206–207.

5. Palisano R, Rosenbaum P, Walter S, Russell D, Wood E, Galuppi B. Development and reliability of a system to classify gross motor function in children with cerebral palsy. *Dev Med Child Neurol* 1997;39(4):214–223.

6. *Guide for the uniform data set for medical rehabilitation* (Adult (FIM) Version 4.0). Buffalo, NY: State University of New York, Buffalo/U.B. Foundation Activities, Inc, 1993.

7. Mahoney FI, Barthel DW. Functional evaluation: the Bathel Index. *Md State Med J* 1965;14:61–65.

8. Bower E, Michell D, Burnett M, Campbell MJ, McLellan DL. Randomized controlled trial of physiotherapy in 56 children with cerebral palsy followed for 18 months. *Dev Med Child Neurol* 2001;43(1):4–15.

9. Carlson WE, Vaughan CL, Damiano DL, Abel MF. Orthotic management of gait in spastic diplegia. *Am J Phys Med Rehabil* 1997;76(3):219–225.

10. Wilson H, Haideri N, Song K, Telford D. Ankle-foot orthoses for preambulatory children with spastic diplegia. *J Pediatr Orthop* 1997;17(3):370–376.

11. Corry IS, Cosgrove AP, Duffy CM, McNeill S, Taylor TC, Graham HK. Botulinum toxin A compared with stretching casts in the treatment of spastic equinus: a randomised prospective trial. *J Pediatr Orthop* 1998;18(3):304–311.

12. Flett PJ, Stern LM, Waddy H, Connell TM, Seeger JD, Gibson SK. Botulinum toxin A versus fixed cast stretching for dynamic calf tightness in cerebral palsy. *J Paediatr Child Health* 1999;35(1):71–77.

13. Bottos M, Benedetti MG, Salucci P, Gasparroni V, Giannini S. Botulinum toxin with and without casting in ambulant children with spastic diplegia: a clinical and functional assessment. *Dev Med Child Neurol* 2003;45(11):758–762.

14. Kay RM, Rethlefsen SA, Fern-Buneo A, Wren TA, Skaggs DL. Botulinum toxin as an adjunct to serial casting treatment in children with cerebral palsy. *J Bone Joint Surg Am* 2004;86-A(11):2377–2384.

15. Ackman JD, Russman BS, Thomas SS et al. Comparing botulinum toxin A with casting for treatment of dynamic equinus in children with cerebral palsy. *Dev Med Child Neurol* 2005;47(9):620–627.

16. Romeiser Logan L, Gaebler-Spira D. Integrating physical and occupational therapy with botulinum toxin treatment in children with cerebral palsy. In: Brashear A, Mayer NH, editors. *Spasticity and other forms of muscle overactivity in the upper motor neuron syndrome: etiology, evaluation, management, and the role of botulinum toxin.* New York: WE MOVE, 2008:193–205.

17. Taub E, Ramey SL, DeLuca S, Echols K. Efficacy of constraint-induced movement therapy for children with cerebral palsy with asymmetric motor impairment. *Pediatrics* 2004;113(2):305–312.

18. Charles JR, Gordon AM. A repeated course of constraint-induced movement therapy results in further improvement. *Dev Med Child Neurol* 2007;49(10):770–773.

19. Charles JR, Wolf SL, Schneider JA, Gordon AM. Efficacy of a child-friendly form of constraint-induced movement therapy in hemiplegic cerebral palsy: a randomized control trial. *Dev Med Child Neurol* 2006;48(8):635–642.

20. Engsberg JR, Ross SA, Park TS. Changes in ankle spasticity and strength following selective dorsal rhizotomy and physical therapy for spastic cerebral palsy. *J Neurosurg* 1999;91(5):727–732.

21. Holt KS. The use of diazepam in childhood cerebral palsy. Report of a small study including electromyographic observations. *Ann Phys Med* 1964;Suppl:16–24.

22. Engle HA. The effect of diazepam (Valium) in children with cerebral palsy: a double-blind study. *Dev Med Child Neurol* 1966;8(6):661–667.

23. Pranzatelli MR. Oral pharmacotherapy for the movement disorders of cerebral palsy. *J Child Neurol* 1996;11 Suppl 1: S13–S22.

24. Denhoff E. Cerebral palsy: a pharmacologic approach. *Clin Pharmacol Ther* 1964;5:947–954.

25. Nogen AG. Medical treatment for spasticity in children with cerebral palsy. *Childs Brain* 1976;2(5):304–308.

26. Gracies JM, Nance P, Elovic E, McGuire J, Simpson DM. Traditional pharmacological treatments for spasticity. Part II: general and regional treatments. *Muscle Nerve Suppl* 1997;6: S92–120.

27. Milla PJ, Jackson AD. A controlled trial of baclofen in children with cerebral palsy. *J Int Med Res* 1977;5(6):398–404.

28. Joynt RL, Leonard JA, Jr. Dantrolene sodium suspension in treatment of spastic cerebral palsy. *Dev Med Child Neurol* 1980;22(6):755–767.

29. Haslam RH WJLP. Dantrolene sodium in children with spasticity. *Arch Phys Med Rehabil* 1974;55:384–388.

30. Baker R, Jasinski M, iag-Tymecka I et al. Botulinum toxin treatment of spasticity in diplegic cerebral palsy: a randomized, double-blind, placebo-controlled, dose-ranging study. *Dev Med Child Neurol* 2002;44(10):666–675.

31. Corry IS, Cosgrove AP, Walsh EG, McClean D, Graham HK. Botulinum toxin A in the hemiplegic upper limb: a double-blind trial. *Dev Med Child Neurol* 1997;39(3):185–193.

32. Fehlings D, Rang M, Glazier J, Steele C. An evaluation of botulinum-A toxin injections to improve upper extremity function in children with hemiplegic cerebral palsy. *J Pediatr* 2000;137(3):331–337.

33. Speth LA, Leffers P, Janssen-Potten YJ, Vles JS. Botulinum toxin A and upper limb functional skills in hemiparetic cerebral palsy: a randomized trial in children receiving intensive therapy. *Dev Med Child Neurol* 2005;47(7):468–473.

34. Steenbeek D, Meester-Delver A, Becher JG, Lankhorst GJ. The effect of botulinum toxin type A treatment of the lower extremity on the level of functional abilities in children with cerebral palsy: evaluation with goal attainment scaling. *Clin Rehabil* 2005;19(3):274–282.

35. Sutherland DH, Kaufman KR, Wyatt MP, Chambers HG, Mubarak SJ. Double-blind study of botulinum A toxin injections into the gastrocnemius muscle in patients with cerebral palsy. *Gait Posture* 1999;10(1):1–9.

36. Wallen MA, O'flaherty SJ, Waugh MC. Functional outcomes of intramuscular botulinum toxin type A in the upper limbs of children with cerebral palsy: a phase II trial. *Arch Phys Med Rehabil* 2004;85(2):192–200.

37. Yang EJ, Rha DW, Kim HW, Park ES. Comparison of botulinum toxin type A injection and soft-tissue surgery to treat hip subluxation in children with cerebral palsy. *Arch Phys Med Rehabil* 2008;89(11):2108–2113.

38. Moore AP, de-Hall RA, Smith CT et al. Two-year placebo-controlled trial of botulinum toxin A for leg spasticity in cerebral palsy. *Neurology* 2008;71(2):122–128.

39. Howell K, Selber P, Graham HK, Reddihough D. Botulinum neurotoxin A: an unusual systemic effect. *J Paediatr Child Health* 2007;43(6):499–501.

40. Gracies JM, Elovic E, McGuire J, Simpson DM. Traditional pharmacologic treatments for spasticity part I: local treatments. In: Mayer NH, Simpson DM, editors. *Spasticity: etiology, evaluation, management, and the role of botulinum toxin.* New York: WE MOVE, 2005: 44–64.

41. Kolaski K, Ajizian SJ, Passmore L, Pasutharnchat N, Koman LA, Smith BP. Safety profile of multilevel chemical denervation procedures using phenol or botulinum toxin or both in a pediatric population. *Am J Phys Med Rehabil* 2008;87(7):556–566.

42. Wong AM, Chen CL, Chen CP, Chou SW, Chung CY, Chen MJ. Clinical effects of botulinum toxin A and phenol block on

gait in children with cerebral palsy. *Am J Phys Med Rehabil* 2004;83(4):284–291.

43. Gooch JL, Patton CP. Combining botulinum toxin and phenol to manage spasticity in children. *Arch Phys Med Rehabil* 2004;85(7):1121–1124.

44. Albright AL, Barron WB, Fasick MP, Polinko P, Janosky J. Continuous intrathecal baclofen infusion for spasticity of cerebral origin. *JAMA* 1993;270(20):2475–2477.

45. Rawlins PK. Intrathecal baclofen therapy over 10 years. *J Neurosci Nurs* 2004;36(6):322–327.

46. Gilmartin R, Bruce D, Storrs BB et al. Intrathecal baclofen for management of spastic cerebral palsy: multicenter trial. *J Child Neurol* 2000;15(2):71–77.

47. Van SP, Nuttin B, Lagae L, Schrijvers E, Borghgraef C, Feys P. Intrathecal baclofen for intractable cerebral spasticity: a prospective placebo-controlled, double-blind study. *Neurosurgery* 2000;46(3):603–609.

48. Gerszten PC, Albright AL, Barry MJ. Effect on ambulation of continuous intrathecal baclofen infusion. *Pediatr Neurosurg* 1997;27(1):40–44.

49. Gerszten PC, Albright AL, Johnstone GF. Intrathecal baclofen infusion and subsequent orthopedic surgery in patients with spastic cerebral palsy. *J Neurosurg* 1998;88(6):1009–1013.

50. Senaran H, Shah SA, Presedo A, Dabney KW, Glutting JW, Miller F. The risk of progression of scoliosis in cerebral palsy patients after intrathecal baclofen therapy. *Spine* 2007;32(21):2348–2354.

51. de LG, Matza LS, Green H, Werner M, Edgar T. Cost-effectiveness of intrathecal baclofen therapy for the treatment of severe spasticity associated with cerebral palsy. *J Child Neurol* 2007;22(1):49–59.

52. Murphy NA, Irwin MC, Hoff C. Intrathecal baclofen therapy in children with cerebral palsy: efficacy and complications. *Arch Phys Med Rehabil* 2002;83(12):1721–1725.

53. Zuckerbraun NS, Ferson SS, Albright AL, Vogeley E. Intrathecal baclofen withdrawal: emergent recognition and management. *Pediatr Emerg Care* 2004;20(11):759–764.

54. Darbari FP, Melvin JJ, Piatt JH, Jr., Adirim TA, Kothare SV. Intrathecal baclofen overdose followed by withdrawal: clinical and EEG features. *Pediatr Neurol* 2005;33(5):373–377.

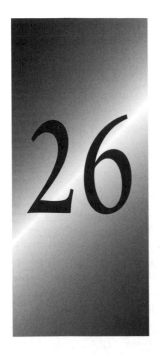

26 Surgical Management of Spasticity in the Child With Cerebral Palsy

Kat Kolaski
John Frino
L. A. Koman

Surgical interventions for the treatment of spasticity are well-accepted treatment options for children with cerebral palsy (CP). However, recommendations for any potential surgical interventions should be considered in the context of optimal medical and rehabilitative management and rational goal setting provided by a multidisciplinary team of health care providers who specialize in CP. The surgical options currently considered for the child with CP include selective dorsal rhizotomy (SDR), chronic administration of intrathecal baclofen (ITB), and orthopedic surgery. This chapter provides a general review of these surgical options; specific topics covered include scientific rationale, indications, evaluation, planning, techniques, adverse events, and outcomes.

SELECTIVE DORSAL RHIZOTOMY

Rationale

Muscle tone is regulated by the output of the alpha motor neurons in the spinal cord. The alpha motor neurons normally are regulated by interneurons in the spinal cord, which, through a balance of competing excitatory and inhibitory influences, exert a net inhibitory influence (1–2). Inhibitory impulses travel in descending corticospinal projections from the cerebellum and basal ganglia. Excitatory influences from the muscle spindles travel to the spinal cord in the sensory or dorsal roots where they mediate the local spinal reflex arc. In CP, early central nervous system (CNS) injury results in a reorganization of corticospinal projections that reduces the descending inhibition on the alpha motor neurons (3). During a rhizotomy procedure, excitatory input from the dorsal roots is attenuated by sectioning of individual rootlets. Theoretically, this selective sectioning results in restoration of the balance of the excitatory and inhibitory influences on the alpha motor neurons.

Sectioning of the dorsal roots to modify spasticity was described in the early 20th century (4); however, because of concerns that this neuroablative procedure resulted in excessive sensory and motor loss, rhizotomy did not receive much attention until the 1970s. Gros et al. (5) introduced the concept of selectivity to the procedure with the use of electromyography (EMG) monitoring to identify rootlets innervating more clinically abnormal muscle groups. Fasano et al. (6) proposed criteria for rootlet sectioning primarily based upon the results of intraoperative electrical stimulation. In North America, this technique was further modified and popularized for the treatment of spasticity in patients with CP by Peacock et al. (7–9). Today, most centers performing SDR continue to use variations of the surgical techniques described in these earlier studies.

Indications for Surgical Treatment of Spasticity

The current patient selection guidelines are based on those described in several early series of patients with CP by Fasano et al. (10, 11) and Peacock et al. (8). The best results were reported in primarily spastic, intelligent, motivated patients who possessed some degree of independent locomotion but who did not have fixed deformity or mass synergy patterns. Peacock et al. (8) emphasized the importance of preoperative assessment and postoperative rehabilitation. In these and subsequent series, less favorable outcomes in terms of both spasticity reduction and function were reported in patients with quadriplegic CP (10–12). The reduction of spasticity after SDR—especially in more severely involved patients—has the potential to unmask significant coexisting movement disorders such as dystonia (8, 10, 12). Greater functional benefits after SDR have been shown in younger patients (13, 14) and patients with spastic diplegia versus quadriplegia (15–19). Chiccoine et al. (20) reported that a better initial gait score and the diagnosis of diplegia versus quadriplegia were the strongest predictors of ability to walk after SDR. Based on a multivariate analysis, Kim et al. (12) found that the diagnosis of spastic diplegia versus quadriplegia was the only variable that predicted a good versus poor outcome after SDR.

The information accumulated about outcomes of SDR over the past few decades has led to the development of rigorous criteria for SDR candidacy at most centers currently offering this treatment option for patients with CP (21–24). Screening of potential SDR candidates typically involves a comprehensive clinical evaluation as described in Chapter 24; videotaping and/or gait analysis are also commonly used (25–27). Good potential candidates are typically ambulatory, intelligent patients 3 to 8 years of age with spastic diplegic CP and a history of prematurity. These children exhibit good proximal strength and selective motor control in the lower extremities with minimal contracture. The ability to participate in and access to a physical therapy program post-SDR must also be considered. Relative contraindications include predominantly nonspastic movement disorders, poor trunk control, severe weakness, and multiple, severe contractures or a history of multiple, previous orthopedic surgeries. Parks and Johnston (28) recommend SDR for ambulatory, motivated adults less than 40 years of age who have mild spastic diplegic CP and minimal orthopedic deformity. In general, ITB is recommended instead of SDR for nonambulatory patients with more severe neurologic impairment (18, 27, 29, 30). However, a recent study comparing nonconcurrent patients treated with SDR or ITB matched by age and functional level found that SDR was more effective in reducing spasticity and improving function (31). Based on these findings, the authors suggest consideration of SDR for spastic patients with more severe functional impairment.

Techniques

The neurosurgical procedure requires general anesthesia without the use of muscle relaxants. With the patient in the prone position, a 1- to 2-in incision along the center of the lower back is made, and the dura is opened. Most commonly, this is done through multiple-level laminectomies or laminotomies from L1 or L2 to L5 or S1 with preservation of the facet joints. Alternatively, a single-level L1 laminectomy offers the advantages of a smaller incision and less dissection but is more technically challenging (28). The segmental levels of the exposed roots are identified with EMG surface or needle recording electrodes placed in 4 to 10 target muscles with L1/2–S2 innervation (32, 33). The L1–S2 posterior roots are separated from the anterior roots and lower sacral roots. The rootlets within each targeted root segment are transected (Figure 26.1).

The neurophysiologic methods used and the criteria applied to identify which rootlets are "abnormal"—that is, contributing most to spasticity—vary among centers performing SDR. Original criteria for an abnormal EMG response as defined by Fasano et al. (6) include a low threshold to a single stimulus, and a sustained response to tetanic stimulation in the stimulated muscles that may spread to other segmental, contralateral, and/or upper extremity and trunk muscles. Over the past few decades, the validity of these criteria has been questioned. In one series of patients with CP, none of the rootlets stimulated met the criteria for a "normal" response (34, 35), whereas another study found that nonspastic patients exhibited sustained contractions that met criteria for an abnormal response (36). In a series of 92 patients with CP, Hays et al. (37) found that the percentage of abnormally responding rootlets sectioned at SDR did not correspond to measures of spasticity or function performed at baseline and post-SDR evaluations. The issue is further confused by the variability that exists in the electrophysiologic techniques used among centers performing SDR (9, 33, 38). In addition, significant intrinsic variability in these responses exists as well (39). Accordingly, a wide range of total rootlets transected are reported in the literature. Peacock et al. (8) reported that 25% to 50% of rootlets tested are sectioned in a typical patient with spastic diplegic CP. In studies published within the last 5 years, the average

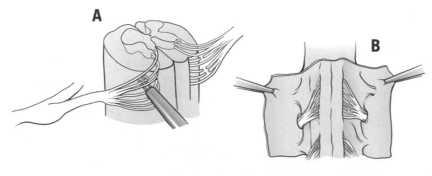

FIGURE 26.1

Techniques for performing SDR. (A) The stimulation of the dorsal roots. (B) The transection of the dorsal roots. (Reproduced with permission from Koman LA, ed. *Wake Forest University School of Medicine Orthopaedic Manual 2001.* Winston-Salem, NC: Orthopaedic Press.)

rootlet transection rate reported is between 40% and 70% (23, 27, 28, 30, 31), but the maximal percentage imposed varies by center.

There is also specific debate in the literature with regard to the inclusion and sectioning of certain dorsal roots. The L1 root is included when hip flexor spasticity is problematic, but typically one half or less of rootlets are sectioned nonselectively (28). Relatively less of the L4 root may be transected to maintain some quadriceps tone (27). Many earlier series excluded the S2 root, presumably because of the potential for injuring functionally normal S2 afferent fibers, which mediate bladder reflexes (8, 10, 16). However, preserving the S2 dorsal roots allows persistence of potentially abnormal reflex circuits that subserve the ankle plantar flexors; thus, exclusion at this level may result in continued ankle plantar spasticity interfering with function. The literature offers inconclusive evidence, with case series showing spasticity reduction in ankle plantar flexors with (25) and without (40) S2 root sectioning. Lang et al. (41) compared retrospective results of SDR in which S2 sectioning was or was not performed. At 6 months post-SDR, they found a significant reduction in ankle plantar flexor spasticity with the addition of the S2 roots but did not evaluate any functional changes. These authors used sensory-evoked potentials to ensure the preservation of bowel and bladder function. Other authors support S2 sectioning with pudendal nerve monitoring and less total percentage of rootlets cut and/or more stringent EMG criteria applied for sectioning (25, 27, 30, 42).

Unfortunately, the ultimate contribution of electrophysiologic monitoring cannot be determined by the available evidence. Only one report compares outcomes after selective versus nonselective rhizotomy, in which a certain percentage of rootlets were transected

randomly. This study found no advantage to electrophysiologically guided SDR in 26 patients compared to a historical cohort at 12 months (43). Although most centers currently performing SDR continue to use some form of intraoperative neurophysiologic monitoring for accurate root identification, different approaches to guide rootlet selection have developed at different centers (9, 19, 27, 30, 33). These typically involve the critical integration of the unfolding results of neurophysiologic monitoring along with clinical information and goals. Although such approaches are rational and based to some extent on objective criteria, they remain nonstandardized. Finally, because the overall clinical results from centers performing SDR are not significantly different, the value of electrophysiologic techniques remains questionable.

Adverse Events

In general, studies of SDR report a low incidence of adverse events and rare occurrence of any serious adverse events resulting in long-term morbidity (44, 45). Intraoperative and perioperative adverse events involving respiratory problems were more common (1.3%–6.9%) as reported in earlier studies (46, 47). Improvements in these rates reported in later series are attributed to refinements in surgical and anesthetic care (45, 46).

In a review by Steinbok (27), perioperative transient urinary retention is a common adverse event, with an incidence of between 1.25% and 24%. One center reports that transient urinary retention was associated with the use of postoperative epidural morphine analgesia, leading to their recommendation that the epidural catheter be removed at postoperative day 3 with maintenance of the Foley catheter an additional 24 hours

(30). Transient dysesthesias are also common (2.5%–40%), but permanent symptoms occur uncommonly (0%–6%) (27). Persistent sensory changes were associated with more rootlet sectioning in one study (47), but this finding was not statistically significant. The lower rate of post-SDR is also attributed to the decreased in the amount (<70%) of sectioning (23, 30).

Late-onset bowel and bladder dysfunction was reported in 5.1% of patients in the series by Steinbok and Schrang (47), and this adverse event was associated with the lack of pudendal nerve monitoring. As described above, the current use of pudendal nerve monitoring techniques and more stringent criteria for sectioning are recommended when the S2 root is included. According to several authors, use of these techniques also has greatly reduced the occurrence of bladder dysfunction (30, 46, 48).

Another important late adverse event is the development of musculoskeletal problems. Development of foot deformities after SDR has been anecdotally reported (49) but not well documented in any retrospective or prospective series. Hip subluxation, another common problem in patients with CP, has been studied more extensively, but many studies are retrospective and do not use consistent definitions of hip pathology. More systematic, prospective studies suggest that the effect of SDR on hip subluxation is likely to be neutral or positive (50–52). One such study found that worsening of hip subluxation after SDR may be more likely to occur in more severely affected patients (52). It has also been suggested that foot deformities and hip subluxation may occur in patients with CP after SDR or other antispasticity interventions more as the result of lever arm dysfunction and growth rather than from spasticity (53–54).

The musculoskeletal area of greatest concern after SDR is the spine. This is because of the association of spinal deformity in patients with CP as well as in children without CP who undergo multiple lumbar laminectomies (55–57). The risk of spinal deformity after SDR has been evaluated in numerous studies; unfortunately, a lack of consistent surgical and radiographic techniques does not allow for accurate comparison. Selective dorsal rhizotomy may increase the incidence of scoliosis, kyphosis, hyperlordosis, and lumbosacral spondylolisthesis (58–65). The increased risk of scoliosis after SDR has been found to be higher for nonambulatory patients with spastic quadriplegia (30, 61, 62, 65), whereas the risk of spondylolisthesis is higher in ambulatory children (58, 60, 61, 65). It has been suggested that the use of a limited laminectomy may reduce the risk of these complications (28, 40). However, this finding has not been demonstrated in any controlled studies.

Overall, lower rates of both early operative and late adverse events in the last 20 years are attributed to a variety of technical improvements and refinements, and currently, SDR is considered to be a very safe procedure. More rigorous studies are needed to determine the long-term influence of SDR on spinal and hip deformities; however, based on the available information, development of hip and/or spinal deformities requiring surgical intervention in ambulatory patients who undergo SDR is probably not significantly increased. Ongoing orthopedic monitoring of the spine and hips is recommended for all patients who undergo SDR (29, 50, 65).

Outcomes of Surgical Treatment of Spasticity

Of all the surgical procedures currently performed on patients with CP, SDR has undergone the most thorough scientific scrutiny. Multiple prospective and retrospective case series document long-term improvements in spasticity and range of motion (ROM). In 2001, Steinbok (66) published an extensive literature review of 63 articles that rated the strength of evidence available for SDR. There was conclusive evidence to support SDR efficacy at the impairment level, including decreased spasticity (Ashworth score) for up to 12 years and increased lower extremity joint ROM for up to 5 years.

The association between SDR and the requirement for orthopedic surgery is another outcome of interest. However, because of the interdependence of spasticity, deformity evolution, and growth, this is a difficult outcome to evaluate, especially without a control group. In the literature review by Steinbok, there was weak evidence to support SDR for decreasing the need for orthopedic procedures (66). Two subsequent studies have evaluated 1- to 2-year outcomes after orthopedic surgery or SDR. Seinko-Thomas et al. (67) found similar improvements in energy costs as well as gait parameters, spasticity, and ROM after either type of intervention. Schwartz et al. (26) report improvements in gait parameters, gait efficiency, and functional skills in ambulatory children with CP after orthopedic surgery, SDR, or a combination of both treatments. However, a lower rate of soft tissue surgery was performed in subjects who underwent a combination of SDR and orthopedic surgery compared to those who underwent orthopedic surgery alone. The 2 procedures are indicated for different purposes and thus should be viewed as complementary options in a comprehensive treatment philosophy (3, 26, 53, 68, 69).

Improvements in function in patients undergoing SDR have been documented in several short- and long-term studies. However, compared to improvements in spasticity and ROM, there is more variability in the reported results. In addition, findings reported in earlier studies are more difficult to evaluate because most of the studies were retrospective and used nonstandardized assessments of function (9–11, 16). Three randomized clinical trials compared results of SDR combined with physical therapy to physical therapy alone in children ages 3 to 18 years with spastic diplegic CP (44, 70, 71). Of the three studies, 2 reported increased Gross Motor Functional Measure (GMFM) scores. A meta-analysis of these 3 studies demonstrated greater functional improvement as represented by a 4- to 5-point gain in the GMFM score in the SDR group (72). In a systematic literature review by Steinbok (66), there was strong evidence to support SDR efficacy for improved motor function based primarily on these same trials and other nonrandomized, prospective studies. The Steinbok review (66) also found evidence of a moderate degree of certainty supporting SDR for improvement in function based on Pediatric Evaluation of Disability Index and wee-Functional Independence Measure scores, improvements in gait including increased stride length and velocity, and improvement in suprasegmental effects including upper limb function and cognition.

Several recent noncontrolled studies describe lasting functional benefits after SDR. Improvements in GMFM scores have been documented at 5 years postoperatively (18, 73, 74), and improvements in Pediatric Evaluation of Disability Index scores have been documented at 5 and 10 years postoperatively (73, 75). Langerak et al. (76) report improvements in sagittal gait analysis parameters 20 years after SDR in 13 patients with spastic diplegic CP. Development of more accurate predictive outcome variables and long-term outcome studies are a focus of current and future SDR research (22, 23, 77).

INTRATHECAL BACLOFEN

Rationale

Direct ITB delivery and continuous infusion via a device delivery system evolved to compensate for the problems associated with the orally administered drug (see Chapter 24). Administration of continuous ITB (CITB) is a nonsurgical, pharmacological treatment that is typically managed by nonsurgical specialists. However, it requires surgical intervention for implantation of the drug delivery system and for correction of later, potential delivery system complications.

Indications

The general indications for CITB in patients with CP and the associated screening process for patient selection are reviewed in Chapter 24. From a surgical perspective, candidates for the CITB must be medically and neurologically stable and free of infection; in addition, candidates must have adequate body mass and abdominal girth to accommodate the pump (78).

Instrumentation

The Medtronic Synchromed Infusion® system is used to treat spasticity with CITB in children with CP. The system components are a surgically implanted, battery-powered pump connected to a flexible, radiopaque intrathecal silicone catheter. The drug dosage and mode of delivery (eg, bolus or continuous) are adjusted to individual needs with an external programmer using radiofrequency telemetry (Figure 26.2). Two pump sizes are available that are both approximately the diameter of a hockey puck; however, the pumps differ in the volume of the drug reservoir (20 or 40 mL) (Figure 26.3). The drug reservoir is accessed percutaneously in the office setting to refill the pump. The 20-mL reservoir pump is thinner and has less volume displacement compared to the 40-mL pump, making it more suitable for smaller and thinner patients (79) (Figure 26.4). The catheter is available as 1- or 2-piece models that are supplied with spinal

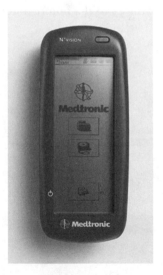

FIGURE 26.2

The 8840 N'Vision programmer uses a touch screen display for data entry, and telemetry for programming drug doses and infusion rates. (Photo courtesy of Medtronic, Inc.)

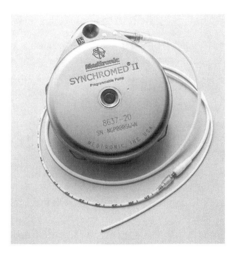

FIGURE 26.3

A SynchroMed II pump showing the catheter access port and the reservoir fill port. (Photos courtesy of Medtronic, Inc.)

needles, guidewires, and the appropriate anchoring devices (Figure 26.5(A) and (B)).

Techniques

Surgical implantation of the ITB delivery system is performed under general anesthesia, typically by a pediatric neurosurgeon. Details of the procedure are described elsewhere (80, 81). The procedure involves 3 basic steps: placement of the catheter in the spine, connection of the catheter to the pump, and implantation

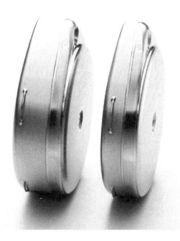

FIGURE 26.4

A lateral view of the 2 SynchroMed II pumps demonstrating the difference in their width to accommodate either 20 or 40 mL of drug. (Photo courtesy of Medtronic, Inc.)

of the pump in the abdomen. All steps are performed with the patient in the lateral decubitus position. First, the spinal needle is placed into the intrathecal space at the L2-3 or L3-4 level. The catheter tubing is introduced through the needle and is advanced through the intrathecal space (Figure 26.6). The catheter tip is positioned under fluoroscopic guidance at a spinal cord level predetermined by clinical information. A longitudinal incision is made at the needle site, and the subcutaneous tissues are dissected to secure the catheter with the appropriate anchoring devices.

The next step involves creation of the abdominal pump implant site. The site and depth of pump placement in the abdomen are determined before surgery. The site and side of abdominal placement depends on the presence of feeding tubes, ventriculoperitoneal shunts, and abdominal scars from previous surgery as well as consideration of the patient's daily positioning and activity level. The pump is placed in either the subcutaneous or subfacial plane. Subfascial placement is recommended in children with CP because it maximizes soft tissue coverage and, theoretically, decreases the risk of skin breakdown and infection (80, 82–85). A transverse skin incision is made, and the subcutaneous or subfacial tissues are dissected to form a pocket for pump implantation (Figure 26.7(A) and (B)). The catheter is tunneled subcutaneously from the spinal incision to the abdominal pump implant site where it is connected to a pump that is prefilled with baclofen. The catheter is then secured to the pump with a sutureless connector. In the final step, the pump is anchored using suture loops or a mesh pouch. A postoperative radiograph is used to confirm the continuity and location of the catheter (Figure 26.8(A) and (B)).

Adverse Events

Adverse events may be related to the surgery, infusion system components, human error, or the drug itself. Surgical adverse events are estimated to occur with a frequency of 25% to 40%, with infections having the greatest morbidity (85). System-related adverse events usually involve issues with the catheter (eg, kinking, migration, occlusion, disconnection, fracture) and occur at rates of 20% to 25% (86). Primary problems with the pump itself occur at rates of less than 10% (86). Catheter problems typically require corrective surgeries but are not associated with significant long-term morbidity (80, 83, 85). Both human error and system failures have the potential to cause abnormally high or low drug levels. The acute ITB withdrawal syndrome can occur after sudden cessation of CITB infusion and is potentially fatal (87). However, all cases of pediatric patients with CP who experienced

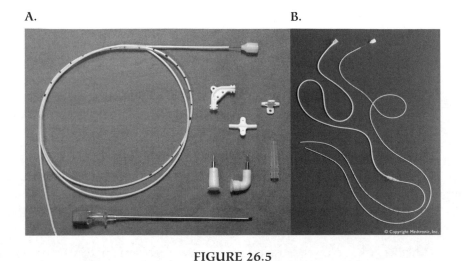

FIGURE 26.5

Various silicone catheters have been developed for use with the SynchroMed infusion system. Catheters are available in 1-piece (A) and 2-piece (B) configurations. (Photos courtesy of Medtronic, Inc.)

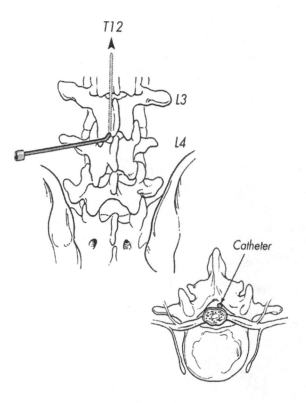

FIGURE 26.6

During the ITB surgical procedure, the catheter is introduced into the intrathecal space and is advanced to the appropriate spinal level. (Reproduced with permission from Koman LA, ed. *Wake Forest University School of Medicine Orthopaedic Manual 2001.* Winston-Salem. NC: Orthopaedic Press.)

CITB withdrawal described in the literature recovered without long-term morbidity (85). In fact, in studies of children with CP, cases of serious overdosage of ITB are described more frequently than cases of withdrawal (85).

Other drug-related adverse events that have reported to occur at presumably appropriate ITB dosages include CNS side effects, reported at rates of 2% to 43%, and problems such as nausea, constipation, and headaches, reported at rates of 11% to 36% (85). In addition, concerns have been raised about an association between CITB and increased frequency and/or severity of 2 problems commonly associated with CP—seizures and scoliosis. One retrospective controlled study concluded that seizure activity was not aggravated or induced by CITB (88). Two retrospective studies with control groups matched for a number of clinical characteristics did not find an increased progression of scoliosis in patients with CP treated with CITB (89, 90). Special techniques must be used in patients who undergo pump implantation before or after spinal fusion or who undergo the procedures concurrently (91). One retrospective study that used a matched control group found that patients with CP treated with CITB who subsequently underwent spinal fusion experienced higher rates of adverse events (92).

In general, CITB is acknowledged to be associated with a relatively high rate of adverse events in children with CP (85). In a multicenter study, Albright et al. report that approximately 50% of patients experience some adverse event within 2 months after implantation, and 50% of patients experience an adverse event during chronic therapy (93). In addition, younger patients and those with more neurologic im-

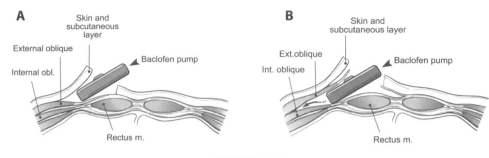

FIGURE 26.7

The pump can be placed under the skin (A) or under the fascia (B). (Reproduced with permission from Koman LA, ed. *Wake Forest University School of Medicine Orthopaedic Manuel 2005*. Winston-Salem, NC: Orthopaedic Press.)

pairment appear to be at higher risk for adverse events (84, 85). Changes in surgical techniques and technologic improvements in the pump and catheter are purported to have decreased rates of adverse events, but to date, such claims have not been substantiated by specific investigations (85). However, there is consensus in the literature that adverse events can be minimized when patients are treated with CITB in a coordinated system of care by a dedicated and experienced team (85, 93–95).

Outcomes

Two systematic reviews considered all published reports of outcomes in patients with CP since ITB was approved for use in patients with spasticity of cerebral origin in 1996 (96, 97). Both reviews use an evidence-based approach (98) and classify outcomes using the International Classification of Functioning, Disability and Health (ICF) model (99). Of the total of 33 articles reviewed, 3 reports provide strong evidence for the efficacy of ITB to reduce spasticity (as measured by the Ashworth or Modified Ashworth scales) or to decrease neurophysiologic reflexes after a single bolus injection of ITB (100–102). Multiple noncontrolled, prospective, or retrospective case series studies report on the effectiveness of chronic ITB for long-term maintenance of decreased muscle tone after pump implantation. Improvements in other aspects of the ICF (eg, decreased need for orthopedic surgery, improved

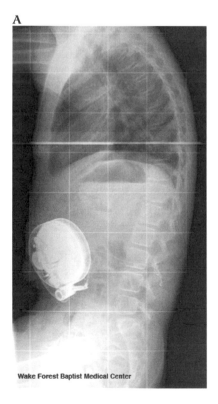

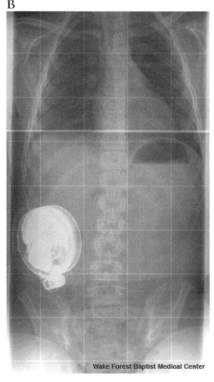

FIGURE 26.8

Postsurgical radiographs after pump placement. (A) anterior-posterior and (B) lateral view. (Wake Forest University Press, with permission.)

function, ease of care, and health-related quality of life) are reported, but efficacy is not well established in the available literature.

ORTHOPEDIC SURGERY

Rationale

Orthopedic procedures have traditionally been—and continue to be—the mainstay of surgical intervention for children with spastic CP. Of the 5 most frequent surgical procedures performed in children with CP in the United States, 3 are orthopedic (103). However, unlike SDR and CITB, orthopedic surgical procedures do not treat spasticity directly; rather, orthopedic surgery is used to address 2 major musculoskeletal consequences of spasticity: (1) soft tissue contractures of muscle, tendon, and/or joint and (2) bony deformities. In the extremities, bony deformities are often referred to as "lever arm dysfunction" and include hip subluxation, torsional deformities of long bones, and foot deformities (104).

Orthopedic surgery for correction of these problems in children with CP must proceed with an understanding of the complex, interdependent processes of deformity evolution, and growth (53, 54). Contractures are initiated by the primary problems of increased and/or imbalanced muscle tone resulting in dynamic abnormalities; these abnormal movements and postures can eventually become fixed with muscles in a shortened position. This contributes to the secondary problem of impaired longitudinal muscle growth relative to bone growth (105, 106). In the development of bony deformity, the abnormal forces around a joint caused by spastic and imbalanced muscles result in malalignment, which then interferes with normal bone and joint structural development (54, 107, 108). The processes of both soft tissue and bony deformity formation are exacerbated in children with impaired mobility due to the lack of normal developmental stimuli from muscle stretch and weight-bearing forces (54, 109).

Evaluation

In patients with CP, the musculoskeletal complications of spasticity present with considerable clinical heterogeneity. This heterogeneity reflects the variation that exists in the type and extent of the primary CNS lesion and also depends on the level of skeletal maturity. The orthopedic assessment typically involves both clinical and radiological evaluations. Clinical examination is necessary to document motor function, sensibility, balance, joint ROM, the extent and severity of spasticity, and the presence of other movement disorders. Because day-to-day variation in spasticity and function is observed in children with CP, a potential surgical candidate may need to be examined several times before a final decision for surgical intervention is made (110, 111). Details on specific orthopedic physical examination techniques are available in several well-known references (106, 112, 113). Clinical and laboratory measurements of spasticity are reviewed in Chapters 5 to 7; the clinical assessment of motor function in patients with CP is reviewed in Chapter 24, including some of the common measures and instruments developed and validated in this population.

Radiographic assessment is usually performed with plain radiographs. Serial radiographs are recommended to monitor common problems such as progressive hip subluxation and scoliosis (114, 115). Useful radiographic indices commonly used for the measurement of these problems are, respectively, the Reimer migration percentage (Figure 26.9) and the Cobb angle (Figure 26.10) (107, 116). Computed tomography, 3-dimensional computed tomography, or magnetic resonance imaging may be indicated to evaluate joint congruency and bony architecture (111, 117). The EMG and diagnostic muscle blocks assist n the identification of muscles with clinically relevant spasticity and weakness.

For ambulatory patients, the walking ability of the child is evaluated. Determination of the causes of gait abnormalities may be performed by observation using a standardized scale such as the Physician's Rating Scale or—when available—the 3-dimensional motion analysis (112, 118, 119). For children with ambulatory diplegic and hemiplegic CP, gait analysis has identified common patterns of muscle overactivity and deformity, which are often used to guide surgical decision making (120, 121).

Indications and Surgical Planning

Orthopedic surgery is designed to prevent fixed deformities that have the potential to cause pain, interfere with function and/or caregiving, or correct such problems after they have developed. Before orthopedic surgery is considered, spasticity management must be optimized using nonsurgical interventions as described in Chapter 24 and, in selected cases, with the use of SDR or ITB. These interventions may prevent the occurrence of fixed deformities or slow their progression (122–124). When surgery is indicated, potential candidates may need referral for a nutritional assessment and evaluation of general medical and neurologic stability (125). Nonsurgical options such as medications,

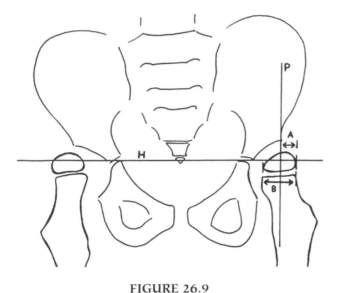

FIGURE 26.9

Reimer migration index for measurement of hip subluxation. (Reproduced with permission from Koman LA, ed. Wake Forest University School of Medicine Orthopaedic Manual (2009). Winston-Salem, NC: Orthopaedic Press.)

bracing, and adaptive devices may be better long-term strategies for patients with significant medical comorbidities.

Specific issues addressed in preoperative planning include the following: (1) timing of surgery; (2) choice, number, and staging of procedures; and (3) postoperative and rehabilitation care. The decision-making process involved can be complex and is often more challenging than the techniques used to

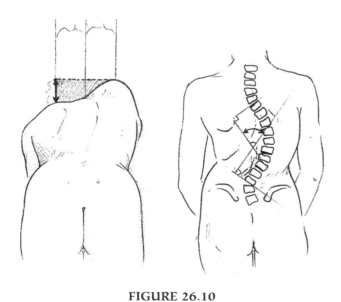

FIGURE 26.10

Cobb angle technique for measurement of scoliosis.

perform the surgery (110, 126). Ideally, both the recommendation for orthopedic intervention for a child with CP—and the associated preoperative decision-making process—are informed by the input of a multidisciplinary team (53, 127, 128).

In general, orthopedic surgery before 4 years of age is not recommended because of the higher risk of deformity recurrence (129–132). In addition, results in younger children may be less predictable because the full spectrum of neurologic impairments and movement disorders may not be apparent, and the child's gait pattern is not fully mature (27, 133, 134). If possible, procedures should be delayed until the patient is close to skeletal maturity, but typically, soft tissue procedures are performed around 5 to 7 years of age and bony procedures after 8 to 10 years (112, 135). This schedule allows for more longitudinal bone growth to occur and improves the available bone stock, thus potentially decreasing the chance of recurrence of soft tissues contractures and improving the stability of bony procedures. However, consideration must also be given to the natural history of specific musculoskeletal deformities. For example, a major exception to this schedule is the treatment of hip subluxation. Soft tissue procedures in younger patients with early hip subluxation will prevent progression to hip dislocation in most cases (107, 115, 136). In addition, surgery in younger patients with fixed deformity may be necessary if function and/or health-related quality of life are significantly compromised.

Another general principle guiding the current practice of orthopedic surgery for patients with CP is the performance of multiple procedures to correct soft tissue and bony deformities in a single session as opposed to intermittent surgical procedures throughout childhood. This type of approach, which has been termed single-event, multilevel surgery (SEMLS), relies on serial clinical examinations and the anticipation of potential structural skeletal problems (130, 137). Because a deformity at one joint can affect the function of others, use of SEMLS potentially decreases the occurrence of complications from interventions performed at a single level (106, 138, 139). In addition, SEMLS potentially decreases the amount of time needed for hospitalization and rehabilitation. Multiple noncontrolled studies document the safety and benefits of SEMLS (130, 137, 140–144). A small, controlled study suggests that this approach may result in stabilization of function and deformity, which represents an improvement over the natural history of CP (145).

Surgical planning should also include preparation for postoperative management, which may be the most important contribution to a successful outcome. Postoperative pain is controlled with epidural, caudal, or local nerve blocks (146). Postoperative spasticity may be addressed with intraoperative chemodenervation with botulinum A toxin intramuscular injection and/or short-term oral medications such as diazepam (110, 126, 147). Patients with CP often have significant underlying weakness and steopenia and may be more susceptible to the deleterious effects of immobilization. To prevent loss of muscle strength and cardiovascular conditioning, patients should be given clearance to return to their preoperative level of activity as quickly as possible (148). To avoid complete joint immobilization, removable splints or short-term casting is utilized. These strategies may also decrease the risk of postoperative pathologic fracture (149). For patients with functional goals, intensive outpatient physical and/or occupational therapy emphasizing strengthening for several months postoperatively is recommended. All postoperative patients and their families should receive instructions for a maintenance home exercise program involving positioning, stretching, splinting, and/or strengthening.

Surgical Techniques

The orthopedic procedures that are performed to correct musculoskeletal deformities in children with CP are individualized based on patient age, level of neurologic impairment, motor disorder, ambulatory status, and goals. Different types of procedures are used for correction of soft tissue versus bony deformity, and a variety of orthopedic surgical techniques options are available for both.

For correction of soft tissue contractures and muscle imbalances without significant joint contracture, the 2 basic categories of surgical procedures include (1) musculotendinous lengthenings and (2) tendon transfers. Neurectomy is another approach included in this category but is rarely indicated because of the risks of excessive weakness and development of new deformities (112, 150).

Musculotendinous lengthening procedures are the most common approach for correction of contractures. The mechanical changes associated with these procedures have physiologic effects that are complex and not fully understood (109, 151–153). There is likely an effect on the stretch reflex that attenuates a spastic muscle's response to stretch (154, 155). Four methods of lengthening are described: (1) tendon lengthening, which is performed with various cuts in the tendon. Common examples include the "Z" lengthening and sliding techniques, which are frequently done in the tendoachilles and medial hamstring tendons (Figure 26.11); (2) Tenotomy, which

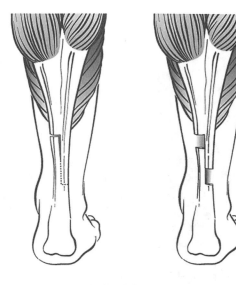

FIGURE 26.11

Sliding lengthening of tendoachilles. (Reproduced with permission from Koman LA, ed. *Wake Forest University School of Medicine Orthopaedic Manual (2009)*. Winston-Salem, NC: Orthopaedic Press.)

involves transection through the tendon, can be done near the muscle origin or insertion (Figure 26.12). The hip adductors, iliopsoas, rectus femoris, and pronator teres are often lengthened using this technique; (3) Intramuscular or fascial lengthening is also referred to as a muscle recession. This technique involves transection—typically with several partial cuts—of the tendinous attachments of the muscle but preserves the muscle fibers (Figure 26.13). Sites conducive to this procedure include the iliopsoas, semimembranosus, biceps femoris, gastrocnemius-soleus, finger flexors, and deltoids; (4) Myotomy involves transection through the muscle belly (Figure 26.14). This procedure is rarely used in patients with CP but may be indicated for treatment of more severe contractures when function is not an issue, for example, the latissimus dorsi muscle in a fixed shoulder joint.

Tendon transfer procedures attempt to restore balance between the overactive transferred agonist muscle and weakness in the antagonist muscle group to which the transferred muscle is attached. Tendon transfers are performed using an intact or "split" tendon (Figure 26.15). Ideally, muscles chosen for tendon transfer procedures are overactive and directly contribute to a spastic deformity but have adequate strength for preserved functioning after transfer. Dynamic motion and EMG analyses may assist in these determinations in both the upper and lower extremities (112, 156, 157). For example, tendon transfer

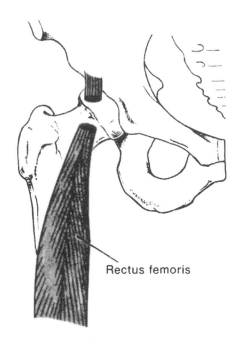

FIGURE 26.12

Tenotomy of rectus femoris.

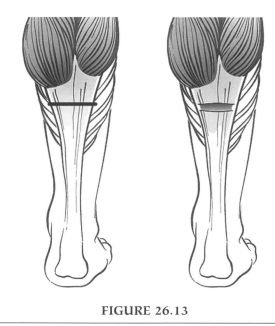

FIGURE 26.13

Intramuscular recession of gastrocnemius. (Reproduced with permission from Koman LA, ed. *Wake Forest University School of Medicine Orthopaedic Manual (2009).* Winston-Salem, NC: Orthopaedic Press.)

procedures for correction of equinovarus contractures include split tendon transfers of either the tibialis anterior or tibialis posterior muscles (158, 159). Both muscles are ankle invertors, but evaluation of their contribution to motion at the ankle joint may not be obvious on clinical examination.

For correction of bony deformities, orthopedic surgery techniques include (1) reduction of subluxed or dislocated joints; (2) fixation or fusion of joints to provide stability; (3) correction of rotational problems; and (4) excision of heterotopic bone. Such procedures may involve osteotomies, placement of various internal—or occasionally external—fixation devices, bone grafting, and adjunctive soft tissue procedures. Common problems addressed are scoliosis, hip subluxation (Figure 26.16), rotational deformities of the lower extremity long bones, and foot and ankle deformities such as equinovarus, equinovalgus, and planovalgus (Figure 26.17).

Review of literature for evidence has not identified any one best technique or combination of procedures; thus, the specific surgical techniques applied will depend to some extent on individual surgeon preference and/or institutional bias. However, some general trends can be described; these reflect the fact that the occurrence of deformities varies by the type and severity of CP. Lower extremity deformities occur

in all types of spastic CP. Patients with spastic diplegia are typically treated with multiple-level soft tissue procedures; bony procedures are performed less often, usually for correction of lower extremity rotational deformities and/or foot and ankle deformity. Patients with spastic quadriplegia are at greatest risk for hip subluxation and scoliosis and frequently undergo corrective procedures to address these problems (103). Patients with hemiplegia tend to have more distal involvement and most commonly undergo surgery at the foot and ankle and in the forearm, wrist, and hand. Compared to the lower extremities, corrective procedures of the upper extremity are, overall, performed far less often and are limited to patients with spastic hemiplegia and quadriplegia (160, 161). Upper extremity procedures are typically performed to improve comfort, hygiene, appearance, self-esteem, and/or function; for the latter, good candidates are those with good sensation, voluntary control, and the ability to participate in postsurgical rehabilitation. In general, orthopedic surgery in patients with predominantly nonspastic movement disorders such as athetosis and dystonia have more unpredicatable results; thus, soft tissue procedures of both the upper and lower extremities—especially tendon transfers—are relatively contraindicated in these patients (110, 111, 135, 162).

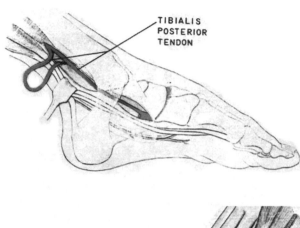

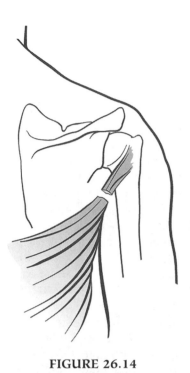

FIGURE 26.14

Myotomy of latissimus dorsi. (Reproduced with permission from Koman LA, ed. *Wake Forest University School of Medicine Orthopaedic Manual (2009)*. Winston-Salem, NC: Orthopaedic Press.)

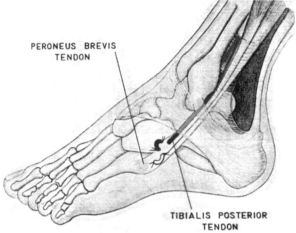

FIGURE 26.15

Tendon transfer using split tibialis posterior tendon.

Adverse Events

Given the variability in patient types and in the types of procedures used to treat them, the frequency of adverse events of orthopedic procedures in patients with CP is difficult to determine. The operative adverse events with the most potential to cause significant morbidity and mortality are most often related to cardiopulmonary issues, neurovascular compromise, and infection. These complications are more frequent in patients who are more neurologically impaired and in procedures which involve greater anesthestic exposure and higher risk of blood loss such as osteotomies and spinal fusion (163, 164). Careful preoperative evaluation and experienced, intensive postoperative management are recommended to minimize complications for higher-risk patients and procedures (125, 165).

Postoperative adverse events related to infection can occur early or late. In several large series of patients with CP undergoing spinal fusion, the wound infection rate was reported to be 2.5% to 19% (166–168). Wound infections occur less often with soft tissue compared to bony procedures, but procedures in the groin area are at higher risk (110, 112, 130). The risk of infection may be lowered in higher-risk situations with the use of careful surgical site preparation and/or prophylactic antibiotics (136, 169, 170).

Neurovascular compromise of the spinal cord resulting in neurologic deficts is a well-recognized complication of spinal fusion in patients with neuromuscular scoliosis (171). Several special surgical and anesthetic techniques for patients with CP are recommended to decrease the risk of neurologic deficits (110, 125, 172, 173). Neurovascular compromise of peripheral nerves can result from changes in alignment and ROM at a joint that cause excessive stretching of nearby nerves and vessels. This adverse event is more common with soft tissue procedures but can occur in bony procedures—for example, correction of more severe torsional deformities and treatment of crouch gait with distal femoral extension osteotomy (174, 175). Symptoms of postoperative nerve palsy—dysesthesia, sensory and/or motor loss—are likely underreported for several reasons. Preoperative and postoperative changes in sensation and strength are often not well documented, and symptoms of nerve injury may be difficult to evaluate in more severely involved patients.

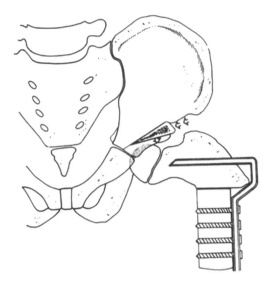

FIGURE 26.16

Correction of hip subluxation with peri-ilial pelvic and femoral osteotomies with blade plate fixation.

In one study, sciatic nerve palsy was documented in 9.6% of patients undergoing hamstring lengthening, but most resolved with treatment. Older patients and those with more neurologic impairment were found to be at higher risk (176).

Often categorized together as surgical "failures," other important postoperative adverse events are the recurrence of treated deformities and the development of new deformities. These types of postoperative adverse events are relatively common and can occur after soft tissue or bony procedures; in addition, they are often associated with long-term morbidity and the need for repeat surgical procedures.

The frequency of recurrence reported after soft tissue procedures varies greatly from 3% to 40% (112, 130–132, 139, 140, 164). In bony procedures for correction of lower extremity deformities, recurrence rates reported ranged from 0% to 33% (158, 164, 177–180). Relatively lower recurrence rates in bony versus soft tissue procedures may reflect the fact that bony procedures are more often performed in older children (164). Thus, deformity recurrence may not represent surgical failure per se (162). Recurrence occurs more often in younger patients because of their growth potential; in addition, some studies have shown that more neurologically impaired patients tend to demonstrate higher rates of recurrence suggesting a relationship to more severe spasticity (132, 181, 182). In some cases, however, undercorrection related to surgical technique may also contribute to recurrence. Nevertheless, review of the literature strongly suggests that undercorrection is preferable to overcorrection, especially at the ankle; in addition, although recurrence occurs frequently, it can be adequately addressed with repeat corrective procedures (110, 126, 183).

The development of new postoperative deformities is attributed to excessive weakness and the exacerbation of existing—or the creation of new—muscle imbalances. New deformities are of particular concern because they can produce worsening of function and/or deformity that may be irreversible or very difficult to correct (110). The most common new postoperative deformities are contractures or bony deformity in the opposite direction of the treated deformity. However, new deformity can also occur in the nontreated extremity. Examples of the former include development of recurvatum after hamstring lengthenings reported in 3% to 28% cases; calcaneus and/or valgus

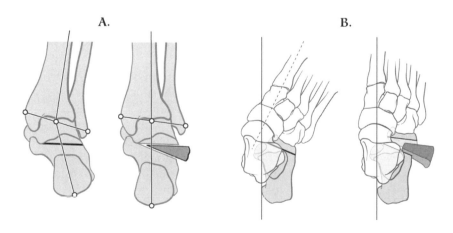

A.   B.

FIGURE 26.17

Techniques for correction of hindfoot valgus deformity. (A) Opening wedge osteotomy; (B) calcaneal lengthening.

deformity after treatment of equinus or equinovarus are reported in 2% to 28% of cases (112, 182, 184–186). An example of the latter is the development of windswept hip deformity after unilateral treatment of hip subluxation. Development of a new deformity usually results from 2 causes: (1) overcorrection and (2) abnormal muscle activity, either from antagonistic muscles acting at the same joint or muscles acting at adjacent joints (109, 112, 187, 188).

Many joint and procedure-specific strategies are described for the prevention of new deformities. For example, intramuscular lengthening of eligible muscles has been shown to maintain strength and is recommended by several authors as the initial soft tissue corrective technique for ambulatory patients in whom muscle weakness is a concern (117, 189, 190). Motion analysis and EMG along with the performance of multilevel procedures are advocated to minimize the risk of problems associated with abnormal muscle activity (53, 54, 114, 127, 139). Guidance for the amount of rotation necessary for correction of torsional deformity may be obtained from the preoperative planning process, including physical examination, gait analysis, and/or radiographic imaging, but should primarily rely on careful intraoperative evaluation of the degree of rotation obtained (110, 112). Consideration of surgery on the opposite limb is recommended in treatment of hip subluxation to prevent windswept deformity (153, 180, 191).

Based on the available information, it is reasonable to conclude that the rate of adverse events is higher in bony compared to soft tissue procedures (164). This is because bony procedures attempt correction of complex decompensated joint pathology, which involves more complicated and lengthier procedures (53). Additional postoperative risks specifically associated with bony surgeries are pseudoarthrosis, malunions, delayed unions, nonunions, loss of fixation, avascular necrosis, osteomyelitis, and fractures. These adverse events are uncommon, and the literature suggests that there has been a decrease in the rates of such complications in recent decades, particularly with more frequently performed procedures for correction of hip subluxation and spinal deformity. This trend has been attributed to various refinements in surgical techniques as well as hardware improvements. For example, in spastic hip deformity, loss of fixation occurs rarely with the use of rigid internal fixation devices compared to the use of pins and cast immobilization (112, 169). In spinal fusion, lower rates of pseudoarthrosis (0–10%) are associated with the replacement of distraction instrumentation by segmental instrumentation along with use of generous bone grafting (110).

Outcomes

The literature contains many retrospective reviews documenting outcomes of different orthopedic techniques for specific deformities. Some studies attempt to compare results using nonconcurrent or historical controls (185, 192–197). Most outcomes reported are assessments of the extent of deformity correction. However, assessment of changes in other ICF dimensions is receiving more attention in recent studies (153, 190, 198, 199). Overall, outcomes of "salvage" versus reconstructive bony procedures are less successful (53, 110, 126). Yet, there has never been a randomized trial in which 2 or more orthopedic operative techniques to manage CP have been compared, nor has there been a randomized trial comparing surgery with observation.

Based on experience, Bleck (112) expects good results after orthopedic surgery in children with CP to be greater than 80% to 90% of cases, provided there is careful preoperative evaluation, correct selection of procedure, proper technique and postoperative care, and clearly defined goals. However, as is true for many of the interventions to treat spasticity in patients with CP, the literature does not contain a high level of evidence to support the use of orthopedic surgery (53, 183, 200). The use of biomechanical and physiologic measures and concurrently gathered multidimensional functional outcomes is advocated to improve the ability to objectively evaluate treatment outcomes (53, 54, 145, 201).

*R*eferences

1. Katz RT, Rymer WZ. Spastic hypertonia mechanisms and measurement. *Arch Phys Med Rehabil.* 1989;70(2):145–55.
2. Young RR. Spasticity: a review. *Neurology.* 1994;44(11 Suppl 9):S12–20.
3. Oppenheim WL. Selective posterior rhizotomy for spastic cerebral palsy. A review. *Clin Orthop Relat Res.* 1990;253: 20–29.
4. Foerster O. On the indications and results of the excision posterior spinal nerve roots in man. *Surg Gynecol Obstet.* 1913; 16: 463–474.
5. Gros C, Ooaknine G, Vlahhovitch B, et al. La radicotomie selective poeteriordans le traitment neurochirurgical de l'hypertonic pyramidale. *Neurochirurgir.* 1967;13:505–518
6. Fasano VA, Barolat-Romana G, Zeme S, et al. Electrophysiological assessment of spinal circuits in spasticity by direct dorsal root stimulation. *Neurosurgery.* 1979;4(2): 146–51.
7. Peacock WJ, Arens LJ. Selective posterior rhizotomy for the relief of spasticity in cerebral palsy. *S Afr Med J.* 1982;62: 119–124.
8. Peacock WJ, Arens LJ, Berman B. Cerebral palsy spasticity. Selective posterior rhizotomy in children with cerebral palsy. *Pediatr Neurosci.* 1987;13:61–66.
9. Staudt LA, Nuwer MR, Peacock WJ. Intraoperative monitoring during selective posterior rhizotomy: technique and patient outcome. *Electroencephalogr Clin Neurophysiol.* 1995;97: 296–309.

10. Fasano VA, Broggi G., Barolat-Romana G, et al. Surgical treatment of spasticity in cerebral palsy. *Childs Brain.* 1978;4(5): 289–305.

11. Fasano VA, Broggi G, Zeme S, et al. Long-term results of posterior functional rhizotomy. *Acta Neurochir.* 1980;30:435–439.

12. Kim HS, Steinbok P, Wickenheiser D. Predictors of poor outcome after selective dorsal rhizotomy in treatment of spastic cerebral palsy. *Childs Nerv Syst.* 2006;22(1):60–6.

13. Arens LJ, Peacock WJ, Peter J. Selective posterior rhizotomy a long-term follow up study. *Childs Nerv Syst.* 1989;5(3): 148–52.

14. O'Brien DF, Park TS, Puglisis JA, et al. Effect of selective dorsal rhizotomy on need for orthopaedic surgery for spastic quadriplegic cerebral palsy; long term outcome analysis. *J Neurosurg.* 2004;101(1):59–63.

15. Russell, D.J., Rosenbaum, P.L. Cadman DT. The gross motor function measure: a means to evaluate the effects of physical therapy. *Dev Med Child Neurol:* 1989;31:341–352.

16. Steinbok P, Reiner A, Beauchamp RD, et al. Selective functional posterior rhizotomy for treatment of spastic cerebral palsy in children review of 50 consecutive cases. *Pediatr Neurosurg.* 1992;18(1):34–42.

17. McLaughlin JF, Bjornson KF, Astley SJ, et al. The role of selective dorsal rhizotomy in cerebral palsy: a critical evaluation of a prospective clinical series. *Dev Med Child Neurol.* 1994; 36(9):755–69.

18. Mittal S, Farmer JP, Al-Attasst B, et al. Long-term functional outcome after selective posterior rhizotomy. *J Neurosurg.* 2002;97:315–325.

19. Nishida T, Thatcher SW, Marty GR. Selective posterior rhizotomy for children with cerebral palsy: a 7-year experience. *Childs Nerv Syst.* 1995;11(7):374–380.

20. Chiccoine MR, Part TS, Vogler GP, Kaufman BA. Predictors of ability to walk after selective dorsal rhizotomy in children with cerebral palsy. *Neurosurgery.* 1996;38(4):711–714.

21. Park TS, Owen JH. Surgical management of spastic diplegia in cerebral palsy. *N Engl J Med.* 1992;326:745–749.

22. Engsberg JR, Ross SA, Collins DR, et al. Predicting functional change from preintervention measures in selective dorsal rhizotomy. *J Neurosurg.* 2007;106(4 Suppl):282–7.

23. Trost J, Schwartz MH, Krach LE, et al. Comprehensive short-term outcome assessment of selective dorsal rhizotomy. *Dev Med Child Neurol.* 2008;50:765–771.

24. Nordmark E, Lundkvist JA, Lagergren, et al. J. Long-term outcomes five years after selective dorsal rhizotomy. *BMC Pediatr.* 2008;8(1):54.

25. Peacock WJ, Staudt LA. Functional outcomes following selective dorsal rhizotomy in children with cerebral palsy. *J Neurosurg.* 1991;74:380–385.

26. Schwartz MH, Viehweger E, Stout J, et al. Comprehensive treatment of ambulatory children with cerebral palsy: an outcome assessment. *J Pediatr Orthop.* 2004;24(1):45–53.

27. Steinbok P. Selective dorsal rhizotomy for spastic cerebral palsy; a review. *Childs Nerv Syst.* 2007;23:981–90.

28. Parks TS, Johnston JM. Surgical techniques of selective dorsal rhizotomy for spastic cerebral palsy. *Neurosurg Focus.* 2006; 21(2):1–6.

29. Von Koch CS, Park TS, Steinbok P, et al. Selective posterior rhizotomy and intrathecal baclofen for the treatment of spasticity. *Pediatr Neurosurg.* 2001;35(2):56–64.

30. Farmer JP, Sabbagh AJ. Selective dorsal rhizotomies in the treatment of spasticity related to cerebral palsy. *Childs Nerv Syst.* 2007;23:991–1002.

31. Kan P, Gooch J, Amini A, et al. Surgical treatment of spasticity in children: comparison of selective dorsal rhizotomy and intrathecal baclofen pump implantation. *Childs Nerv Sys.* 2008; 24:239–243.

32. Nelson KR, Phillip LH. Neurophysiologic monitoring during surgery of peripheral and cranial nerves, and in selective dorsal rhizotomy. *Semin Neurol.* 1990;10(2):141–9.

33. Newberg NL, Gooch JL. Walker ML. Intraoperative monitoring in selective dorsal rhizotomy. *Pediatr Neurosurg.* 1991–1992; 17(3):124–7.

34. Fasano VA, Barolat-Romana G, Zeme S, et al. Electrophysiological assessment of spinal circuits in spasticity by direct dorsal root stimulation. *Neurosurgery.* 1979;4(2):146–51.

35. Cohen AR, Webster HC. How selective is selective posterior rhizotomy. *Surg Neurol.* 1991;35(4):267–72.

36. Steinbok P, Langill L, Cochrane DD, et al. Observations on electrical stimulation of lumbosacral nerve roots in children with and without lower limb spasticity. *Childs Nerv Syst.* 1992;8(7) 376–82.

37. Hays RM, McLaughlin JF, Bjornson KF, et al. Electrophysiological monitoring during selective dorsal rhizotomy and spasticity and GMFM performance. *Dev Med Child Neurol.* 1998;40(4):233–8.

38. Steinbok P, Kestle JR. Variation between centers in electrophysiologic techniques used in lumbosacral selective dorsal rhizotomy for spastic cerebral palsy. *Pediatr Neurosurg.* 1996; 25(5):233–9.

39. Weiss IP, Schiff SJ. Reflex variability in selective dorsal rhizotomy. *J Neurosurg.* 1993;79(3):346–53.

40. Lazareff JA, Mata-Acosta AM, Garcia-Mendez MA, Limited selective posterior rhizotomy for the treatment of spasticity secondary to infantile cerebral: a preliminary report. *Neurosurgery.* 1990;27(4):535–538.

41. Lang FF, Deletis V, Cohen HW, et al. Inclusion of the S2 dorsal rootlets in functional posterior rhizotomy for spasticity in children with cerebral palsy. *Neurosurgery.* 1994;34(5):847–853.

42. Abbott R. Complications with selective posterior rhizotomy. *Pediatr Neurosurg.* 1992;18(1):43–47.

43. Steinbok P, Tidemann A, Miller S, et al. Electrophysiologically guided vs non electrophysiologically guided selective dorsal rhizotomy for spastic cerebral palsy—a comparison of outcomes. *37th Annual Meeting of the AANS/CNS Section on Pediatric Neurological Surgery.* Spokane, Washington, Dec. 2–5, 2008.

44. McLaughlin JF, Bjornson KF, Astley SJ, et al. Selective dorsal rhizotomy efficacy and safety in an investigator-masked randomized clinical trial. *Dev Med Child Neurol.* 1998;40(4): 220–32.

45. Van de Wiele BM, Staudt LA, Rubinstien EH, et al. Perioperative complications in children undergoing selective posterior rhizotomy: a review of 105 cases. *Paediatr Anaesth.* 1996; 6(6):479–86.

46. Abbott R, Johann-Murphy M, Shiminski-Maher T, et al. Selective dorsal rhizotomy: outcome and complications in treating spastic cerebral palsy. *Neurosurgery.* 1993;933(5):851–857.

47. Steinbok P, Schrang C., Complications after selective posterior rhizotomy for spasticity in children with cerebral palsy. *Pediatr Neurosurg.* 1998;28:300–13.

48. Deletis V, Vodusek DB, Abbott R, et al. Intraoperative monitoring of the dorsal sacral roots: minimizing the risk of iatrogenic micturition disorders. *Neurosurgery.* 1992;30(1): 72–75.

49. Mooney JF III, Koman LA. Acquired vertical talus after selective dorsal rhizotomy. *American Academy for Cerebral Palsy and Developmental Medicine,* 1994.

50. Heim RC, Park TS, Vogler GP, et al. Changes in hip migration after selective dorsal rhizotomy for spastic quadriplegia in cerebral palsy. *J Neurosurg.* 1995;82(4):567–71.

51. Park TS, Vogler GP, Phillips LH2nd, et al. Effects of selective dorsal rhizotomy for spastic diplegia on hip migration in cerebral palsy. *Pediatr Neurosurg.* 1994;20(1):43–9.

52. Hicdonmcz T, Steinbok P, Beauchamp R, et al. Hip joint sub luxation after selective dorsal rhizotomy. *J Neurosurg.* 2005; 103(Suppl 1):10–6.

53. Graham HK, Selber P. Musculoskeletal aspects of cerebral palsy. *J Bone Joint Surg.* 2003;85:157–166.

54. Novacheck TF, Gage JR. Orthopedic management of spasticity in cerebral palsy. *Childs Nerv Syst.* 2007;23:1015–1031.

55. Fraser RD, Paterson DC, Simpson DA. Orthopaedic aspects of spinal tumors in children. *J Bone Joint Surg Br.* 1977;59(2): 143–51.

56. Madigan RR, Wallace SL. Scoliosis in the institutionalized cerebral population. *Spine.* 1981;6(6):583–90.

57. Saito N, Ebara S, Ohotsuka K, et al. Natural history of scoliosis in spastic cerebral palsy, *Lancet.* 1998;351:1687–1692.

58. Johnson MB, Goldstein L, Thomas SS, et al. Spinal deformity after selective dorsal rhizotomy in ambulatory patients with cerebral palsy. *J Pediatr Orthop.* 2004;24:529–536.

59. Peter JC, Hoffman EB, Arens LJ, et al. Incidence of spinal deformity in children after multiple level laminectomy for selective posterior rhizotomy. *Childs Nerv Syst.* 1990;6(1): 30–2.

60. Peter JC, Arens LJ. Selective posterior lumbosacral rhizotomy for the management of cerebral palsy spasticity. A ten year experience. *S Afr Med J.* 1993;83(10):745–7.

61. Spiegal DA, Loder RT, Alley KA, et al. Spinal deformity following selective dorsal rhizotomy, *J Pediatr Orthop.* 2004; 24(1):30–6.

62. Steinbok P, Hicdonmez T, Sawatzky B, et al. Spinal deformities after selective dorsal rhizotomy. *J Neurosurg.* 2005;102 (Suppl 4):363–373.

63. Turi M, Kalen V. The risk of spinal deformity after selective dorsal rhizotomy. *J Pediatr Orthop.* 2000;20(1):104–7.

64. Li Z, Zhu J, Liu X. Deformity of lumbar spine after selective dorsal rhizotomy for spastic cerebral palsy. *Microsurgery.* 2008;28:10–12.

65. Golan JD, Hall JA, O'Gorman G, et al. Spinal deformities following selective dorsal rhizotomy. *J Neurosurg.* 2007; 106(Suppl 6):441–9.

66. Steinbok P. Outcomes after selective dorsal rhizotomy for spastic cerebral palsy. *Childs Nerv Syst.* 2001;17(1-2):1–18.

67. Seinko-Thomas SS, Buckon CE, Piatt JH, et al. A 2-year follow-up of outcomes following orthopedic surgery or selective dorsal rhizotomy in children with spastic diplegia. *J Pediatr Orthop.* 2004;13(6):358–66.

68. Marty GR, Dias LS, Gaebler-Spira D. Selective posterior rhizotomy and soft-tissue procedures for the treatment of cerebral diplegia. *J Bone Joint Surg.* 1995;77-A(5):713–718.

69. O'Brien DF, Park TS. A review of orthopaedic surgeries after selective dorsal rhizotomy. *Neurosurg Focus.* 2006;21(2):e2.

70. Steinbok P, Reiner AM, Beauchamp R, et al. A randomized clinical trial to compare selective posterior rhizotomy plus physiotherapy with physiotherapy alone in children with spastic diplegic cerebral palsy. *Dev Med Child Neurol.* 1997; 39(3):178–84.

71. Wright FV, Sheil EM, Drake JM, et al. Evaluation of selective dorsal rhizotomy for the reduction of spasticity in cerebral palsy: a randomized controlled trial. *Dev Med Child Neurol.* 1998;40(4):239–47.

72. McLaughlin J, Bjornson K, Temkin N, et al. Selective dorsal rhizotomy: meta-analysis of three randomized controlled trials. *Dev Med Child Neurol.* 2002;44(1):17–25.

73. Nordmark E, Lundkvist JA, Lagergren, et al. J. Long-term outcomes five years after selective dorsal rhizotomy. *BMC Pediatr.* 2008;8(1):54.

74. Parolin M, Saluja R, Gibis J, et al. Long term functional outcome after selective rhizotomy. *37th Annual Meeting of the AANS/CNS Section on Pediatric Neurological Surgery,* Spokane, Washington, Dec. 2–5, 2008(A).

75. Parolin M, Saluja R, Montpetit MS, et al. Functional performance following selective posterior rhizotomy: long-term results determined using a validated evaluative measure. *37th Annual Meeting of the AANS/CNS Section on Pediatric Neurological Surgery,* Spokane, Washington, Dec. 2–5, 2008(B).

76. Langerak NG, Lamberts RP, Fieggen AG, et al. A prospective gait analysis study in patients with diplegic cerebral palsy 20 years after selective dorsal rhizotomy. *J Neurosurg Pediatr.* 2008;1(3):180–186.

77. Albright AL, Selective dorsal rhizotomy and the challenge of monitoring its long-term sequelae. *J Neurosurg Pediatr.* 2008; 1(3):178–179.

78. Kolaski K. Patient selection. In: Koman LA, Smith BP, eds. *Management of spasticity in cerebral palsy: the role of intrathecal baclofen.* Towson, Maryland: Date Trace Publishing Company, 2005.

79. Albright AL, Awaad Y, Muhonen M, et al. Performance and complications associated with the synchromed 10-ml infusion pump for the intrathecal baclofen administration in children. *J Neurosurg.* 2004, 101(1Suppl):64–68.

80. Albright Al, Ferson SS. Intrathecal baclofen therapy in children. *Neurosurg Focus.* 2006; 21(2):e3.

81. Follett KA, Burchiel, K, Deer T, et al. Prevention of intrathecal drug delivery catheter-related complications. *Neuromodulation.* 2003;6(1):32–41.

82. Kopell BH, Sala D, Doyle WK, et al. Subfascial implantation of intrathecal baclofen pumps in children: technical note. *Neurosurgery.* 2001;49(3):753–756.

83. Vendor JR, Hester S, Waller Jl., et al. Identification and management of intrathecal baclofen pump complications: a comparison of pediatric and adult patients. *J Neurosurg.* 2006; 104(1):9–15.

84. Motta F, Buonaguro V, Stignani C. The use of intrathecal baclofen pump implants in children and adolescents: safety and complications in 200 consecutive cases. *J Neurosurg.* 2007(Suppl 1):32–5.

85. Kolaski K, Logan LR, A reviews of the complications of intrathecal baclofen in patients with cerebral palsy. *NeuroRehabilitation.* 2007;22(5):383–395.

86. Kolaski K. Complications of ITB: overdosage and withdrawal. In: Koman LA, Smith BP, editors. *Management of spasticity in cerebral palsy: the role of intrathecal baclofen.* Towson, Maryland: Date Trace Publishing Company, 2005.

87. Coffey RJ, Edgar TS, Francisoc GE, et al. Abrupt withdrawal from intrathecal baclofen: recognition and management of a potentially life threatening syndrome. *Arch Phys Med Rehabil.* 2002;83(6):735–741.

88. Buonaguro V, Scelsa B, Curci D. et al. Epilepsy and intrathecal baclofen therapy in children with cerebral palsy. *Pediatr Neurol.* 2005;33(2):110–113.

89. Senaran H, Shah SA, Presedo A, et al. The risk of progression of scoliosis in cerebral palsy patients after intrathecal baclofen therapy. *Spine.* 2007;32(21):2348–2354.

90. Shilt JS, Lai LP, Frino J, et al. The impact of intrathecal baclofen on the natural history of scoliosis in cerebral palsy. *J Pediatr Orthop.* 2008;28(6):684–7.

91. Borowski A, Shah S, Littleton AG, et al. Baclofen pump implantation and spinal fusion in children. *Spine.*2008;33(18):1995–2000.

92. Caird MS, Palanca AA, Garton H, et al. Outcomes of posterior spinal fusion and instrumentation in patients with continuous intrathecal baclofen infusion pumps. *Spine.* 2008;15(33):E94–9.

93. Albright AL, Gilmartin R, Swift D, et al. Long term intrathecal baclofen therapy for severe spasticity of cerebral origin. *J Neurosurg.* 2003;98(2):291–295.

94. Ridley B, Rawlins PK. Intrathecal baclofen therapy: ten steps toward best practice. *J Neurosci Nurs.* 2006;38(2):72–82.

95. Brennan PM, Whittle IR. Intrathecal baclofen therapy for neurological disorders: a sound knowledge base but many challenges remain. *Br J Neurosurg.* 2008;22(4):508–19.

96. Butler C, Campbell S. Evidence of the effects of intrathecal baclofen for spastic and dystonic cerebral palsy. AACPDM treatment outcomes committee review panel. *Dev Med Child Neurol.* 2000;42(9):634–645.

97. Kolaski K, Logan L. Intrathecal baclofen in cerebral palsy. A decade of treatment outcomes. *J Pediatr Rehabil Med.* 2007; 1(3):3–32.

98. Sackett DL. Rules of evidence and clinical recommendations for the management of patient. *Can J Cardiol.* 1993, 9(6):487–489.

99. World Health Organization. *International classification of functioning, disability and health,* 2001. Geneca: World Health Organization

100. Albright AL, Cervi A, Singletary J. Intrathecal baclofen for spasticity in cerebral palsy. *JAMA.* 1991;265(11):1418–1422.

101. Gilmartin R, Bruce D, Storrs BB, et al. Intrathecal baclofen for management of spastic cerebral palsy: multicenter trial. *J Child Neurol.* 2000;15(2):71–7.

102. Hoving MA, van Kranen-Mastenbroek VH, van Raak EP, et al. Placebo controlled utility and feasibility study of the H-reflex and flexor reflex in spastic children treated with intrathecal baclofen. *Clin Neurophysiol.* 2006;117(7):1508–1517.

103. Murphy NA, Hoff C, Jorgensen T, et al. A national perspective of surgery in children with cerebral palsy. *Pediatr Rehabil.* 2006;9(3):293–300.

104. Gage JR, DeLuca PA, Renshaw TS, Gait analysis principle and applications with emphasis on its use in cerebral palsy. *Instr Course Lect.* 1996;45:491–507.

105. Ziv I, Rang M, et al. Muscle growth in normal and spastic mice. *Dev Med Child.* 1984;26:94–95.

106. Rang M. Cerebral palsy. In: Morrissy RT, ed. *Pediatric orthopedics.* Philadelphia: JB Lippincott, 1990:465–506.

107. Reimers J. The stability of the hip in children. A radiological study of the results of muscle surgery in cerebral palsy. *Acta Orthop Scand Suppl.* 1980;184:1–100.

108. Brown JK, Minns RA. Mechanisms of deformity in children with cerebral palsy. *Seminars in Orthopedics.* 1989;14(40):236–55.

109. Moseley CF. Physiologic effects of soft-tissue surgery. In: Sussman MD, ed. *The diplegic child: evaluation and management.* 1992;259–269.

110. Miller F et al. Complications in cerebral palsy. 1995. In: Epps CH and Bowen JR, editors. *Complications in pediatric surgery.* Philadelphia: JB Lippincott, pages 477–544.

111. Koman LA, Li Z, Smith BP. Orthopaedic intervention in the upper extremity in the child with cerebral palsy: musculoskeletal surgery. In: Eliasson A, Burtner PA eds, *Improving hand function in children with cerebral palsy: theory, evidence and intervention,* Clinics in Developmental Medicine No. 178, London:Mac Keith Press 2008: 198–212.

112. Bleck EE. *Orthopaedic management in cerebral palsy.* Philadelphia: MacKeith Press, 1987:65–105.

113. Sussman M, Cusick B. Early mobilization of patients with cerebral palsy following muscle release surgery. *Orthopaedic Transactions.* 1992;5:193.

114. DeLuca PA, The musculoskeletal management of children with cerebral palsy. *Pediatr Clin North Am.* 1996;43(5):1135–50.

115. Miller F, Bagg MR. Age and migration percentage as risk factors for progression in spastic hip disease. *Dev Med Child Neurol.* 1995;37(5):449–455.

116. Cobb JR. Outline for the study of scoliosis. *Am Acad Orthop Surg Inst Course Lect.* 1948;5:261–75.

117. Abel MF, Wenger DR, Mubarak SJ, et al. Quantitative analysis of hip dysplasia in cerebral palsy: a study of radiographs and 3-D reformatted images. *J Pediatr Orthop.* 1994;14(3):283–9.

118. Koman LA, Mooney JR 3rd, Smith B, et al. Management of cerebral palsy with botulinum-a toxin preliminary investigation. *J Pediatr Orthop.* 1993;13:489–95.

119. DeLuca PA, Davis RB 3rd, Ounpuu S, et al. Alterations in surgical decision making in patients with cerebral palsy based on three-dimensional gait analysis. *J Pediatr Orthop.* 1997; 17(5):608–614.

120. Winters TF, Gage JR, Hick R. Gait patterns in spastic hemiplegia in children and young adults. *J Bone Joint Surg Am.* 1987; 69(3):437–41.

121. Roddy J, Graham HK. Classification of gait patterns in spastic hemiplegia and spastic diplegia: a basis for a management algorithm. *Eur J Neurol.* 2001;8(Suppl. 5):98–108.

122. Hagglund G, Andersson S, Duppe H, et al. Prevention of severe contractures might replace multilevel surgery in cerebral palsy: results of a population based health care programme and new techniques to reduce spasticity. *J Pediatr Orthop B.* 2005;14(4):269–73.

123. Ruiz FJ, Guest JF, Lehmann A, et al. Cost and consequences of botulinum toxin type a use. Management of children with cerebral palsy in Germany. *Eur J Health Econ.* 2004;5(3):227–235.

124. Molenaers G, Desloovere K, Fabry G, et al. The effects of quantitative gait assessment and botulinum toxin a on musculoskeletal surgery in children with cerebral palsy. *J Bone Joint Surg Am.* 2006;88(1):161–70.

125. Hod-Feins R, Anekstein Y, Mirovsky Y, et al. Pediatric scoliosis surgery the association between preoperative risk factors and postoperative complications with emphasis on cerebral palsy children. *Neuropediatrics.* 2007;38(5):239–43.

126. Graham HK. The orthopaedic management of cerebral palsy. A textbook of pediatric orthopedics. 1997;101–14.

127. Dabney KW, Lipton GE, Miller F. Cerebral palsy. *Curr Opin Pediatr.* 1997;9(1):81–8.

128. Sharan D. Recent advances in management of cerebral palsy. *Indian J Pediatr.* 2005;72(11):969–73.

129. Lee CL, Bleck EE. Surgical correction of equinus deformity in cerebral palsy. *Dev Med Child Neurol.* 1980;22(3): 287–92.

130. Norlin R, Tkaczuk H. One session surgery for correction of lower extremity deformities in children with cerebral palsy. *J Pediatr Orthop.* 1985;5(2):208–11.

131. Dhawlikar SH, Root L, Mann RL. Distal lengthening of the hamstrings in patients who have cerebral palsy. Long term retrospective analysis. *J Bone Joint Surg Am.* 1992;74(9).1385–91.

132. Rattey TE, Leahey L, Hyndman J, et al. Recurrence after Achilles tendon lengthening in cerebral palsy. *J Pediatr Orthop.* 1993;13(2):184–7.

133. Samilson RL, Hoffer MM. Problems and complications in orthopaedic management of cerebral palsy. In: Samilson, RL ed. *Orthopaedic aspects of cerebral palsy. clinics in development medicine,* Nos. 52/53. 1975. London: S.I.M.P. with Heinemann Medical; Philadelphia, PA: JB Lippincott, 258–274.

134. Sutherland DH, Olshen R, Cooper L, et al. The development of mature gait. *J Bone Joint Surg Am.* 1980;62(2):336–53.

135. Renshaw TS, Green NE, Griffin PP, et al. Cerebral palsy: orthopaedic management. *Instr Course Lect.* 1996;45:475–490.

136. Smith JT, Stevens PM. Combined adductor transfer iliopsoas release and proximal hamstring release in cerebral palsy. *J Pediatr Orthop.* 1989;9(1):1–5.

137. Browne AO, McManus F. One-session surgery for bilateral correction of lower limb deformities in spastic diplegia. *J Pediatr Orthop.* 1987;7(3):259–261.

138. Gage JR. Surgical treatment of knee dysfunction in cerebral palsy. *Clin Orthop Relat Res.* 1990;253:45–54.

139. Karol LA. Surgical management of lower extremity in ambulatory children with cerebral palsy. *J Am Acad Orthop Surg.* 2004;12(3):196–203.

140. Norlin, R, Tkaczuk H. One session surgery on the lower limb in children with cerebral palsy. A five-year follow up. *Int Orthop.* 1992;16(3):291–3.

141. Nene AV, Evans GA, Patrick JH. Simultaneous multiple operations for spastic diplegia. *J Bone Joint Surg.* 1993;75-B: 488–494.

142. Saraph V, Zwick E, Zwick GP, et al. Multilevel surgery in spastic diplegia: evaluation by physical examination and gait analysis in 25 children. *J Pediatr Orthop.* 2002;22(2):150–157.

143. Kokavec M. Long term results of surgical treatment of patients suffering from cerebral palsy. *Bratisl Lek Listy.* 2006;107(11-12):430–4.

144. Khan MA, Outcome of single-event multilevel surgery in untreated cerebral palsy in a developing country. *J Bone Joint Surg.* 2007;89:1088–91.

145. Gough M, Eve LC, Robinson RO, et al. Short-term outcome of multilevel surgical intervention in spastic diplegic cerebral palsy compared with the natural history. *Dev Med Child Neurol.* 2004;46:91–97.

146. Nolan J, Chalkiadis GA, Low J, et al. Anaesthesia and pain management in cerebral palsy. *Anaesthesia.* 2000;55: 32–41.

147. Barwood S, Baillieu C, Boyd R, et al. Analgesic effects of botulinum toxin a: a randomized, placebo-controlled clinical trial. *Dev Med Child Neurol.* 2000;42:116–121.

148. Sussman M, Cusick B. Early mobilization of patients with cerebral palsy following muscle release surgery. *Orthopaedic Transactions.* 1981;5:193.

149. Ko CH, Tse PW, Chan AK. Risk factors of long bone fracture in non ambulatory cerebral palsy children. *Hong Kong Med J.* 2006;12(6):426–31.

150. Samilson RL, Carson JJ, James P, et al. Results and complications of adductor tenotomy and obturator neurectomy in cerebral palsy. *Clin Orthop Relat Res.* 1967;53:61–73.

151. Tardieu G, Tardieu C. Cerebral palsy. Mechanical evaluation and conservative correction of limb joint contractures. *Clin Orthop Relat Res.* 1987;219:63–69.

152. Delp SL, Zajac FE. Force and moment generating capacity of lower extremity muscle before and after tendon lengthening, *Clin Orthop Relat Res.* 1992;11(284):247–59.

153. Abel MF, Damiano DL, Pannunzio M, et al. Muscle-tendon surgery in diplegic cerebral palsy: functional and mechanical changes. *J Pediatr Orthop.* 1999;19(3):366–75.

154. Chambers HG. The surgical treatment of spasticity. *Muscle Nerve.* 1997;209 (Supp 6):128–135.

155. Arnold AS, Liu MQ, Schwartz MH. Do the hamstrings operate at increased muscle-tendon lengths and velocities after surgical lengthening? *J Biomech.* 2006;39(8):1498–1506.

156. Perry J, Hoffer MM. Preoperative and postoperative dynamic electromyography as an aid in planning tendon transfers in children with cerebral palsy. *J Bone Joint Surg.* 1977;59-A(4):531–537.

157. Hoffer MM, Perry J, Melkonian G. Postoperative electromyographic function of tendon transfers in patients with cerebral palsy. *Dev Med Child Neurol.* 1990;32(9): 789–91.

158. Hoffer MM, Barakat G, Koffman M. A 10-year follow-up of split anterior tibial tendon transfer in cerebral palsy patients with spastic equinovarus deformity. *J Pediatr Orthop.* 1985; 5(4):432–434.

159. Green NE, Griffin PP, Shiavi R. Split posterior tibial-tendon transfer in spastic cerebral palsy. *J Bone Joint Surg.* 1983;65-A (6):748–754.

160. Manske PR. Cerebral palsy of the upper extremity. *Hand Clin.* 1990; 6(4):697–709.

161. Koman LA, Gelberman RH, Toby EB, et al. Cerebral palsy management of the upper extremity. *Clin Orthop Relat Res.* 1990;253, 62–74.

162. Phelps WM. Complications of orthopaedic surgery in the treatment of cerebral palsy. *Clin Orthop Relat Res.* 1967;53: 39–46.

163. Kalen V, Conklin MM, Sherman FC. Untreated scoliosis in severe cerebral palsy, *J Pediatr Orthop.* 1992;12(3):337–40.

164. Tis JE, Sharif S, Shannon B, et al. Complications associated with multiple sequential osteotomies for children with cerebral palsy. *J Pediatr Orthop B.* 2006;15(6):408–13.

165. McCarthy RE. Management of neuromuscular scoliosis. *Orthop Clin North Am.* 1999;30(3):435–449, viii. Review.

166. Sponseller RD, LaPorte DM, Hungerford MW, et al. Deep wound infections after neuromuscular surgery: a multicenter study of risk factors and treatment outcomes. *Spine.* 2000; 25(19):2461–6.

167. Comstock CP, Leach J, Wenger DR. Scoliosis in total-body-involvement cerebral palsy: analysis of surgical treatment and patient and caregiver satisfaction. *Spine.* 1998;23(12):1412–1424.

168. Tsirikos A, Lipton G, Chang WN, et al. Surgical correction of scoliosis in pediatric patients with cerebral palsy using the rod instrumentation. *Spine.* 2008;33(10):1133–1140.

169. Beauchesne R, Miller F, Moseley C. Proximal femoral osteotomy using the fixed angle blade plate. *J Pediatr Orthop.* 1992, 12(6):735–40.

170. Transfeldt EE, et al. Wound infections in reconstructive spinal surgery. *Orthop Transactions.* 1985;9:128–9.

171. Murphy NA, Firth S, Jorgensen T, et al. Spinal surgery in children with idiopathic and neuromuscular scoliosis, what's the difference?. *J Pediatr Orthop.* 2006;26(2):216–20.

172. Rinsky LA. Surgery of spinal deformity in cerebral palsy. Twelve years in the evolution of scoliosis management. *Clin Orthop Relat Res.* 1990;4(253):100–9.

173. Lipton GE, Miller F, Dabney KW, et al. Factor predicting postoperative complications following spinal fusions in children with cerebral palsy. *J Spinal Disord.* 1999;12(3):197–205.

174. Slawski DP, Schoenecker PL, Rich MM. Peroneal nerve injury as a complication of pediatric osteotomies; a review of 255 osteotomies. *J Pediatr Orthop.* 1994;14(2): 166–72.

175. Stout JL, Gage JR, Schwartz MH, et al. Distal femoral extension osteotomy and patellar tendon advancement to treat persistent crouch gait in cerebral palsy. *J Bone Joint Surg.* 2008; 90:2470–2484.

176. Karol LA, Chambers C, Popejoy D, et al. Nerve palsy after hamstring lengthening in patients with cerebral palsy. *J Pediatr Orthop.* 2008;28(7):773–776.

177. Ounpuu S, DeLuca P, Davis R, et al. Long term effects of femoral derotation osteotomies; an evaluation using three dimensional gait analysis. *J Pediatr Orthop.* 2002;22(2): 134–45.

178. Ryan DD, Rethlefsen SA, Skaggs DL et al. Results of tibial rotational osteotomy without concomitant fibular osteotomy in children with cerebral palsy. *J Pediatr Orthop.* 2005; 25(1):84–8.

179. Kim H, Aiona M, Sussman M. Recurrence after femoral derotational osteotomy in cerebral palsy. *J Pediatr Orthop.* 2005; 25(6):739–43.

180. Oh CW, Presedo A, Dabney KW et al. Factors affecting femoral varus osteotomy in cerebral palsy a long term result over 10 years. *J Pediatr Orthop B.* 2007;16(1):23–30.

181. Elmer EB, Wenger DR, Mubarak SJ, et al. Proximal hamstring lengthening in the sitting cerebral palsy patient, *J Pediatr Orthop.* 1992;12(3):329–36.

182. Chang CH, Albarracin JP, Lipton GE, et al. Long-term follow-up of surgery for equinovarus foot deformity in children with cerebral palsy. *J Pediatr Orthop.* 2002;22: 792–799.

183. Goldstein M, Harper DC. Management of cerebral palsy: equinus gait. *Dev Med Child Neurol.* 2001;43:563–569.

184. Damron T, Breed AL, Roecker E. Hamstring tenotomies in cerebral palsy: long term retrospective analysis. *J Pediatr Orthop.* 1991;11(4):514–9.

185. Damron TA, Greenwald TA, Breed AL. Chronologic outcome of surgical tendo-achilles lengthening and natural history of gastroc-soleus contracture in cerebral palsy. a two-part study. *Clin Orthop Relat Res.* 1994;(301):249–255.

186. Snyder M, Kumar SJ, Stecyk MD. Split tibialis posterior tendon transfer and tendo-achilles lengthening for spastic equinovarus feet. *J Pediatr Orthop.* 1993;13(1):20–3.

187. Segal LS, Thomas SF, Mazur JM, et al. Calcaneal gait in spastic diplegia after heel cord lengthening: a study with gait analysis. *J Pediatr Orthop.* 1989;9(6):697–701.

188. Sutherland DH, Cooper L. The pathomechanics of progressive crouch gait in spastic diplegia. *Orthop Clin North Am.* 1978; 9(1):143–54.

189. Rose SA, DeLuca PA, Davis PB 3rd, et al. Kinematic and kinetic evaluation of the ankle after lengthening of the gastrocnemius fascia in children with cerebral palsy. *J Pediatr Orthop.* 1993; 13(6):727–732.

190. Novacheck TF, Trost JP, Schwartz MH. Intramuscular psoas lengthening improves dynamic hip function in children with cerebral palsy. *J Pediatr Orthop.* 2002;22:158–164.

191. Carr C, Gage JR. The fate of the nonoperated hip in cerebral palsy. *J Pediatr Orthop.* 1987;7(3):262–7.

192. Sharrard WJ, Allen JM, Heaney SH. Surgical prophylaxis of subluxation and dislocation of the hip in cerebral palsy. *J Bone Joint Surg Br.* 1975;57(2):160–6.

193. Hoffer MM. Management of the hip in cerebral palsy. *J Bone Joint Surg Am,* 1986;68(4):629–31.

194. Bagg MR, Farber J, Miller F. Long-term follow-up of hip subluxation in cerebral palsy patients. *J Pediatr Orthop.* 1993; 13(1):32–36.

195. Ounpuu S, Muik E, Davis RB 3rd, et al. Rectus femoris surgery in children with cerebral palsy. Part II: a comparison between the effect of transfer and release of the distal rectus femoris on knee motion. *J Pediatr Orthop.* 1993;13(3):331–335.

196. Yngve DA, Chambers C. Vulpius and z-lengthening. *J Pediatr Orthop.* 1996;16(6):759–64.

197. Dobson F, Boyd RN, Parrott J, et al. Hip surveillance in children with cerebral palsy. Impact on the surgical management of spastic hip disease. *J Bone Joint Surg Br.* 2002;84(5):720–6.

198. Buckon CE, Thomas SS, Piatt JH, et al. Selective dorsal rhizotomy versus orthopedic surgery: a multidimensional assessment of outcome efficacy. *Arch Phys Med Rehabil.* 2004;85(3):457–65.

199. Cuomo AV, Gamradt SC, Kim CO, et al. Health-related quality of life outcomes improve after multilevel surgery in ambulatory children with cerebral palsy. *J Pediatr Orthop.* 2007;27(6):653–657.

200. Patrick JH, Roberts AP, Cole GF. Therapeutic choices in the locomotor management of the child with cerebral palsy-more luck than judgment. *Arch Dis Child.* 2001;85(4):275–9. Review.

201. Boyd RN, Gage JR, Hicks R. Management of upper limb dysfunction in children with cerebral palsy: a systematic review. *Eur J Neurol.* 2001;8(Suppl 5):156–66.

V

BASIC SCIENCE OF SPASTICITY

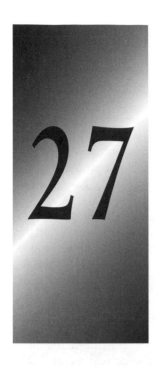

Animal Models of Spasticity

27

Patrick Harvey Kitzman

WHY USE ANIMAL MODELS FOR EXAMINING SPASTICTIY

To evaluate a technique designed to reduce impairment or to facilitate recovery, it is important to appreciate fully the physiological and behavioral impact of the lesion before treatment or repair (1). The ideal model for examination of the impact of injury on the central nervous system (CNS) should be able to correlate physiological and behavioral changes to the size and position of the lesion. The presentation of spasticity differs based on its etiology, and it is widely accepted that the different CNS insults (eg, spinal cord injury [SCI], stroke, cerebral palsy, multiple sclerosis) lead to different presentations and pathophysiological origins. This has necessitated the development and refinement of multiple different animal models that mimic aspects of spasticity as seen in humans to better understand the underlying pathology involved with the development of this impairment.

In contradistinction to the clinical world, the use of animal models allows for the production of reproducible deficits that are appropriate for examining the relationship between structures within the CNS and their function. For example, hemisection of the midthoracic spinal cord in both felines and rodents leads to the destruction of the fiber tracts that provide the descending motor control of spinal reflexes. In these animals, there is an increased magnitude of

lumbar monosynaptic reflexes ipsilateral to the injury compared to the intact side (2–4). This is an example of how animal models can mimic at least one of the features of altered reflex activity that is characteristic of human spasticity. This chapter will review several of the most common animal models that are used to examine spasticity induced by a variety of CNS insults and discuss the potential underlying pathologies that may be responsible of each type of spasticity.

TYPES OF ANIMAL MODELS FOR EXAMINING SPASTICITY

The animal models most commonly used to examine spasticity can be broken down into 4 main categories. Although this is not an exhaustive list of the models being developed, these are the ones that have been studied in the greatest detail. Although there are differences in the underlying pathology of spasticity based on etiology, there are also some similarities that may be applied between them.

Spinal Cord Injury Models of Spasticity

Of the different models that have been developed and refined to examine spasticity with respect to upper motor neuron lesions, the SCI model was examined in the greatest detail. Four main categories of SCI that lead to the onset of spasticity will be described.

Hemisection Model. Hemisection refers to the process of surgically cutting one half or part of one half of the spinal cord. Studies have shown that after hemisection of the lower lumbar spinal cord (L_5), the monosynaptic response to stimulation below the level of the injury is increased between 2 to 5 times on the side ipsilateral to the injury as compared to the contralateral side or to the response seen in control (uninjured) animals (1). However, other physiological components associated with reflex activity, such as rise times and latencies of the responses, do not appear to be affected by hemisection. Rise time refers to the time it takes from the start of the pulse (baseline) to reach the peak amplitude, and latencies refer to the time (milliseconds) required to activate the nerve and initiate an action potential. In addition to changes in monosynaptic responses, hemisection induces a progressive increase in both deep tendon reflexes and cutaneous flexion reflexes. The progressive increase in these reflex responses mimics what is observed clinically in humans after SCI.

It is well documented that each level of the spinal cord contains both subtle and not so subtle differences in circuitry. This is not surprising because each level of the spinal cord subserves different functions. Because of these differences in circuitry, it is important to determine if injury at different spinal levels leads to similar or different alterations in reflex activity. This has been addressed as multiple hemisection studies have been performed in the lower thoracic and upper lumbar spinal regions in felines (2, 5, 6) and have demonstrated similar enhanced monosynaptic and polysynaptic spinal reflexes.

Although lateral hemisection of the spinal cord can produce many symptoms that correlate to spasticity (eg, hypertonia, clasp-knife, exaggerated reflexes), these changes appear to be time depended in that they diminish over time in long-term injured animals, with many animals eventually regaining motor function (1–3). In addition, in many cases, hemisection leads to only mild hyperreflexia, which differs from what is typically seen clinically, where SCI-induced spasticity (SCIID) in humans is a chronic issue, especially in cases of incomplete SCI. There is a body of evidence that suggest that in many cases spinal hemisection may not reliably induce signs of spasticity that mirror the clinical presentation seen in humans (1, 2). For example, animals who undergo a T12 hemisection appear behaviorally normal and only detailed testing reveal differences in reflexes between the hind limbs and the gait abnormalities (2). As a result of these findings, additional models of SCIID that more reliably reproduce the behavioral and electrophysiological signs and symptoms of this impairment have been developed.

Complete Spinal Transection. Studies that use complete spinal transection in animal models appear to consistently duplicate spastic activity that can be observed long term. Transection at the lower lumbar (L_5) spinal level is associated with enlarged monosynaptic excitatory postsynaptic potentials (EPSPs) in extensor motoneurons that can be observed for at least 4 months after injury (7, 8). The enhanced monosynaptic reflexes were also observed in a series of experiments by Hochman and McCrea (9–11) that examined the effects of complete transection at the upper lumbar (L_1–L_2) level in the cat. These studies demonstrated that 6 weeks after spinal cord transection, EPSPs evoked by low-strength nerve stimulation of the Ia primary sensory afferents have increased amplitudes as well as decreased rise times and half-widths. It is of interest that the changes in reflex activity were not consistent among different motoneuron pools involved with the activation of ankle extensors. For example, in chronically injured animal's, stimulation of Ia afferents evoked larger EPSPs in motoneurons innervating the lateral gastrocnemius compared to those in motoneurons that innervate the medial gastrocnemius. The observed disparity among different extensor motoneuron pools with respect to Ia-evoked EPSPs appears to involve differences in motor unit type and motoneuron class. Specifically, the greatest increase in Ia EPSP amplitude and decrease in rise time occur in fast-twitch fatigue-resistant motoneurons associated with the lateral gastrocnemius motoneurons.

With respect to the time course for the onset of enhanced reflex activity postinjury, several studies have demonstrated that spinal transection in both lower thoracic and upper lumbar regions can lead to increase reflex activity within hours or a few days of injury (12, 13). However, several aspects of the increased reflex activity as well as the development of behavioral changes may require longer periods of time (ie, weeks) (8, 12, 13). Although complete spinal transection of the thoracic spinal cord produces many signs normally associated with spasticity (14–16), these animals require twice daily bladder and bowel expression and are at significant risk of developing bladder infections and pressure. Therefore, an animal model that leads to the development of spasticity while preserving bowel and bladder function as well as hind limb function could be advantageous.

Low Sacral Transection Model. The earliest study that described the use of complete transection of the spinal cord that produced signs of spasticity while maintaining bowel and bladder function as well as hind limb function was conducted by Ritz et al. (17) These researchers demonstrated that complete transaction of the sacral (S_2) spinal cord in the cat leads to hypertonia, hyperactive reflexes, and clonus in the tail muscles that can be measured for at least 2 years postinjury. This animal model allows for studies of long-term chronic spasticity. Although the spastic behavior that is seen in tail muscles may not completely mimic the spastic behavior seen in the lower extremities, this model is very appropriate for examining spasticity in the axial postural muscles (which are responsible for the maintenance of posture). The trunk muscles are important for the control, in both animals and humans of the complex instruction between the lower extremities, hips and trunks. Of the postural muscle groups, the trunk musculature is important for providing the proximal stability required for efficient and effective movement of the limbs, head and neck movement, and respiration. Thus, animal models that can examine the potential pathophysiology of spasticity within these muscle groups are clinically relevant. In addition, comparison of the behavioral aspects of spasticity induced by transaction at the L_5 spinal level versus those observed after S_2 spinal transaction suggests that tail spasticity may in fact be comparable to that seen in the hind limbs (1).

Because most SCI studies use the rodent model, Bennett et al. (19) modified Ritz's protocol and demonstrated that similar to the cat model, S_2 transection in the rat reliably produced spasticity in the tail muscles with many of the same characteristics found in the human spastic syndrome, including muscle hypertonus, hyperreflexia both to muscle stretch and cutaneous stimulation, clonus, flexor spasms, paraesthesia, and clasp-knife responses (19–27). Behaviorally, cutaneous stimulation significantly increased muscle activation in both amplitude and duration. Specifically, in animals that have undergone S_2 spinal injury, application of a brief pinch (noxious) stimulus to the tip of the tail induced a burst of electromyographic (EMG) activity in the tail musculature that remains significantly elevated for approximately 6 seconds post-stimulus (27). The same stimulus applied to the tail of control (uninjured) animals produces an increased EMG activity lasting only approximately 1 second. The significantly prolonged duration of EMG activity, as seen in the SCI animals, would be considered a clinically relevant time period that would result in functional restrictions.

Recently, an in vitro version of the S_2 transection model has been developed in which spinal cords are removed from injured animals and maintained in special recording chambers (21, 23, 28). This in vitro preparation has allowed researchers to examine the membrane characteristics of spinal motoneurons, such as persistent inward currents (PICs) and plateau potentials (see below).

Contusion/Compression Model. A limitation of the hemisection and complete transection injury models is that the lesions produced by these approaches are different from those commonly encountered clinically in patients with SCI. Most human SCIs are caused by contusion or compression of the spinal cord produced by acceleration-related fracture/dislocation of the spine. Because of this, multiple groups of researchers have worked at refining experimental approaches that yield reproducible compression/contusion injuries in animals (29–33), which lead to multiple permanent changes in reflex excitability (spasticity) (30, 34–36).

Although newer models of spinal compression/contusion continue to be developed, the most widely used method of inducing a contusion injury to the spinal cord in animals involves variations on the weight drop method described by Wrathall et al. (32) Thompson et al. (34) demonstrated that after midthoracic contusion of the spinal cord, the threshold for reflex initiation fell progressively subsequent to the injury. In addition, the Hoffman reflex (H reflexes; a measure of monosynaptic spinal reflex activity) elicited in spinal cord–injured animals was progressively less sensitive to rate depression after injury. Rate-sensitive depression is a fundamental rate-modulatory process that normally attenuates reflex magnitude during repetitive afferent stimulation. This work suggests that spinal contusion significantly changes spinal reflex excitability. Spasticity was originally defined by Lance (37) as a velocity-dependent increase in tone. Until relatively recently, this characteristic of spasticity has been difficult to measure in animal models of SCI. However, Bose et al. (38) demonstrated that a midthoracic spinal contusion in the rat induces a progressive velocity-dependent increase in ankle torque that is consistent with the expression of spastic hyperreflexia, as seen clinically.

Although the weight-drop method has been the predominate method for reliably inducing compression/contusion injury, a newer model for spinal compression injury has recently been described (30). This model involves implantation of a wax ball at the cervical spinal level to induce compression of the spinal cord. Animals that receive this compression type of injury display spastic behavior within 4 days of implantation, and this spastic behavior lasts for at least 8 weeks postsurgery.

Ischemic SCI Model. Not all spasticity of spinal origin results from traumatic injury to the spinal cord. A sudden loss of blood flow to the spinal cord can lead to an ischemic insult similar to that seen with cerebral vascular accidents. Like cerebral vascular accidents, ischemic events within the spinal cord can lead to damage to the spinal cord and significant changes in spinal circuitry function. Multiple studies have demonstrated induction of spinal ischemia using an intra-aortic balloon catheter, which leads to the development of long-term spasticity in both rats and rabbits (39–45). This occlusion injury model causes permanent hind limb extensor and flexor hypertonus (39) and exaggerated EMG activity after activation of either nociceptive or proprioceptive afferents as well as a velocity-dependent increase in muscle resistance (40). One unique feature of the study by Marsala et al. (40) was that spasticity was measured using a newly developed limb flexion resistance meter that permitted a semi-automated, computer-controlled measurement of peripheral muscle resistance in the lower extremities during forced flexion of the ankle in the awake rat. This type of velocity-dependent measurement of tone is similar to isokinetic measurement techniques (eg, Biodex) that have been used for both research and clinical applications to measure changes in tone in humans. In addition to changes in the velocity-dependent characteristic of the limb muscles, an increase in tonic EMG activity with a variable degree of rigidity can be seen within the first week after ischemic injury (42). Assessment of H reflex activity reveals a significant increase in Hmax/Mmax ratio as well as a significant loss of rate-dependent inhibition. Therefore, the ischemia injury animal model appears to provide a reproducible model to examine multiple aspects of spasticity in a non–trauma-induced SCI system.

Rodent Model of Multiple Sclerosis

Multiple sclerosis is another disease that can cause the upper motoneuron syndrome, and individuals often present clinically with signs and symptoms of spasticity. Recently, an animal model that mimics many of the signs of multiple sclerosis has been developed. Chronic relapsing experimental allergic encephalomyelitis (CREAE) is an autoimmune model in which animals demonstrate repeated neurological insults that are associated with increasing primary demyelination and axonal loss in the CNS (46–49). Approximately 50% to 60% of CREAE animals develop a form of relapsing-remitting multiple sclerosis. Between 60 and 80 days postinduction of the encephalomyelitis, these animals develop clinical signs of upper motor neuron syndrome, which include unilateral or bilateral forelimb and hind limb tremor and hind limb spasticity (46–49). Although the exact cause of spasticity in this model remains to be clarified, it appears that alterations in the balance between excitatory and inhibitory

neural circuits may play a key role in the pathophysiology (49).

Rodent Model of Cerebral Palsy

Cerebral palsy is characterized as a movement and postural disorder caused by premature, nonprogressive damage of the developing brain. Because of the difficulties in inducing controlled perinatal damages to the developing animal, this injury model has only recently been successfully reported in rabbits and rodents (50–54). Prenatal uterine ischemia (21, 22 days gestation) in rabbits produces pups that display significant motor impairments, including increased tone of the limbs at rest (as measured by a version of the Ashworth Scale) and with active flexion and extension (50). This study describes one of the first animal models in which prenatal insult during development of the immature CNS results in hypertonic deficits at term birth that are consistent with those clinically observed in children with cerebral palsy. A major advantage to using rabbits for this model is that motor development and white matter development in the rabbit progress in a manner similar to that seen in humans. Since the publication of this initial study, additional work has also been published that continues to characterize the resultant hypertonia after perinatal ischemic injury (51–53). In addition to the rabbit model of cerebral palsy, a rodent model of perinatal asphyxia has recently been developed in which spasticity can be measured in the hind limbs (54).

The Spastic, Spasmotic, and Oscillator Mutant Mouse Models

Naturally occurring mutations in the glycine receptor have been identified in both humans (55) and mice (56–60). All of these mutations produce a phenotype with an exaggerated startle response to auditory or tactile stimuli. The final animal model of spasticity that will be discussed involves 3 lines of mutant mice (spastic, spasmodic, and oscillator) that have naturally occurring glycine receptor mutations, which manifest as motor deficits and an exaggerated "startle response." (61) The *spastic* mutant mouse is characterized by muscle rigidity and a fine tremor that becomes more prominent when the animals are disturbed or picked up by the tail (62). These homozygous animals appear normal at birth but by 2 weeks postnatal display muscle rigidity, tremors, myoclonic jerks, and a pronounced startle reaction (57, 59, 63–66). The complex motor disorders associated with this mutant mouse model result from a reduction of the adult form of the glycine receptor, leading to a decrease in the inhibitory control of spinal reflex activity.

The second mutant mouse model that demonstrates exaggerated startle reflexes and neonatal hypertonia is the *spasmodic* mutant mouse model of hereditary startle disease (57). Similar to the *spastic* mutant mouse, *spasmotic* mutant mice begin to display motor deficits around 2 weeks postnatal, at which time they demonstrate an exaggerated acoustic startle reflex and develop rigidity with tremor and impaired righting reflexes. The *spasmodic* mouse is a recessive mutation that affects the glycine receptor, which leads to a reduction in sensitivity of the glycine receptors to this inhibitory neurotransmitter. The ultimate result is a decreased ability to control spinal reflex activity.

Finally, the third mutant mouse model that demonstrates several aspects of the spastic syndrome is the lethal *oscillator* mutation. As with the *spastic* and *spasmodic* mutant mouse models, this mutation leads to a heightened startle response, muscle rigidity, and tremor by 2 weeks postnatal (61, 67). In addition, like the *spastic* mutant mouse model, the *oscillator* mouse has a naturally occurring autosomal recessive mutation of the glycine receptor.

PATHOPYSIOLOGY OF SPASTICITY IN ANIMAL MODELS

As discussed previously, spasticity is a complex collection of clinical conditions, and it is widely accepted that though different types of insult to the CNS can lead to the development of spasticity, each form of spasticity has a different underlying cause (pathophysiology). Over the past 2 to 3 decades, the underlying pathophysiology behind the development of spasticity in each of the animal models has been the focus of intense examination. Because the animal models of SCIIS contribute the largest amount of information with respect to the underlying pathology related to the development of spasticity, the majority of the following section will focus on results gained from the examination of animal models of SCI.

Pathophysiology of Spasticity Arising From SCI

Changes in Spinal Motoneuron Morphology. One essential component to understanding the development of SCIIS is determining changes in spinal cord neuronal morphology that occur over a time course that parallels that of the observed behavior. A great deal of evidence exists that demonstrates that particular features of motoneuron morphology significantly influence motoneuron excitability. These include the size of the cell body (soma), dendritic architecture, and dendritic branching. The size of the cell body directly influences the membrane characteristics that determine the threshold at which a neuron can be activated. The neuronal dendrites are that portion of the neuron that receives the enormous amount of synaptic input that arises from spinal, supraspinal, and potentially peripheral nervous system sources. Therefore, dendrites provide the conduit by which information is transmitted to the cell body. Under normal circumstances, soma size has been shown to correlate with the overall size of the dendritic arbor, dendritic length, and amount of branching (68–76). Therefore, as the number or length of dendritic branches changes, so should the size of the soma. It has been demonstrated in multiple regions of the CNS that excitatory synaptic stimulation promotes the elaboration of dendrites and that the loss of synaptic input leads to atrophy (77–82). Consequently, the loss of excitatory drive to motoneurons mediated by descending cortical and brainstem inputs after SCI would be expected to influence motoneuron dendritic structure and subsequently motoneuronal soma size.

The final major morphological component of a neuron is the axon, which is that portion of the neuron that conducts signals away from the cell body, thus allowing the neuron to transmit information to other targets throughout the nervous system. Neuronal morphology has been shown to be intimately involved with neuronal function (68–70). For example, of the 3 types of neurons electrophysiologically examined in the dorsal commissural nucleus of the lumbosacral spinal cord, each type of neuron has a characteristic dendritic morphology and extended its axon collaterals to distinct regions of the sacral spinal segments (68). The distinct anatomy of each of these neurons is consistent with each having discrete functional roles as interneurons participating in segmental, intersegmental, or supraspinal reflexes. Changes in dendritic or axonal morphology would directly affect the neuron's ability to receive and/or transmit information, which would ultimately affect the neuron's overall function. Therefore, changes in neuronal morphology after SCI or disease states could be indicative of the physiological changes involved with the onset of spasticity.

Although alpha motoneurons are only one component of the spinal reflex circuitry, the fact that these are the neurons that ultimately activate skeletal muscles has made them an attractive target for investigation. In addition, due to the relative ease in which the motoneuronal population can be visualized and thus studied, the majority of studies that have examined

SCI-induced changes in neuronal morphology have focused on this neuronal population. Initially, animal studies that examined changes in motoneuronal morphology caudal to the injury site utilized hemisection, partial transection, or reversible cold block injury models (71–73). However, these initial injury models do not consistently induce spastic behavior. More recently, studies have examined changes in the morphology of motoneurons, caudal to the injury, after either complete spinal transection or contusion (24, 74). Both of these models of SCI have been shown to produce more reliable, long-term changes in reflex behavior.

After a complete S_2 spinal transection, sacrocaudal motoneuronal somal size remains unchanged over the first 2 weeks postinjury (24). During this first 2-week period, there is an increase in the length of both primary and secondary dendrites. However, there is an overall decease in the number of dendritic branches. The increase in the primary and secondary

dendritic lengths could be responsible for maintaining the overall size of the dendritic arborization, which in turn maintains the somal size at a preinjury level. In chronically injured animals (4–12 weeks postinjury), a reduction in the length of both primary and secondary dendrites to control levels as well as a significant loss in the number of secondary and tertiary dendrites is observed (Figure 27.1, Table 27.1). As would be predicted, a decrease in somal size is also observed in these chronically injured animals. It is of interest that during the time period in which there is an overall progressive loss of dendritic arborization and corresponding decrease in somal size, there is an increase in spastic behavior in the tail muscles.

Although there appears to be a correlation between changes in sacral motoneuron morphology and the onset of spasticity, differences in neuronal morphological response to injury can be seen depending upon the type of spinal injury and the level of

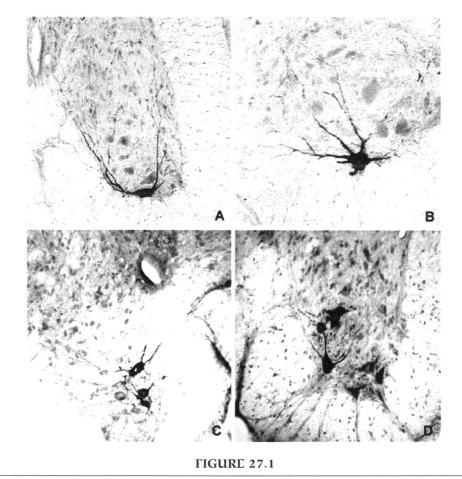

FIGURE 27.1

CTB labeling of sacrocaudal motoneurons in control and transected spinal cords. (A) Cholera toxin-β labeled motoneuron from a control spinal cord. (B)-(D) Labeling of motoneurons from 2-week (A), 4-week (B), and 12-week (C) posttransected spinal cords, respectively. (From: Kitzman P. Alteration in axial motoneuronal morphology in the spinal cord injured spastic rat. *Exp Neurol.* 2005;192:100–108.)

TABLE 27.1

Analysis of Dendritic Arborization in the Sacrocaudal Motoneurons After Spinal Transection

Group	Average No. of Dendrites Per Neuron	Average No. of Primary Dendrites Per Neuron	Average No. of Secondary Dendrites Per Neuron	Average No. of Tertiary Dendrites Per Neuron
Control	10.38/neuron	3.86/neuron	4.9/ neuron	1.58/neuron
1 week postinjury	9.92/neuron (5.5% decrease)	3.5/neuron (9% decrease)	4.86/neuron (2% decrease)	1.56/neuron (no change)
2 weeks postinjury	8.24/neuron (21% decrease)	3.6/neuron (7% decrease)	3.4/neuron (31% decrease)	1.16/neuron (27% decrease)
4 weeks postinjury	7.44/neuron (28% decrease)	3.5/neuron (8% decrease)	3.4/neuron (31% decrease)	0.5/neuron (69% decrease)
12 weeks postinjury	6.86/neuron (34% decrease)	3.4/neuron (12% decrease)	2.96/neuron (40% decrease)	0.5/neuron (69% decrease)

The table depicts the number of primary, secondary, and tertiary dendrites on motoneurons at each experimental time point. In addition, the values in parentheses are the percentage of change in the number of dendrites, at each experimental time point, as compared to controls. (From: Kitzman P. Alteration in axial motoneuronal morphology in the spinal cord injured spastic rat. *Exp Neurol.* 2005;192:100–108.)

the spinal cord examined. For example, it has been demonstrated that midthoracic (T_8) spinal contusion leads to changes in soleus motoneuron morphology (74). Specifically, spinal contusion leads to a decrease in the overall motoneuronal dendritic arborization, including primary, secondary, and tertiary dendrites. These changes in motoneuronal morphology are similar to those seen in sacrocaudal motoneuron after spinal transection. However, the response of sacral motoneurons to spinal transection differs from spinal contusion at the same level. After spinal transection, there is an initial increase in the length of the primary dendrites at 1 and 2 weeks postinjury followed by a return to control levels by 4 weeks postinjury. Spinal contusion, on the other hand, leads to an increase in primary dendrite length in soleus motoneurons that is sustained for at least 4 months postinjury. In addition to differences in the responses of the primary dendrites to different forms of SCI, the neuronal soma also appears to respond differently depending upon the injury type and the spinal level examined. Whereas sacrocaudal motor neurons demonstrate an overall decrease in somal size over time after spinal transection, soleus motoneurons display a different response pattern after spinal contusion. Specifically, after spinal contusion, there is a significant decrease in the number of small- and medium-sized soleus motoneurons but a significant increase in the number of larger neurons in injured animals compared with uninjured animals. Therefore, while the dendritic tree gets smaller, the soleus motoneuron soma appears to actually get bigger.

The differences between how sacral and soleus motoneurons respond to injury may reflect some innate differences in these motoneuron pools because they are located at different levels of the spinal cord. Additionally, the difference in responsiveness to injury by these different subsets of motoneurons may be reflective of the type of injury used (transection versus contusion). Thus, as with all critical examination of research data, it is important to know at what level within the spinal cord each study is evaluating and what type of injury model is being employed when trying to correlate anatomical changes with changes in behavior.

Relationship Between Changes in Motoneuronal Morphology and Physiology. The size of the neuronal soma directly affects the membrane characteristics that determine the threshold at which that cell can be activated. A change in the size of the soma would directly affect its activation threshold and consequently impact its overall function. It has been shown that presynaptic inhibition and recurrent inhibition can decrease with increasing cell size. Therefore, theoretically, an increase in the number of larger motoneurons might result in an overall decrease in presynaptic inhibition, which in turn might produce spastic activity in the muscles innervated by these enlarged motoneurons.

The size and complexity of the dendritic arbor relate directly to the number of synaptic inputs received by the neuron (83, 84) and are intimately connected to neuronal identity and the electrophysiological response properties of neurons (68–70). By correlating morphological features with action potential propagation,

Vetter et al. (70) demonstrated that the number of dendritic branch points is a critical variable for determining propagation efficacy. Dendritic spines are also extremely important in regulating action potential propagation in dendrites (85, 86). Because dendritic spines can contribute more than 50% to the total dendritic membrane area, the relationship between membrane area and propagation efficacy suggests that changes in spine density that occur during development and with synaptic plasticity will also modulate the extent of propagation (87, 88). Dendritic morphological features act in concert with dendritic voltage-gated ion channels to generate a diversity of neuronal activities (69, 70). An increase in dendritic complexity will reduce neuronal activity unless accompanied by a compensatory increase in voltage-gated ion channel densities. Conversely, a progressive decrease in dendritic complexity, as seen after SCI, without a compensatory decrease in voltage-gated channels could lead to an increase in motoneuronal activity, which could theoretically lead to the development of spastic activity.

Anatomical Changes in Excitatory Inputs and Spasticity. Because the function of each neuron is a reflection of the type of information (inputs) it receives (excitatory and inhibitory), changes in the overall numbers of each of these inputs, changes of ratio of excitatory to inhibitory inputs, or changes in the frequency at which each type of input fires will directly influence the activity level of the target neuron and ultimately its output. With respect to spinal motoneurons, the output refers to the direct activation of skeletal muscles. Spinal motoneurons receive excitatory (glutamatergic) input from primary sensory afferents that originate in the periphery and that provide information to the spinal cord with respect to touch, proprioception, mechanoreception, and nociception. In addition to excitatory inputs from peripheral sources, motoneurons receive excitatory inputs from cortical (corticospinal), brain stem (bulbospinal), and spinal interneuron (propriospinal) connections that communicate with and integrate information from one level of the CNS with another. When discussing excitatory inputs within the CNS, especially within the spinal cord, glutamate is the prevalent excitatory neurotransmitter.

The circuitry involved with reflex activity to a great extent is wired into the spinal cord, and under normal circumstances, external stimuli are capable of evoking reflex behavior. Spinal reflexes allow for coordinated movements of multiple muscles and muscle groups. Normally, these reflexes are tonically controlled by descending inhibitory connections from the brainstem. However, after SCI, there is a loss of these descending connections that allows spinal reflexes to be activated by any external stimuli (eg, stretch, noxious stimuli) of sufficient strength or duration. In addition, SCIIS may involve an alteration in how primary sensory information is processed within the spinal cord itself. Primary sensory inputs can influence spinal output either by direct activation of spinal motoneurons through monosynaptic inputs from large myelinated Ia afferents or by integrating first within the spinal cord dorsal horn and then projecting to the motoneurons through polysynaptic spinal connections.

With respect to changes in monosynaptic connections to motoneurons after spinal injury, it has been shown that complete spinal cord transection in the low sacral cord leads to minimal changes in the number of glutamatergic inputs arising from myelinated afferents, labeling sacrocaudal motoneurons (26). Thus, anatomical changes in monosynaptic glutamatergic inputs to this population of motoneurons do not appear to be involved with the development of spasticity in the tail musculature. Similarly, thoracic level transection leads to an apparent increase in myelinated and unmyelinated primary afferent labeling in the dorsal horn and middle laminae but not in the ventral horn of the lumbar spinal cord (89, 90).

Unlike the lack in apparent SCI-induced changes in glutamatergic inputs to the motoneuron pool arising from myelinated primary afferents, SCI appears to significantly increase in the number of glutamatergic inputs to sacrocaudal motoneurons arising from spinal interneuronal (polysynaptic) sources (25). This increase in glutamatergic labeling is especially evident in animals that display significant spasticity in the tail musculature. The results from these anatomical studies would suggest that the interaction between sensory afferents and polysynaptic glutamatergic inputs to sacrocaudal motoneurons plays a greater role in the development of SCIIS in the tail musculature than monosynaptic inputs. This would appear to fit with the results of current physiological studies that demonstrate excessive flexor and extensor reflexes in spinal cord–injured individuals appear to be triggered by afferents that utilize polysynaptic interneuronal circuitry more than by monosynaptic activation of motoneurons (91–95). One caveat with respect to interpreting the results of anatomical studies is that an increase in immunological labeling of excitatory inputs to the motoneurons does not necessarily demonstrate an actual increase in the release of glutamate at those synapses, only that there is the potential of increased neurotransmitter release.

Another line of evidence that would suggest that an increased release in glutamate plays a role in SCI SCIIS comes from a study that demonstrated the administration of the antiepileptic agent gabapentin

(Neurontin®) significantly reduces SCI-induced exaggerated responses to a quick stretch, noxious (pinch), and nonnoxious (light touch) cutaneous stimulation of the tail muscles in animals with chronic sacral spinal transection (27). Although gabapentin possesses multiple cellular mechanisms, recent work has suggested that an inhibition of glutamatergic transmission may be preeminent in mediating its therapeutic effects in epilepsy, neuropathic pain, and perhaps spasticity (96). Specifically, gabapentin reduces presynaptic glutamate release (97–99) in a large part via binding to the $\alpha_2\delta$ subunit of presynaptic voltage-sensitive calcium channels (100–103). In animals that receive low sacral spinal injury, application of a pinch stimulus to the tip of the tail induces a burst of EMG activity in the tail musculature that remains significantly elevated for approximately 6 seconds poststimulus (27). The same stimulus applied to the tail of control (uninjured) animals produces an increase in EMG activity lasting only approximately 1 second. The significant increase in the duration of EMG activity in the SCI animals would be considered a clinically relevant time period that could result in functional restriction. Administration of gabapentin effectively reduces the level of EMG activity to control levels and maintains this decreased level of activity for 3 to 6 hours postinjection. The therapeutic window for gabapentin in this animal model is similar to that seen clinically after administration of gabapentin to control epilepsy and neuropathic pain.

Anatomical Changes in Inhibitory Inputs and Spasticity. In addition to glutamatergic inputs, spinal cord neurons also receive substantial inhibitory inputs, mainly in the form of GABAergic and glycinergic inputs. These inhibitory inputs control the ability of a neuron to be activated by excitatory inputs and thus control (modulate) neuronal output. One theory of spasticity predicts that a decrease in the number of GABAergic and/or glycinergic inhibitory inputs leads to decreased inhibitory control of spinal segments, caudal to the injury, and thus an increase in spinal reflex activity (104–106). However, anatomical studies have demonstrated that the number of both GABAergic and glycinergic inputs to sacrocaudal motoneurons actually increases slightly after spinal transection (25, 26). In addition, several studies have demonstrated an up-regulation of the GABAergic inhibitory system after complete thoracic spinal transection in both rats and felines (107, 108). This increase in the inhibitory system may serve a general role in preventing premature activity after injury. This would fit with the observations that at 1-week postinjury, when the animals displayed a decrease in reflex activity, there was an increase in inhibitory input labeling without

TABLE 27.2
Ratio of VGLUT2 Labeling to VGAT Labeling

TIME POSTINJURY	SOMA	PROXIMAL DENDRITE	OVERALL
Control	1 to 1.2	1 to 1.02	1 to 1.1
1 Week	1 to 1.47	1 to 1.16	1 to 1.3
2 Weeks	1 to 0.65*	1 to 0.64	1 to 0.64***
4 Weeks	1 to 0.57**	1 to 0.56**	1 to 0.57***
12 Weeks	1 to 1.03	1 to 0.71	1 to 0.87

Ratio of VGLUT2-IR labeling to VGAT-IR labeling of CTB-labeled sacrocaudal motoneurons after complete transection of the S_2 spinal cord. At 1 week postinjury, there is a significant increase in the ratio of VGLUT2 to VGAT, suggesting an increased inhibitory on influence on sacrocaudal motoneurons at this time point. From 2 to 12 weeks postinjury, a decrease in the ratio of VGLUT2 to VGAT labeling was observed, suggesting and increase in the excitatory influence on sacrocaudal motoneurons at these time points. One-way analysis of variance was used to compare the mean size of immunoreactive boutons for all experimental groups with post hoc comparison by the Dunnett many-to-one t test. Data are presented as the mean ± SEM; *$P < .05$; **$P < .01$; ***$P < .001$. (From: Kitzman P. Changes in vesicular glutamate transporter 2, vesicular GABA transporter and vesicular acetylcholine transporter labeling of sacrocaudal motoneurons in the spastic rat. *Exp Neurol.* 2006;197:407–419, Table 1, p. 414.)

a change in excitatory labeling. However, over time, when animals demonstrate increased reflex behavior, the increase in inhibitory input labeling appears to be surpassed by the increase in excitatory glutamatergic inputs (25, 26) (Table 27.2). Thus, the normal suppressive activity of the inhibitory inputs may not be sufficient to prevent the development of spasticity in more chronically injured animals.

Physiological Changes in Spinal Activity and Spasticity

Thompson et al. (34) evaluated spinal cord–injured rats at 6, 28, and 60 days after contusion injury at the T_8 level. In this study, specific attention was given to neurophysiological measures that may be related to the development of enhanced excitability of hind limb reflexes because segmental hyperreflexia is a hallmark of transection-type lesions in animals and of spinal trauma in humans (109, 110). Accordingly, 4 aspects of reflex excitability were tested: (1) reflex thresholds (2), slope of the reflex recruitment curve (an estimate of reflex gain) (3), maximal plantar H reflex/maximal plantar M response rations, and (4) rate-sensitive depression, which is a fundamental rate-modulatory process that normally attenuates reflex magnitude during repetitive afferent stimulation. At 6 days after contusion injury, H reflex magnitude, as a function of reflex repetition rate, was not significantly different from that recorded in normal animals. However, the H reflex in these animals displayed substantial decrease in slope of the recruitment curve, suggesting a decrease in the gain of reflex excitability. Collectively, these observations indicated that at 1-week postinjury, lumbar reflex excitability was significantly depressed. When H reflex activity was examined in chronically injured animals (28 and 60 days postcontusion), the rate sensitivity of H reflex magnitude was significantly decreased. In the absence of the normal pattern of rate-sensitive depression, the relative reflex magnitude in both 28- and 60-day postcontusion animals was increased compared with normal animals. The changes in motoneuron excitability, below the level of a spinal injury, would suggest that initially spinal injury results in a substantial depression of reflex excitability. During the first few weeks postinjury, progressive changes occur that result in an increase in the reflex excitability of motoneurons.

The results demonstrated in the H reflex study were built upon subsequent studies of reflex activity after SCI. In particular, in addition to a significant decrease in rate depression, posttetanic potentiation, another rate-modulatory process that increases excitability, is altered after contusion (36). Analysis of monosynaptic reflexes after spinal contusion demonstrates a significant increase in reflex amplitude, whereas the posttetanic potentiation of the tibial monosynaptic reflexes significantly decreases. Because the monosynaptic reflexes include muscle stretch reflexes, the results of this study suggest that a larger proportion of the motoneuron pool is recruited by segmental stimulation in postcontusion rats than in normal animals. This type of exaggerated response is consistent with the increased reflex excitability associated with conditions of spasticity (111). The origin of the altered monosynaptic spinal reflex to contusion appears to differ from that after spinal hemisection, in which enhanced monosynaptic reflex responses may reflect an increased activity of a single population of motoneurons rather than recruitment of multiple separate populations responding with different time courses (1).

One key aspect of the definition of spasticity has always been the velocity dependency of muscle response to a stretch. This aspect of spasticity has been difficult to measure in animals until recently. Tests of velocity-dependent ankle torques and extensor EMGs in rodents at 2 months after midthoracic contusion injury reveal that the development of significant levels of spasticity is present in the ankle extensor muscles (38, 112). Bose et al. (38) demonstrated that after spi-

nal contusion, there is an initial transient pattern of tonic spasticity that is displayed as a significant increased stiffness that is independent of velocity. This pattern was followed by a period of decreased or suppressed velocity-sensitive excitability. Finally, a pattern of spasticity appears that is velocity dependent. In these animals, the ankle torques and the ankle extensor EMG magnitudes are significantly increased only when tested at the upper range of ankle rotation velocities. Collectively, these observations indicate that 1 month after midthoracic contusion injury, a velocity-dependent exaggeration of the stretch reflexes can be demonstrated in the rat that is consistent with the clinical assessment of spasticity.

It is important to note that, as in previous studies, (3) spasticity has not been reliably detected in the ankle extensor muscles using manual examination of the hind limbs. However, spasticity can be demonstrated using instrumentation that produces ankle rotation across a broad range of velocities. The literature supports the role of the rat spinal contusion injury model as a useful model to investigate SCI-induced velocity-dependent spasticity and that demonstration of spasticity requires a comparison of lengthening resistance across a broad range of muscle-lengthening velocities. The contusion injury–associated increase in the velocity-dependent ankle torque is consistent with the expression of a spastic hyperreflexia that develops over time and is of lasting duration.

Low-Sacral Transaction Model. Two weeks after S_2 spinal transection, low-level stimulation that would not evoke an EMG reflex in a normal or acute spinal rat now evokes long-lasting reflexes that are (1) very low threshold, (2) evoked from rest without prior EMG activity, (3) of polysynaptic latency with more than 6 millisecond central delay, (4) about 2 seconds long, and (5) enhanced by repeated stimulation (windup) (113, 114). These long-lasting reflexes in chronic spinal cord–injured rats have greater excitability and demonstrate a lower threshold to initiate the response, which is similar to the exaggerated flexor withdrawal reflexes seen chronically in spastic humans after SCI (106, 113).

Input from polysynaptic excitatory postsynaptic potentials (pEPSPs) to motoneurons is normally inhibited by descending control. After SCI, these pEPSPs are released from inhibition immediately after injury. However, in the low sacral injury model, the release of polysynaptic potentials does not initially produce long-lasting reflexes due to an overall loss in motoneuron excitability (114). In more chronically injured animals, both in vitro and in vivo studies demonstrate that the same low-threshold polysynaptic inputs to the motoneurons are greatly amplified and prolonged by calcium and sodium PICs (20–22). The development of SCI-induced amplified and prolonged low-threshold polysynaptic inputs has been confirmed clinically in humans (115, 116). These low-threshold polysynaptic EPSPs are NMDA dependent (21, 117) and are especially important in triggering spasms in chronic injured animals. A single EPSP becomes sufficiently long (>200 milliseconds) to evoke the slowly activating PICs in motoneurons, which in turn induce prolonged motoneuron discharges. The exaggerated activity of the motoneurons can last for several seconds and is partially the result of the initiation of plateau potentials by the PICs (20, 23, 114). Consequently, normally harmless stimulation such as gentle rubbing of the skin can evoke pEPSPs, which in turn can trigger PICs and plateau potentials that ultimately cause exaggerated long-lasting reflex responses.

In addition to changes in PIC discharge after SCI, the normal depression of monosynaptic and polysynaptic reflexes with repeated stimulation is also lost after injury (34, 118), and cutaneous polysynaptic reflexes are instead enhanced with repeated stimulation (23, 117, 119). Thus, repeated inputs can summate to produce sufficiently long EPSPs to trigger PICs (23). These PICs enable motoneurons to produce vigorous discharges in response to brief inputs that, without the normal descending inhibitory control, ultimately produce the exaggerated spasms seen with chronic injury. (20, 28, 115, 116)

The Role of Plateau Potentials in the Development of Spasticity. During the last 2 decades, research has shown that multiple active membrane properties shape the motoneuronal output. Voltage-dependent PICs are an important intrinsic property of spinal motoneurons. After SCI, the reemergence of these PICs is hypothesized to play a significant role in the development of spasticity. One mechanism by which PIC plays a role in the development of spasticity is through the activation of plateau potentials. With the motoneuron already active, plateau potentials are able to produce a distinct jump to a higher firing rate and produce firing that outlasts the stimulation (self-sustained firing) in animals and humans, which can contribute substantially to long-lasting reflexes and spasticity (20, 21, 28, 120, 121).

Overall, there have been 2 categories of PICs that have been examined with respect to the generation of plateau potentials: the Ca^{2+} PIC (Ca PIC) and the sodium PIC (Na PIC). Of these 2 categories, it is the Ca PICs that have been shown to be more involved with generating the long-lasting reflexes that are characteristic of spasticity (21, 22). However, the Na PICs and the sodium spike properties also appear to be crucial for enabling sustained firing of motoneurons as well

as significantly interact with the neuromodulators serotonin and noradrenalin (122–124).

With respect to the Ca PICs, it is the postsynaptically located L-type voltage-sensitive Ca^{2+} channels that significantly contribute to this active membrane property. These L-type voltage-sensitive calcium channels can be divided into Cav1.2 and Cav1.3 L-type channels depending upon the α_1 subunit that is present. In rodent spinal motoneurons, both Cav1.2 and Cav1.3 channels are localized in the cell body and dendritic processes (125–129), with almost all spinal motoneurons expressing Cav1.3 (128). Experimentally, the induction of PICs associated with spinal motoneurons has been shown to be due in a large part to Cav1.3 L-type calcium channels (22, 130). While the presence of the Cav1.3 channel is important for PIC formation, its presence alone is not sufficient for producing plateau potentials; there must also be an appropriate neuromodulation to enable their function (121, 131). Specifically, the behavior of Cav1.3 channels has been shown to be dependent on input from axons that originate in the brainstem and release monoamines, such as serotonin (5-HT) and norepinephrine (NE) (121, 132, 133). Although the role of the Cav1.3 channels in the development of PICs has been established, the role of Cav1.2 channels is less well known. Recent studies in a variety of CNS neurons have shown that, like the Cav1.3 channels, Cav1.2 channels are influenced by the modulatory effects of monoamines (134, 135).

After S_2 spinal transaction, a significant increase in Cav1.2 α_1 subunit expression in the motoneuron pool caudal to the injury can be observed (136). However, there is no apparent change in the expression of the Cav1.3 α_1 subunit expression. This lack of change in the Cav1.3 α_1 subunit is surprising because it has been hypothesized that the Cav1.3 channels play a greater role in the production of PICs, which are implicated in the onset of spasticity after spinal transection. One possible explanation may be that although the overall level of expression of the Cav1.3 channels do not change, the distribution of this calcium channel subtype along the soma and dendrites may change, which would lead to an alteration in neuronal function (136). Subsequently, an alteration in the distribution of these channels could partially account for motoneurons developing hypersensitivity to monoamines after SCI (28).

The Role of Neuromodulators in Spasticity. Although excitatory (glutamatergic) or inhibitory (GABAergic and glycinergic) inputs control the overall firing rate of neurons, it is the influence of various neuromodulators that ultimately shapes the activity of the neurons. With respect to the spinal cord, the predominate neuromodulators of neuronal activity are serotonin (5-HT) and NE. Anatomically, it has been demonstrated that the spinal cord in general and the spinal motoneurons specifically are densely innervated by terminals of 5-HT and NE neurons arising from brain stem sources as well as a small population arising from spinal neurons. Complete SCI eliminates all but a very small percentage of the 5-HT content within the spinal cord (137–139), with approximately 10% of 5-HT and NE inputs remaining caudal to the injury long after spinal transection (123). Administration of low doses (20–100 mg/kg) of the serotoninergic agonist 5-hydroxtryptophan increases spontaneous and evoked muscle activity in chronically spinalized rats but not in uninjured animals (138, 139). The results from these studies suggest that the release of 5-HT from residual spinal sources could contribute to the development of spastic activity in chronically injured animals, possibly through the induction of large PICs. This idea has been partially verified when it was demonstrated that Na PICs are supersensitive to 5-HT$_2$ receptor activation (122). Low doses of 5-HT significantly lower the threshold and increase the amplitude of Ca PICs in sacrocaudal motoneurons from chronically transected animals (140). These Ca PICs demonstrate approximately a 30-fold increased sensitivity to 5-HT in chronic spinal rats when compared to uninjured animals. Thus, after spinal injury, the development of 5-HT super sensitivity in the motoneurons appears to more than compensate for the lost brainstem 5-HT inputs.

In addition to modulating PICs, 5-HT also significantly modulates H reflex activity in spinal cord–injured animals (141). At 4 weeks postinjury, H reflex recordings from the hind paw plantar muscles of contused rats show twice the H reflex amplitude of that in uninjured and transected animals. In animals that receive contusion injury, the 5-HT$_2$ receptor antagonist significantly reduces H reflex amplitude, whereas the 5-HT$_2$ agonist significantly increases reflex amplitude. In addition, immunohistochemical analysis demonstrates increased 5-HT$_2$ receptor immunoreactivity in plantar muscle motoneurons compared with uninjured control animals. The results from this study suggest that increased expression of the 5-HT$_2$ receptor is likely involved in the enhanced H reflex that develops after contusive SCI. The increased H reflex amplitude observed at 4 weeks after different severities of contusive SCI in rats is positively correlated with 5-HT immunoreactivity around motoneurons involved in the reflex (142). That is, the greater their apparent 5-HT innervation, the more abnormally elevated their reflex activation. The clinical relevance to this work is that

many individuals with SCI develop depression and are prescribed serotoninergic antidepressants. In cases of incomplete SCI, where descending 5-HT fibers are preserved (142), these antidepressants may cause an increase in the local concentration of 5-HT in the spinal cord. If this increase occurs at a time when increased sensitivity to 5-HT has developed due to receptor upregulation, exaggerated reflexes and spasticity may actually be promoted in these individuals (141). In addition, administration of 5-HT and NE agonist can both facilitate and inhibit SCI-induced long-lasting reflexes depending upon the dosage (23) and that activation of select subsets of 5-HT receptors improves locomotor function in the spinal-injured rat (143, 144).

The super sensitivity of spinal motoneurons to residual 5-HT may result in part from an SCI-induced increase in the expression of 5-HT receptors below the level of injury (145, 146). After T$_{13}$ spinal cord transection in the feline, there is a significant increase in the expression of the 5 HT$_{1A}$ receptor in lamina II, III, and X of the lumbar spinal cord at 15 and 30 days postinjury (145). Although spinal injury induces a compensatory increase in 5-HT receptor expression in several lamina of the spinal gray matter, there is no apparent change in 5-HT$_{1A}$ receptor labeling of lumbar motoneurons. However, a lack of change in expression of the 5-HT$_{1A}$ receptor subtype does not preclude the lumbar motoneurons from up-regulating the expression of another 5-HT receptor subtype to compensate for the loss of descending 5-HT input after spinal injury. In the phrenic motoneuron pool, immunohistochemical analysis reveals that 5-HT$_{2A}$ receptor expression significantly increases on phrenic motoneurons as well as in the surrounding gray matter 2 weeks after C$_2$ spinal hemisection (146).

Norepinephrine is another neuromodulator that normally regulates spinal activity and continues to do so even in chronically spinal-injured animals. Administration of amphetamine leads to an increase in long-lasting reflexes in the tail muscles of spinal-injured rats, which is believed to be mediated by in part by the activation of Ca PICs (124). Similarly, earlier studies demonstrated that the administration of amphetamine enhances flexor reflex activity in chronically spinal-injured animals (147, 148). Amphetamine is known to specifically enhance the release of NE as well as inhibit its reuptake (147, 149). Thus, the increase in reflex activity in spinal-injured animals induced by the application of amphetamine most likely involves the release of intraspinal NE. In addition, administration of L-dopa, a drug that leads to the synthesis and release of NE, leads to increased flexor reflexes elicited by a noxious stimulus in acute spinal rats (150). Multiple studies have demonstrated an up-regulation of the $NE_{\alpha1}$ receptors in the spinal cord of chronically transected rats (145, 151, 152). As with serotonin, an up-regulation in the expression of NE receptors would indicate the potential for super sensitivity of spinal neurons to the release of NE from the spinal sources that remain after spinal injury, and that this super sensitivity to NE likely plays a role in the development of SCIID.

In addition to serotoninergic and noradrenergic inputs, motoneurons receive innervation from cholinergic inputs. Acetylcholine (Ach) is a powerful modulator of spinal motoneuronal activity that has been shown to facilitate rhythmic activity in motoneurons in the neonatal rat spinal cord (153, 154). Cholinergic inputs arise from collateral branches from the axons of motoneurons themselves. These inputs help synchronize the firing patterns of functional groups of motoneurons and allow for a coordinated activation of muscle groups. Low sacral spinal transection has been shown to cause to a progressive loss of the vesicular Ach transporter (VAChT; a marker for cholinergic terminals) labeling of sacrocaudal motoneurons (25). At 1 week postinjury, when the animals display decreased tail reflexes, there is an almost complete loss of cholinergic labeling of motoneurons. However, over time, a more complex pattern of labeling emerges in which VAChT labeling moderately increases at 2 weeks postinjury and then progressively decreases over the next 2 TO 3 months postinjury. The almost complete loss of VAChT labeling at 1 week postinjury may be reflective of a decreased motoneuron activity that has been demonstrated postspinal transection (20). While, at later time points, when the spinal cord begins to recover from spinal shock and motoneuron activity increases, the production of VAChT from spinal inputs to these motoneuronal pools may be partially reestablished. Because the cholinergic inputs help in coordinating the firing pattern of groups of muscles, the loss of these inputs would lead to a disorganization of muscle firing patterns.

In addition to serotonin, NE, and Ach, another neuromodulator that has been examined with respect to the development of spasticity after spinal injury is dynorphin. Dynorphin is a member of the opioid family that is endogenously produced within the CNS and is typically associated with the control of somatosensation. after spinal compression in the cervical region, animals display spasticity within 4 days of surgery that persists for at least 8 weeks (30). Radioimmunoassay results demonstrated that at 1 week after compression injury, dynorphin-A immunoreactivity is significantly decreased in thoracic and lumbar spinal segments. Physiologically, administration of a dynorphin κ-receptor agonist significantly reduces the level of spasticity in these animals. These results suggest that a reduction of endogenous dynorphin might play an important role in the pathogenesis of spinally induced muscle spasticity, which fits with the results of a previous physiological study that demonstrated that administration of an analogue of dynorphin successfully relives spasticity induced in the rabbit by cervical compression injury (155).

Changes in Response to Ischemic SCI. While traumatic SCI models remain the predominate models for examining pathology underlying the development of spasticity, other studies have examined the pathophysiology involved with ischemic spinal injury-induced spasticity (41, 44, 45, 156, 157). Physiologically ischemic SCI leads to a clear increase in EMG activity measured from gastrocnemius muscles in response to noxious stimulus (40). In addition, simultaneous measurement of EMG activity in gastrocnemius and muscle resistance during ankle rotation shows a clear appearance of increased EMG activity during the muscle stretch, and the increase in muscle resistance is velocity dependent. Together, these observations demonstrate the presence of spasticity in the ischemic model. However, the ischemia injury model also leads to muscle rigidity, which needs to be considered when interpreting electrophysiological data.

Biochemical studies indicate that ischemic SCIID appears to involve a decrease in the level of spinal glycine. Because glycine has been established as 1 of the 2 main inhibitory neurotransmitters in the spinal cord and is closely associated with the modulation of segmental efferent activity within the ventral horn and afferent activity within the dorsal horn, a decrease in the level of this neurotransmitter would effectively release spinal reflexes from inhibitory control. In animals displaying spinal shock, the glycine levels have been shown to be 2 to 3 times higher than spastic or control (uninjured) animals (158). Thus, during the time frame in which animals display decreased reflex activity, there is an elevated level of inhibition. Administration of glycine or closely related compounds is able to suppress spastic activity, whereas blockade of glycine-mediated chloride channels amplifies spastic activity (44).

The decrease in the level of glycine (and GABA) that is seen in ischemic injured spasticity animals can be linked to the loss of spinal neurons that produce these inhibitory interneurons (41) Specifically, increased motor tone after spinal ischemia may be a result of a loss of small-sized and medium-sized inhibitory glycine and GABAergic interneurons, which are known to provide the principle local modulation of motoneuron excitability (156, 159–161). In addition to changes within the inhibitory component of the spinal cord, ischemic spinal injury also appears to induce changes in the excitatory circuitry. Specifically, spastic animals demonstrated a significant increase in GluR1 but a decrease in GluR2 and GluR4 proteins (162). These results suggest that ischemia-induced spinal injury differentially effects the expression of the different AMPA receptor subtypes, which would impact the responsiveness of spinal neurons to glutamate. Pharmacologically blocking the GluR1 receptor significantly reduces the manifestation of spasticity and rigidity as well as down-regulates the expression of neuronal and astrocytic GluR1 expression in the lumbar spinal cord. These results suggest that the injury-induced increase in GluR1 receptor expression contributes to the expression of spasticity in these animals.

Pathophysiology in the Rodent Model of Multiple Sclerosis

As with SCI, animal models of multiple sclerosis demonstrate signs and symptoms of upper motor neuron lesions, including the development of spasticity. The CREAE is an autoimmune model of multiple sclerosis that has become the predominate animal model for studying this disease. It has been proposed that spasticity in CREAE mice is associated with changes in the expression of endocannabinoids because endocannabinoids are up-regulated locally in areas of CREAE-induced damage. For this reason, most studies that have examined the pathophysiology of spasticity in CREAE animals have focused on the role of the cannabinoid system. Physiological studies have shown that cannabinoid receptor agonists significantly decrease tremor and spasticity, whereas administration of cannabinoid receptor antagonists significantly exacerbates spasticity in these animals (46). More recently, it has been demonstrated that inhibitors of endocannabinoid reuptake significantly inhibit limb spasticity in mice with CREAE (48). Gene knockout technology has also been combined with this animal model to examine the effects of removing (knocking out) the expression of the cannabinoid type-1 (CB$_1$) receptor subtype on the manifestation of spasticity (49). Loss of CB$_1$ receptor subtype expression leads to an attenuation of the antispastic effects of CB agonists, suggesting that the cannabinoid system in general and the CB$_1$ receptor subtype specifically may be very appropriate targets for interventions aimed at managing the expression of CREAE-induced spasticity.

Pathophysiology in Rodent Models of Cerebral Palsy

Of the different animal models of spasticity that have been examined, the most recent models to be developed involve either a hypoxia-ischemia or anoxia-induced form of cerebral palsy in the rabbit or rodent, respectively (50–52, 54). However, very little work has been conducted with respect to determining the anatomical or physiological aspects of the pathophysiology behind the hypertonia in either of these animal models. Magnetic resonance imaging analysis demonstrates that in animals that underwent hypoxia-ischemia injury and demonstrate pronounced hypertonia, there is white matter damage especially in the corpus callosum and the internal capsule (51, 52). With respect to anoxia-injured rodents, mild increases in muscular tone paralleled a modest disorganization of the primary motor cortices (54). These initial studies represent the first steps in the evolution of animal models of cerebral palsy that can be used to elucidate the pathophysiology involved with the onset of spasticity.

Pathophysiology in Spastic, Spasmotic and Oscillator Mutant Mouse Models

Spastic, spasmodic, and oscillator mutant mice have naturally occurring glycine receptor mutations that manifest as motor deficits and an exaggerated "startle response" similar to animal models of multiple sclerosis; it appears that changes in the glycinergic system play a significant role in the development of spasticity in these mutant animals (57, 59, 61, 63, 64, 162). Adult homozygotic *spastic* mutants exhibit a severe reduction of adult isoform of glycine receptors in the spinal cord and brain (59, 63). Specifically, it appears that the onset of spastic symptoms coincides with a developmental switch from the neonatal isoform of glycine receptor to the adult isoform glycine receptor (63). The adult glycine receptor isoform is composed of ligand-binding α_1 and structural β subunits. In spastic mice, there is an aberrant splicing of the β subunit (59). Therefore, during the development stage in which glycine receptors normally switch from their immature to adult forms, the spastic mutants are unable to make this transition.

Physiologically, a reduction in glycine receptor-mediated neurotransmission in spastic mice correlates with the severity of the neurological symptoms. Specifically, the abnormal motor output of the spastic mutant mouse appears to be related to a dramatic reduction in chloride-dependent glycine-mediated synaptic conductance (64). In addition, the amplitudes of glycine receptor-mediated inhibitory postsynaptic currents are significantly reduced in the severe phenotype when compared to the wild type and mild phenotype mutants, suggesting a release of reflex activity from its normal inhibitory control (162). Along with the documented alterations in the glycinergic neurotransmitter system, physiological assessment has determined that the amplitudes of the $GABA_A$ receptor-mediated Inhibitory post-synaptic potential (IPSP) which is a local hyperpolarization of the post-synaptic membrane. It becomes more negative and therefore less likely to be activated are also significantly reduced in the spastic mutant mice. This attenuation of GABAergic inputs would continue to reduce the amount of inhibition present in the spinal cord, thus allowing for uncontrolled activation of spinal reflexes.

The spasmodic genetic disorder, like the spastic mutation, is caused in part to a mutation in spinal glycine receptors, resulting in neurons having a reduced sensitivity to glycine (57). Specifically, the spasmodic mutation affects the α_1 subunit of the adult glycine receptor. This alteration in the α_1 subunit leads to a 6-fold reduction in glycine sensitivity by the adult glycine receptor. In addition, glycine receptor kinetics are faster in spasmodic mutant mice compared with wild-type animals (61). The faster inhibitory postsynaptic current rise and decay times would suggest that the main effect of the spasmodic mutation is to increase the rate of glycine unbinding from its receptor, thereby shortening the time these inhibitory receptors remain activated (163). As with other mutant mouse models, the oscillator mutant mice also demonstrate naturally occurring mutations to the glycine receptor (61, 67). Specifically, these animals appear to have a complete absence of the α_1-containing glycine receptors.

Finally, in the spastic mouse model of human hyperekplexia, researchers have observed a developmental loss of glycinergic presynaptic terminals but an increase in the density of GABAergic presynaptic terminals during the first 2 postnatal weeks (66). In addition, whereas spastic mice display a strong impairment in glycine receptor aggregation postsynaptically, the proportion of inhibitory presynaptic terminals facing diffuse $GABA_A$ receptors significantly increases during development. These results suggest that while GABAergic neurotransmission may increase in these mutant mice, it does not compensate for defects in glycine receptor postsynaptic aggregation.

Overall, the results of studies that have examined mutant mice models of spasticity have all demonstrated different mutations that disrupt glycine and GABA receptor-mediated inhibition via different physiological mechanisms. Each of these mutations would allow excitatory inputs within the spinal cord to go relatively unchecked by the inhibitory system and therefore potentially allow for exaggerated reflex responses (164).

CONCLUSION

As we have shown throughout this chapter, different insults to the CNS (eg, SCI, stroke, cerebral palsy, multiple sclerosis) lead to spasticity with different pathophysiology. This has necessitated the need to develop and refine multiple animal models that mimic aspects of spasticity and the upper motor neuron syndrome that are seen in humans to better understand the underlying pathology involved with the development of this impairment. The use of animal models allows for the production of reproducible deficits that are appropriate for examining the relationship between structures within the CNS and their function. As our understanding of the underlying causes of spasticity increases and new research techniques become available, the use of animal models will also evolve and will continue to play a significant role in our understanding of the underlying pathology of spasticity as well as a role in the development of new interventions for the treatment of this complex impairment.

References

1. Carter RL, Ritz LA, Shank CP, Scott EW, Sypert GW. Correlative electrophysiological and behavioral evaluation following L5 lesions in the cat: a model of spasticity. *Exp Neurol* 1991;114:206–15.
2. Hultborn H, Malmsten J. Changes in segmental reflexes following chronic spinal cord hemisection in the cat. II. Conditioned monosynaptic test reflexes. *Acta Physiol Scand* 1983;119:423–33.
3. Malmsten J. Time course of segmental reflex changes after chronic spinal cord hemisection in the rat. *Acta Physiol Scand* 1983;119:435–43.
4. Hultborn H. Changes in neuronal properties and spinal reflexes during development of spasticity following spinal cord lesions and stroke: studies in animal models and patients. *J Rehabil Med* 2003:46–55.
5. Cavallari P, Pettersson LG. Tonic suppression of reflex transmission in low spinal cats. *Exp Brain Res* 1989;77:201–12.
6. Eidelberg E, Nguyen LH, Deza LD. Recovery of locomotor function after hemisection of the spinal cord in cats. *Brain Res Bull* 1986;16:507–15.
7. Munson JB, Foehring RC, Lofton SA, Zengel JE, Sypert GW. Plasticity of medial gastrocnemius motor units following cordotomy in the cat. *J Neurophysiol* 1986;55:619–34.
8. Nelson SG, Mendell LM. Enhancement in Ia-motoneuron synaptic transmission caudal to chronic spinal cord transection. *J Neurophysiol* 1979;42:642–54.
9. Hochman S, McCrea DA. Effects of chronic spinalization on ankle extensor motoneurons. III. Composite Ia EPSPs in motoneurons separated into motor unit types. *J Neurophysiol* 1994;71:1480–90.
10. Hochman S, McCrea DA. Effects of chronic spinalization on ankle extensor motoneurons. II. Motoneuron electrical properties. *J Neurophysiol* 1994;71:1468–79.

11. Hochman S, McCrea DA. Effects of chronic spinalization on ankle extensor motoneurons. I. Composite monosynaptic Ia EPSPs in four motoneuron pools. *J Neurophysiol* 1994; 71:1452–67.

12. Bailey CS, Lieberman JS, Kitchell RL. Response of muscle spindle primary endings to static stretch in acute and chronic spinal cats. *Am J Vet Res* 1980;41:2030–6.

13. Nelson SG, Collatos TC, Niechaj A, Mendell LM. Immediate increase in Ia-motoneuron synaptic transmission caudal to spinal cord transection. *J Neurophysiol* 1979;42:655–64.

14. Naftchi NE, Schlosser W, Horst WD. Correlation of changes in the GABA-ergic system with the development of spasticity in paraplegic cats. *Adv Exp Med Biol* 1979;123:431–50.

15. Sherrington CS. On secondary and tertiary degenerations in the spinal cord of the dog. *J Physiol* 1885;6:177–292 10.

16. Ashby P, Mailis A, Hunter J. The evaluation of "spasticity". *Can J Neurol Sci* 1987;14:497–500.

17. Ritz LA, Friedman RM, Rhoton EL, Sparkes ML, Vierck CJ, Jr. Lesions of cat sacrocaudal spinal cord: a minimally disruptive model of injury. *J Neurotrauma* 1992;9:219–30.

18. Bouisset S, Zattara M. Biomechanical study of the programming of anticipatory postural adjustments associated with voluntary movement. *J Biomech* 1987;20:735–42.

19. Bennett DJ, Gorassini M, Fouad K, Sanelli L, Han Y, Cheng J. Spasticity in rats with sacral spinal cord injury. *J Neurotrauma* 1999;16:69–84.

20. Bennett DJ, Li Y, Harvey PJ, Gorassini M. Evidence for plateau potentials in tail motoneurons of awake chronic spinal rats with spasticity. *J Neurophysiol* 2001;86:1972–82.

21. Bennett DJ, Li Y, Siu M. Plateau potentials in sacrocaudal motoneurons of chronic spinal rats, recorded in vitro. *J Neurophysiol* 2001;86:1955–71.

22. Li Y, Bennett DJ. Persistent sodium and calcium currents cause plateau potentials in motoneurons of chronic spinal rats. *J Neurophysiol* 2003;90:857–69.

23. Li Y, Harvey PJ, Li X, Bennett DJ. Spastic long-lasting reflexes of the chronic spinal rat studied in vitro. *J Neurophysiol* 2004;91:2236–46.

24. Kitzman P. Alteration in axial motoneuronal morphology in the spinal cord injured spastic rat. *Exp Neurol* 2005;192:100–8.

25. Kitzman P. Changes in vesicular glutamate transporter 2, vesicular GABA transporter and vesicular acetylcholine transporter labeling of sacrocaudal motoneurons in the spastic rat. *Exp Neurol* 2006;197:407–19.

26. Kitzman P. VGLUT1 and GLYT2 labeling of sacrocaudal motoneurons in the spinal cord injured spastic rat. *Exp Neurol* 2007;204:195–204.

27. Kitzman PH, Uhl TL, Dwyer MK. Gabapentin suppresses spasticity in the spinal cord-injured rat. *Neuroscience* 2007; 149:813–21.

28. Li Y, Gorassini MA, Bennett DJ. Role of persistent sodium and calcium currents in motoneuron firing and spasticity in chronic spinal rats. *J Neurophysiol* 2004;91:767–83.

29. Black P, Markowitz RS, Cooper V, et al. Models of spinal cord injury: part 1. Static load technique. *Neurosurgery* 1986; 19:752–62.

30. Dong HW, Wang LH, Zhang M, Han JS. Decreased dynorphin A (1-17) in the spinal cord of spastic rats after the compressive injury. *Brain Res Bull* 2005;67:189–95.

31. Kerasidis H, Wrathall JR, Gale K. Behavioral assessment of functional deficit in rats with contusive spinal cord injury. *J Neurosci Methods* 1987;20:167–79.

32. Wrathall JR, Pettegrew RK, Harvey F. Spinal cord contusion in the rat: production of graded, reproducible, injury groups. *Exp Neurol* 1985;88:108–22.

33. Bresnahan JC, Beattie MS, Todd FD, 3rd, Noyes DH. A behavioral and anatomical analysis of spinal cord injury produced by a feedback-controlled impaction device. *Exp Neurol* 1987;95:548–70.

34. Thompson FJ, Reier PJ, Lucas CC, Parmer R. Altered patterns of reflex excitability subsequent to contusion injury of the rat spinal cord. *J Neurophysiol* 1992;68:1473–86.

35. Thompson FJ, Reier PJ, Parmer R, Lucas CC. Inhibitory control of reflex excitability following contusion injury and neural tissue transplantation. *Adv Neurol* 1993;59:175–84.

36. Thompson FJ, Parmer R, Reier PJ. Alteration in rate modulation of reflexes to lumbar motoneurons after midthoracic spinal cord injury in the rat. I. Contusion injury. *J Neurotrauma* 1998;15:495–508.

37. Lance JW. The control of muscle tone, reflexes, and movement: Robert Wartenberg Lecture. *Neurology* 1980;30:1303–13.

38. Bose P, Parmer R, Thompson FJ. Velocity-dependent ankle torque in rats after contusion injury of the midthoracic spinal cord: time course. *J Neurotrauma* 2002;19:1231–49.

39. Coston A, Laville M, Baud P, Bussel B, Jalfre M. Aortic occlusion by a balloon catheter: a method to induce hind limb rigidity in rats. *Physiol Behav* 1983;30:967–9.

40. Marsala M, Hefferan MP, Kakinohana O, Nakamura S, Marsala J, Tomori Z. Measurement of peripheral muscle resistance in rats with chronic ischemia-induced paraplegia or morphine-induced rigidity using a semi-automated computer-controlled muscle resistance meter. *J Neurotrauma* 2005;22:1348–61.

41. Marsala M, Kakinohana O, Yaksh TL, Tomori Z, Marsala S, Cizkova D. Spinal implantation of hNT neurons and neuronal precursors: graft survival and functional effects in rats with ischemic spastic paraplegia. *Eur J Neurosci* 2004;20: 2401–14.

42. Kakinohana O, Hefferan MP, Nakamura S, et al. Development of GABA-sensitive spasticity and rigidity in rats after transient spinal cord ischemia: a qualitative and quantitative electrophysiological and histopathological study. *Neuroscience* 2006;141:1569–83.

43. Matsushita A, Smith CM. Spinal cord function in postischemic rigidity in the rat. *Brain Res* 1970;19:395–410.

44. Simpson RK, Jr., Gondo M, Robertson CS, Goodman JC. The influence of glycine and related compounds on spinal cord injury-induced spasticity. *Neurochem Res* 1995;20:1203–10.

45. Simpson RK, Jr., Robertson CS, Goodman JC. The role of glycine in spinal shock. *J Spinal Cord Med* 1996;19: 215–24.

46. Baker D, Pryce G, Croxford JL, et al. Cannabinoids control spasticity and tremor in a multiple sclerosis model. *Nature* 2000;404:84–7.

47. Baker D, Pryce G, Croxford JL, et al. Endocannabinoids control spasticity in a multiple sclerosis model. *FASEB J* 2001;15:300–2.

48. Ligresti A, Cascio MG, Pryce G, et al. New potent and selective inhibitors of anandamide reuptake with antispastic activity in a mouse model of multiple sclerosis. *Br J Pharmacol* 2006;147:83–91.

49. Pryce G, Baker D. Control of spasticity in a multiple sclerosis model is mediated by CB1, not CB2, cannabinoid receptors. *Br J Pharmacol* 2007;150:519–25.

50. Derrick M, Luo NL, Bregman JC, et al. Preterm fetal hypoxia-ischemia causes hypertonia and motor deficits in the neonatal rabbit: a model for human cerebral palsy? *J Neurosci* 2004;24:24–34.

51. Derrick M, Drobyshevsky A, Ji X, Tan S. A model of cerebral palsy from fetal hypoxia-ischemia. *Stroke* 2007;38:731–5.

52. Drobyshevsky A, Derrick M, Wyrwicz AM, et al. White matter injury correlates with hypertonia in an animal model of cerebral palsy. *J Cereb Blood Flow Metab* 2007;27:270–81.

53. Tan S, Drobyshevsky A, Jilling T, et al. Model of cerebral palsy in the perinatal rabbit. *J Child Neurol* 2005;20:972–9.

54. Strata F, Coq JO, Byl N, Merzenich MM. Effects of sensorimotor restriction and anoxia on gait and motor cortex organization: implications for a rodent model of cerebral palsy. *Neuroscience* 2004;129:141–56.

55. Floeter MK, Hallett M. Glycine receptors: a startling connection. *Nat Genet* 1993;5:319–20.

56. Buckwalter MS, Cook SA, Davisson MT, White WF, Camper SA. A frameshift mutation in the mouse alpha 1 glycine

receptor gene (Glra1) results in progressive neurological symptoms and juvenile death. *Hum Mol Genet* 1994;3: 2025–30.

57. Ryan SG, Buckwalter MS, Lynch JW, et al. A missense mutation in the gene encoding the alpha 1 subunit of the inhibitory glycine receptor in the spasmodic mouse. *Nat Genet* 1994;7:131–5.

58. Kingsmore SF, Giros B, Suh D, Bieniarz M, Caron MG, Seldin MF. Glycine receptor beta-subunit gene mutation in spastic mouse associated with LINE-1 element insertion. *Nat Genet* 1994;7:136–41.

59. Mulhardt C, Fischer M, Gass P, et al. The spastic mouse: aberrant splicing of glycine receptor beta subunit mRNA caused by intronic insertion of L1 element. *Neuron* 1994;13: 1003–15.

60. Saul B, Schmieden V, Kling C, et al. Point mutation of glycine receptor alpha 1 subunit in the spasmodic mouse affects agonist responses. *FEBS Lett* 1994;350:71–6.

61. Graham BA, Schofield PR, Sah P, Margrie TW, Callister RJ. Distinct physiological mechanisms underlie altered glycinergic synaptic transmission in the murine mutants spastic, spasmodic, and oscillator. *J Neurosci* 2006;26:4880–90.

62. Chai CK, Roberts E, Sidman RL. Influence of aminooxyacetic acid, a gamma-aminobutyrate transaminase inhibitor, on hereditary spastic defect in the mouse. *Proceedings of the Society for Experimental Biology and Medicine Society for Experimental Biology and Medicine* (New York, NY 1962;109:491–5.

63. Becker CM, Schmieden V, Tarroni P, Strasser U, Betz H. Isoform-selective deficit of glycine receptors in the mouse mutant spastic. *Neuron* 1992;8:283–9.

64. Biscoe TJ, Duchen MR. Synaptic physiology of spinal motoneurones of normal and spastic mice: an in vitro study. *J Physiol* 1986;379:275–92.

65. Heller AH, Hallett M. Electrophysiological studies with the spastic mutant mouse. *Brain Res* 1982;234:299–308.

66. Muller E, Le Corronc H, Scain AL, Triller A, Legendre P. Despite GABAergic neurotransmission, GABAergic innervation does not compensate for the defect in glycine receptor postsynaptic aggregation in spastic mice. *Eur J Neurosci* 2008;27:2529–41.

67. Graham BA, Schofield PR, Sah P, Callister RJ. Altered inhibitory synaptic transmission in superficial dorsal horn neurones in spastic and oscillator mice. *J Physiol* 2003;551:905–16.

68. Lu Y, Inokuchi H, McLachlan EM, Li JS, Higashi H. Correlation between electrophysiology and morphology of three groups of neuron in the dorsal commissural nucleus of lumbosacral spinal cord of mature rats studied in vitro. *J Comp Neurol* 2001;437:156–69.

69. Mainen ZF, Sejnowski TJ. Influence of dendritic structure on firing pattern in model neocortical neurons. *Nature* 1996;382:363–6.

70. Vetter P, Roth A, Hausser M. Propagation of action potentials in dendrites depends on dendritic morphology. *J Neurophysiol* 2001;85:926–37.

71. Castro-Moure F, Goshgarian HG. Morphological plasticity induced in the phrenic nucleus following cervical cold block of descending respiratory drive. *Exp Neurol* 1997;147:299–310.

72. Hirakawa M, Kawata M. Influence of spinal cord hemisection on the configurational changes in motor and primary afferent neurons and the chemical messenger alterations in the rat lumbar segments. *J Hirnforsch* 1992;33:419–28.

73. Sperry MA, Goshgarian HG. Ultrastructural changes in the rat phrenic nucleus developing within 2 h after cervical spinal cord hemisection. *Exp Neurol* 1993;120:233–44.

74. Bose P, Parmer R, Reier PJ, Thompson FJ. Morphological changes of the soleus motoneuron pool in chronic midthoracic contused rats. *Exp Neurol* 2005;191:13–23.

75. Ulfhake B, Cullheim S. A quantitative light microscopic study of the dendrites of cat spinal gamma-motoneurons after intracellular staining with horseradish peroxidase. *J Comp Neurol* 1981;202:585–96.

76. Zwaagstra B, Kernell D. Sizes of soma and stem dendrites in intracellularly labelled alpha-motoneurones of the cat. *Brain Res* 1981;204:295–309.

77. Benes FM, Parks TN, Rubel EW. Rapid dendritic atrophy following deafferentation: an EM morphometric analysis. *Brain Res* 1977;122:1–13.

78. Deitch JS, Rubel EW. Changes in neuronal cell bodies in N. laminaris during deafferentation-induced dendritic atrophy. *J Comp Neurol* 1989;281:259–68.

79. Deitch JS, Rubel EW. Rapid changes in ultrastructure during deafferentation-induced dendritic atrophy. *J Comp Neurol* 1989;281:234–58.

80. Deitch JS, Rubel EW. Afferent influences on brain stem auditory nuclei of the chicken: time course and specificity of dendritic atrophy following deafferentation. *J Comp Neurol* 1984;229:66–79.

81. Gazula VR, Roberts M, Luzzio C, Jawad AF, Kalb RG. Effects of limb exercise after spinal cord injury on motor neuron dendrite structure. *J Comp Neurol* 2004;476:130–45.

82. Soha JM, Herrup K. Abnormal Purkinje cell dendrites in lurcher chimeric mice result from a deafferentation-induced atrophy. *J Neurobiol* 1996;29:330–40.

83. Hume RI, Purves D. Geometry of neonatal neurones and the regulation of synapse elimination. *Nature* 1981;293: 469–71.

84. Purves D, Hume RI. The relation of postsynaptic geometry to the number of presynaptic axons that innervate autonomic ganglion cells. *J Neurosci* 1981;1:441–52.

85. Baer SM, Rinzel J. Propagation of dendritic spikes mediated by excitable spines: a continuum theory. *J Neurophysiol* 1991;65:874–90.

86. Jaslove SW. The integrative properties of spiny distal dendrites. *Neuroscience* 1992;47:495–519.

87. Engert F, Bonhoeffer T. Dendritic spine changes associated with hippocampal long-term synaptic plasticity. *Nature* 1999; 399:66–70.

88. Maletic-Savatic M, Malinow R, Svoboda K. Rapid dendritic morphogenesis in CA1 hippocampal dendrites induced by synaptic activity. *Science* (New York, NY 1999;283:1923–7.

89. Krenz NR, Weaver LC. Sprouting of primary afferent fibers after spinal cord transection in the rat. *Neuroscience* 1998; 85:443–58.

90. Wong ST, Atkinson BA, Weaver LC. Confocal microscopic analysis reveals sprouting of primary afferent fibres in rat dorsal horn after spinal cord injury. *Neurosci Lett* 2000;296: 65–8.

91. Knikou M, Kay E, Rymer WZ. Modulation of flexion reflex induced by hip angle changes in human spinal cord injury. *Exp Brain Res* 2006;168:577–86.

92. Schmit BD, McKenna-Cole A, Rymer WZ. Flexor reflexes in chronic spinal cord injury triggered by imposed ankle rotation. *Muscle Nerve* 2000;23:793–803.

93. Schmit BD, Benz EN. Extensor reflexes in human spinal cord injury: activation by hip proprioceptors. *Exp Brain Res* 2002;145:520–7.

94. Schmit BD, Benz EN, Rymer WZ. Afferent mechanisms for the reflex response to imposed ankle movement in chronic spinal cord injury. *Exp Brain Res* 2002;145:40–9.

95. Valero-Cabre A, Fores J, Navarro X. Reorganization of reflex responses mediated by different afferent sensory fibers after spinal cord transection. *J Neurophysiol* 2004;91:2838–48.

96. Wheeler G. Gabapentin. Pfizer. *Curr Opin Investig Drugs* 2002;3:470–7.

97. Maneuf YP, McKnight AT. Block by gabapentin of the facilitation of glutamate release from rat trigeminal nucleus following activation of protein kinase C or adenylyl cyclase. *Br J Pharmacol* 2001;134:237–40.

98. Maneuf YP, Hughes J, McKnight AT. Gabapentin inhibits the substance P-facilitated K(+)-evoked release of [(3)H] glutamate from rat caudial trigeminal nucleus slices. *Pain* 2001;93:191–6.

99. Maneuf YP, Blake R, Andrews NA, McKnight AT. Reduction by gabapentin of K+-evoked release of [3H]-glutamate from

the caudal trigeminal nucleus of the streptozotocin-treated rat. *Br J Pharmacol* 2004;141:574–9.

100. Bayer K, Ahmadi S, Zeilhofer HU. Gabapentin may inhibit synaptic transmission in the mouse spinal cord dorsal horn through a preferential block of P/Q-type Ca2+ channels. *Neuropharmacology* 2004;46:743–9.

101. Fink K, Dooley DJ, Meder WP, et al. Inhibition of neuronal Ca(2+) influx by gabapentin and pregabalin in the human neocortex. *Neuropharmacology* 2002;42:229–36.

102. Fink K, Meder W, Dooley DJ, Gothert M. Inhibition of neuronal Ca(2+) influx by gabapentin and subsequent reduction of neurotransmitter release from rat neocortical slices. *Br J Pharmacol* 2000;130:900–6.

103. Luo ZD, Calcutt NA, Higuera ES, et al. Injury type-specific calcium channel alpha 2 delta-1 subunit up-regulation in rat neuropathic pain models correlates with antiallodynic effects of gabapentin. *J Pharmacol Exp Ther* 2002;303:1199–205.

104. Calancie B, Broton JG, Klose KJ, Traad M, Difini J, Ayyar DR. Evidence that alterations in presynaptic inhibition contribute to segmental hypo- and hyperexcitability after spinal cord injury in man. *Electroencephalogr Clin Neurophysiol* 1993;89:177–86.

105. Heckman CJ. Alterations in synaptic input to motonerons during partial spinal cord injury. *Med Sci Sports Exerc* 1994;26:1480–90.

106. Hornby TG, Rymer WZ, Benz EN, Schmit BD. Windup of flexion reflexes in chronic human spinal cord injury: a marker for neuronal plateau potentials? *J Neurophysiol* 2003;89:416–26.

107. Edgerton VR, Leon RD, Harkema SJ, et al. Retraining the injured spinal cord. *J Physiol* 2001;533:15–22.

108. Tillakaratne NJ, de Leon RD, Hoang TX, Roy RR, Edgerton VR, Tobin AJ. Use-dependent modulation of inhibitory capacity in the feline lumbar spinal cord. *J Neurosci* 2002;22:3130–43.

109. Landau WM. Editorial: Spasticity: the fable of a neurological demon and the emperor's new therapy. *Arch Neurol* 1974;31:217–9.

110. Burke D. Spasticity as an adaptation to pyramidal tract injury. *Adv Neurol* 1988;47:401–23.

111. Katz RT, Rymer WZ. Spastic hypertonia: mechanisms and measurement. *Arch Phys Med Rehabil* 1989;70:144–55.

112. Thompson FJ, Parmer R, Reier PJ, Wang DC, Bose P. Scientific basis of spasticity: insights from a laboratory model. *J Child Neurol* 2001;16:2–9.

113. Roby-Brami A, Bussel B. Long-latency spinal reflex in man after flexor reflex afferent stimulation. *Brain* 1987;110 (Pt 3):707–25.

114. Bennett DJ, Sanelli L, Cooke CL, Harvey PJ, Gorassini MA. Spastic long-lasting reflexes in the awake rat after sacral spinal cord injury. *J Neurophysiol* 2004;91:2247–58.

115. Gorassini MA, Knash ME, Harvey PJ, Bennett DJ, Yang JF. Role of motoneurons in the generation of muscle spasms after spinal cord injury. *Brain* 2004;127:2247–58.

116. Gorassini M, Bennett DJ, Kiehn O, Eken T, Hultborn H. Activation patterns of hindlimb motor units in the awake rat and their relation to motoneuron intrinsic properties. *J Neurophysiol* 1999;82:709–17.

117. Clarke RW, Eves S, Harris J, Peachey JE, Stuart E. Interactions between cutaneous afferent inputs to a withdrawal reflex in the decerebrated rabbit and their control by descending and segmental systems. *Neuroscience* 2002;112:555–71.

118. Mailis A, Ashby P. Alterations in group Ia projections to motoneurons following spinal lesions in humans. *J Neurophysiol* 1990;64:637–47.

119. Gozariu M, Roth V, Keime F, Le Bars D, Willer JC. An electrophysiological investigation into the monosynaptic H-reflex in the rat. *Brain Res* 1998;782:343–7.

120. Theiss RD, Kuo JJ, Heckman CJ. Persistent inward currents in rat ventral horn neurones. *J Physiol* 2007;580:507–22.

121. Heckmann CJ, Gorassini MA, Bennett DJ. Persistent inward currents in motoneuron dendrites: implications for motor output. *Muscle Nerve* 2005;31:135–56.

122. Harvey PJ, Li X, Li Y, Bennett DJ. 5-HT2 receptor activation facilitates a persistent sodium current and repetitive firing in spinal motoneurons of rats with and without chronic spinal cord injury. *J Neurophysiol* 2006;96:1158–70.

123. Harvey PJ, Li X, Li Y, Bennett DJ. Endogenous monoamine receptor activation is essential for enabling persistent sodium currents and repetitive firing in rat spinal motoneurons. *J Neurophysiol* 2006;96:1171–86.

124. Rank MM, Li X, Bennett DJ, Gorassini MA. Role of endogenous release of norepinephrine in muscle spasms after chronic spinal cord injury. *J Neurophysiol* 2007;97:3166–80.

125. Westenbroek RE, Hoskins L, Catterall WA. Localization of Ca2+ channel subtypes on rat spinal motor neurons, interneurons, and nerve terminals. *J Neurosci* 1998;18:6319–30.

126. Carlin KP, Jones KE, Jiang Z, Jordan LM, Brownstone RM. Dendritic L-type calcium currents in mouse spinal motoneurons: implications for bistability. *Eur J Neurosci* 2000;12:1635–46.

127. Jiang Z, Rempel J, Li J, Sawchuk MA, Carlin KP, Brownstone RM. Development of L-type calcium channels and a nifedipine-sensitive motor activity in the postnatal mouse spinal cord. *Eur J Neurosci* 1999;11:3481–7.

128. Zhang M, Moller M, Broman J, Sukiasyan N, Wienecke J, Hultborn H. Expression of calcium channel CaV1.3 in cat spinal cord: light and electron microscopic immunohistochemical study. *J Comp Neurol* 2008;507:1109–27.

129. Zhang M, Sukiasyan N, Moller M, et al. Localization of L-type calcium channel Ca(V)1.3 in cat lumbar spinal cord—with emphasis on motoneurons. *Neurosci Lett* 2006;407:42–7.

130. Alaburda A, Perrier JF, Hounsgaard J. Mechanisms causing plateau potentials in spinal motoneurones. *Adv Exp Med Biol* 2002;508:219–26.

131. Hultborn H, Brownstone RB, Toth TI, Gossard JP. Key mechanisms for setting the input–output gain across the motoneuron pool. *Prog Brain Res* 2004;143:77–95.

132. Rekling JC, Shao XM, Feldman JL. Electrical coupling and excitatory synaptic transmission between rhythmogenic respiratory neurons in the preBotzinger complex. *J Neurosci* 2000;20:RC113.

133. Hultborn H. Plateau potentials and their role in regulating motoneuronal firing. *Adv Exp Med Biol* 2002;508:213–8.

134. Day M, Olson PA, Platzer J, Striessnig J, Surmeier DJ. Stimulation of 5-HT(2) receptors in prefrontal pyramidal neurons inhibits Ca(v)1.2 L type Ca(2+) currents via a PLCbeta/IP3/calcineurin signaling cascade. *J Neurophysiol* 2002;87:2490–504.

135. Kasim S, Egami K, Jinnah HA. Self-biting induced by activation of L-type calcium channels in mice: serotonergic influences. *Dev Neurosci* 2002;24:322–7.

136. Anelli R, Sanelli L, Bennett DJ, Heckman CJ. Expression of L-type calcium channel alpha(1)-1.2 and alpha(1)-1.3 subunits on rat sacral motoneurons following chronic spinal cord injury. *Neuroscience* 2007;145:751–63.

137. Anden NE, Haeggendal J, Magnusson T, Rosengren E. The time course of the disappearance of noradrenaline and 5-hydroxytryptamine in the spinal cord after transection. *Acta Physiol Scand* 1964;62:115–8.

138. Hadjiconstantinou M, Panula P, Lackovic Z, Neff NH. Spinal cord serotonin: a biochemical and immunohistochemical study following transection. *Brain Res* 1984;322:245–54.

139. Newton BW, Hamill RW. The morphology and distribution of rat serotoninergic intraspinal neurons: an immunohistochemical study. *Brain Res Bull* 1988;20:349–60.

140. Li X, Murray K, Harvey PJ, Ballou EW, Bennett DJ. Serotonin facilitates a persistent calcium current in motoneurons of rats with and without chronic spinal cord injury. *J Neurophysiol* 2007;97:1236–46.

141. Lee JK, Johnson CS, Wrathall JR. Up-regulation of 5-HT2 receptors is involved in the increased H-reflex amplitude after contusive spinal cord injury. *Exp Neurol* 2007;203: 502–11.

142. Lee JK, Emch GS, Johnson CS, Wrathall JR. Effect of spinal cord injury severity on alterations of the H-reflex. *Exp Neurol* 2005;196:430–40.

143. Antri M, Mouffle C, Orsal D, Barthe JY. 5-HT1A receptors are involved in short- and long-term processes responsible for 5-HT-induced locomotor function recovery in chronic spinal rat. *Eur J Neurosci* 2003;18:1963–72.

144. Landry ES, Guertin PA. Differential effects of 5-HT1 and 5-HT2 receptor agonists on hindlimb movements in paraplegic mice. *Prog Neuropsychopharmacol Biol Psychiatry* 2004;28:1053–60.

145. Giroux N, Rossignol S, Reader TA. Autoradiographic study of alpha1- and alpha2-noradrenergic and serotonin1A receptors in the spinal cord of normal and chronically transected cats. *J Comp Neurol* 1999;406:402–14.

146. Fuller DD, Baker-Herman TL, Golder FJ, Doperalski NJ, Watters JJ, Mitchell GS. Cervical spinal cord injury up-regulates ventral spinal 5-HT2A receptors. *J Neurotrauma* 2005;22:203–13.

147. Nozaki M, Bell JA, Martin WR. Noradrenergic action of amphetamine following degeneration of descending monoaminergic fibers in the spinal cord. *Psychopharmacology* 1980;67:25–9.

148. Nozaki M, Bell JA, Vaupel DB, Martin WR. Responses of the flexor reflex to LSD, tryptamine, 5-hydroxytryptophan, methoxamine, and d-amphetamine in acute and chronic spinal rats. *Psychopharmacology* 1977;55:13–8.

149. de la Torre R, Farre M, Navarro M, Pacifici R, Zuccaro P, Pichini S. Clinical pharmacokinetics of amfetamine and related substances: monitoring in conventional and non-conventional matrices. *Clin Pharmacokinet* 2004;43:157–85.

150. Austin JH, Nygren LG, Fuxe K. A system for measuring the noradrenaline receptor contribution to the flexor reflex. *Med Biol* 1976;54:352–63.

151. Roudet C, Mouchet P, Feuerstein C, Savasta M. Normal distribution of alpha 2-adrenoceptors in the rat spinal cord and its modification after noradrenergic denervation: a quantitative autoradiographic study. *J Neurosci Res* 1994;39:319–29.

152. Roudet C, Savasta M, Feuerstein C. Normal distribution of alpha-1-adrenoceptors in the rat spinal cord and its modification after noradrenergic denervation: a quantitative autoradiographic study. *J Neurosci Res* 1993;34:44–53.

153. Cowley KC, Schmidt BJ. A comparison of motor patterns induced by N-methyl-D-aspartate, acetylcholine and serotonin in the in vitro neonatal rat spinal cord. *Neurosci Lett* 1994;171:147–50.

154. Cowley KC, Schmidt BJ. Regional distribution of the locomotor pattern-generating network in the neonatal rat spinal cord. *J Neurophysiol* 1997;77:247–59.

155. Yuan Y, Yan SC, Chen XH, Han JS. 66A-078:a kappa-opiate receptor agonist for amelioration of spinal spasticity. *Chin Med J* 1994;107:192–5.

156. Taira Y, Marsala M. Effect of proximal arterial perfusion pressure on function, spinal cord blood flow, and histopathologic changes after increasing intervals of aortic occlusion in the rat. *Stroke* 1996;27:1850–8.

157. Homma S, Suzuki T, Murayama S, Otsuka M. Amino acid and substance P contents in spinal cord of cats with experimental hind-limb rigidity produced by occlusion of spinal cord blood supply. *J Neurochem* 1979;32:691–8.

158. Simpson RK, Jr., Robertson CS, Goodman JC. Glycine: an important potential component of spinal shock. *Neurochem Res* 1993;18:887–92.

159. Marsala J, Sulla I, Santa M, Marsala M, Mechirova E, Jalc P. Early neurohistopathological changes of canine lumbosacral spinal cord segments in ischemia-reperfusion-induced paraplegia. *Neurosci Lett* 1989;106:83–8.

160. Ornung G, Ottersen OP, Cullheim S, Ulfhake B. Distribution of glutamate-, glycine- and GABA-immunoreactive nerve terminals on dendrites in the cat spinal motor nucleus. *Exp Brain Res* 1998;118:517–32.

161. Jankowska E. Spinal interneuronal systems: identification, multifunctional character and reconfigurations in mammals. *J Physiol* 2001;533:31–40.

162. Hefferan MP, Kucharova K, Kinjo K, et al. Spinal astrocyte glutamate receptor 1 overexpression after ischemic insult facilitates behavioral signs of spasticity and rigidity. *J Neurosci* 2007;27:11179–91.

163. von Wegerer J, Becker K, Glockenhammer D, Becker CM, Zeilhofer HU, Swandulla D. Spinal inhibitory synaptic transmission in the glycine receptor mouse mutant spastic. *Neurosci Lett* 2003;345:45–8.

164. Legendre P. The glycinergic inhibitory synapse. *Cell Mol Life Sci* 2001;58:760–93.

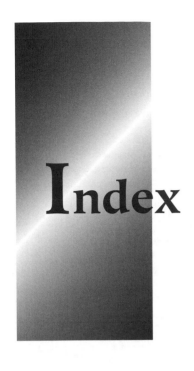

Index